NUTRITION IN THE INFANT

Problems and Practical Procedures

NUTRITION IN THE INFANT
Problems and Practical Procedures

Edited by

Victor R Preedy
Department of Nutrition
School of Life Sciences
King's College London
Franklin-Wilkins Building
London

George Grimble BSc PhD
Honorary Senior Lecturer
Department of Clinical Biochemistry
Kings College Hospital Medical School
Reader in Clinical Nutrition
School of Life Sciences
University of Surrey, Roehampton
Whitelands College
London
UK

Ronald Watson PhD
Department of Family and Community Medicine
University of Arizona School of Medicine
Tucson
Arizona
USA

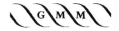

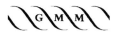

© 2001

GREENWICH MEDICAL MEDIA LTD
137 Euston Road
London
NW1 2AA

ISBN 1 90015162 6

First published 2001

Visit our website at:
www.greenwich-medical.co.uk

Distributed worldwide by Plymbridge Distributors Ltd

Typeset by Phoenix Photosetting, Chatham, Kent
Printed by MPG Books Ltd, Bodmin, Cornwall

CONTENTS

CHAPTER 16

CHAPTER 17

CHAPTER 18

CHAPTER 19

CHAPTER 20

CHAPTER 21

CHAPTER 22

CHAPTER 23

CONTRIBUTORS

David Adamkin, MD
Professor of Pediatrics
University of Louisville
Louisville KY
USA

Marcel Johannes Ivo Jacques
Albers, MD
Paediatrician Intensivist
Paediatric Surgical Intensive Care Unit
Department of Paediatric Surgery
Sophia Children's
Hospital/University of Rotterdam
The Netherlands

Gema Ariceta, MD
Nefrologia Pediatrica
Depto de Pediatria
C.H.U.S
C/Galeras s/n
Santiago de Compostela
Spain

Isabel T. Avencena, MD
Associate Acute Consultant
Pediatric Gastroenterology,
Idepatology and Nutrition
Makati Medical Centre
Makati City
Philippines

Ruth Ayling, PhD, MRCP,
MRCPath
Consultant Chemical Pathologist and
Honorary Senior Lecturer
Department of Chemical Biochemistry
Kings College Hospital
London
UK

Roberta L. Babbitt, PhD
Director, Program Research and
Development
Department of Behavioral Psychology
The Kennedy Krieger Institute
Assistant Professor
Department of Psychiatry and
Behavioural Sciences
Johns Hopkins University School of
Medicine
USA

Alastair J. Baker, MB ChB,
FRCP (UK), FRCPCH
Consultant Paediatric Hepatologist
Paediatric Liver Service
King's College Hospital
Denmark Hill
London
UK

Howard I. Baron, MD, FAAP
Chemical Associate Professor
Department of Pediatrics
University of Nevada School of
Medicine
Las Vegas, Nevada
USA

R. M. Beattie, FRCPCH,
MRCP, BSc
Paediatric Medical Unit
Southampton General Hospital
Tremona Road
Southampton
UK

Katja Becker-Brandenburg, MD
Professur fur Biochemie der Ernahrung
Interdisziplinares Forchungszentrum
Germany

Marilyn Bernard, MS, RD
Clinical Dietitian
Children's Hospital
Boston, Massachusetts
USA

Carol L. Berseth, MD
Associate Professor of Pediatrics
Baylor College of Medicine
Dept of Pediatrics, Section of
Neonatology
One Baylor Plaza
Houston
USA

Martin W. Bloem, MD, PhD
Regional Director Asia Pacific
Helen Keller International
Division of Helen Keller Worldwide
Country Director Indonesia
Jakarta
Indonesia

Ian Booth, BSc, MSc, MD,
FRCP, FRCPCH, DObst
RCOG, DCH
Leonard Parsons Professor of
Paediatrics & Child Health
Honorary Consultant Paediatric
Gastroenterologist
Institute of Child Health
University of Birmingham
Clinical Teaching Block
UK

Arlene M. Butz, ScD
Associate Professor of Nursing
Johns Hopkins University
USA

Geoffrey Cleghorn, MBBS, FRDCP, FACG
Associate Professor and Academic Head
Dept of Paediatrics and Child Health
University of Queensland
Clinical Director
The Childrens Nutrition Research Centre
Royal Childrens Hospital
Brisbane
Australia

Tim J. Cole, MA, PhD
Professor of Medical Statistics
Institute of Child Health, London
UK

Christine E. Cronk, ScD
Adjunct Associate Professor
Department of Pediatrics
Medical College of Wisconsin
Milwaukee
USA

Patricia Davidson, MB ChB, Muirhead Adward (General Medicine), Ure Prize (General Medicine), MD, MRCP, FRCS, FRACS, FRCP
Director of Surgery
John Hunter Children's Hospital
Locked Bag 1, Newcastle Mail Centre
Newcastle
Australia

Sean P. Devane, MD, DCH, FRCP(Irl), FRCPCH
Consultant Paediatrician
Ruskin Wing
King's College Hospital
London
UK

Christopher Duggan, MD, MPH
Children's Hospital
Boston
USA

Ellen B. Fung, PhD, RD
Assistant Research Scientist
Division of Gastroenterology and Nutrition
Children's Hospital Oakland
USA

Lauren Furuta, MOE, RD
Clinical Dietitian
Childrens Hospital
Boston, Massachusetts
USA

Michael Green, MBBS, MRCP, FRCPCH
Consultant Paediatrician
Leicester Royal Infirmary NHS Trust
Infirmary Square
Leicester
UK

Stephen Gromer, MD, PhD
Biochemiezentrum
Universitat Heidelberg
Heidelberg
Germany

Rainer Gross, MD
Postgraduate Program Coordinator
National Agricultural University
La Molina
Peru

Robin A. Henderson, PhD, RD
Assistant Professor of Pediatrics
John Hopkins Children's Center
Gastroenterology and Nutrition
N Wolfe Street
Baltimore, Maryland
USA

J. Iglesias
Boul. Levesque West
Laval (QC)
Canada

Dierdre Kelly MD, FRCP, FRCPI, FRCPCH
Reader in Paediatric Hepatology
The Liver Unit
Birmingham Children's Hospital
NHS Trust
Reader in Paediatric Hepatology
University of Birmingham
UK

Caleb K. King, MD, PhD
Pediatric Gastroenterologist
McLeod Regional Medical Centre
South Carolina
USA

Samuel Kocoshis, MD
Professor of Pediatrics
University of Cincinnati
Children's Hospital Medical Centre
Division of Pediatric Gastroenterology
Cincinnati, Ohio
USA

Cheryl Levitt, MBBCh, CCFP, FCFP
Professor and Chair
Faculty of Health Sciences
Department of Family Medicine
McMaster University
Hamilton, Ontario
Canada

Carlos Lifschitz, MD
Associate Professor
Baylor College of Medicine
Children's Nutrition Research Center
Houston, Texas
USA

Clifford Lo, MD, MPH SC.D
Assistant Professor of Pediatrics
Harvard Medical School
Lecturer in Nutrition
Harvard School of Public Health
Member
Nutrition Support Service
Children's Hospital Boston
Massachusetts
USA

Thomas T. MacDonald, PhD, PRCPath
Professor of Immunology and Director of the Centre for Infection Allergy, Inflammation and Repair University of Southampton School of Medicine Southampton UK

Maura MacPhee, RN, PhD
Assistant Professor of Nursing The University of Colorado School of Nursing, Denver, Colorado Education Specialist The Children's Hospital of Denver Colorado USA

Robin Meyers, MPH, RD
Clinical Nutritionist Children's Hospital of Philadelphia Home Care USA

Graham Neale, MA, BSc, MB, FRCP
Research Fellow Clinical Risk Unit University College London UK

Christine Northrop-Clewes, BSc, PhD
Research Fellow Northern Ireland Centre for Diet and Health University of Ulster Coleraine Northern Ireland

Yoshikazu Ohtsuka, MD
Clinical Research Fellow Department of Paediatric Gastroenology St Bartholomew's and the Royal London School of Medicine and Dentistry London UK

Akira Okada, MD, PhD, FACS
Professor and Chief Dept of Paediatric Surgery Osaka University Medical School Osaka Japan

Beth Olsen, PhD
Senior Nutrition Scientist Kellogg Company Porter Street Battle Creek USA

Alexandra Papadopoulou, MD
Senior Specialist in Paediatrics First Department of Paediatrics Faculty of Nursing University of Athens Greece

Susan M. Protheroe, MD, MBCP, MRCP, MRCPH
Consultant Paediatric Gastroenterologist, Honorary Senior Clinical Lecturer in Paediatrics & Child Health Department of Gastroenterology & Nutrition, Birmingham UK

John William Lambert Puntis, BM (Hons), DM, FRCP, FRCPCH
Senior Lecturer in Paediatrics and Child Health University of Leeds Consultant Paediatric Gastroenterologist The Children's Centre The General Infirmary Leeds Leeds UK

Philip E. Putnam
Associate Professor of Pediatrics University of Cincinnati Division of Gastroentrology and Nutrition Childrens Hospital Medical Centre Cincinnati, Ohio USA

J. Rodríguez-Soriano, MD
Division of Paediatric Nephrology Department of Paediatrics Hospital de Cruces and Basque University School of Medicine Bilbao Spain

Ian R. Sanderson, MD
Professor of Paediatric Gastroenology Department of Paediatric Gastroenology St Bartholomew's and the Royal London School of Medicine and Dentistry London UK

Kinya Sando, MD
Dept of Pediatric Surgery Osaka Medical School Yamadaoka Osaka Japan

Rolf Heiner Schirmer, MD
Biochemiezentrum Universitat Heidelberg Heidelberg USA

Barbara O. Schneeman, PhD
Professor of Nutrition University of California USA

Werner Schultink, MD

Deutcher Gasellschaft, Fur Technische, Zusammenarbistt (GTZ) c/o Southeast Asians Minister of Education Centre for Community Nutrition University of Indonesia Jakarta Indonesia

Alan Shenkin, BSc, PhD, FRCP, PRCPath

Professor of Chemistry The University of Liverpool Liverpool UK

Roger Shrimpton, SRD, BSc, MSc, PhD

Honorary Senior Research Fellow Centre for International Child Health Institute of Child Health University College London UK

Virginia Stallings, MD

Chief, Nutrition Section Professor of Pediatrics The Children's Hospital Philadelphia University of Pennsylvania School of Medicine Philadelphia USA

Richard D. Stevenson, MD

Associate Professor of Pediatrics Kluge Children's Rehabilitation Center and Research Institute University of Virginia School of Medicine Charlottesville USA

Dick Tibboel, MD, PhD

Paediatrician Intensivist Professor of Experimental Paediatric Surgery Paediatric Surgical Intensive Care Unit, Department of Paediatric Surgery Sophia Children's Hospital/University Hospital Rotterdam The Netherlands

Jitka Vobecky, PhD

Boul. Levesque West Laval (QC) Canada

Fiona Watson, MSc, BSc

Institute of Child Health London University London UK

Keith E. Williams, PhD

Director, Feeding Program Hershey Medical Centre Assistant Professor Department of Paediatrics Penn State College of Medicine Philadelphia USA

Ray Yip, MD, MPH

Chief Health and Nutrition Section UNICEF Beijing People's Republic of China

PREFACE

The infant is particularly vulnerable to the effects of malnutrition, with long-term consequences for tissue maturation and intellectual impairment. In addition, malnutrition increases the susceptibility to infections and post-operative recovery is compromised. Traditionally, some practical aspects of nutritional disorders have been placed in the third world context, such as repeated episodes of diarrhoea, tropical infections; precipitated by changes in agricultural proficiency, social cohesion or civil conflict. However, malnutrition may also arise as a consequence of organ pathologies, metabolic derangement, operational stress as well as overt nutrient deficiencies. These need to be diagnosed either in the general population setting, or in the individual.

After diagnosis, the appropriate therapeutic regimen needs to be instigated which may take the form of specific formulations or more subjective treatment protocols such as educational strategies. In the book Nutrition in The Infant: Practice and Procedures all these facets of nutrition and nutritional therapy are covered in a precise and practical way. The book includes the latest developments in diagnostic procedures and nutritional support. The authors are International experts in their field and the book is recommended for all those involved or interested in infant nutrition.

Victor R Preedy
March 2001

1

The nature and extent of
malnutrition in children

Isabel T. Avencena and Geoffrey Cleghorn

Introduction

Malnutrition is an important contributing factor in up to 40–60% of deaths amongst under-5-year-old children in developing countries (Schroeder & Brown 1994). *Protein-energy malnutrition* (PEM), the term used to describe a deficiency in carbohydrate, protein and fat, now also can include deficiencies in vitamins, minerals and trace elements. PEM may range in severity from mild to severe, and severe forms may present as any of the following syndromes:

- A visceral attrition state or kwashiorkor-like syndrome accompanied by oedema, skin, hair, liver and affective disorders;
- A marasmus-like syndrome in which the patient is visibly underweight with depleted muscle and fat stores. Serum proteins are maintained until late in the course; or
- An acute state combining both kwashiorkor and marasmus often caused by severe trauma and stress in mildly-undernourished individuals (Waterlow1973).

Pathophysiology

Malnutrition is usually a result of starvation but may occur also in response to an injury or illness. During starvation, reserve nutrients are consumed with consequent erosion of body mass. Energy metabolism is then aimed towards: 1) maximum use of endogenous energy reserves; 2) preservation of body protein, which constitutes the vital structures; 3) reduction in energy consumption to prolong reserves; and 4) maintenance of blood glucose for glucose-dependent tissues (McMahon & Bistrian 1990).

In the absence of an exogenous supply of glucose but with a continued endogenous requirement, circulating glucose levels decrease. The hormonal response is a reduction in insulin production and an increase in glucagon. In turn, this induces consumption of the already limited amount of stored glycogen, stored fatty acids and ketones as the main source of energy (Cahil 1981).

The body attempts to use the major fuel storage form, fat, to meet the needs of obligate glucose consumption until the brain can make the transformation to a system using ketone bodies and free-fatty acids and to minimize breakdown of visceral protein (McMahon & Bistrian 1990).

Reduction in energy consumption is achieved through a decrease in physical and metabolic activity at all levels. At the cellular level, the most important adaptive reduction is in the activity of the sodium-potassium pump. This results in an increase in intra-cellular sodium from approximately 109 mmol/kg to 185 mmol/kg of dry residue, with a concomitant drop in intracellular potassium from 367 to 327 mmol/kg of dry residue. This increase in body sodium may explain the increase in total body fluid that is common in malnourished states (Patrick & Golden 1977).

Malnutrition can evolve also as a result of the body's response to inflammation or to the increased energy requirements seen in some specific disease states. The mechanisms of adaptation in these situations can be different from that of starvation states. Endogenous host responses are concentrated on recovery and decreasing the extent of injury with hormones and monokines as modulators of this process. The response is characterized by: 1) an increase in basal metabolic rate (catecholamines); 2) increased use of fatty acid as fuel; 3) increased production of glucose from proteins; and 4) unaltered ketone body production (McMahon & Bistrian 1990).

Many of the components of the injury response (e.g., fever, neutrophilia, acute-phase protein production) are beneficial if the accompanying semi-starvation does not exceed 10–14 days. If the injury stimulus persists beyond this, nitrogen losses of up to 20–30 g daily can occur; over a 2-week period this can result in a loss of 300–400 g of nitrogen. Energy reserves are depleted and body protein is consumed rapidly (McMahon & Bistrian 1990).

Practice and procedures

Nutritional assessment

There are five major components of a nutritional assessment:

1. Anthropometry;
2. Clinical assessment;
3. Biochemistry;
4. Dietary assessment;
5. Behavioural and feeding-skill development.

Anthropometry

Single measurements of weight and height (or length) may be sufficient for an initial nutritional assessment.

These measurements as well as head circumference (for children < 2 years) should be plotted on a standardized growth chart (e.g., those of the National Centre for Health Statistics). Any weight or height (or length) measurement that falls below the fifth centile or crosses two major centile lines is considered to represent an abnormal growth pattern. However, serial measurements confirm whether this growth pattern is truly abnormal or secondary to constitutional growth delay.

In a research setting, height and weight measurements can be converted to *Z-scores* (i.e., values that represent standard deviations (SD) from the mean height and weight values for age). Any child more than 2SD below the mean is considered to have significant growth abnormalities.

The degree of acute or chronic malnutrition can be assessed using *Waterlow (1973) criteria* (Table 1.1). This approach assumes that during periods of nutritional deprivation, a weight deficit is the first abnormality noted followed by a length or height deficit. The Waterlow criteria assume also that the expected height and weight measurements of the child follow the fiftieth centile of the growth curves. This assumption is necessary because prior height or weight measurements may not be available.

Acute malnutrition (i.e., wasting) measured in terms of weight deficit by Waterlow criteria can be determined by the following equation:

$$\text{Weight deficit (\%)} = (\text{Actual weight (kg)}/\text{Expected weight (kg) for actual height}) \times 100$$

Chronic malnutrition (i.e., stunting) measured in terms of height or length deficit by the Waterlow criteria can be determined by the following equation:

$$\text{Height deficit (\%)} = (\text{Actual height (cm)}/\text{Expected height (cm) at 50th centile for chronological age}) \times 100$$

Alternative techniques that can also be useful for nutritional assessment include the *mid-upper-arm circumference* (MUAC) and the *triceps skinfold thickness* (TSF). A single cut-off value for MUAC is simple but has been shown to correlate poorly with wasting. It has been proposed by the World Health Organization (WHO) that MUAC-for-height and MUAC-for-age Z-scores prove to be better predictors for wasting (de Onis et al 1997, Mei et al 1997).

Clinical assessment

As defined by Jelliffe (1966), the physical examination looks at 'those changes, believed to be related to inadequate nutrition, that can be seen or felt in superficial epithelial tissue, especially the skin, eyes, hair and buccal mucosa, or in organs near the surface of the body (parotid, thyroid glands)'.

As a technique for nutritional assessment the physical examination has several limitations however:

1. Non-specificity of physical signs—some physical signs may be produced by more than one nutrient deficiency;

2. Multiple physical signs, coexisting nutrient deficiencies;

3. Bi-directional signs—signs may occur during the development and/or recovery from a deficiency (e.g., hepatomegaly occurs in PEM and during its treatment);

4. Examiner inconsistencies;

5. Variation in pattern of physical signs.

Taking these limitations into consideration, bipedal oedema and visible signs of wasting are useful clinical indicators of significant malnutrition especially when used in conjunction with anthropometric measurements (Bern et al 1997) or another marker.

Biochemistry

The ideal nutritional biochemical marker should have the following characteristics (Goldsmith 1996):

• Short circulation half-life (<2 days);
• Responds rapidly to improved nutrient intake;
• Reflects a moderately-decreased intake early;
• Indicates current nutritional status;
• Accurately reflects degree of deficiency and is not affected by non-nutritional factors.

Tests for protein status are one of the most useful in assessing nutritional status because skeletal and visceral proteins comprise the majority of the metabolically-active body-cell mass. Laboratory indices of protein

Table 1.1 — Waterlow classification of malnutrition

	Normal	Mild	Moderate	Severe
Height for age (%)	95	90–95	85–90	85
Weight for age (%)	90	80–90	70–80	70

Decreased height for age suggests chronic malnutrition (stunting);
Decreased weight for age suggests acute malnutrition (wasting).
Adapted from Waterlow (1973).

status include: 1) somatic protein status; 2) visceral protein status; 3) metabolic changes; 4) muscle function; and 5) immune function.

Somatic protein status can be determined using the creatinine-height index and 3-methylhistidine. The *creatinine-height index* assesses the amount of creatinine excreted in the urine and compares it with the standard levels expected for the patient's height. Urinary elimination of muscle metabolites (i.e., creatinine and 3-methylhistidine) reflects the degree of muscle mass and its variations. This degree correlates, in turn, with fat-free mass measured by anthropometry. However, this correlation is of limited value because it does not take into account the rate of muscle-protein turnover and the metabolic consequences of the patient's illness (Goldsmith 1996).

To assess *visceral protein status*, it has been proposed to use concentrations of plasma proteins, which reflect synthetic function, as markers. The four proteins most commonly assayed are albumin, thyroxin-binding pre-albumin (TBPA), retinol-binding protein (RBP) and transferrin (Table 1.2). Serum albumin and transferrin are most useful for monitoring long-term changes during convalescence because they have long half-lives. The TBPA-RBP combination is an early and sensitive index of malnutrition and can be used to monitor the efficacy of re-nutrition (Gibson 1990).

Fibronectin, a cold insoluble globulin, has also been proposed as a nutritional marker for mild to moderate nutritional deficiency. Fibronectin levels have been shown to decrease after 4–5 days in adults and sharply increase in 2–3 weeks after nutritional therapy (Hassanein et al 1998).

Insulin-like growth factor-1 (IGF-1) is an anabolic hormone associated with growth hormone and has a half-life of 2–4 h. It has been proposed as a marker for nitrogen balance, increased catabolism and linear growth. It is a reliable marker of malnutrition and can

Table 1.2 — Common plasma proteins used as nutritional parameters

Plasma protein	Pool size and half-life	Plasma level	Factors of variation
Albumin	Large pool size Half-life: 15–20 days	36–45 g/L At birth: 80% of adult level	PEM Liver failure Protein-losing enteropathy Protracted infectious state
Thyroxin-binding pre-albumin	Small pool size Half-life: 2–3 days	0.32–0.35 g/L At birth: 80% of adult level	PEM Liver disease (hepatitis, cirrhosis, cancer) Hyperthyroidism Inflammatory disease
Retinol-binding protein	Small pool size Half-life: 12 h	60 ± 16 mg/L 0–10 years, 60% of adult level Rapid increase at puberty	PEM Inflammatory disease Vitamin A, zinc deficiency Liver disease (hepatitis, cirrhosis, cancer) Glomerulonephritis and renal tubular defect increase level
Transferrin	Large pool size Half-life: 8 days	2–4 g/L (age dependent) Wide variation in plasma levels	PEM Liver failure Protein-losing enteropathy Glomerulopathy Inflammatory disease Iron deficiency

be used in children, providing it is measured in an experienced laboratory. IGF-1 levels fall during the course of malnutrition and return to normal after a few days of re-nutrition (Minuto et al 1989).

Nitrogen balance studies measure the difference between nitrogen intake and excretion. These studies are difficult to perform in clinical practice. In field surveys, 24-h urine collections are impractical. Instead, the urinary urea nitrogen:creatinine ratio on random urine samples can be calculated to assess the adequacy of protein intake (Goulet et al 1993).

Immunocompetence is affected by malnutrition, especially cellular immunity, with a risk of infectious complications. Lymphopenia, delayed hypersensitivity tests and the fall in CD4:CD8 cell ratio are the main indices of cellular immunity, humoral immune responses being preserved (Chandra 1991). These markers are helpful in prognostic assessments but have no value in detection of protein calorie malnutrition (PCM).

Clinical expression of deficiency states of most water-soluble vitamins has been identified in children. Biochemical assays may be used for objective analysis but their significance remains questionable.

The assessment of fat-soluble vitamin deficiencies is also possible. Vitamin A status may be measured directly by the serum level of its binding protein, RBP. Measuring the level of 25-OH-cholecalciferol and the 1,25-diOH-cholecalciferol using liquid chromatography assesses Vitamin D. Vitamin E status is estimated from tocopherol plasma or serum levels. Vitamin K status is measured indirectly by prothrombin time and its correction with parenteral administration of vitamin K1.

Assessment of minerals and trace elements is impractical for clinical use. Only plasma levels of the minerals or their storage form in the body fluids or tissues are measurable (Goulet 1998). These may not be clinically relevant.

Dietary assessment

Analysis of a child's dietary pattern can predict and prevent nutrient deficiencies. It may range from a simple screening by food groups of a 24-h dietary recall to a computer-facilitated nutrient analysis.

In the 24-h recall method, the parents or caretakers are asked by a nutritionist who has been trained on interviewing techniques to recall the patient's exact food intake during the preceding day. The foods consumed are usually estimated in household measures and entered on a data sheet.

The dietary history method attempts to estimate usual food intakes over a relatively-long period of time. The interview is made up of three components: 1) 24-h recall of actual intake and collection of general information on overall eating pattern of the child; 2) questionnaire on the frequency of consumption of specific food items; and 3) 3-day food record using household measures. This method is labour-intensive and generally provides qualitative and not quantitative data on usual food intake.

Other methods for assessing nutritional intake include a weighed-food record, an estimated-food record and a food-frequency questionnaire (Gibson 1990).

It is also helpful to enquire about the child's level of activity, dietary supplements and/or medications, unusual food habits or inappropriate feeding behaviours, and the cultural/economic constraints of the family's diet.

Feeding skill-development

Delays in development of feeding skills may be due to neuromuscular dysfunction, resulting in the persistence of primitive reflexes or muscle inco-ordination, which makes positioning, chewing, or hand-to-mouth movement difficult. It also may be due to cognitive delays in the neurologically-intact child that lead to caregivers treating him as a younger child. Assessment of the child's developmental level and the child-feeder interaction as well as behavioural problems is essential to developing an intervention strategy.

Discussion

Management of severe malnutrition

The median case fatality of children suffering from severe malnutrition has remained unchanged over the last 50 years. It is typically in the range 20–30% with an even higher mortality of 50–60% in those with oedematous malnutrition (Schofield & Ashworth 1996).

This high mortality has been attributed to the following practices:

- Inappropriate diets that are high in protein and energy given in the acute phase of management;
- Diuretics given to treat oedema;

- No distinction between 'acute' and 'rehabilitation' phases of management;
- High-dose vitamin A not given;
- Anaemia treated immediately with iron supplements;
- Intravenous albumin and amino acids administered;
- Broad-spectrum antibiotics not given;
- Use of high-sodium oral-rehydration solutions and intravenous fluids;
- Failure to monitor food intake;
- Lack of feeding at night;
- Lack of provision of blankets when hypothermia is at risk.

Management of severe malnutrition can be achieved in 3 phases (Khanum et al 1994, Ahmed et al 1999, WHO 1999):

1. **Phase 1: Resuscitation of the acutely-ill mal-nourished and or infected child, prevention of hypoglycaemia and hypothermia, and prevention of further tissue catabolism**. Functional capacity of the intestine, liver and other organs during this phase is limited and the physician must guard against metabolic imbalances that may occur during re-nutrition. Energy intake should be restricted to 75 mg/kg/day and provided (in developing countries) as a special feed (F75, Table 1.3), which contains 75 kcal and 0.9 g protein/100 ml and consists of dried skimmed milk, sugar, rice starch or dextromaltose, vegetable

oil, and mineral and vitamin mixes. This can be formulated to give a diet of 1 kcal/ml and fed at a rate of 132 ml/kg/day in multiple frequent or even continuous feeds (if necessary by nasogastric tube) throughout a 24-h period. This initial phase may last for 1–2 days and the use of intravenous rehydration and of standard WHO oral rehydration solutions (ORS) is best avoided because of the high risk of precipitating heart failure.

Instead, an ORS with lower sodium (45 mmol/L) and higher potassium (40 mmol/L) with added magnesium, zinc, copper and selenium (ReSoMal, Table 1.4) should be used. Physical signs of mal-nutrition (e.g., sunken eyes and poor skin elasticity) may be misleading and treating these children with large volumes of intravenous fluids may prove disastrous. Additionally, there is now a consensus that prophylactic broad-spectrum antibiotics are essential as the physical signs of infection may be absent. Severe anaemia with haemoglobin < 50g/L may be treated with careful blood transfusion. Treatment with iron supplements should be delayed until the rehabilitation phase because it has been shown clearly that iron provision can precipitate fatal infection.

2. **Phase 2: Stabilization phase**. A return of appetite heralds the correction of metabolic imbalances and the need to increase the nutrient density gradually to 100 kcal/kg/day to promote rapid catch-up. Another formulation of the basic diet known as F100 (see Table 1.3) is used. It contains 2.9 g protein/100 ml. Continued careful monitoring of intake is essential to ensure adequacy but not over-loading. This phase may last up to 10 days.

3. **Phase 3: Rehabilitation phase**. The child is encouraged to take increasing amounts of F100.

Table 1.3 — Recipes for F-75 and F-100 feeds

	F-75	F-100
Dried skimmed milk (g)	25	80
Sugar (g)	100	50
Vegetable oil (g)	30	60
Electrolyte/mineral solution (ml)	20	20
Water: make up to	1000 ml	1000 ml
Contents per 100 ml		
Energy kcal	75	100
Protein (g)	0.9	2.9
Lactose (g)	1.3	4.2
Potassium (mmol)	4	6.3
Sodium (mmol)	0.6	1.9
Magnesium (mmol)	0.43	0.73
Zinc (mg)	2	2.3
Copper (mg)	0.25	0.25
% Energy from protein	5	12
% Energy from fat	36	53
Osmolarity (mOsmol/L)	413	419

Table 1.4 — Recipe for electrolyte mineral solution[a]

	Quantity (g)	Molar content of 20 ml
Potassium chloride: KCl	224	24 mmol
Tripotassium citrate	81	2 mmol
Magnesium chloride	76	3 mmol
Zinc acetate	8.2	300 µmol
Copper sulphate	1.4	45 µmol
Water: to make up to	2500 ml	

[a]Weigh ingredients and make up to 2500 ml. Add 20 ml of electrolyte/mineral solution to 1000 ml milk feed.

Regular meals of modified porridge or family foods interspersed with F100 should be continued until discharge. This process may take 2–6 weeks when 90% of the expected weight for height should be attained. Weight gain should be in the order of 5–20 g/kg/day. In addition, it is also essential to provide child-orientated care as well as psychological stimulation through play and exercise to overcome the psychological trauma of severe illness and hospitalization and the adverse effects of malnutrition on cognitive development.

Complications of refeeding

The history of the *refeeding syndrome* goes back to the 1940s when prisoners of war were noted to develop cardiopulmonary and neurological complications after being re-nourished. This syndrome was then rediscovered in the 1970s and 1980s with the introduction of parenteral nutrition for chronically-ill, essentially-starved hospitalized patients.

The refeeding syndrome describes the metabolic and physiological consequences of the depletion, repletion and compartmental shifts and inter-relationships of phosphorus, potassium, magnesium, glucose metabolism, vitamin deficiency and fluid resuscitation (Soloman & Kirby 1990).

As refeeding is initiated, there is a rapid reversal in the insulin, thyroid and adrenergic endocrine systems. Basal metabolic rate increases, and glucose becomes the predominant cellular fuel. The body immediately begins the process of rebuilding lost tissue. Positive balances of intracellular minerals accompany anabolism. As these minerals shift to the intracellular spaces, serum levels plummet. Body fluid compartments redistribute as the intracellular fluid level increases; extracellular fluid volume may increase or decrease depending on the previous intake, the persistent digestive losses and the refeeding regimen. The refeeding syndrome becomes most evident around the third day of treatment and needs to be looked for specifically. These rapid changes in metabolic status can create life-threatening complications, so the nutritional regimen must be chosen wisely and monitored closely. Several potential metabolic complications of the refeeding syndrome are listed in Table 1.5.

Parenteral nutrition in severely-malnourished children

Parenteral nutrition (PN) should always be used

Table 1.5 — Metabolic disorders associated with refeeding syndrome

Hypophosphataemia
Cardiac: altered myocardial function, arrhythmia, congestive heart failure, sudden death.
Haematological: altered red blood cell morphology, haemolytic anaemia, white blood cell dysfunction, thrombocytopenia, depressed platelet function, haemorrhage.
Hepatic: liver dysfunction (especially in cirrhotics).
Neuromuscular: acute areflexic paralysis, confusion, coma, cranial nerve palsies, diffuse sensory loss, Guillain-Barré-like syndrome, lethargy, paraesthesias, rhabdomyolysis, seizures, weakness.
Respiratory: acute ventilatory failure.
Skeletal (occurs with long-term hypophosphataemia): osteomalacia.

Hypokalaemia
Cardiac: arrhythmias, cardiac arrest, increased digitalis sensitivity, orthostatic hypotension, EKG changes (T-wave flattening or inversion, U-waves, ST segment depression).
Gastrointestinal: constipation, ileus, exacerbation of hepatic encephalopathy.
Metabolic: glucose intolerance, hypokalaemic metabolic alkalosis.
Neuromuscular: areflexia, hyporeflexia, paralysis, paraesthesias, respiratory depression, rhabdomyolysis, weakness.
Renal: decreased urinary concentrating ability, polyuria and polydipsia, nephropathy with decreased glomerular filtration rate, myoglobinuria (secondary to rhabdomyolysis).

Hypomagnesemia
Cardiac: arrhythmias, tachycardia, torsade de pointes.
Gastrointestinal: abdominal pain, anorexia, diarrhoea, constipation.
Neuromuscular: ataxia, confusion, fasciculations, hyporeflexia, irritability, muscle tremors, painful paraesthesias, personality changes, positive Trousseau's sign, seizures, tetany, vertigo, weakness.

Abbreviation: EKG electrocardiograph

cautiously in malnourished patients and only if the gastrointestinal tract is unable to meet the protein-energy requirements.

Nitrogen intake

Paediatric solutions are better suited for use in newborns, premature babies and malnourished infants.

They have a higher percentage of branched-chain amino acids, a modified aromatic amino acid content (a $\frac{1}{3}$ reduction in phenylalanine) and a modified sulphur amino acid content; methionine is reduced by 50% and cysteine is increased. The solutions also contain taurine, which is absent in standard solutions and an increased lysine level.

Excessive nitrogen intake may lead to hyper-ammonaemia and/or acidosis by exceeding renal clearance capacity for H^+ and phosphate ions. An intake of 0.5–1 g/kg parenteral amino acids is sufficient to maintain the plasma amino acid pool (Goulet 1998).

Energy intake

Glucose infusion rates should be kept constant without exceeding 1 g or 1.5 g/kg per h. A constant infusion is required to maintain blood glucose homeostasis as glucose reserves are very low. Under these conditions, the appearance of glycosuria indicates either a technical problem with the infusion or stress, particularly an infection. Energy intake is correlated closely with that of nitrogen. In infants, it varies from 100–120 kcal/kg per day, but the intake is reduced to 60–80 kcal/kg per day in older children.

Intravenous fat emulsions (IVFE) provide a highly-concentrated source of calories with a reduction of hepatic consequences of excessive glucose supply. The concentrated calories as well as the low osmolality make them ideal for peripheral PN. Despite these advantages, there are restrictions on the administration of lipids to malnourished infants. Malnutrition reduces lipoprotein lipase activity but this reappears with the onset of anabolism. Thus it is recommended that IVFE should not be administered until a few days after the start of PN (Goulet 1998).

Optimum glucose:fat ratio

A study in malnourished infants and young children has shown a maximum lipid utilization rate of about 3.3–3.6 g/kg per day. Above these values, there is an increased risk of fat deposition secondary to the incomplete metabolic utilization of the infused lipid. It is suggested that 2–3 g/kg/day lipid is required as soon as the clinical situation permits. This represents about 30% of non-protein energy intake. Slow infusions at a rate of 0.1–0.2 g/kg/h allows the best metabolic utilization and avoids fat overload and reticulo-endothelial system involvement (Goulet 1998).

Fluid and maintenance requirements

Following the initial phase of refeeding, water and electrolyte intake should be adjusted according to the child's age, degree of malnutrition and water electrolyte status. Infants require 120–140 ml/kg/day and older children 80–100 ml/kg/day. All normal infants and children need about 3–5 mmol chloride, sodium and potassium/kg/day.

When there are losses because of vomiting or gastric aspiration, 8 mmol sodium, 1 mmol potassium, 6 mmol H^+ and 12 mmol chloride should be added to each 100 ml water. In the case of an enterostomy, 15 mmol sodium, 1 mmol potassium, 10 mmol chloride and 5 mmol bicarbonate should be added to each 100 ml water.

Vitamins and trace elements should be provided also as a function of intake of respective nutrients. Adherence to recommendations may prevent depletion or excess. These intakes however, can be adjusted in situations of catabolic stress, infection or intestinal losses (Goulet 1998).

References

Ahmed, T., Ali, M., Ullah, M.M., Choudhury, I.A., Haque, M.E. et al. (1999) Mortality in severely malnourished children with diarrhoea and use of a standardised management protocol. *Lancet*, 353, 1919–1922.

Bern, C., Zucker, J.R., Perkins, B.A., Otienno, J., Oloo, A.J., Yip, R. (1997) Assessment of potential indicators for protein-energy malnutrition in the algorithm for integrated management of childhood illness. *Bulletin of the World Health Organization*, 75(Supplement 1), 87–96.

Cahill, G.F. (1981) Ketosis. *J of Parent Ent Nutr*, 5, 281–287.

Chandra, R.K. (1991) 1990 McCollum Award Lecture. Nutrition and Immunity: Lessons from the past and new insights into the future. *Amer J Clin Nutr*, 53, 1087–1101.

de Onis, M., Yip, R., Mei, Z. (1997) The development of MUAC-for-age reference data recommended by a WHO Expert Committee. *Bulletin of the World Health Organization*, 75; 11–18.

Gibson, R.S. (1990) Clinical Assessment. In: *Principles of Nutritional Assessment*, Oxford University Press pp. 577–586.

Goldsmith, B. (1996) Nutritional assessment in pediatric patients: How can the laboratory help? *Pediatric Pathology and Laboratory Medicine*, 16, 1–7.

Goulet, O. (1998) Assessment of nutritional status in clinical practice. *Baillière's Clinical Gastroenterology*, 12, 647–669.

Goulet, O. (1998) Nutritional support in malnourished paediatric patients. *Baillière's Clinical Gastroenterology*, 12, 843–876.

Goulet, O., de Potter, S., Salas, J. et al. (1993) Leucine metabolism at graded amino acid intakes in children receiving parenteral nutrition. *Amer J Physiol*, 265, E540–E546.

Hassanein, E.A., Assem, H.M., Rezk, M.M., El-Maghraby, R.M. (1998) Study of plasma albumin, transferrin, and firbonectin in children with mild to moderate protein-energy malnutrition. *J Tropical Pediatrics*, 44, 363–364.

Jelliffe, D.B. (1966) The assessment of the nutritional status of the community. *World Health Organization Monograph*, 53. Geneva: World Health Organization.

Khanum, S., Ashworth, A., Huttly, S.R. (1994) Controlled trial of three approaches to the treatment of severe malnutrition. *Lancet*, 344, 1728–1732.

McMahon, M.M., Bistrian, B.R. (1990) The physiology of nutritional assessment and therapy in protein calorie malnutrition. *Disease a Month*, 36, 385–417.

Mei, Z., Grummer-Strawn, L.M., de Onis, M., Yip, R. (1997) The development of MUAC-for-height reference including a comparison to other nutritional status screening indicators. *Bulletin of the World Health Organization*, 75, 333–341.

Minuto, F., Barreca, A., Adami, F. et al. (1989) Insulin-like growth factor I in human malnutrition relationship with some body composition and nutritional parameters. *J Parent Enter Nutr*, 113, 392–396.

Patrick, J., Golden, M.H.N. (1977) Leukocyte electrolytes and sodium transport in protein-energy malnutrition. *Amer J Clin Nutr*, 30, 1478–1481.

Schofield, C., Ashworth, A. (1996) Why have mortality rates for severe malnutrition remained so high? *Bulletin of the World Health Organization*, 74, 223–229.

Schroeder, D.G., Brown, K.H. (1994) Nutritional status as a predictor of child survival: Summarizing the association and quantifying its global impact. *Bulletin of the World Health Organization*, 72, 569–579.

Solomon, S.M., Kirby, D.F. (1990) The refeeding syndrome: A review. *J Parent Enter Nutr*, 14, 90–97.

Waterlow, J.C. (1973) Note on the assessment and classification of protein-energy malnutrition in children. *Lancet*, 2, 87–89.

WHO. (1999) Management of severe malnutrition: Manual for physicians and other senior health workers. Geneva: WHO.

2

Severe malnutrition in infancy and childhood

Graham Neale

Introduction

We are all familiar with the photographs of malnourished children in developing coutnries. The growing child needs a balanced diet containing all the nutrients. Clearly millions of children do not get this. Deficiencies of certain individual nutrients give highly-characteristic clinical pictures such as the anaemia of iron deficiency or the scorbutic rash of vitamin C deficiency. However, these pictures do not explain the appearance of the miserable starved-looking child who has been fed insufficient quantities of a poor quality diet for months or years. Famine and war are the two most potent causes of generalized malnutrition. Infectious disease is a highly-important contributory and modifying factor. Many authorities classify children with generalized malnutrition as suffering from marasmus or kwashiorkor (Table 2.1), often including an intermediate term, '*marasmic-kwashiorkor,*' to describe the child who is markedly underweight but also oedematous. As this is a book about practices and procedures we should be careful about definitions. Generalized undernutrition in infancy and childhood gives rise to three classical clinical pictures: marasmus, kwashiorkor and stunting.

Definitions

Marasmus

Clinicians interested in disorders of infancy and early childhood have used the term *marasmus* for more than a century. It is derived from the Greek 'marasmus,' which means a dying away. At the end of the nineteenth century it was applied to severe wasting occurring especially in the first year of life. Now it is used to describe the nutritional state of millions of infants and children living in developing countries. Often, especially in the early phases of marasmus, afflicted infants have good appetites and appear remarkably alert. Anthropomorphic indices show severe wasting with little subcutaneous fat and markedly-reduced skeletal muscle (see Table 2.1). In contrast, simple blood tests often give remarkably normal values, especially of circulating albumin, although such children are often anaemic because of associated deficiencies of iron and folic acid. The child with not-too-severe uncomplicated marasmus responds to refeeding.

Areas of the world that have short food supplies are often also plagued with infectious disease. The health of many children who appear to have uncomplicated marasmus is compromised by infection of the gut, especially with helminths, *Giardia*, *Cryptosporidia* and overgrowth of the small intestine by colonic bacteria. Moreover, intercurrent infection with malaria, schistosomiasis and other tropical infections is common as well. In addition, infection with the human immunodeficiency virus (HIV) is a major cause of extreme wasting (i.e., 'slim' disease). Thus the response to simple refeeding is unpredictable. A lively infant with a good appetite is likely to have a good prognosis. Anorexia and irritability often point to a slow uncertain recovery, especially if the child has persistent diarrhoea.

Stunting

With prolonged semi-starvation, the child fails to grow normally. On casual observation, an affected child may look quite normal except that the head and facial appearance may look older than the body. Puberty is delayed and the adolescent is slow to develop secondary sex characteristics. If height and weight is plotted against age the degree of stunting can be appreciated immediately (Fig. 2.1).

Kwashiorkor

The term *kwashiorkor* is used when the malnourished infant has pitting oedema of the extremities. Unfortunately, it is used in two quite different contexts and this leads to confusion in the literature. The word was introduced in 1931 when Cicely Williams wrote in the annual medical report of the Gold Coast colony

Table 2.1 — Wellcome classification for infants with generalized malnutrition

Weight for age (% median for NCHS★ standard)	Without oedema	With oedema
60–80	Undernutrition	Kwashiorkor
<60	Marasmus ★★	Marasmic-kwashiorkor

★ NCHS: American National Centre for Health Statistics; ★★ Includes both wasting and stunting

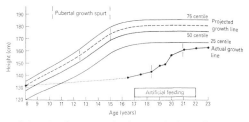

Figure 2.1 — Catch-up growth. The growth chart of a young man with Crohn's disease. The inflammatory condition of the bowel began in his ninth year. He was given various anti-inflammatory agents including corticosteroids. The symptoms were held in check but his pattern of growth was accepted as part of the disease process. Over 8 years he gained only 8 cm in height. The normal pre-pubertal growth rate is 5 cm per annum.

At age 17, he showed only early signs of puberty (stage 2). He had marked ileocolonic Crohn's pathology and was treated with a regimen of 'bowel rest'. For a few months he was fed a standard 2000 kcal parenteral diet by a central venous catheter and subsequently he was weaned onto an oral elemental diet. He had a normal but seriously delayed pubertal growth spurt. Sexual development was also delayed but normal. The graph shows that he did not make up the additional 10 cm he should have grown in the first four years of his illness. (With kind permission of Cambridge University Press from Tomlinson, Hegarty and Westman (eds) Mechanisms of Disease 1997, pp 431 and 438)

(now Ghana) about her studies in malnourished children.

The classical description

To try to improve understanding, the original publication is quoted:

'It (kwashiorkor) occurs in children between the ages of 1–4 years in whom there is a history of deficient breast feeding. The only supplementary food used is a preparation of maize. The disease takes from 4–12 months to express itself. The lesions of the skin are extensive, well marked and characteristic. They may be accompanied by oedema of the extremities. The mucus membranes are often inflamed and ulcerated. There is a tendency to vomiting and in chronic cases wasting may be severe. Diarrhoea occurs and may become persistent. The stools show undigested food but no ova or parasites. The child is extremely irritable and may die in a few days if not treated. It has been impossible to conduct a scientific investigation into the cause or to make controlled experiments into the nature of the cure. But the similarity of this condition with other deficiency diseases suggests that the remedy should be dietetic. My general impression is that cod liver oil and a good brand of tinned milk are the most important elements of treatment. Cod liver oil seems to delay the onset of the fulminating phase; but only

with in-patients for whom an adequate supply of good milk can be assured, is a cure established. At post-mortem nothing characteristic is found except a very fatty almost diffluent liver. Several aetiological factors may play a part in this syndrome. As maize is the only source of food some amino acid or protein deficiency cannot be excluded as a cause.… Maize is deficient in tryptophan, lysine and glycine.'

Cicely Williams took the term kwashiorkor from the language of the Ga tribe who lived around Accra. It has been interpreted variously but it was the word used for the sickness befalling the older child when the next baby was born. It is clear that Williams believed kwashiorkor to be due to the feeding of inappropriate food after weaning and indeed her classical article is headed Nutritional (Maize) Disease (Williams 1933). Curiously, her observations were ignored for 20 years. Some nutritionists confused the condition with pellagra and in many developing countries oedematous malnutrition did not appear to be closely related to specific diets.

Kwashiorkor and oedematous malnutrition – classifications

In 1952, the Food and Agricultural Organization of the United Nations/World Health Organization (FAO/WHO) Expert Committee on Nutrition commissioned an enquiry into the distinctive features of severe malnutrition. It was clear that the classical definitions took no account of overlap with other nutritionally-determined illnesses. As well, they paid no attention to the effect of other factors that affect growth, development and general well being such as infection, deficiency of specific nutrients and social deprivation. Gomez (1956) introduced a simple classification of generalized malnutrition based on weight for age, but this has little clinical value. The Wellcome Trust working party (Editorial 1970) added the presence or absence of oedema to the Gomez classification thereby giving four categories of generalized malnutrition: undernutrition, marasmus, kwashiorkor and marasmic-kwashiorkor (see Table 2.1). These terms appear in most textbooks. So defined, kwashiorkor is a term to be applied to any child who is malnourished and who has oedema.

The problem of defining kwashiorkor was not resolved by the Waterlow classification of generalized malnutrition (Waterlow 1972). However, this classification is useful because it incorporates the concept of stunting by using deficits of weight for height and of weight for age (Table 2.2). In the Wellcome

Table 2.2 — Waterlow classification for infants with generalized malnutrition

	Normal	Mild★	Moderate★	Severe★
Weight/height (% median NCHS standard★★) -measure of degree of wasting	90–120	80–89	70–79	<70
Height/age (% median NCHS standard ★★) -measure of degree of stunting	95–110	90–94	85–89	<85

★Without oedema; infants with oedema are classified as severe malnutrition (kwashiorkor); ★★ NCHS: American National Centre for Health Statistics

classification, malnutrition is classified as mild, moderate or severe (see Table 2.1). This may be fine for epidemiological studies but it is not satisfactory for defining the clinical state of an individual infant. It seems better to use Waterlow variables to define nutritional states in all three characteristics. Thus a child may be moderately wasted, mildly stunted and have oedema (the cause of which may be uncertain).

Dietary kwashiorkor

Perhaps the term kwashiorkor is best limited to those infants in whom the pathogenesis is clearly related to the sort of diet Cicely Williams describes. The infants she described in Ghana were weaned onto maize 'pap' that was deficient in the essential amino acids typtophan and lysine. Dietary kwashiorkor appears to be common in Central Africa where the dietary staples are cassava or plantain (which contain poor quality protein) (Trowell et al 1954) but rare in the Gambia were rice and millet are the principal foods (Whitehead et al 1977). Although the pathogenesis of dietary kwashiorkor is not applicable to oedematous malnutrition as a whole, the three other reasons for thinking that diets containing poor-quality protein and a high-carbohydrate content relative to protein may cause kwashiorkor without the effect of other agents are:

1. A similar condition can be produced experimentally by feeding an appropriate diet to baboons (Coward and Whitehead 1972);

2. In affluent countries, kwashiorkor has been described in infants taking extraordinary diets (often based on sugar drinks) over several months (Lunn et al 1998);

3. A similar condition may occur in patients with severe malabsorption in which the uptake of amino acids is much more severely affected than that of monosaccharides. This is seen occasionally in infants with cystic fibrosis (Philips et al 1993) and after gastric resection in adults who also have bacterial overgrowth in the small intestine or chronic pancreatic insufficiency (Neale et al 1967).

Oedematous malnutrition

Oedema is not uncommon in the malnourished. That it is not always due to kwashiorkor is clear from wartime studies that describe its appearance after severely-malnourished people started eating normal diets (i.e., 'war oedema', 'refeeding oedema'). The cause is not clear, but impaired integrity of the microvasculature due to the effect of circulating free radicals and a decrease in the activity of the cellular-sodium pump have been postulated. Similarly, many nutritionally-deprived oedematous infants labelled as having kwashiorkor do not have the clinical signs described by Cicely Williams and do not respond promptly to refeeding. In many countries, no differences can be found in the protein content of the diets of malnourished children with oedema and those without. Moreover there is no close correlation of oedema with hypoalbuminaemia. Many of these sick oedematous infants have infections, have possibly ingested toxins from contaminated food (e.g., aflatoxins) (Hendrickse 1998) and have eaten diets that do not contain sufficient antioxidants (such as vitamins C and E, lycopene in tomatoes, catecins in berries and carotenoids in carrots) to prevent damage by free radicals to key tissues. Cytokines and leukotrienes generated by inflammatory cells are also believed to be a cause of tissue damage in oedematous malnutrition (Mayakepek E. et al 1993). Often affected infants become oedematous quite suddenly (over a few days). This has been described especially after an outbreak of measles. The response of such infants to refeeding is variable (Golden 1998). The question is whether to label these children as having kwashiorkor.

Practice and procedures

Examination of the malnourished child

In assessing the malnourished infant, clinical examination remains very important (Trowell et al 1954).

Initial impressions should be noted. An emaciated but alert infant who is ravenous for food nearly always does well. On the other hand, a listless child with a pathetic cry needs a lot of help. A kwashiorkor infant who is swollen with oedema is usually apathetic and irritable. But if the problem is primarily that of protein-calories malnutrition careful feeding with a good diet (usually milk-based) leads to steady improvement.

Next the physician should undertake a careful clinical examination, noting the condition of the skin (integrity, rashes and pigmentation including the presence or absence of pitting oedema), the hair (colour, texture and quantity), the nails (quality and signs of dystrophy) and mucous membranes. The abdomen should be examined carefully and the size of the liver and spleen assessed. In classical kwashiorkor the liver is enlarged but the edge may be quite soft and difficult to feel.

The physician needs methods of measuring weight and height accurately and recording these against age on appropriate charts. Next, fluid retention should be noted by assessing the presence or absence of oedema. Anthropomorphic indices such as skinfold thickness (especially the tricep which is usually oedema-free) and mid-arm circumference provide simple estimates of body fat and body muscle. Thus it is possible to build up a simple picture of the infant's nutritional state with respect to the major nutrients.

The next step is to look for evidence of concomitant disease, especially infection and infestation, discussion of which is outside the scope of this chapter. Some illnesses can be shown clinically (e.g., infections of the skin or pneumonia); others require simple investigations such as thick-blood film for malaria and examination of the faeces for gut pathogens.

Finally some simple blood tests to assess haematological indices need to be done. Renal and hepatic function as well as antibodies to serious infections such as hepatitis B and HIV are necesary to complete the initial assessment. The measurement of circulating proteins throws an interesting light on the condition of the infant and these may be supplemented by more specific tests.

Circulating proteins

Most circulating proteins are produced in the parenchymal cells of the liver and they can be measured quite easily. Serum albumin is often used as a nutritional marker but it is important not to equate this measurement with protein-energy malnutrition (PEM) or worse still the amount of

Disease related to major nutrients

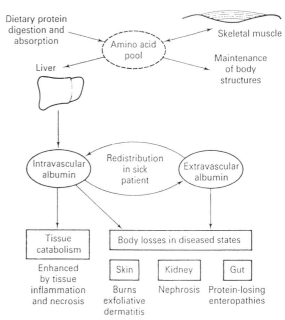

Figure 2.2— Factors influencing the concentration of circulating albumin. (With kind permission from Cambridge University Press from Tomlinson, Hegarty and Westman (eds) Mechanisms of Disease. 1997, pp 431 and 438)

protein in the diet. The concentration of circulating albumin reflects not only its synthetic rate but also the distribution of albumin in body pools, tissue catabolism of protein and losses from the body (Fig. 2.2).

More than half the albumin in the body is extravascular. It transfers from the intravascular pool continuously and is returned to circulation by the lymphatic system. With severe pathology (e.g., major infection) there is usually an increased proportion of albumin in the extravascular pool. This contrasts with the effect of simple starvation, which is associated with a preferential preservation of the intravascular albumin mass. Thus, the concentration of plasma albumin is well maintained in otherwise fit infants who are losing weight. Albumin has a half-life of 12–20 days but this is considerably shortened in the presence of inflammatory disease. Thus, the concentration of plasma albumin falls with any serious illness. It is also low in patients who are losing protein from the skin (e.g., severe weeping conditions), from the kidneys (nephrosis) or the gut (protein-losing enteropathy).

In uncomplicated malnutrition, significant hypo-albuminaemia appears to occur only under special circumstances. Usually it occurs when the diet has a low protein:energy ratio and especially if the protein is not of first-class quality. The starved child breaks down fat for energy and muscular protein to maintain the essential protein structure of the body, including circulating proteins. In contrast, the infant with dietary kwashiorkor may gain sufficient calories from its diet, which elevates blood glucose and promotes hyperinsulinaemia. In turn, this encourages the synthesis of muscle protein, increasing the requirement for essential amino acids. If these are in short supply (as they will be in a diet deficient in first-class quality protein) the body muscle competes with the liver and other structures requiring a good supply of well-balanced amino acids (such as the skin, the gut and the bone marrow). Thus the hepatic synthesis of 'export' proteins, such as albumin and the lipoproteins, is reduced; the infant becomes hypoalbuminaemic and develops a profoundly fatty liver (Coward & Lunn 1981).

Other circulating proteins are sometimes measured but the significance of abnormal concentrations is just as difficult to assess (Neale 1997). Pre-albumin, transferrin and retinol-binding protein (RBP) all fall with acute starvation but are also low in inflammatory conditions and in patients with liver disease. RBP is also low in patients with zinc deficiency and vitamin A deficiency. On the other hand, transferrin is increased in patients who are iron deficient. In contrast, ferritin is increased in patients with inflammatory disease (and iron overload) and reduced in those who are iron deficient.

Other laboratory tests

Special tests have been used in the assessment of dietary kwashiorkor but there is no good data on their sensitivity and specificity.

Concentration of circulating amino acids

It might be expected that the free-circulating amino acids mirror dietary deficiencies. This has proved not to be the case (Holt et al 1963). In dietary kwashiorkor, the aminogram shows a remarkable uniformity with a reduction in the concentration of essential amino acids such as methionine, tryptophan and the three branded-chain amino acids (isoleucine, leucine, valine), contrasting with the maintenance or even elevation of values for the nonessential amino acids such as glycine, serine, glutamine and taurine. Four nonessential amino acids also tend to be low. A simple method of determining the ratio of leucine, isoleucine, valine and

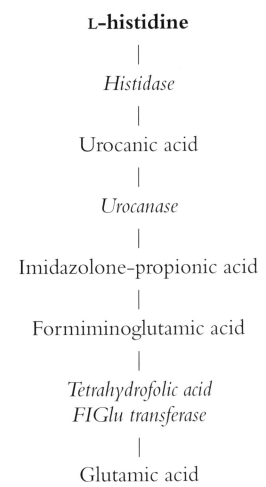

L-histidine

|

Histidase

|

Urocanic acid

|

Urocanase

|

Imidazolone-propionic acid

|

Formiminoglutamic acid

|

Tetrahydrofolic acid
FIGlu transferase

|

Glutamic acid

Figure 2.3 — Metabolic pathway for the metabolism of L-histidine.

methionine to glycine, serine, taurine and glutamine has been used as a marker for early kwashiorkor (Whitehead 1964), but its specificity remains uncertain.

Metabolic pathways

The metabolic pathways of amino acids that are not used in protein synthesis have been studied in some detail in kwashiorkor. Histidine is of peculiar interest because in the 1960s it was used as a marker of folate deficiency (FIGlu test). The main metabolites in the degradation of L-histidine are shown in Figure 2.3. After loading with L-histidine, folate-deficient subjects excrete formiminoglutamic acid (FIGlu). Urocanic acid, which is further up the metabolic pathway, was first detected in human urine in patients with intrinsic liver disease (Merritt et al 1960). Then it was detected in subjects with severe malnutrition (kwashiorkor), especially in the tropics (Whitehead and Arnstein

1961). Occasionally, it is found in the Western world (Hoffbrand et al 1966). It seems that severe impairment of urocanase activity occurs not only with serious liver pathology but also with severe generalized malnutrition. Whether or not it can be used to help distinguish between the various types of malnutrition that have been described in this chapter is not clear. However, with successful appropriate refeeding the abnormality in the metabolism in L–histidine is reversed within a few days (Hoffbrand et al 1966, Antener et al 1983). In severely-malnourished infants persistence of a high urocanic acid excretion in urine indicates a bad prognosis (Antener et al 1983).

Principles of management

Most infants with mild to moderate malnutrition (Waterlow classification) respond to refeeding with a good diet, correction of specific nutrient deficiencies and treatment of infection/infestation. Those with severe malnutrition (including all infants with oedema and those not taking food well by mouth) need specialist-monitored care in a residential unit.

The first step is a careful assessment, treatment of infection, restoration of plasma volume with balanced electrolytes and management designed to support vital functions of heart, lungs, kidney and liver. On admission, it is usual to give a course of broad-spectrum antibiotics and folic acid together with additional vitamins to cover any suspected specific deficiencies. Rehabilitation is begun by giving small quantities of oral rehydration fluid and then by providing a well-balanced liquid diet in increasing quantities by mouth or by nasogastric tube every 2–3 h. The diet must contain all essential nutrients but the most appropriate composition of the diet appears to depend on the stage of treatment (Badaloo et al 1999).

Infants with straightforward dietary kwashiorkor or uncomplicated marasmus usually respond quite quickly to any well-balanced diet. On the other hand, very sick infants showing signs of toxic shock with a low blood pressure, poor peripheral circulation, watery diarrhoea and deteriorating renal and liver function need very careful management. Such infants lose the ability to control body temperature (they are poikilothermic) and blood glucose (they develop hypoglycaemia). Almost certainly they have cerebral oedema. They require skilful restoration of plasma volume and inotropic support with maintenance of blood glucose before effective refeeding can begin. They often have to be kept warm and may need correction of a severe anaemia and treatment for heart failure. Hepatic, renal and intestinal function improve with adequate circulatory support.

The return of appetite and increasing physical activity are good signs. For about 7–10 days infants may need encouragement to eat as much as possible and thereafter they usually make good progress. They all need psycho-social support in addition to nutritional rehabilitation as they frequently show mental and psychological immaturity as well as physical stunting. Such infants are often said to be recovered when they achieve an appropriate weight for height. However, the scars of malnutrition remain. If the infant is to make optimal progress then the home environment needs to be assessed carefully and the family has to be equipped to prevent a recurrence of disease. All too often such children have been abandoned or come from social and economic conditions that cannot be corrected. In such cases, appropriate community care must be attempted.

References

Antener, I., Verwilghen, A.M., Van Geert, C., Mauron, J. (1983) Biochemical study of malnutrition. Part VI: Histidine and its metabolites. *Int J Vit Nut Res*, 53, 199–209.

Badaloo, A., Boyne, M., Reid, M., Persaud, C., Forrester, T., Millward, D.J., Jackson, A.A. (1999) Dietary protein, growth and urea kinetics in severely-malnourished children and during recovery. *J Nut*, 129, 969–979.

Coward, W.A., Whitehead, R.G. (1972) Experimental protein-energy malnutrition in baby baboons. *Br J Nutr*, 28, 223–237.

Coward, W.A., Lunn, P.G. (1981) The biochemistry and physiology of kwashiorkor and marasmus. *Brit Med Bull*, 37, 19–24.

Editorial. (1970) Classification of infantile malnutrition. *Lancet*, 2, 302–303.

Golden, M.H. (1998) Oedematous malnutrition (Review). *Brit Med Bulletin*, 54, 433–444.

Gomez F., Galvan R.R., Frenk S., Munoz Jc., Chavez R., Vazquez J. (1956) Mortality in second and third degree malnutrition. *J. Trop. Pediat*, 2, 77–83.

Hendrickse, R.G. (1998) Of sick turkeys, kwashiorkor, malaria, perinatal mortality, heroin addicts and food poisoning: Research on the influence of aflatoxins on child health in the tropics (Review). *Ann Trop Med Parasit*, 91, 787–793.

Holt, L.E., Snyderman, S.E., Nortin, P.N., Roitman, E.,

Finch, J. (1963) The plasma aminogram in kwashiorkor. *Lancet*, 2, 1343–1348.

Hoffbrand, A.V., Neale, G., Hines, J.D., Mollin, D.L. (1996) The excretion of FIG1u and urocanic acid after partial gastrectomy. *Lancet*, 1, 1231–1235.

Lunn, P.G., Morley, C.J., Neale, G. (1998) A case of kwashiorkor in the UK. *Clin Nut*, 17, 131–133.

Mayakepek, E., Becker K., Gana, L., Hoffman G.L., Leichsenring M. (1993) Leukotrienes in the pathophysiology of kwashiorkor. *Lancet*, 342, 958–960.

Merritt, A.D., Rucknagel, D.L., Gardiner, R.C., Silverman, M. (1960) The identification of urocanic acid in human urine and a comparison of N-forminoglutamic acid (FGA) with urocanic acid (UA) excretion following L-histidine loading. *Clin Res*, 8, 213.

Neale, G. (1997) Diet and disease. In: Tomlinson, S., Heagerty A.M., Weetman A.P. (eds.) *Mechanisms of Disease*, ch. 15, pp. 412–456 Cambridge: Cambridge University Press.

Neale, G., Antcliffe, A.C., Welbourn, R.J., Mollin, D., Booth, C.C. (1967) A syndrome resembling kwashiorkor after partial gastrectomy. *QJ Med*, 36, 469–475.

Philips, R.J., Crock, C.M., Dillon, M.J., Clayton, P.J., Curren, A., Harper, J. (1993) Cystic fibrosis presenting as kwashiorkor with florid skin rash. *Arch Dis Childh*, 69, 446–448.

Trowell, H.C., Davies, J.N.P., Dean, R.F.A. (1954) *Kwashiorkor* London: Edward Arnold.

Waterlow, J.C. (1972) Classification and definition of protein-calorie malnutrition. *BMJ*, 3, 566–569.

Waterlow, J.C. (1992) Protein-energy malnutrition. London: Edward Arnold.

Whitehead, R. (1964) Rapid determination of some plasma amino acids in subclinical kwashiorkor. *Lancet*, 1, 250–252.

Whitehead, R.G., Arnstein, H.R.V. (1961) Imidazole acrylic acid excretion in kwashiorkor. *Nature*, 190, 1105–1106.

Whitehead, R.G., Coward, W.A., Lunn, P.G., Rutishauser, I.H.E. (1977) A comparison of the pathogenesis of protein-energy malnutrition in Uganda and the Gambia. *Trans R Soc Trop Med Hyg*, 71, 189–195.

Williams, C.D. (1933) A nutritional disease of childhood associated with a maize diet. *Arch Dis Childh*, 8, 423–433.

3

Nutritional screening methods during emergencies

Fiona Watson

Abbreviations

CDC	Center for Disease Control
IDP	Internally Displaced Person
MUAC	Mid-Upper-Arm Circumference
NCHS	National Centre for Health Statistics
PEM	Protein-Energy Malnutrition
UNHCR	United Nations High Commissioner for Refugees
UNICEF	United Nations Children's Fund
WHO	World Health Organisation

Introduction

Whilst the large-scale food emergencies of the 1970s and 1980s were largely confined to Africa and to a lesser extent Asia, an increasing number of emergencies have occurred in eastern Europe (notably the former Yugoslavia) since the ending of the Cold War. The term *complex emergency* has been adopted to reflect the complex interaction of factors that trigger many of today's emergencies. These factors include: war and civil conflict; political, economic and social instability; and natural disasters such as drought and floods. Currently, the most severe emergencies in terms of widespread food insecurity, starvation, and excess mortality are linked to war and conflict. These emergencies are frequently protracted (lasting for more than 1 year) and accompanied by massive population movements.

Three population groups who are adversely affected during a complex emergency can be distinguished: refugees who have fled their country of origin; internally displaced people (IDPS) who have migrated within their country; and residents who have either remained in their homes within the emergency area or who are members of a host population that is affected by a population influx with whom resources must be shared. At the beginning of the millennium, there were more than 11 million refugees around the world and between 20–25 million IDPs (UNHCR 2000). About half of all emergency-affected people live in Africa.

Mass migration during an emergency frequently leads to settlements of large populations in either camps or as free-living individuals within a host community. Settlements differ greatly in character. The image which leaps to mind is of thousands of people crowded into temporary shelters (tents or home-made shacks), and this describes the living conditions of many refugees and IDPs in Africa. During the conflicts in the former Yugoslavia, however, less than one third of refugees and IDPs were housed in camps and

collective centres, while the majority either shared accommodation with host families or occupied empty properties. Long-term refugees may build permanent shelters and develop their own 'villages'. This is the case in the Gaza Strip, for example, where the refugee population has been resident since 1948.

The health and nutritional status of populations in large settlements and the basic services accessible to them vary enormously. Conditions also change over time. In the initial stages of an emergency, there may be large population influxes arriving in settlements that are ill-equipped to cater to their needs. Health and nutritional may suffer as a consequence and soaring crude mortality rates have been reported (Toole & Waldman 1988). Conditions may improve as settlements become established and aid is organized, but the situation is likely to fluctuate in response to relief-aid flows and changing populations.

Overcrowding, lack of food and clean water, inadequate sanitation and health care characterize the sudden displacement and settlement of large populations, and lead too often to epidemics, famine and death. A major concern therefore is to prevent and treat malnutrition whether this arises from inadequate protein-energy or micronutrient intake, and/or from repeated infections. This chapter describes procedures for screening the nutritional status of young children in large settlements during the acute phase of a food emergency through anthropometric (body) measurements and clinical examination. The chapter aims to present some of the general principles concerning screening in emergencies and should not be used as a guideline. Specific guidelines for nutritional screening are included in the references at the end of the chapter.

Practice and procedures

What is nutritional screening?

Nutritional screening during an emergency usually refers to the assessment of nutritional status of an at-risk population. Screening implies that all individuals within the population are assessed rather than just a sample of the population as for a survey. In the acute stage of an emergency, nutritional screening will generally be confined to anthropometric (body) measurement and physical examination to identify clinical signs of protein-energy malnutrition (PEM) and micronutrient deficiency. Information can, therefore, be collected about the prevalence and severity of malnutrition, but not about the causes of malnutrition within the population.

Nutritional screening differs from medical screening in that the goal of medical screening is the early detection of a disease in asymptomatic patients while nutritional screening only identifies individuals who are already exhibiting signs of malnutrition.

Why carry out nutritional screening?

Beaton et al (1990) state that 'the prime objective of nutritional screening in an emergency is to identify those individuals requiring immediate intervention to prevent deterioration of nutrition and risk of death, and to ensure survival until longer-term help is available'. Studies have shown that mortality risk rises sharply below a certain threshold of nutritional status (Tomkins & Watson 1989, Young & Jaspars 1995). The threshold varies between populations and age groups but in most cases severe PEM indicates life-threatening risk. Some micronutrient deficiencies such as vitamin A deficiency are also associated with increased mortality (Sommer et al 1983, Sommer et al 1986), whereas malnutrition (both PEM and micronutrient deficiency) is strongly associated with infection (Tomkins & Watson 1989). The prevention and treatment of malnutrition will therefore reduce rates of both mortality and morbidity. In the emergency context, the aim of nutritional screening is to identify individuals who are at immediate and gravest risk, and who will benefit most from intervention.

When should nutritional screening be carried out?

A number of criteria can be applied to determine when nutritional screening should be carried out.

Functioning interventions

Screening should only be carried out if it results in appropriate intervention. The priority of any emergency food relief programme is to provide a general ration in sufficient quantity and quality in terms of macro- and micronutrients to prevent malnutrition. Where this fails, however, and where malnutrition rates are high and rising, it may be necessary to open targeted feeding programmes. Two types of emergency targeted feeding programmes can be distinguished: 1) therapeutic feeding in which severely malnourished individuals receive intensive medical and nutritional treatment; and 2) supplementary feeding in which extra foods are provided to moderately malnourished individuals

(Shoham 1994). Targeted feeding programmes are best implemented in tandem with basic health care and public health interventions, which aim to reduce the spread of infection.

Control strategies for micronutrient deficiencies include: 1) changing the composition and quantity of the general ration; 2) food fortification; and 3) mass supplementation. Because of the increased risk of mortality and morbidity from some sub-clinical micronutrient deficiencies (e.g., vitamin A), mass supplementation to at-risk groups may be implemented as a prophylactic measure. Individuals who are admitted to targeted feeding programmes receive treatment for existing or potential micronutrient deficiencies.

As the essential element of screening is the identification of individuals for intervention, it should only be conducted when intervention programmes such as targeted feeding programmes have been established which have the capacity to cope with the new referrals identified through screening.

High prevalence of malnutrition

The benefits of screening will be outweighed by the costs in terms of time and expense if the prevalence of malnutrition is low. Representative nutrition surveys are usually conducted in the initial stages of an emergency to establish the prevalence of malnutrition. Existing guidelines all recommend that the results of nutrition surveys should be used in conjunction with other information to determine the need for targeted feeding programmes. When prevalence rates are high, screening is justified to identify individuals for entry into targeted feeding programmes. Although it is difficult to specify exactly what prevalence rate is considered high as situations differ, prevalence of malnutrition amongst children of between 15–20% would justify the opening of targeted feeding programmes in most situations.

Costs and feasibility

Screening entire populations is a costly and time-consuming business. Where health referral systems are functioning, unnecessary extra costs are incurred by mass screening. This may be the case in established settlements in more developed countries such as Palestinian refugee camps. A further constraint concerns logistics and security. Affected populations may be almost inaccessible due to distance, terrain or danger. The resources, time and security risks may be judged to be too great to warrant screening. The costs and feasibility of mass screening therefore have to be weighed against potential benefits.

Who should be screened?

High-risk populations

Populations may be at-risk of malnutrition during an emergency due to their socio-economic or physiological vulnerability. Socio-economic vulnerability implies that the resources normally available to a household have been eroded. Access to food (food security) is limited and households are forced to adopt 'coping strategies' in order to survive which further undermining their resource base. Socio-economically vulnerable households are at increased risk of malnutrition. The entire population of large settlements may be at risk of malnutrition in an emergency or certain population groups (e.g., refugees) may be at particular risk and therefore targeted for screening.

The major physiologically vulnerable groups are young children and pregnant and lactating women. Young children below the age of 5 years in developing countries suffer from higher levels of morbidity and mortality than other age groups. Whilst exclusively breast fed babies are largely protected against infection and malnutrition up until 6 months of age, weaning-age children (6 months to 3 years) are at increased risk. Babies who are not exclusively breast fed or who are born with low birth weight as a result of maternal malnutrition or ill health are also a high-risk group. Children under 5 years of age are therefore a priority group for nutritional screening. Nutrient needs during pregnancy and lactation are increased and women caring for young children frequently forego food in favour of their children. For these reasons, mothers are sometimes nutritionally screened.

It should be noted that malnutrition and mortality rates among adults are sometimes higher than those for children in the later stages of famine when large numbers of young children have already died (Collins 1995). In more industrialized countries where chronic diseases are the major public health problem, the elderly may be at greatest nutritional risk (Vespa & Watson 1995). In these cases, nutritional screening of all age groups is advisable. The techniques used to assess nutritional status in adults and the elderly differ from those used to assess children and will not be covered in this chapter.

Screening procedures

Screening implies that all members of the population group are covered. It is therefore essential that all children are screened and none are missed. In practical terms, this means that trained fieldworkers need to go to different areas of a large settlement to find the children rather than depend on mothers to bring children to a central point as the weakest are the least likely to attend. Nutritional screening is often implemented in conjunction with preventative interventions such as mass immunization or mass micronutrient (e.g., vitamin A) distribution.

Anthropometric measurement of children

Acute or recent malnutrition resulting in 'wasting' (i.e., thinness) is the major concern in emergencies. It can be measured in children using the indices of weight-for-height or mid-upper-arm circumference (MUAC). Weight-for-height compares a child's weight with the average weight of a reference population of children of the same height while MUAC is a quicker measure to take as it only involves a measurement around the upper arm. Weight-for-height and MUAC measures are not directly comparable, and MUAC tends to give larger estimates of the percentage of malnourished children. Children with oedema who cannot be anthropometrically measured are automatically classified as malnourished. Generally, MUAC is used for quick screening in the acute stages of an emergency when there are large populations of children to screen while weight-for-height is used in surveys and is carried out on children who have been selected through MUAC screening as a second check to assess their eligibility to enter a targeted feeding programme.

Procedures for measuring weight-for-height and MUAC in children are shown in Table 3.1. Weight-for-height cannot be calculated for children under 49 cm or for those with oedema. Length should be measured in children < 85 cm and those unable to stand. When the length of a child > 85 cm is measured, 1 cm should be subtracted from their length to give the equivalent height measurement. At least two people are needed to measure the weight, height and length of children and a third should record the results. MUAC can only be measured on children between 1–5 years old. One person can carry out the measuring while a second records the measurements.

Interpretation of anthropometric scores

The weight-for-height of a child is best expressed as a Z-score (equivalent to one standard deviation (SD) from the mean). The weight-for-height of each child

Table 3.1 — Methods for measuring the weight, height, length and MUAC of children

Weight	*Using 25 kg hanging Salter or CMS scales:* • Use a piece of rope to secure the scales to a tree ceiling or from a strong pole supported on the shoulders of two people. The dial should be at eye level; • Before each weighing session, check scales with a standard weight (use a stone or jerrycan of sand which has been accurately measured beforehand). In case of inaccuracies, have a spare set of scales available; • Remove all of the child's clothing (including nappies). In exceptionally cold climates, children should keep on underwear and be weighed as quickly as possible; • Place small babies and infants in either hanging pants, a sling, or local basket, and attach to the scales. Older children are able to hold on to the bar attached to the scales and lift themselves off the ground; • Ensure that nothing is touching the child. Stand directly in front of the dial and read the measurement to the nearest 0.1 kg; • Record the weight. *Using electronic scales:* • Check scales are recording accurately by weighing a standard weight; • Weigh mother or caretaker alone. Read the measurement to the nearest 0.1 kg; • Weigh mother with undressed child in her arms. Read the measurement to the nearest 0.1 kg; • Record both weights and calculate child's weight alone.
Height	*Using fixed statometer or portable stadiometer with spirit level:* • Position portable stadiometers against a wall or straight vertical surface with footplate flat on the ground. Fixed statometers can stand alone; • Stand the child up straight with heels and knees together but without leaning on the back of the measuring instrument; • Position head so that it is not tipped back and with eyes looking forward; • Lower the horizontal measuring block to rest gently on the head. Ensure that block is horizontal using spirit level; • Read the height to the nearest 0.5 cm; • Record the height.
Length	*Using a wooden length board or plastic baby-measuring mat:* • Lie the child on the board with the head towards the base board. Hold the child's head against the base of the board with the eyes looking straight up; • Gently hold knees to keep them straight; • Adjust measuring block until it rests flat against the soles of the child's feet, which should be flat; • Read measurement to the nearest 0.5 cm; • Record the length.
MUAC	*Using a MUAC insertion tape:* • Find the mid-point of the upper left arm by standing the child facing you and asking the child to bend the left arm at the elbow at a right angle and placing the left hand flat on the stomach. Use the MUAC tape to measure from the tip of the shoulder to the tip of the elbow. Mark the mid-point with a pen; • Wrap the tape closely round the arm at the mid-point. Do not pull tightly or leave loose; • Read the measurement to the nearest 0.1 cm; • Record MUAC.

has to be calculated and then, following WHO (1986) recommendations, compared with international reference values that are based on growth curves developed by NCHS (Dibley et al 1987). The process can be carried out by hand using NCHS reference tables, or calculations can be carried out automatically using the EpiNut component of the Epinfo computer programme (CDC & WHO 1994).

A Z-score between −3 and < −2 signifies moderate

Table 3.2 — Clinical signs of micronutrient deficiencies commonly found among populations in large settlements during an emergency

Vitamin A (Xeropthalmia)	Vitamin A deficiency is one of the three most common micronutrient deficiencies found in developing countries. There is a high risk of vitamin A deficiency during emergencies and vitamin A supplements are routinely given prophylatically to children. Vitamin A deficiency results in xeropthalmia which affects the eyes and frequently follows an episode of measles in children. The signs in order of presentation are: • Night blindness - inability to see in poor light (after sunset, inside huts); • Conjunctival xerosis – areas on the surface of the eyeball (conjunctiva) become dry and dull; • Bitots spots - dryness accompanied by foamy accumulations on the conjunctiva often near the outer edge of the iris; • Corneal xerosis - dryness, dullness or clouding (milky appearance) of the cornea; • Keratomalacia - softening and ulceration of the cornea. This is sometimes followed by perforation of the cornea, which leads to the loss of eye contents and permanent blindness. Ulceration and perforation may occur alarmingly fast (within a matter of hours).
Vitamin C (Scurvy)	Vitamin C deficiency is not common in stable situations but can arise when there is heavy dependence on an emergency ration which lacks sufficient vitamin C-rich foods. Scurvy usually develops gradually with progressive fatigue and pain in the limbs. Typical signs include: • Swollen and bleeding gums leading to loss of teeth; • Swollen, painful joints (in particular the hips and knees) that reduce mobility; • Minute haemorrhages around the hair follicles spreading to sheet haemorrhage on limbs; • Brittle hair; • Slow healing of wounds; • Infants tend to be fretful and scream on being handled because of tenderness of the limbs. They may lie on their backs in a characteristic 'frog's legs' position.
Vitamin D (Rickets)	Rickets is still endemic in some areas of the world. As the main source of vitamin D is sunlight, rickets in children could arise in war situations where a population has to seek shelter from bombardment during the day. Signs include: • Skeletal deformity (bowed legs); • Bone pain or tenderness; • Muscle weakness; • Rachitic children show reduced bone growth, are anaemic, and prone to respiratory infections.
Niacin (Pellagra)	Pellagra is uncommon in stable situations but can occur in maize eating populations (when the maize is untreated) or when an emergency ration lacks legumes, such as peanuts. Pellagra affects the skin, gastro-intestinal tract and nervous systems. For this reason, it is sometimes called the 3Ds: dermatitis, diarrhoea and dementia. Dermatitis is the most distinctive feature and shows the following signs: • Redness and itching on all areas of the skin exposed to sunlight resembling sunburn; • The redness develops into a distinctive 'crazy pavement' pattern; • Where dermatitis affects the neck, it is sometimes termed 'Casal's necklace'. Complaints of the digestive system include: • Nausea and sometimes constipation. • Disturbances of the nervous system include: • Weakness, tremor, anxiety, depression and irritability in mild cases; • Delirium in acute cases; • Dementia in chronic cases.
Thiamin (Beri-beri)	Populations who consume non-parboiled polished rice as a staple are at risk of beri-beri, particularly where the rice is contaminated with moulds. There are eight clinically recognisable syndromes of beri-beri; five in adults and three in children. Only four forms are commonly due to low intake in developing

Table 3.2 — (cont'd)

	countries: wet beri-beri; dry beri-beri; infantile acute cardiac beri-beri; and aphonic beri-beri. A variety of symptoms including anorexia, oedema, neuropathy, heart failure and muscle wasting characterize beri-beri.
Iron (Anaemia)	Iron-deficiency anaemia is the most common micronutrient deficiency world wide. Signs and symptoms of anaemia are vague but can include: • Fatigue and listlessness; • Breathlessness; • Pale conjunctiva, tongue and finger nails; • Impaired intellectual performance; • Resistance to infection; • Impaired thermoregulation.
Iodine (Goitre)	Iodine deficiency still occurs in populations living in mountainous areas. Goitre is characterized by: • Swelling of the thyroid gland in the neck. Cretinism (in children of mothers who suffered from iodine deficiency during the first trimester of pregnancy) is characterized by: • Mental retardation; • Deaf-mute; • Impaired motor coordination; • Spastic or ataxic gait; • Squint.

Adapted from Young 1992

malnutrition and a Z-score below −3 or oedema signifies severe malnutrition (WHO 1986). A MUAC of less than 13.5 cm signifies moderate malnutrition and below 12.5 cm or oedema signifies severe malnutrition.

Examination for clinical signs of micronutrient status and PEM

Before taking measurements, each child should be examined for clinical signs of protein-energy malnutrition (PEM) and micronutrient deficiencies. Some micronutrient deficiencies such as iron deficiency anaemia, vitamin A deficiency and iodine deficiency are widely prevalent in poor communities and represent major public health problems. Other deficiency diseases (e.g., scurvy, pellagra, and beriberi) do not commonly arise in non-emergency situations but outbreaks have occurred among refugee and displaced populations when relief programmes have failed to provide the minimum recommended daily allowances in food rations (Toole 1992). Correct diagnosis of micronutrient deficiency through clinical examination can be difficult and care should be taken to ensure that fieldworkers are properly trained and that identified cases are verified. The most common mineral and vitamin deficiencies found among populations in large settlements during an emergency are shown in Table 3.2. Kwashiorkor and marasmus are covered Chapters 1 and 2.

Interventions after screening

An example of the steps taken for screening and follow-up action according to recommended cut-off points is shown in Figure 3.1 (Beaton et al 1990). Children admitted to therapeutic and supplementary feeding centres will automatically be treated for infections and will receive vitamin and mineral supplements either to treat an existing deficiency or as a prophylactic measure.

Staff training and 'quality control'

Personnel who carry out nutritional screening do not need to be health professionals. Anyone in the community can be selected and trained as long as they can read and write. At least 1 day is required for training in measuring techniques while training combined with experience is important for correct identification of micronutrient deficiencies. Regular supervision of personnel should be carried out to ensure that standards are being observed.

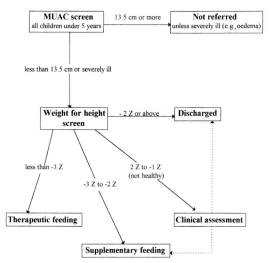

Figure 3.1 — Example of a possible screening procedure in large settlements during an emergency. Adapted from UNICEF 1986.

Discussion

Nutritional screening is a useful tool in identifying individuals for immediate interventions in emergency situations but suffers from a number of limitations. Firstly, nutritional screening alone provides no information about the causes of malnutrition in the population and so wide-scale preventative action cannot be taken. The causes of malnutrition are complex. The immediate causal factors are usually a combination of inadequate dietary intake and disease. These are, in turn affected by: 1) insufficient household food security; 2) inadequate maternal and child care practices; and 3) insufficient health services and an unhealthy environment. Information from a wide variety of sources needs to be collected and carefully interpreted to identify the under-lying causes of malnutrition before appropriate preventative strategies can be initiated. Secondly, nutritional screening provides point prevalence data and must be repeated at regular intervals to ascertain changes in the level of malnutrition and at-risk groups.

Nutritional screening is only one element in a range of strategies needed to prevent and treat malnutrition in large settlements during a food emergency. The nutrition issues of concern in food emergencies are extremely complex and broad based. Nutritional screening is thus only one small part of nutrition-related activities in emergency situations.

Acknowledgments

The advice of Jeremy Shoham, Helen Young and Matthew Law has been most useful in the preparation of this chapter.

References

AICF (1993) Prevenir la denutrition dans les populations à risque. Module iv. Paris: AICF.

Beaton, G., Kelly, A., Kevany, J., Martorell, R., Mason, J. (1990) Appropriate uses of anthropometric indices in children. ACC/SCN State-of-the-Art Series. Nutrition Policy Discussion Paper No. 7. ACC/SCN.

CDC, WHO. (1994) Epi Info 6. A word processing, database and statistics program for public health.

Collins, S. (1995) The limit of human adaptation to starvation. *Nature Medicine*, 1, 810–814.

Dibley, M.J., Goldsby, J.B., Staehling, N.W., Trowbridge, F.L. (1987) Development of normalized curves for the international growth reference: Historical and technical considerations. *Am J Clin Nutr*, 46, 736–748.

ICRC (1986) ICRC policies in emergency situations. Geneva: ICRC.

Lusty, T., Diskette, P. (1984) Selective feeding programmes. Oxfam Practical Health Guide No 1. Oxford: Oxfam.

MSF (1995) Nutrition guidelines. Paris: MSF.

Shoham, J. (1994) *Emergency Supplementary Feeding Programmes. Relief and Rehabilitation Network.* London: ODI.

Sommer, A., Tarwotjo, I., Hussaini, G., Susanto, D. (1983) Increased mortality in children with mild vitamin A deficiency. *Lancet*, 2, 585–588.

Sommer, A., Tarwotjo, I., Djunaedi, E., West, K.P., Loeden, A.A., Tilden, R. (1986) Impact of vitamin A supplementation on childhood mortality. *Lancet*, 1, 1169–1173.

Tomkins, A., Watson, F. (1989) Malnutrition and infection: A review. ACC/SCN State-of-the-Art Series. Nutrition Policy Discussion Paper No. 5. ACC/SCN.

Toole, M.J., Waldman, R.J. (1988) An analysis of mortality trends among refugee populations in Somalia, Sudan and Thailand. *WHO Bull*, 66, 237–247.

Toole, M.J. (1992) Micronutrient deficiencies in refugees. *Lancet*, 339, 1214–1216.

UNHCR (1982) United Nations high commissioner for refugees handbook for emergencies. Geneva: INHCR.

UNHCR (2000) UNHCR and refugees. Geneva: UNHCR Public Information Section.

UNICEF. (1986) Assisting in emergencies: A resource hand-book for UNICEF field staff. New York: UNICEF.

Vespa, J., Watson, F. (1995) Who is nutritionally vulnerable in Bosnia-Hercegovina? *BMJ*, 311, 652–654.

WHO working group. (1986) Use and interpretation of anthropometric indicators of nutritional status. *WHO Bull*, 64, 929–941.

Who (1995) The management of nutritional emergencies in large populations Geneva: WHO.

Young, S., Jaspars, S. (1995) Nutrition matters. People, food and famine. London: Intermediate Technology Publications Ltd.

4

Body composition in children with special health care needs

Christine Cronk, Ellen Fung and Virginia Stallings

Introduction

In the past, the term 'handicap' has been used to define an impairment of a particular kind of social and psychological behaviour or a disadvantage in a particular situation, sometimes caused by a disability. In the United States, Public Law 94–142 (Education of All Handicapped Children Act, 1975), is intended to include children who are mentally retarded, hard of hearing, deaf, speech impaired, visually handicapped, seriously emotionally impaired or multi-handicapped. Present day terminology refers to children with limitations in functional abilities, such as walking, sitting, eating, dressing, reading and learning as: 'Children with Special Health Care Needs.' These children may have functional limitations because of a physically based disorder of prenatal (genetic, disruption of fetal development), perinatal (problem in late pregnancy or delivery) or postnatal origin, and are likely to have accompanying alterations of metabolism, growth, and activity that in turn result in body composition that differs from the healthy child.

This chapter discusses two contrasting models of altered-body composition in children with cerebral palsy (CP) and in children with Down's syndrome (DS). The two conditions are prevalent disorders that cause handicaps, but each has a different aetiology and impact on growth, body composition and nutritional status. These differences require separate approaches to accurate clinical assessment and management.

In the following sections, the backgrounds of each disorder, growth and body composition, and related characteristics are discussed. A discussion of growth is included because of the strong association between increases in body size and changes in fat-free mass (FFM). Finally, recommendations for clinical evaluations of body composition and growth in children with these disorders are presented.

Cerebral palsy

Background

Cerebral palsy is a disorder of movement and posture secondary to a static encephalopathy, with the insult to the brain occurring pre-natally, perinatally or in early childhood. The term refers to the motor components of the underlying disorder, and is defined as specifically non-progressive (Blair and Stanley 1997). This disorder may occur in as many as 1 in 400 live births, with the most common aetiology

being anoxia around the time of birth, which is often due to difficulties at delivery. Handicaps in CP range widely depending upon the extent and motor systems affected. The three main types of CP are *spastic* (stiff and difficult movement), *athetoid* (involuntary and uncontrolled movement) and *ataxic* (disturbed sense of balance and depth perception). The disorder may affect one limb (*monoparesis*), two limbs (*hemiparesis*, *diplegia*), three limbs (*triplegia*) or all four limbs (*quadriplegia*). It is estimated that over 100,000 children in the United States under age 18, manifest one or more of the symptoms of CP and at least 5000 babies are diagnosed with the condition each year in the United States (Cummins, 1993).

Growth characteristics

Increases in body size are highly correlated with increases in FFM therefore, body weight may serve as a rough indicator of changes in FFM when studies using direct-body-composition measures are unavailable. By measuring height or a limb length, studies of children with CP indicate that growth is compromised throughout their lives and that the more severe the motor deficit, the greater the degree of growth retardation. Early studies assumed that growth failure was due to the underlying disorder, some set of factors linked to it (e.g., central nervous system (CNS) damage, lack of normal activity, altered energy expenditure, limb atrophy, scoliosis), or chronic malnutrition (Cronk and Stallings 1977). Recent studies (Stallings et al 1993 ab, 1995, 1996 Samson-Fang and Stevenson, 2000) have strongly implicated malnutrition as a frequent cause of growth failure, particularly among severely-affected children. Because of the heterogeneity found in children with CP, growth delays vary greatly.

A summary of studies which have used traditional anthropometic tools to assess stature suggest that children with quadriplegic CP are about 1.5 standard deviations (SD) below average (between fifth and tenth centiles) for body size; those with hemi or diplegia are reduced by less than 0.5 SD (between twenty-fifth and fiftieth centiles). Because accurate height is difficult or impossible to measure in this population of children, alternative measures (upper-arm or lower-leg lengths) are used to assess growth (Spender et al 1989, Stallings 1996a, Stevenson 1995). Among children with quadriplegic CP, size is usually less than the third centile with significantly greater deficits in lower-leg than upper-arm length. Hemiplegic and diplegic children have proportionate reductions in each dimension of around 0.5 SD (near the twenty-fifth centile).

Based on cross-sectional studies (where children of different ages are evaluated), children with severe CP show progressively-greater growth retardation with age probably owing to the cumulative effects of nutritional factors, CNS factors, contractures and scoliosis among others. In the studies of Spender et al (1989), Stallings et al (1993a), and Krick et al (1996), age specific measures of growth were closer to normal in infancy and toddlerhood (around tenth centile), but substantially less than third centile by mid-childhood. During adolescence, the degree of growth retardation is increased by a small pubertal growth spurt. By the oldest pre-adult ages, body size is sometimes reduced by as much as 3 SD below the average.

Among children with milder CP, those < 6 years of age may have slightly greater linear growth deficiency than older children (Stallings 1993b). Improvements with age appear to be associated with better nutritional status and higher levels of body fat, and this may arise from improved oral motor functioning as feeding milestones are achieved.

As indicated above, children with more severe disease including those with the greatest degree of hyper-tonicity, seizure disorders, and where all four limbs are involved, demonstrate both the most substantial growth failure and the greatest compromise in body fat and FFM. However, feeding difficulties associated with poor oral-motor functioning almost inevitably affect these children and contribute to under-nutrition (Thommessen et al 1991, Krick 1984, Dahl & Gebre-Medhin 1993). Thus nutritional compromise and disease severity confound each other. A substantial number of studies have demonstrated an association between poor growth and feeding abnormalities. Stallings et al (1993a) separated effects of disease severity and other factors (i.e., age, gender and ethnicity) contributing to growth failure in children 2–18 years of age with quadriplegic CP using a two-step regression procedure. For children < 8 years, the impact of nutritional status (assessed by body-fat measures) on growth was larger than in children > 8 years. This age difference probably reflects the irremediable effects of long-term under-nutrition on growth of older children who ultimately reach skeletal maturation (i.e., loss of growth potential) in spite of chronic malnutrition. Nutritional status may also contribute to the milder growth deficiency in children with hemiplegia and diplegia with significant correlations between size, fat

and muscle measurements in these children (Stallings et al 1993b).

Body composition and nutritional status

In general, children with CP have reduced body fat and FFM, though the differences are small for children with milder forms of CP. Children with severe CP have been found to be deficient in both fat mass (FM) and FFM by various measures (Azcue 1996, Spender et al 1989, Stallings et al 1993ab, Stallings et al 1995). Anthropometric measures of body fat (e.g., triceps and other skinfolds, percent body fat computed from skinfolds) indicate that body-fat stores are reduced by 0.5–1 SD (between tenth and twenty-fifth centiles) for children with quadriplegic CP and by about 0.3 SD (between twenty-fifth and fiftieth centiles) for children with less severe CP (Stallings et al 1993ab). Arm-muscle area (an indicator of muscle mass (Frisancho 1990)) is around tenth centile for quadri-plegic CP children, but near the median on average for children with hemiplegic and diplegic CP.

Age changes in anthropometric indicators of body composition in severe CP

Changes with age are of interest for children with severe CP because of the increasing risk of malnutrition in these children (Stallings et al 1993a). Figure 4.1 shows age trends for subscapular and triceps fat and arm-muscle area for children with quadriplegic CP. In the earliest age intervals, both measures of body fat are < 100% of the normal median value, with triceps skinfold being more reduced (around 60% of the median) than subscapular skinfolds (about 80% of the median). By later adolescence, average values in the two skinfold sites are similar; each are about 65% of the median, suggesting that truncal body fat stores are slowly depleted with age. Arm-muscle area is similar to the normal median at the earlier ages, but is reduced to around 60% of the normal median by

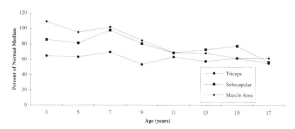

Figure 4.1 — Age trends for subscapular and triceps fat folds and arm-muscle area in children with spastic quadriplegic CP.

adolescence, suggesting that FFM may also be sacrificed over time in severe CP.

Estimates of body composition in severe CP

Stallings et al (1995) evaluated relative FFM and FM in pre-pubertal children with quadriplegic CP compared with a group of normal control children. FM in these children was reduced to about 60% of the control value (2.9 kg versus 4.6 kg in control), and FFM was reduced to about 75% of the control value (13.5 kg versus 17.6 kg) using deuterium oxide dilution (D_2O). Anthropometric estimates of FM and FFM (Slaughter et al 1988) yielded even lower estimates (47% for FM, 69% for FFM). Regression analyses indicated that black children were at risk for even lower fat stores (on average, 1.8 kg < white children) and that children with gastrostomy tubes had higher fat stores (on average 1.7 kg > those without tubes). The reduced fat stores in black children may be in part an artifact of the expected greater bone density and lower body fat levels seen in otherwise normal black children (Frisancho, Bell et al 1991). FFM showed an expected significant impact from age in both the CP and control children. Figure 4.2 shows the regression line for FFM fitted to age for children with severe CP and normal children. At 2 years of age, the FFM for controls and children with severe CP is similar. Increases in FFM with age (the slope of the lines) are significantly smaller in children with severe CP (1.06 kg/year) than controls (2.16 kg/year).

Centripetal fat pattern

As with other conditions associated with chronic nutritional deprivation, children with severe CP have a centripetal fat pattern (i.e., the fat on the arm (at the triceps-fat site) is differentially more depleted than that on the body (at the subscapular-fat site)). This was first documented in the study by Spender et al (1988)

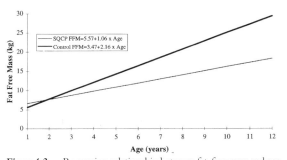

Figure 4.2 — Regression relationship between fat-free mass and age in children with spastic quadriplegic CP.

and replicated by Stallings et al (1995). Thus, exclusive use of the triceps-fat site may underestimate FM in these children. Simple correlations showed that the best estimator of percent body fat in children with CP (measured using D_2O) is the Slaughter equation (Slaughter et al 1988), which uses triceps and subscapular skinfold measurements (Stallings et al 1995) (see below).

Clinical assessment in children with cerebral palsy

Growth assessment for children with CP should follow many of the procedures used in a standard paediatric examination, including accurate and re-producible measurements of recumbent length or height and weight, head circumference in younger children and measurement of one (triceps) or more (biceps, subscapular and suprailiac) skinfolds when possible to determine body-fat stores more directly. These measures should be made accurately (Lohman et al 1988) using standard equipment and the National Centre for Health Statistics (NCHS) growth charts (Hamill et al 1979) or other comparable reference data that are based on a large national sample that reflects the growth of normal children. If only height and weight are measured, Krick et al (1996) have provided a special set of reference charts for height, weight and weight-for-height for children with quadriplegic CP to assist in identifying children who are aberrant compared to other children with quadriplegic CP. These charts were developed using tools of unknown reliability and malnourished children were not subtracted from the sample, therefore they are of questionable utility.

However, because measurement accuracy for height is usually poor in children with severe CP, special approaches to growth assessment should also be instituted (Stevenson 1996). Spender et al (1989) first suggested using upper-arm and/or lower-leg length as alternatives to height measures for difficult-to-measure children. These measures have a high correlation with height in normal children (around 0.8), and are particularly useful for children > 3–4 years of age. Stevenson (1995) evaluated a convenient sample of younger children with CP using these same measures and knee height, using only children with CP whose height/recumbent length could be measured. The correlation between height and each of the three measurements was around 0.97, indicating that such measures are an excellent proxy for height.

Stallings and Zemel (1996) present reference charts for upper-arm and lower-leg length drawn from a sample of normal children 3–18 years old on which measurements of children with CP can be plotted. Using these charts, the clinician can compare linear growth of a child with CP to that of normal, same-aged children as well as arrive at a proxy for height-age that might be used to assess the child's weight-for-height. In contrast, Stevenson recommended use of either lower-leg length (measurable with a steel tape) or knee height (measurable with a modestly-priced device) and computation of height using the following equations:

Upper-arm length	stature (cm) = 21.8 + (4.35 × upper-arm length)
Lower-leg (tibial) length	stature (cm) = 30.8 + (3.26 × lower-leg length)
Knee height	stature (cm) = 24.2 + (2.69 × knee height)

The computed values can then be plotted on the widely-available NCHS or another growth chart. This approach has the advantage of allowing weight-for-height determinations to be made. The equations, however, are only valid for children 12 years and under. Equations developed to estimate height from knee height in a normal, healthy population (Chumlea et al 1994) are recommended to be used for estimating height in adolescents and adults with CP.

Nutritional status assessment should help identify children who are over- or undernourished. Approaches to dietary intake are reviewed in Stallings & Zemel (1995). Body fat may be assessed in children with CP by measurement of triceps and subscapular skinfold thickness (described in Lohman et al 1988). Percent body fat can then be calculated using the equations from Slaughter et al (1988) as follows:

All females: % body fat = 1.33(triceps + subscapular) − 0.013(triceps + subscapular)^2 − 2.5

Prepubescent White males: % body fat = 1.21(triceps + subscapular) − 0.008(triceps + subscapular)^2 − 1.7

Prepubescent Black males: % body fat = 1.21(triceps + subscapular) − 0.008(triceps + subscapular)^2 − 3.2

In overweight subjects, when the sum of triceps and subscapular skinfolds is > 35 mm, the following equations are used:

All females: % body fat = 0.546(triceps + subscapular) + 9.7

All males: % body fat = 0.783(triceps + subscapular) + 1.6

Values for summed triceps and subscapular skinfolds can also be used and compared to reference data from the National Health and Nutrition Examination surveys I and II provided in Frisancho (1990). However, estimation of percentage body fat by use of skinfold measures should be made with caution in severely affected children because of the dis-proportionality of total body fat compared to healthy, physically active children from which the estimation equations were developed. (Van den Berg-Emons et al 1998).

Down's syndrome

Background

Down's syndrome (DS) is a relatively common disorder caused by the presence of an extra chromosome (number 21) in all of the cells of the body that usually results from a non-disjunction during meiotic cell division in the gametes. Approximately 4000 children with DS are born in the United States each year, or about 1 in every 800–1000 live births. DS is characterized by a wide range of phenotypic abnormalities including altered head and facial growth, disproportionately-short proximal-limb growth and organ abnormalities (including heart defects in up to 40% of affected children). These children are usually hypotonic and hyper-reflexic, though these abnormalies are ameliorated, to some extent, with age. Mental retardation occurs almost inevitably and is usually moderate. However, in the United States with the growth of early intervention, individual programming and mainstreaming, many children can reach more normal developmental accomplishments.

Growth characteristics

Post-natal growth retardation is a clearly identified feature of DS (Cronk 1993). Birth length and weight are slightly reduced from normals (≤ 1 cm in both genders), but progressive reduction in average length compared to normals is apparent with mean values 2 cm < normal at 3 months and 3.5 cm < normal by 3 years. There is, however, great variability with some children that is well within the range of normal variation, whereas other children are reduced by several SD. These size reductions are manifest in reduced growth velocities (rates), with the average child with DS growing 38 cm in 3 years compared with 46 cm of growth typical for healthy children. Similar reduction in weight and weight velocity are apparent during early infancy, reflecting reduced FFM accretion during this period. Velocity of weight gain is reduced by as much as

22% < normal children. Between 18–36 months, weight velocity is not different from normal.

From early childhood until about 11 or 12 years of age for girls and 15 or 16 years of age for boys, the difference in body height between children with DS and normal children is similar, reflecting relatively more normal changes in FFM. However, there is continued slow growth velocity in height (between third and twenty-fifth centiles compared to normals). Weight velocities for this same period show a more normal pattern (between twenty-fifth and fiftieth centiles), again indicating overweight relative to height. After these ages, the distance between the normal and DS growth curves increases.

During adolescence, height is reduced by 2–4 SD below the normal mean. By the end of adolescence, height is reduced by −3.5 and −4 SD. Peak pubertal growth spurts range from 5 to about 13 cm/year (similar or low compared to normal), and these spurts occur at ages similar to those of normals. Final height may be reached earlier than in normal children (15 years in boys, 14.3 years in girls). Boys with DS may have more-greatly-reduced pubertal growth spurts than girls.

Body composition

As indicated above, overweight is a commonly noted problem in children with DS beginning in late infancy and early childhood. Analyses of weight-for-height and body-mass index (Cronk et al 1985, Cronk 1993) indicate that between 2–12 years of age measures of body fatness for children with DS are above normal. Values of weight-for-height are clearly above those for normal children beginning at about the 100 cm interval for height (around 4–6 years of age) and remain above the normal mean for all the remaining intervals.

Median values for body-mass index (weight/height^2) are < those for normal children from about 3 months to 2 years of age. Thereafter, they are > normal, usually between seventy-fifth and ninety-fifth centiles throughout childhood and adolescence. Pseudo-velocities (i.e., growth velocities estimated from the difference of average weights at successive ages) for weight are between twenty-fifth and seventy-fifth centiles for normals throughout childhood but increase to ninetieth centile during adolescence. Because height velocities during this age interval are often below normal for adolescents with DS, the percentage of these children who are overweight or the degree of overweight probably increases during adolescence.

In a study on institutionalized children from Hungary,

Buday (1990) reported distributions for six skinfold sites in individuals 4 years of age through adulthood. Children with DS showed higher values only at the subscapular site. The differences increased with age, particularly in girls. The other sites (triceps, biceps, suprailiac and abdominal) did not differ from the normal control group.

Direct measurements of body composition

Few studies directly measuring body composition have been conducted on children with DS. A small sample of prepubescent children aged five to eleven years were assessed for body composition, dietary intake and energy expenditure and compared to a control group of healthy children (Luke et al 1994). Unfortunately, comparisons of body composition between the two groups is confounded by the fact that the control group was selected so that their percentage of ideal body weight would be similar to that of the DS group. Despite similarities between the two groups in BMI, percentage body fat, % ideal body weight and FFM, resting energy expenditure was reduced in the children with DS compared to the control group. These investigators speculate that this reduction is due in part to the characteristic hypotonicity of these children.

Clinical assessment in children with DS

As with children with CP, growth and body composition assessment for children with DS should follow the procedures used in a standard paediatric exam. Careful and accurate measurements of recumbent length or height and weight, head circumference in younger children, and measurement of one (triceps) or more (biceps, subscapular and suprailiac) skinfolds where possible to determine body fat stores more directly should be taken. These measures should be made accurately (Lohman et al 1988) using standard equipment and NCHS growth charts (Hamill et al 1979). In addition, height/recumbent length and weight should be plotted on growth charts specifically for children with DS (Cronk et al 1988). Reference data for weight-for-height (Cronk et al 1985) or body-mass index can also be used to evaluate relative body fatness.

References

Azcue, M.P., Zello, G.A., Levy, L.D., Pencharz, P.B. (1996) Energy expenditure and body composition in children with spastic quadriplegic cerebral palsy. *J Pediatr*, 129, 870–876.

Bell, W.H., Shary, J., Stevens, J., Garza, M., Gordon, L., Edwards, J. (1991) Demonstration that bone mass is greater in black than in white children. *J Bone Miner Res*, 6, 719–723.

Blair, E., Stanley, F.J. (1997) Issues in the classification and epidemiology of cerebral palsy. *Mental Retard Develop Disab Res Rev*, 3, 184–193.

Buday, J. (1990) Growth and physique in Down syndrome children and adults. Budapest, Humanbiologia Budapestinensis.

Chumlea, W.C., Guo, S.S., Steinbaugh, M. (1994) Prediction of stature from knee height for black and white adults and children with application to mobility-impaired or handicapped persons. *J Am Diet Assoc*, 94, 1385–1388.

Cronk, C.E. (1993) Growth Retardation in Children with Down Syndrome. In: Castells, S., Wisniewski, H. (eds.) *Growth Hormone Treatment in Down Syndrome: Proceedings of an International Conference*, pp. 13–32. New York: John Wiley & Sons.

Cronk, C.E., Chumlea, W.C., Roche, A.F. (1985) Assessment of overweight in children with trisomy 21. *Am J Ment Defic*, 89, 433–436.

Cronk, C.E., Crocker, A.C., Pueschel, S.M., Shea, A.M., Zackai, E., Pickens, G., Reed, R.B. (1988) Growth charts for children with Down syndrome: 1 month to 18 years of age. *Pediatrics*, 81, 102–110.

Cronk, C.E., Stallings, V.A. (1997) Growth in children with cerebral palsy. Mental Retardation Developmental Disabilities Research Reviews. 3, 129–137.

Cummins, S.K., Nelson, K.B., Grether, J.K., Velie, E.M. Cerebral Palsy in four northern California counties, births 1983 through 1985. *J Pediatr* 1993; 123, 230–237.

Dahl, M., Gebre-Medhin, M. (1993) Feeding and nutritional problems in children with cerebral palsy and myeloemningocoele. *Acta Paediatr*, 82, 816–820.

Frisancho, A.R. (1990) *Anthropometric Standards for The Assessment of Growth And Nutritional Status*. Ann Arbor: University of Michigan Press.

Hamill, P.V.V., Drizd, T.A., Johnson, C.L., Reed, R.B., Roche, A.F. (1979) Physical growth: National Center for Health Statistics percentiles. *Am J Clin Nutr*, 32, 607–629.

Krick, J., VanDuyn, M.A.S. (1984) The relationship between oral motor involvement and growth: a pilot study in a pediatric population with cerebral palsy. *J Am Diet Assoc*, 84, 555–559.

Krick, J., VanDuyn, M.A.S. (1996) Pattern of growth in children with cerebral palsy. *J Am Diet Assoc*, 96, 680–685.

Lohman, T.G., Roche, A.F., Martorell, R. (1988) *Anthropometric Standardization Reference Manual*. Champaign, IL: Human Kinetics Books.

Luke, A., Raoizen, N.J., Sutton, M., Schoeller, D.A. (1994)

Energy expenditure in Children with Down syndrome: Correcting metabolic rate for movement. *J Pediatr*, 125, 829–838.

Samson-Fang, L., Stevenson, R.D. (2000) Identification of malnutrition in children with CP: Poor performance of weight and height centiles. *Devel Med Child Neurol*, 42, 162–168.

Slaughter, M.H., Lohman, T.G., Boileau, R.A., Horswill, C.A., Stillman, R.J., VanLoan, M.D., Bemben, D.A. (1988) Skinfold equations for estimation of body fatness in children and youth. *Human Biol*, 60, 709–724.

Spender, Q.W., Cronk, C.E., Charney, E.B., Stallings, V.A. (1989) Assessment of linear growth of children with cerebral palsy: use of alternative measures to height or length. *Devel Med Child Neurol*, 31, 206–214.

Spender, Q.W., Hediger, M.L., Cronk, C.E., Stallings, V.A. (1988) Fat distribution in children with cerebral palsy. *Ann Hum Biol*, 15, 191–195.

Stallings, V.A., Charney, E.B., Davies, J.C., Cronk, C.E. (1993a) Nutrition-related growth failure of children with quadriplegic cerebral palsy. *Devel Med Child Neurol*, 35, 126–138.

Stallings, V.A., Charney, E.B., Davies, J.C., Cronk, C.E. (1993b) The relationship of growth and nutrition status in children with diplegic and hemiplegic cerebral palsy. *Devel Med Child Neurol*, 35, 997–1006.

Stallings, V.A., Cronk, C.E., Zemel, B.S., Charney, E.B. (1995) Body composition in children with spastic quadriplegic cerebral palsy. *J Pediatr*, 126, 833–839.

Stallings, V.A., Zemel, B.S. (1996a) Nutritional Assessment of The Disabled Child. In: Sullivan, P.B., Rosenbloom, L. (eds.) *Feeding the Disabled Child. Clin Dev Med*, 140, 62–76.

Stallings, V.A., Zemel, B.S., Davies, J.C., Cronk, C.E., Charney, E.B. (1996) Energy expenditure of children and adolescents with severe disabilities: A cerebral palsy model. *Amer J Clin Nutr*, 64, 627–634.

Stevenson, R.D. (1995) Use of segmental measures to estimate stature in children with cerebral palsy. *Arch Pediatr Adolesc Med*, 149, 658–662.

Stevenson, R.D. (1996) Measurement of growth in children with developmental disabilities. *Dev Med Child Neurol*, 38, 855–860.

Thommessen, M., Heiberg, A., Kase, B.F., Larsen, S., Riis, G. (1991) Feeding problems, height and weight in different groups of disabled children. *Acta Paediatr Scand*, 80, 527–533.

van den Berg-Emons, R.J.G., van Baak, M.A., Westerterp K.R. (1998) Are skinfold measurements suitable to compare body fat between children with spastic cerebral palsy and healthy controls? *Devel Med Child Neurol*, 40, 335–339.

5

Use and abuse of centile curves for BMI

T.J. Cole

Introduction

BMI is a simple index of weight adjusted for height. It has been used as such in adults for several decades, and published cut-offs are used to define underweight, overweight and obesity. There is some debate as to whether the cut-offs should increase with age, reflecting the known trend of BMI over life, or whether a single cut-off should be applied at all ages.

The application of BMI to children is a relatively recent event. Its statistical justification was first provided by Cole (1979), who pointed out the need to adjust it for age in the same way as for weight and height. Rolland-Cachera et al (1982) published the first BMI centile charts for French children, and these have since been followed by American, Swedish, Scottish, British and Hong Kong charts.

Historical background

The *body mass index* or BMI, defined as weight/height^2 in units of kg/m^2, was first described by Quetelet in 1869. Subsequently it was re-invented by Kaup, and so is alternatively known as the *Quetelet index* or the *Kaup index*.

Practice and procedures

BMI centile charts

BMI centiles for British boys and girls in 1990 are shown in Figures 5.1 and 5.2 (Cole et al 1995). The nine centiles are spaced two-thirds of a standard deviation score apart. The highest and lowest centiles identify the most extreme 4/1000 fat and thin individuals. The centiles are broadly the same shape in the two sexes, with a steep rise in BMI during the first year. There is a peak just before 12 months, followed by a period when BMI falls, reaching a minimum at about 6 years. Then, the BMI increases into adulthood. Compared to boys, girls' centiles fall less fast, then rise more steeply, and after puberty flatten off earlier. As a result, at age 20 years, median BMI is very similar in the two sexes, but rising more steeply in boys.

The second rise in BMI has been named the *adiposity rebound*, and the age when it occurs in individuals is predictive of later fatness (Rolland-Cachera et al 1984) — an earlier age is associated with greater adult fatness. It is noticeable (see Figs 5.1 and 5.2) that this age of adiposity rebound occurs earlier on the higher

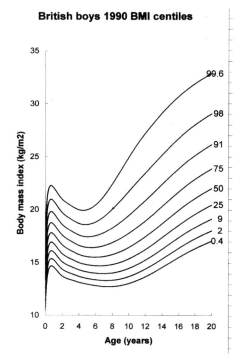

British boys 1990 BMI centiles

Figure 5.1 — BMI centile curves for British boys in 1990. The nine centiles are spaced two-thirds of a standard deviation score apart.

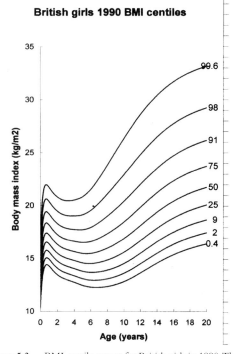

British girls 1990 BMI centiles

Figure 5.2 — BMI centile curves for British girls in 1990. The nine centiles are spaced two-thirds of a standard deviation score apart.

centiles than on the lower, though at similar ages in the two sexes. On the 99.6th centile, the age at adiposity rebound is soon after 4 years, whereas on the 0.4th centile it is at least 3 years later, between 7 and 8 years. This supports the idea that an early age at adiposity rebound is associated with greater fatness later.

Apart from the shape of the centiles, the other striking feature of the chart is the evidence of skewness in the centiles. The upper centiles are much further apart than the corresponding lower centiles, which shows that the BMI distribution skews to the right. Specially developed statistical methods (Cole et al 1998) are required to estimate the chart centiles when such skewness is present.

Use of the chart to assess obesity

The BMI chart is used in just the same way as conventional weight or height charts. An individual child's measurements are plotted on the chart, and if they show an extreme centile or marked centile crossing over time, then the child may need referral to a specialist. In contrast to height, where there is usually concern over low or falling centiles, the danger signs for BMI are more likely to be high or rising centiles. Being underweight is obviously a possibility, but with the current secular trends to increasing weight and fatness, patients are more likely to be above the top centile than below the bottom one.

Growth charts are designed to provide a screening aid for single measurements, with the false-positive rate fixed in advance. For example, using the 98th BMI centile as a cut-off for referral means that 2% of the reference population are above the centile. Therefore, the false-positive rate is set at 2% by definition. This principle can be used to decide which centile cut-off to use to define obesity — the less extreme the centile the larger the number of children that will be identified. When applied to the reference population, the choice of centile defines the prevalence of obesity.

The American BMI reference (Must et al 1991) uses the 85th centile for overweight and the 95th centile for obesity, implying rates for overweight and obesity of 15% and 5%, respectively. The British reference (Cole et al 1995) suggested using the 98th centile for overweight and the 99.6th for obesity, giving corresponding rates of 2.3% and 0.4%. The different definitions lead to more than a six-fold difference in the prevalence of overweight and a twelve-fold difference for obesity between the two countries, even if the reference populations are the same.

This highlights the need for a standardized definition of obesity. Unfortunately, there is no international consensus about which cut-off to use to define obesity in children. Unlike adults, the link between child obesity and later ill health is weak and poorly documented, and therefore cannot be used as a basis for defining the cut-off. A more pragmatic justification for the cut-off is needed, and this is currently being sought by a World Health Organisation sponsored task force. It involves linking the absolute cut-offs used in adults (e.g., BMI over 25 or 30) with corresponding centiles of BMI in late adolescence.

A related problem arises with the updating of BMI charts. If a cut-off for obesity is defined as a given BMI centile, for example the 95th, then 5% of the reference population lies above the cut-off. However, as more children become obese, the prevalence of obesity is seen to increase above 5%. This may well be interpreted as a need to update the BMI charts, but this would be a mistake. If the charts were updated, the prevalence of obesity based on the 95th centile would revert to 5%, and the obesity problem would, quite wrongly, appear to have gone away. The only way to avoid this happening is to 'freeze' the BMI chart, and agree not to update it. In this way it can continue to act as a baseline against which future changes in obesity prevalence can be measured (Power et al 1997).

Centile crossing

A recurring difficulty with growth charts is that they give no guidance about how to interpret centile crossing. No child stays on the same centile over a period of time, yet the chart does not indicate how much centile crossing is acceptable and how much is not. In addition, the trend to centile crossing can be shallow and long-lasting or, alternatively, steep and short-lived, which may have different implications for interpretation.

What determines the degree of centile crossing is the strength of the correlation between BMIs in the same children at different ages. For height, children exhibit a high degree of 'tracking,' that is staying close to their chosen centile, except during infancy and puberty. For weight, the tracking is less and the correlations are correspondingly weaker. BMI is equivalent to weight adjusted for height, and so is likely to show even less tracking. The clinical significance is that children can be expected to show quite large changes in BMI centile over time, and this should not necessarily be interpreted as unusual or sinister.

Weaknesses of BMI

An important aspect of the management of child obesity lies in the prediction of adult obesity, which is a risk factor for a wide range of chronic diseases. A high BMI centile in childhood and/or an early age of adiposity rebound are both risk factors for later fatness, but it is important to realize that child obesity does not predict adult obesity particularly well. Although fat children tend to remain fat as adults, it is also true that most fat adults were not fat as children (Power et al 1997). This is probably the main weakness of the child BMI chart: it does identify the many subjects who become obese in early adulthood.

The appeal of BMI is its simplicity, which is an easily calculated index of weight for height. In many circumstances, a high BMI is indicative of overweight due to an excess of body fat. However its simplicity is also its weakness, in that BMI does not measure body fat directly. A child with a high BMI may be fat, but alternatively he may simply be muscular. It has often been observed that athletes or similarly muscular subjects tend to screen false-positive for obesity based on the BMI. Clinically, this mis-classification can be avoided by using a measure of skinfold thickness to confirm the presence of excess body fat.

Recently, this mis-classification of muscle as fat has become important epidemiologically. Studies in the United States have found that obesity in adolescence, as assessed by BMI, shows little evidence of increasing over time, whereas obesity assessed by triceps skin-fold thickness in the same age group is increasing dramatically (Flegal 1993). This may be because the increase in body fat, as shown by skinfold thickness, is matched by a reduction in muscle mass, so that the net effect on weight, and hence on BMI, is minimal. This means that secular increases in BMI are likely to under-estimate the scale of the underlying problem of obesity.

Discussion

In summary, child BMI charts are a useful addition to the paediatric armamentarium, providing the clinician with a simple but adequate quantitative measure of overweight for height which is valid throughout childhood. Due to the relatively recent introduction of such charts, experience with them is necessarily limited, so that the behaviour of individual children followed for long periods, or the choice of a cut-off for screening purposes, are not well established. However it is clear that such charts are popular, and are likely to be used more and more in the future.

References

Cole, T.J. (1979) A method for assessing age-standardized weight-for-height in children seen cross-sectionally. *Ann Hum Biol*, 6, 249–268.

Cole, T.J., Freeman, J.V., Preece, M.A. (1995) Body Mass Index reference curves for the UK, 1990. *Arch Dis Child*, 73, 25–29.

Cole, T.J., Freeman, J.V., Preece, M.A. (1998) British 1990 growth reference centiles for weight, height, body mass index and head circumference fitted by maximum penalized likelihood. *Stat Med*, 17, 407–429.

Cole, T.J., Bellizzi, M.C., Flegal, K.M., Dietz, W.H. (2000) Establishing a standard definition for child overweight and obesity: international survey. *BMJ* 320, 1240–1243.

Flegal, K.M. (1993) Defining obesity in children and adolescents: Epidemiologic approaches. *Crit Rev Food Sci Nutr*, 33, 307–312.

Kaup, J. (1921) Munchener Mediziner Wochen Schrift; 68: 976.

Must, A., Dallal, G.E., Dietz, W.H. (1991) Reference data for obesity: 85th and 95th percentiles of body mass index (wt/ht^2) and triceps skinfold thickness. *Amer J Clin Nutr*, 53, 839–846.

Power, C., Lake, J.K., Cole, T.J. (1997) Measurement and long-term health risks of child and adolescent fatness. *Int J Obes*, 21, 507–526.

Rolland-Cachera, M.F., Sempé, M., Guilloud-Bataille, M., Patois, E., Pequignot-Guggenbuhl, F., Fautrad, V. (1982) Adiposity indices in children. *Amer J Clin Nutr*, 36, 178–184.

Rolland-Cachera, M.F., Deheeger, M., Bellisle, F., Sempé, M., Guilloud-Bataille, M., Patois, E. (1984) Adiposity rebound in children: A simple indicator for predicting obesity. *Amer J Clin Nutr*, 39, 129–135.

Quetelet L.A.J. (1969) Physique sociale. Brussels: C. Muquardt.

6

Behavioural aspects of feeding disorders

Roberta L. Babbitt and Keith E. Williams

Introduction

Most attempts at classifying paediatric feeding disorders have focused primarily on creating dichotomous groupings of children, differentiating between physiological and behavioural/environmental aetiologies. In the past, children who failed to gain weight were labelled as *failure-to-thrive* (FTT), then further differentiated as being either *organic* or *non-organic* FTT (Drotar 1988). Their failure to gain weight was attributed to either inadequate intake, retention or utilization of caloric nutrients. In the absence of organic findings, and often without a thorough intake assessment, many children were diagnosed with non-organic FTT. Non-organic FTT has been attributed to multiple factors, including childhood psychiatric disorders such as Reactive Attachment Disorder, caregiver psychopathology such as maternal depression, and environmental conditions such as social isolation or family stresses (Drotar 1989).

Unfortunately, the use of these types of dichotomous diagnoses is limiting, does not adequately reflect the clinical presentation of many children with feeding problems, and does not include the wide range of potential contributing and maintaining variables (Kerwin & Berkowitz 1996). Because of recent advances in medical science, there is a growing population of infants and children who live beyond the neonatal period and infancy despite their prematurity and complicated medical conditions. Children who have complicated developmental or medical histories usually have interrupted feeding histories and often have long histories of dysfunctional interactions surrounding feeding. All of these factors may bring about and maintain a feeding problem even when their medical conditions have resolved. Additionally, results of research that has attempted to identify variables that consistently differentiate children with organic versus non-organic feeding problems is mixed.

Because the clinical value and validity of the afore-mentioned diagnostic classification systems have not yet been proven (Budd et al 1992), an alternative more pragmatic approach is recommended, namely a behavioural system of diagnosis, assessment and treatment of paediatric feeding disorders. In this system, *feeding disorders* are defined as the child's inability or refusal to eat (or drink) sufficient quantities or types of food to sustain weight, meet nutritional needs or grow, regardless of aetiology (Babbitt et al 1994a). The focus of this functional approach is on the overt behaviours exhibited by the child and caregiver during mealtimes. Applied behaviour analysis based on empirically-verified principles of learning is a viable treatment option for children with feeding problems regardless of aetiology. It is based upon a science that identifies a behaviour and its environmental influences, develops an intervention strategy to change the behaviour, and measures the behaviour before, during and after intervention to evaluate effectiveness.

The purpose of this chapter is to provide an overview of the paediatric behavioural feeding literature and to acquaint the reader with basic behavioural assessment and treatment procedures demonstrated to be effective. Rather than provide an exhaustive, critical analysis of previous work in this field, we refer interested readers to excellent reviews in the literature (Babbitt et al 1994, Palmer et al 1975, Riordan et al 1980, Iwata et al 1982b, Blackman & Nelson 1987, Sisson & Van Hasselt 1989, O'Brien et al 1991).

Incidence/prevalence

A wide range of prevalence figures has been reported for children with varying degrees of feeding and growth-related problems. Berwick (1980) reported that between 1–5% of all paediatric admissions to hospital were for infants with FTT. Feeding problems that have been brought to the attention of a health care professional have been estimated to affect between 20–45% of infants/children at some point in their development (Kanner 1957, Bentovim 1970, Palmer & Horn 1978). For children with developmental disabilities, these reported figures can be even higher, from 13–80% (Coffey & Crawford 1971, Perske et al 1977, Palmer & Horn 1978, Jones 1982). Regardless of aetiology, these feeding and growth-related problems can lead to undesirable consequences for physical, intellectual, social and academic development as well as place excessive stress on the child's family (Christophersen & Hall 1978, Linscheid 1978, Riordan et al 1980, Finney 1986, Sisson & Van Hasselt 1989, Budd et al 1992).

Classification of feeding problems

Historically, feeding problems have been classified by aetiologies, physical topographies or even related behaviours and medical conditions (Illingworth & Lister 1964, Christophersen & Hall 1978, Linscheid 1978, Palmer & Horn 1978, Budd et al 1992). Although these systems may be useful, attention must be paid to observable behavioural topographies and their functions in order to develop effective interventions.

Table 6.1 — Operational definitions

Target feeding behaviours

Accept — the child allows a bite/drink to be deposited in the mouth within 5 seconds.

Expel — presence of any food/drink beyond the lip or chin area that had previously been in the child's mouth.

Gag — gagging or choking sounds emitted or facial grimacing.

Interruption — any behaviour that precludes acceptance within 5 seconds of presentation, e.g. turning the head, batting the spoon.

Negative vocalization — any crying, whining, screaming, or stating that one does not like the food, does not want to eat, and so forth.

Swallow — no piece of food larger than a pea is visible in the child's mouth prior to the next bite. A swallow is not scored unless the empty mouth is visible.

Behavioural terminology

Baseline — period of time prior to treatment during which behaviours are observed and measured; serves as an objective basis for evaluating treatment.

Continuous reinforcement — a schedule in which a reinforcer is delivered each time that a desired behaviour occurs.

Extinction — withholding a reinforcer that has been maintaining or increasing a behaviour.

Fading — a procedure in which the physical dimension(s) of a stimulus is (are) gradually changed to increase the likelihood that a desired behaviour will occur, e.g. systematically reducing the amount of prompting required for scooping a bite of food.

Food refusal — accepting an insufficient amount of food to maintain appropriate weight.

Food selectivity by type — accepting only a limited variety of food; often eating only one or two foods from an entire food group.

Food selectivity by texture — accepting a texture lower than age appropriate, typically one that does not require chewing.

Portion consumed — the amount of food measured before the meal minus the amount measured after the meal (controlling for amount spilled, expelled, or otherwise lost).

Reinforcement — an event that maintains or increases the probability of a response when it follows that response.

Shaping — a procedure in which behaviours not previously in the person's repertoire are systematically developed by providing positive reinforcement for successive approximations to the desired behaviour.

Swallowing skill deficit — inability to swallow or difficulty with swallowing, synonymous with oral-phase dysphagia.

Self-feeding skill deficit — inability to self-feed independently.

Target behaviour — a behaviour that has been selected for change, e.g. accept, expel, mouth clean.

Feeding behaviour is actually a complex, developmental chain of behaviours that need to be taught sequentially. A typical sequence of and definitions for common feeding target behaviours are presented in the first part of Table 6.1.

Practice and procedures

Assessment

In the behavioural literature, there is increasing emphasis on precisely specifying problem behaviours and then determining controlling variables (Iwata et al 1982a, Northrup et al 1991). Standardized and objective operational definitions of behaviours are critical for establishing treatment goals and evaluating outcomes, but alone do not indicate what factors account for target behaviours that should be addressed by treatment (Babbitt et al 1994). For this reason, there is a growing consensus that environmental factors that maintain a feeding problem should be isolated and systematically manipulated to optimize treatment (Shore & Piazza In press). Identifying environmental factors permits a better understanding of the ways in which these problem behaviours function in the environment (e.g., maintaining parental attention or avoiding texture changes and non-preferred foods). Comprehensive evaluation of a feeding problem involves medical, nutritional, oral motor and behavioural assessments as well as semi-structured caregiver interviews and standardized observations of feeding under baseline conditions (see Table 6.1).

Medical assessment

A comprehensive assessment of a child with a feeding

problem should begin with a medical assessment to identify any underlying conditions that may be amenable to therapeutic intervention. The physician/gastroenterologist should interview the caregivers and record the child's and family's medical history. When necessary, the child's neuro-developmental status is determined. Chronic medications should be reviewed to determine if any have adverse effects contributing to the feeding problem. Diagnostic laboratory testing should be performed to search for underlying abnormalities, such as metabolic or renal disease. In addition, diagnostic assessments of the gastrointestinal (GI) tract (e.g., upper GI, upper endoscopy) and swallowing mechanism (e.g., cinesophagram) should be performed to identify or rule out structural and functional problems as well as to ensure that the child can protect his/her airway while swallowing. If any abnormalities (e.g., acid peptic injury, gastro-oesophageal reflux) exist, then these conditions can be treated prior to entering an intensive treatment programme. Evaluation of suspected food allergies is also important during assessment. Finally, a gastric emptying scan should be performed to evaluate GI tract motility and function. Motility dysfunction can affect the appetite and definitely affects the development of future interventions.

Related allied health disciplines

Results of other disciplines' evaluations provide necessary information for the delineation of target goals and the development of treatment programmes. For example, a nutrition evaluation helps determine daily fluid and caloric intake goals, and an oral-motor assessment can recommend target food textures and appropriate feeding utensils.

Caregiver interview

Behavioural assessment frequently begins with an interview in which caregivers detail the child's behavioural and medical histories. The goal of the interview is to collect basic information to guide subsequent data collection. Information is gathered on the natural course of the child's feeding problem, the current status of the problem(s), previous and ongoing strategies that have or have not helped manage the child's eating, foods and textures that are now and were previously consumed or rejected consistently, meal duration, amounts consumed and caregivers' reports of environment-behaviour relations surrounding feeding (Luiselli 1989, Singer et al 1991, Babbitt et al 1994). Furthermore, information is gathered on other reported behavioural concerns, as well as the child's daily routine and family-home structure to provide a perspective in which to view the feeding problem. The emphasis is not one of treating symptoms and causes, but rather of identifying functional relationships between the feeding problem and its solution by identifying and manipulating those environmental variables that maintain the problem (Linscheid 1978, Shore & Piazza In press).

Direct observation

In order to develop and implement an effective intervention, objective measures of the target behaviours must be made (Kazdin 1982). Repeated observations are critical to determine stability and trend of the target behaviours over time, as any one meal could yield unrepresentative data (Palmer & Horn 1978, Iwata et al 1982b). Target behaviours must be operationally defined in terms of their quantifiable, physical characteristics such as topography, intensity and latency so that two independent observers would agree that a specific response occurred. Examples of operational definitions are presented in Table 6.1. Initial direct observations are made under a series of pre-treatment baseline conditions. The first is labelled a *home condition*, in which the caregiver is instructed to feed as he/she would at home, determining the type, amount and order of foods as well as the duration of the meal. The second phase, called *standard baseline assessment*, is individually tailored to each child, depending primarily on whether the child is a non-self-feeder or self-feeder. For a non-self-feeding child, a bite of food/drink is presented approximately once every 30 seconds, simultaneous with an instruction to take a bite/drink. This is repeated about 50 times in a meal, rotating through all food groups and the drink. No differential consequences follow any behaviour and the meal terminates only after the fiftieth bite has been presented or a maximum time limit for the meal has been reached. In the standard baseline procedure for a self-feeding child, a pre-measured, age-appropriate portion-sized meal is placed before the child. The child is given a verbal prompt about once every 30 seconds to take a bite/drink. No differential consequences follow any behaviour and the meal is ended after either the entire meal is consumed or 20 minutes have elapsed. Consumption data are recorded as frequency counts of bites/drinks taken of each food/drink per minute, as these are typically discrete events with readily observable starting and ending points. Pre- and post-meal weights of foods, drinks, clothing, bibs, napkins, and emesis are recorded. From this information, the number of grams

Table 6.2 — Progression of behavioural feeding treatment goals

1. **Refusal to accept**
   a) Have child sit in high chair/meal environment with minimal distress
   b) Have the child accept an empty spoon/cup
   c) Have the child accept small amounts of food

2. **Refusal to swallow**
   a) Have the child decrease expulsion
   b) Have the child accept and swallow small amounts of food without a time criterion
   c) Have the child accept and swallow small amounts of food within 30 seconds

3. **Limited volume**
   a) Have the child accept and swallow an increased volume of food, gradually increasing to age-appropriate portions

4. **Selectivity by type and texture**
   a) Have the child increase the variety of food consumed to an age-appropriate number
   b) Have the child increase the texture of foods consumed to one appropriate for his/her oral-motor status

5. **Self-feeding skill deficit**
   a) Have the child increase self-feeding skills to a level commensurate with his/her fine motor status

6. **Generalization**
   a) Have the child eat for different persons and/or eat in various settings under treatment conditions
   b) Gradually eliminate the treatment procedures from the meal, e.g. systematically fade the schedule of reinforcement

and percentage of each portion consumed are calculated for each food/drink. Also, the percentage of bites/drinks taken independently or with prompting can be determined.

Frequently, treatment effects can be facilitated by using foods and textures that the child is already likely to consume. Identifying these foods based solely on child or caregiver reports may not produce valid data (Parsons & Reid 1990). Direct observation of the child's food preferences is a more reliable and valid method. A detailed description of these assessment procedures can be found elsewhere (Babbitt et al 1994, Munk et al 1994).

Analysis of child and caregiver interaction

Assessment of the interaction between a caregiver's feeding and a child's eating behaviours provides information on interpersonal variables that may contribute to the feeding disorder. Specifically, the assessment delineates caregiver behaviours that serve as antecedents and consequences for the child's feeding behaviours and thus contribute to the maintenance of the feeding problems (Linscheid 1978, Luiselli 1989). Data are collected on the caregiver's correct use of antecedent stimuli (e.g., providing verbal instructions to eat accompanied by the presentation of a bite), prompts (e.g., in a spoken-gestural-physical prompt sequence unless instructed otherwise, re-presenting expelled food) and consequences (providing positive reinforcement for accepting and/or consuming the food and providing neutral consequences after other behaviours, unless instructed to do otherwise) (Iwata et al 1982b). This interaction analysis is conducted both inside and outside of meals to assess the caregiver's skills using a specific treatment protocol as well as general behaviour management skills (Riley et al 1989, Babbitt et al 1994).

Treatment

Once target behaviours, their function and the environmental variables maintaining them are identified, specific treatment procedures can be developed. Decisions regarding treatment development also include current medical status and intellectual functioning level. Treatment usually begins with the least intrusive yet most effective intervention possible, with additional treatment components added as necessary. Other important factors to consider when choosing treatment procedures include caregiver perceptions of acceptability, caregiver input and ease and pragmatism of implementation for the chosen interventions. Individual treatment procedures are discussed in the following sections. Treatment packages should be based upon the results of the child's assessment and individually tailored to meet his/her needs.

Table 6.3 — Treatment procedures

1. **Refusal to accept**
   a) Graduated exposure — the child is gradually exposed to the meal environment, first reinforced for sitting quietly, then accepting an empty spoon or cup, and then for accepting small amounts of food
   b) Continuous reinforcement — the child is reinforced immediately after each acceptance of a food/drink presentation
   c) Non-removal of the spoon — continue to present a small amount of food until the child allows the food into the mouth, ignoring crying or inappropriate behaviour

2. **Refusal to swallow**
   a) Representation — after the child expels a bite of food, replace the expelled food back into the child's mouth or give the child another bite of the same food until it is no longer expelled
   b) Differential reinforcement for swallowing — praise the child for accepting food and provide toy play or other more powerful reinforcers only after the child swallows the food accepted
   c) Swallow induction — a swallow is elicited and paired with reinforcement. The swallow elicitation is faded when the child begins to swallow

3. **Selectivity by type**
   a) Contingent preferred foods — preferred foods are offered immediately after a bite of a non-preferred food is accepted
   b) Fading preferred foods — preferred and non-preferred foods are mixed together and the preferred foods are systematically faded out of the non-preferred foods

4. **Selectivity by texture**
   a) Texture fading — the texture of the food is systematically increased and the child is reinforced for consumption of the higher texture foods

5. **Self-feeding skill deficit**
   a) 3-step guided compliance — a least-to-most prompting procedure used to teach self-feeding by providing an increasing amount of assistance until the child self-feeds a bite of food

A review of common behavioural terminology is provided in Table 6.1. These learning principles form the basis for all of the treatment procedures briefly described below. The progression of behavioural feeding treatment goals, based upon the logical sequence of feeding-skills development, is presented in Table 6.2. Treatment procedures designed to achieve these goals are presented in Table 6.3.

Acceptance

Reinforcement for oral acceptance and consumption of food has been widely demonstrated to be effective in treating food refusal (Riordan et al 1984, Singer et al 1991). Typically, acceptance is followed by reinforcement, while competing behaviours receive neutral consequences. If the child becomes too distressed in a feeding situation (conditioned aversion) and does not emit any behaviours to reinforce, the use of graduated exposure is recommended to introduce sytematically and gradually feeding demands to the child. Many children have successfully terminated any attempts to feed them, learning that a tantrum and clamping their mouths shut

result in escaping the meal. Therefore, there are too few opportunities for reinforcement to occur in a timely manner. These children may require an additional treatment component, that is non-removal of the spoon, whereby their behaviour to avoid being fed is placed on extinction. Thus, the probability that acceptance will occur is maximized and the child can receive reinforcement (Hoch et al 1994, Cooper et al 1995, Kerwin et al 1995, Ahearn et al 1996).

Swallowing/consumption

Although the child may be accepting food, most likely he/she spits the accepted food out. Consequently, an extinction procedure, *re-presentation*, may be used to decrease expelling (Coe et al 1997) and differential reinforcement can be delivered contingent on swallowing (Cooper et al 1995, Ahearn et al 1996). Dysphagia was treated successfully using a swallow induction procedure and reinforcement (Lamm & Greer 1988).

Selectivity by type

Although most children select and consume a

nutritionally-balanced diet (Birch & Deysher 1986), many children with limited oral feeding histories or neophobia self-limit their intake and become more than just 'picky eaters'. This problem occurs even more frequently among children with developmental disabilities. Food selectivity can be treated by making preferred foods (or other reinforcers) contingent on consuming non-preferred foods or mixing preferred and non-preferred foods and gradually fading out the amount of preferred foods in the mixture (Thompson & Palmer 1974, Finney 1986).

Selectivity by texture

Food selectivity by texture is another commonly encountered problem, especially among children with delayed oral feeding or poor oral-motor skills. Gradually fading up in texture by mixing lower- and higher-textured foods systematically and manipulating the ratio between the two textures (e.g., 80% low: 20% high, 60% low:40% high) has been used successfully to increase acceptance of higher textures (Luisielli & Gleason 1987). It is important to prompt (either verbally or by model) the child to chew to decrease the possibility of gagging and choking.

Self-feeding skill deficit

For many children, learning to feed themselves can be problematic. This is especially true for children with physical handicaps, neuromuscular deficits or developmental disabilities. After initially resolving the food refusal and/or selectivity, a guided compliance prompting procedure can be used to teach self-feeding and utensil use (Linscheid 1978).

Generalization and procedural fading

Although the above procedures can produce effective

Table 6.4 — Factors that may affect oral feeding

Organic
  Gastro-oesophageal reflux
  Anatomical defects
  Neuromotor dysfunction
  Impaired pulmonary status

Associated with chronic illness
  Cystic fibrosis
  Metabolic disorders
  Allergies
  AIDS

Secondary to treatment of illness
  Respiratory support
  Parenteral or enteral feeding
  Nausea-inducing treatment

Functional
  Environmental deprivation
  Behavioural and/or emotional problems
  Maintained by environment

changes in the clinical setting, the ultimate goal for most feeding interventions is for the child to eat well for any caregiver and in all settings (Luiselli 1989). Therefore, it is essential to programme generalization across settings, caregivers, foods and so forth by systematically adding distractions and changing aspects of the feeding setting to approximate more closely the child's community environments (Babbitt et al 1994). Another end goal is for the child to eat well with as little structure and prompts as necessary. Treatment should be faded gradually and systematically (e.g., fading the frequency of reinforcement and prompts, transferring control to more naturally occurring reinforcers like dessert) (Iwata et al 1982b).

Table 6.5 — Physician's screening form for paediatric feeding disorders

One or more 'Yes' answers could indicate the need for further evaluation of a feeding disorder.		
Yes	No	Does the child regularly refuse food at meals?
Yes	No	Does the child only eat certain textures?
Yes	No	Does the child only eat a few, highly-preferred foods? Does the parent prepare separate meals for this child?
Yes	No	Does the child often spit food out?
Yes	No	Does the child frequently vomit during or after meals?
Yes	No	Does the child have difficulty chewing?
Yes	No	Does the child usually finish his/her meal after the rest of the family?
Yes	No	Does the child often cry, scream or throw food during meals?
Yes	No	Does the child eat little at meals and snack throughout the day or subsist primarily on formula/supplements?
Yes	No	Is the child (over 18 months) unable to self-feed using fingers or utensils?

Table 6.6 — Consumer's form for screening treatment programs

Have you worked with children with similar feeding problems and medical conditions?

How many children with feeding problems have you served this year?

What is your rate of success? What are your typical outcomes and how long will each goal take?

What are the admission criteria for your program?

What is the typical length of admission?

What is the typical intensity of service?

Does your program use a multi-disiplinary approach?

Which disciplines will be working with my child?

What types of follow-up services are provided?

What type of caregiver training is provided?

Caregiver training

Finally, caregiver training is critical for the generalization and maintenance of treatment gains and long-term success (Shore & Piazza In press). Competency-based training packages reported in the literature include educational information, instruction in general child-behaviour management strategies, observation of therapist-fed meals, role-playing, behaviour rehearsal, feedback and fading into the meal situation (Linscheid 1978, Werle et al 1993, Babbitt et al 1994).

When to refer?

Health care providers are frequently inundated with parents' concerns about their childrens' eating and growth, sometimes even in the absence of observable weight and growth problems. A battery of medical tests may be ordered to identify possible organic aetiologies. Organic factors associated with feeding and growth disturbances are presented in Table 6.4. Clearly, when the feeding problem results in quantifiable medical conditions such as aspiration, frequent dehydration, constipation, emesis or vitamin deficiencies, the path of medical treatment appears straightforward. In contrast, non-organic factors including behavioural mismanagement, inadequate practice or stimulation, trauma or feeding problems secondary to emotional problems can also impede normal feeding development and growth. When these psychosocial factors interfere with family or school functioning, the reported problem needs to be addressed by trained and experienced feeding specialists. Table 6.5 presents a form for assisting primary health care providers in discriminating when to refer a case

to feeding specialists. To assist caregivers with finding appropriate and effective treatment for their child's feeding problem(s), a Consumer's Screening Form has been provided in Table 6.6, including recommended questions to pose to potential treatment providers.

Discussion and future directions

The application of behaviour analysis to the assessment and treatment of paediatric feeding disorders is burgeoning. Yet this wealth of information rarely reaches beyond the academic community or specialists. Much work still needs to be done to reach health care providers in primary care in order to educate them about the existence and effectiveness of this technology, about how to decide when to make an appropriate referral, and about how to identify suitable treatment programmes.

Acknowledgement

The authors thank and commend the clinicians, trainees and medical staff of the Pediatric Feeding Disorders Program for their efforts.

References

Ahearn, W.H., Kerwin, M.L., Eicher, P.S., Shantz, J., Swearingin, W. (1996) An alternating treatments comparison of two intensive interventions for food refusal. *J App Beh Anal*, 29, 321–332.

Babbitt, R.L., Hoch, T.A., Coe, D.A. (1994a) Behavioral Feeding Disorders. In: Tuchman, D.N., Walters, R. (eds.) *Pediatric Feeding and Swallowing Disorders: Pathophysiology, Diagnosis, and Treatment*, ch. 5, pp. 77–95. San Diego: Singular Publishing Group.

Babbitt, R.L., Hoch, T.A., Coe, D.A., Cataldo, M.F., Kelly, K.J., Stackhouse, C., Perman, J.A. (1994) Behavioral assessment and treatment of pediatric feeding disorders: Review article. *J Dev Behav Pediatr*, 15, 278–291.

Bentovim, A. (1970) The clinical approach to feeding disorders of childhood. *J Psychosomatic Res*, 14, 267–276.

Berwick, D.M. (1980) Non-organic failure to thrive. *Pediatric Review*, 1, 265–270.

Birch, L.L., Deysher, M. (1986) Conditioned and unconditioned caloric compensation: Evidence for self-regulation of food intake by young children. *Learning and Motivation*, 16, 341–355.

Blackman, J.A., Nelson, C.L.A. (1987) Rapid introduction

of oral feedings to tube-fed parents. *J Dev Behav Pediatr*, 8, 63–67.

Budd, K.S., McGraw, T.E., Farbisz, R., Murphy, T.B., Hawkins, D., Heilman, N., Werle, M. (1992) Psychosocial concomitants of children's feeding disorders. *J Pediatr Psychol*, 17, 81–94.

Christophersen, E.R., Hall, C.L. (1978) Eating patterns and associated problems encountered in normal children. *Issues Compr Pediatr Nurs*, 3, 1–16.

Coe, D.A., Babbitt, R.L., Williams, K.E., Hajimihalis, C., Snyder, A.M., Ballard, C.J., Efron, L.A. (1997) Use of extinction and reinforcement contingencies to increase food consumption and reduce expulsion. *J App Beh Anal*, 30, 581–583.

Coffey, K., Crawford, J. (1971) Nutritional Problems Commonly Encountered in The Developmentally Handicapped. In: Smith, M.A. (ed.) *Feeding the Handicapped Child*. Memphis, TN: University of Tennessee Child Development Center.

Cooper, L.J., Wacker, D.P., McComas, J.J., Brown, K., Peck, S.M., Richman, D., Drew, J., Frischmeyer, P., Millard, T. (1995) Use of component analysis to identify active variables in treatment packages for children with feeding disorders. *J App Beh Anal*, 28, 139–153.

Drotar, D. (1988) Failure to Thrive. In: Routh, D.K. (ed.) *Handbook of Pediatric Psychology*. New York: Guilford Press, pp. 71–107.

Drotar, D. (1989) Behavioral diagnosis in nonorganic failure-to-thrive: A critique and suggested approach to psychological assessment. *J Dev Behav Pediatr*, 10, 48–55.

Finney, J.W. (1986) Preventing common feeding problems in infants and young children. *Pediatr Clin North Am*, 33, 775–788.

Hoch, T.A., Babbitt, R.L., Coe, D.A., Krell, D.M., Hackbert, L. (1994) Contingency contacting. *Beh Mod*, 18, 106–128.

Illingworth, R.S., Lister, J. (1964) The critical or sensitive period, with special reference to certain feeding problems in infants and children. *J Pediatr*, 65, 839–848.

Iwata, B., Dorsey, M., Slifer, K., Bauman, K., Richman, G. (1982a) Toward a functional analysis of self-injury. *Anal Intervent Dev Disabil*, 2, 3–20.

Iwata, B.A., Riordan, M.M., Wohl, M.K., Finney, J.W. (1982b) Pediatric Feeding Disorders: Behavioral Analysis and Treatment. In: Accardo, P.J. (ed.) *Failure to Thrive in Infancy and Early Childhood*, ch. 13, pp. 297–329. Baltimore, MD: University Park Press.

Jones, T.W. (1982) Treatment of Behavior-Related Eating Problems in Retarded Students: A Review of The Literature. In: Hollis, J.H., Meyers, C.E. (eds.) *Life Threatening Behavior: Analysis and Intervention*, pp. 3–26, Washington DC: American Association on Mental Deficiency.

Kanner, L. (1957) *Child Psychiatry*. Springfield, IL: Charles C Thomas.

Kazdin, A.E. (1982) *Single Case Research Design: Methods for Clinical and Applied Settings*. New York: Oxford University Press.

Kerwin, M.L.E., Ahearn, W.H., Eicher, P.S., Burd, D.M. (1995) The costs of eating: A behavioral economic analysis of food refusal. *J App Beh Anal*, 28, 245–260.

Kerwin, M.L.E., Berkowitz, R.I. (1996) Feeding and eating disorders: Ingestive problems of infancy, childhood, and adolescence. *Schl Psychol Rev*, 25, 316–328.

Lamm, N., Greer, R.D. (1988) Induction and maintenance of swallowing responses in infants with dysphagia. *J App Beh Anal*, 21, 143–156.

Linscheid, T.R. (1978) Disturbances of Eating and Feeding. In: Magrab, P.R. (ed.) *Psychological Management of Pediatric Problems: Early Life Conditions & Chronic Diseases*, ch. 7, pp. 191–218, Baltimore, MD: University Park Press.

Luiselli, J.K. (1989) Behavioral Assessment and Treatment of Pediatric Feeding Disorders in Developmental Disabilities. In: Hersen, M., Eisler, R.M., Miller, P.M. (eds.) *Progress in Behavior Modification*, pp. 91–131. Newberry Park, CA: Sage Publications.

Luiselli, J.K., Gleason, D.J. (1987) Combining sensory reinforcement and texture fading procedures to overcome chronic food refusal. *J Beh Ther & Exp Psych*, 18, 149–155.

Munk, D.D., Repp, A.C., Karsh, K.G. (1994) Behavioral assessment of feeding problems of individuals with severe disabilities. *J App Beh Anal*, 27, 241–250.

Northrup, J., Wacker, D., Sasso, G. et al. (1991) A brief functional analysis of aggressive and alternative behavior in an outclinic setting. *J Appl Behav Anal*, 24, 509–522.

O'Brien, S., Repp, A.C., Williams, G.E., Christophersen, E.R. (1991) Pediatric feeding disorders. *Beh Mod*, 15, 394–418.

Palmer, S., Horn, S. (1978) Feeding Problems in Children. In: Palmer, S., Ekvalt, S. (eds.) *Pediatric Nutrition in Developmental Disorders*, ch. 13, pp. 107–129. Springfield, IL: Charles S. Thomas.

Palmer, S., Thompson, R.J. Jr., Linscheid, T.R. (1975) Applied behavior analysis in the treatment of childhood feeding problems. *Dev Med Child Neurol*, 17, 333–339.

Parsons, M.B., Reid, D.H. (1990) Assessing food preference among persons with profound mental retardation: Providing opportunities to make choices. *J Appl Behav Anal*, 23, 183–195.

Perske, R., Clifton, A., McClean, B.M., Stein, J.I. (eds.) (1977) *Mealtimes for Severely and Profoundly Mentally-*

Handicapped Persons: New Concepts and Attitudes. Baltimore, MD: University Park Press.

Riley, A.W., Parrish, J.M., Cataldo, M.F. (1989) Training Parents to Meet the Needs of Children with Medical or Physical Handicaps. In: Schaefer, C.E., Briesmeister, J. (eds.) *Handbook of Parent Training: Parents as Co-therapists for Children's Behavior Problems*, ch. 12, pp. 305–336. New York: John Wiley & Sons.

Riordan, M.M., Iwata, B.A., Finney, J.W., Wohl, M.K., Stanley, A.E. (1984) Behavioral assessment and treatment of chronic food refusal in handicapped children. *J App Beh Anal*, 17, 327–341.

Riordan, M.M., Iwata, B.A., Wohl, M.K., Finney, J.W. (1980) Behavioral treatment of food refusal and selectivity in developmentally disabled children. *Appl Res Ment Retard*, 1, 95–112.

Shore, B., Piazza, C. (In press) Pediatric Feeding Disorders. In: Konarski, E.A., Favell, J.E. (eds.) *Manual for the Assessment and Treatment of the Behavior Disorders of People with Mental Retardation*. London: MacKeith Press.

Singer, L.T., Nofer, J.A., Benson-Szekeley, L.J., Brooks, L.J. (1991) Behavioral assessment and management of food refusal in children with cystic fibrosis. *J Dev Behav Pediatr*, 12, 115–120.

Sisson, L.A., Van Hasselt, V.B. (1989) Feeding Disorders. In: Luiselli, J.K. (ed.) *Behavioral Medicine and Developmental Disabilities*, ch. 3, pp. 45–73. New York: Springer-Verlag.

Thompson, R.J. Jr., Palmer, S. (1974) Treatment of feeding problems—A behavioral approach. *J Nutr Educ*, 6, 63–66.

Werle, M.A., Murphy, T.B., Budd, K.S. (1993) Treating chronic food refusal in young children: Home-based parent training. *J App Beh Anal*, 26, 421–433.

7

Minimal enteral nutrition in infants and children

Carol L. Berseth

Historical background

Three parallel aspects in neonatology history have converged to create controversy concerning the use of enteral feedings for the pre-term infant who is admitted to the Newborn Intensive Care Unit or the Intermediate Care Unit. They are: 1) the evolution of medical technology and understanding; 2) the increasing rates of survival of pre-term infants; and 3) the emergence of necrotizing enterocolitis (NEC).

Technical advancements

Until the 1950s simple devices such as incubators and orogastric tubes were not available. Thus, many infants died as a result of metabolic derangements and/or starvation. The introduction of adequate technology permitted the use of early enteral feedings in the early 1960s (Bauman 1960, Smallpiece & Davies 1964). In addition, techniques to provide parenteral nutrition (PN) to infants were developed in the late 1960s (Wilmore & Dudrick 1968). Simultaneously, more scientific knowledge was gained concerning the specific nutritional needs of pre-term infants, and amino acid and lipid solutions were refined and modified for use in pre-term infants. As each of these technologies became available, common neonatal practice shifted pendulously from exclusive enteral feeding and the emergence of NEC to exclusive PN and the emergence of cholestatic jaundice, thrombotic complications and infectious morbidity. A more recent practice entails the use of small enteral feedings to supplement PN support. This newer approach utilizes the technical and scientific understanding of both aspects of feeding.

Increasing survival rates

When neonatology was established as a separate medical discipline in the early 1960s, survival rates were quite low among infants born less than 34–36 weeks gestation and virtually nil among those born < 32 weeks gestation. Over the past 3 decades, however, two epidemiological changes have occurred. First, the survival rates of pre-term infants have dramatically increased such that 85–90% of infants who are born at 28–36 weeks gestation now survive. In addition, the limit of viability has been receding such that 50–80% of infants born at gestational ages of 24–28 weeks gestation now survive. This increased viability has resulted in the presence of patients in newborn intensive care units who require prolonged hospitalizations (2–4 weeks in the 1960s vs. 3–4 months in the 1990s) and who have hospital courses complicated by immaturity of multiple organ systems. Neonatal gastrointestinal function is immature with respect to absorption, host defense and motor function. In addition, immaturity of other organ systems prompts in the use of medications and/or therapies that impair optimal gastrointestinal function. The use of methyl-xanthanes to treat apnoea of prematurity, for example, may cause decreased lower oesophageal-sphincter tone. In addition, these more immature infants often develop bronchopulmonary dysplasia and/or NEC, each of which result in complex nutritional issues that must be placed in the context of the limited abilities of the immature neonatal gastrointestinal tract.

Necrotizing enterocolitis

Outbreaks of NEC were first reported in the 1960s. Although the cause of this entity remains to be elucidated, specific epidemiological characteristics that place infants at risk for NEC have been identified. NEC occurs rarely in term infants, but is predominantly a disease seen in the pre-term infant. Rates of NEC vary from 10–40% of pre-term infants, and significantly the incidence is inversely related to gestational age (Stoll 1994). As a result, the incidence of NEC is increasing because more immature infants are surviving. The incidence of NEC is ten-fold higher among infants who have been fed compared to those who have not. Furthermore, there is an increased risk of NEC among infants whose daily feeding volumes are increased rapidly. In the 1960s, the use of hyper-osmolar formulas also was associated with an increased incidence of NEC. Thus, it is a common practice among neonatologists to use small volumes of iso-osmolar formulas for enteral feeding. The two concerns that arise with respect to NEC and feeding practices are: 1) whether it is advisable to give enteral feedings to pre-term infants; and 2) feeding management in the pre-term infant who has recovered from NEC with or without shortened bowel length (discussed below).

Practice and procedure

Feeding the pre-term infant

There is little consensus amongst neonatologists concerning the optimal way to initiate, advance or maintain feedings in pre-term infants (Churella et al 1985). Indeed there are numerous risks and benefits associated with the exclusive use of enteral nutrition

Table 7.1 — Advantages and disadvantages of early enteral feedings

Advantages

Stimulation of intestinal mucosal growth; release of gastrointestinal hormones and peptides

Improved maturation of gastrointestinal motor function

Better transition to enteral feeding

Less TPN - related Morbidity

Inexpensive

Reduced bacterial translocation

Disadvantages

Increased incidence of NEC

Aspiration of gastric contents

Less efficient caloric intake with respect to fluid intake

Potential exposure to allergies, foreign protein

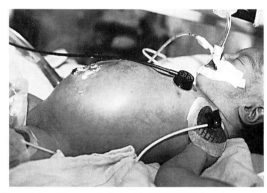

Figure 7.1 — Pre-term infant with NEC. This baby who was born at 30 weeks gestation received small enteral feedings on post-natal day 7. On post-natal day 14 he developed abdominal distention, haematochezia and profound hypotension. His abdominal X-ray demonstrated the presence of pneumatosis intestinal and pneumopesitoneum. At laporotomy the intestine was perforated at 3 sites.

(EN) or PN, as shown in Table 7.1 and Figure 7.1. In addition, there is significant individual variation amongst pre-term infants of similar gestational ages with respect to functional maturation of all of their organ systems including the gastrointestinal system. Finally, superimposed upon these issues is a variation in clinical practices that may result in the exposure of some infants to pharmacological agents that may alter intestinal function (e.g., antenatal steroids, opioids, antibiotics etc.). As well, variations in patient demographics and clinical experience may influence practice styles. For example, the incidence of NEC is often higher in NICU's that provide care for a population of babies who are out-born than in NICU's that provide care for a population of babies who are in-born. Thus, neonatologists who care for babies in the latter hospital may use a more aggressive feeding schedule.

The major benefit of the use of PN is that the physician can provide adequate caloric and nutrient intake quite early in life without concern for immaturity of the gastrointestinal tract. This benefit is important for the infant whose intestinal tract may not be fed because of the presence of an uncuffed endotracheal tube or the reluctance of the neonatologist to feed an infant who is receiving indomethacin. In fact, many studies have now demonstrated that the early use of TPN results in enhanced weight gain, positive nitrogen balance and improved long-term growth. However, there are several disadvantages for the exclusive use of TPN. First, it is expensive as it requires specialized mixing of solutions, the use of monitoring equipment, the insertion of intravenous catheters and frequent laboratory testing. In addition, the risks with TPN are high as infants may develop cholestatic jaundice, osteopenia, bleeding and metabolic derangements as a result of mixing errors. Thrombus formation may also occur resulting in superior vena caval syndrome or migration of small emboli to peripheral capillary beds. Long-term use of central lines may also result in infection by drug-resistant bacteria or fungus.

The exclusive use of EN also has numerous risks and benefits. First, it is inexpensive and technically easier to use; however, its use is often delayed because neonatologists are reluctant to initiate feedings within the first few days of life or to advance feeding volumes rapidly. Therefore, few enterally-fed infants can reliably establish positive nitrogen balance within the first week of life. Because the sucking mechanism is not present until 32–34 weeks gestation, enteral nutrients are often infused through orogastric, nasogastric or transpyloric tubes, which can become dislodged or perforate the stomach, oesophagus or intestine. For the infant who requires fluid restriction because of the presence of chronic lung disease or congenital heart disease, EN provides far less efficient caloric intake (2.81–3.36 J/ml) than does PN (4.2–5.04 J/ml). Moreover, sick premature infants who receive EN are at a significantly-greater risk of developing NEC, particularly when the volume of EN is advanced rapidly. Nevertheless, two recent randomized control trials have failed to confirm an association of NEC with the use of EN (LaGamma et al 1985, Ostertag et al 1986).

In an attempt to balance these risks and benefits, the

concept of minimal EN in sick neonates has evolved over the past several years. PN is used to supply the majority of the infant's nutrient intake while small-volume enteral feedings are given simultaneously to stimulate the gastrointestinal tract. Several regimens for providing minimal EN have been reported. In general, feeding volumes varying from 1.3–24 ml/kg/d of EN have been used.

Bronchopulmonary dysplasia

Another group of neonates who are often given minimal EN are those with bronchopulmonary dysplasia (BPD). Patients who develop BPD require complex medical care directed toward pulmonary care; however, these infants also have a high incidence of gastrointestinal problems and poor growth. The causes for these two issues are multi-factorial. Babies who have BPD often require greater nutritional intake because they have greater work of breathing and their lungs are undergoing rapid growth and healing. In addition, they often experience poor growth because of the catabolic effects of steroids used to treat BPD and the presence of poor tissue oxygenation. The need for increased caloric intake for these infants must be balanced by the need to restrict their fluid intake. Acquisition of sucking skills may be delayed by the presence of an endotracheal tube, and gastro-oesophageal reflux may result from the use of methylxanthines. As a result, many of these infants may require TPN to provide more efficient consistent caloric intake. Small volumes of EN are used to supplement the calories provided by TPN in order to maintain the health of the intestinal tract until it can be used reliably for caloric intake.

Short-gut syndrome

The most common cause of short-gut syndrome in the neonate is surgical resection for NEC. As for infants with BPD, the caloric needs of these infants are exceedingly high because of the rapid healing that occurs post-operatively. Because this caloric intake can not be provided enterally, TPN is the mainstay of nutritional support of these infants post-operatively. When the intestine is exposed to intraluminal nutrients 2–3 weeks post-operatively, extensive mucosal hypoplasia and dysfunction often inhibits efforts to use EN alone. In these infants, the role of minimal enteral feedings is not only to provide maintenance of mucosal function but also to stimulate healing and adaptation of the remaining gut. A more detailed description of the treatment of these patients is provided in Chapter 28. Briefly, these infants often require prolonged TPN support, as complete bowel adaptation may require 1–2 years. These infants are often given small volumes of enteral feedings that lack complex sugars until sufficient mucosal growth and gut hyperplasia permits a greater reliance on EN.

Mucosal and non-mucosal effects of enteral feeding

The use of enteral feedings has been shown to enhance intestinal mucosal growth and function as well as overall metabolic function. Although many studies have been conducted in animals, more recent evidence has been obtained from human adults and neonates.

Mucosal effects

The presence of intraluminal food provides a profound stimulus for growth of the intestinal mucosa. Prolonged starvation produces a thinning of the intestinal mucosa accompanied by villus shortening, loss of deoxyribonucleic acid (DNA) and protein content, and reduction in enzymatic activity (Brown et al 1963). When newborn animals are given early feedings for 48 h they demonstrate a twofold to three-fold increase in the mass of their intestinal mucosa as compared to animals that are not fed (Widdowson et al 1976, Berseth et al 1983, Heird et al 1984). This trophic effect of enteral nutrients appears to be a direct one rather than one mediated by an indirect mechanism of action. If PN is used to provide adequate nutrients to sustain somatic growth, gastrointestinal growth is still impaired morphologically, biochemically and functionally unless enteral nutrients are also provided (Greene et al 1974, Orenstein 1986). This direct trophic effect of enteral nutrients can be influenced by the composition of the feeding as well as its route of delivery (Morin et al 1980, Young et al 1982).

Trophic effects of enteral feedings also may be amplified by the presence of a variety of growth factors in foods. For example, the addition of fresh breast milk to intestinal cells can result in an increase in DNA synthesis (Klagsbrun 1978). The trophic effect of breast milk on intestinal mucosa is attributed to the presence of growth factors such as insulin, epidermal growth factor and other peptides known to exert direct trophic effects (Klagsbrun 1978, Berseth et al 1983, Dembinski et al 1984, Read et al 1984, Koldovsky & Thornburg

Table 7.2 — Growth factors in the gastrointestinal tract

Factor	Effects on growth	Effects on host defence
Glutamine	better intestinal morphology better feeding tolerance	↓ bacterial travel location ↓ incidence of sepsis
Epidermal growth factor	↑ intestinal growth better ulcer healing	
Transforming growth factor	better gastric healing	↑ IgA production by lymphoid cells
Insulin and IGF	↑ growth, maturation	↓ uptake of bacterial endotoxin
Growth hormone	↑ growth	
Glucocorticoids	↑ enzyme activity	
Bombesin	↑ epithelial proliferation	↓ bacterial translocation
PYY	↑ duodenal weight and DNA content	
Polyamines	↑ gut growth	↑ immune function

Adapted from Carver; Abbreviations: IgA, Immunoglobulin A; IGF – Insulin-like Growth Factor, PPY – Peptide YY.

1987). In addition, other bovine milk peptides such as bombesin are known to have trophic effects as they survive commercial processing of milk (Jahnke & Lazarus 1984). Other growth factors do not affect mucosal growth directly per se, but play an important role in enhancing host defence systems as outlined in Table 7.2. Many of these studies have been performed in animal models, however, and clinical application of these capacities in the neonates has been limited. The trophic effects of enteral nutrients on the intestinal mucosa can also be mediated indirectly as specific nutrients trigger the release of endogenous peptides such as gastrin and cholecystokinen, both of which in turn exert direct trophic effects on the gut mucosa (Berseth 1992, Lucas et al 1983, Meetze 1992).

Muscle effects

Three muscle layers that surround the muscoal surface are responsible for mixing and churning nutrients with digestive juices and for moving these nutrients distally through the intestine. In adults, the growth and function of these layers can be altered by the presence of specific nutrients in the intestinal lumen. This effect of intraluminal nutrients in motor function has been seen also in pre-term infants. Motor activity in the pre-term infant is immature compared to that of the term infant or adult. However, its maturation can be increased when the infant is given minimal enteral feedings. In an initial study, Berseth et al (1992) gave minimal enteral nutrition to pre-term infants being

treated for respiratory distress syndrome (RDS) so that by 2 weeks of post-natal age one group had received small enteral feedings and the other had not. All infants received parenteral nutrition during the study. At 2 weeks of age, infants who had received enteral nutrition had: 1) greater migrating motor activity, which is responsible for the forward movement of nutrients; 2) greater motor quiescence, which is reflective of greater inhibitory regulation; and 3) a detectable change in motor activity in response to feeding. In contrast, infants who had received only PN exhibited very few episodes of migrating activity, a paucity of motor quiescence, and an absence of change in motor activity in response to feeding. The differences in motor functions seen in these two groups of infants was clinically significant as the unfed infants experienced slower somatic growth and more frequent episodes of feeding intolerance during the first 5 post-natal weeks than did the group who received minimal EN (Fig. 7.2). Because neonatologists often feed babies sterile water, a second study was then performed to determine whether the maturational changes induced by small enteral feedings were due to the presence of nutrients in the intestine. In this study, 32 pre-term infants received *priming feedings* of 24 ml/kg/d from the third to the fourteenth day of life. Sixteen infants were fed infant formula, and the remaining 16 were fed sterile water. As in the first study, infants who had received minimal enteral feedings displayed more mature motor activity by the second post-natal week than did

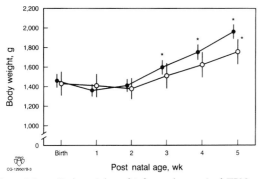

Figure 7.2 — Body weights of infants who received TPN and began small enteral feedings on post-natal day 3 (solid circles) and post-natal day 12 (open circles). Babies who received small enteral feedings had better weight gain during post-natal weeks 3–5 (see Berseth 1992 for full data).

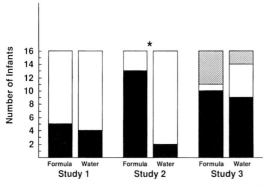

Figure 7.3 — Incidence of migrating motor activity amongst babies fed small volumes of formula and sterile water. At study one, approximately 25% of babies in both groups had migrating activity (black); the others did not (white). The shaded area represents babies who were not evaluated on the third occasion. After 10 days (study 2) of feeding, 3 times as many infants receiving formula had migrating activity compared to those receiving sterile water. After (study 3) water-fed infants' migrating activity was equally present in both groups of infants. From Berseth & Nordyke (1993), with permission.

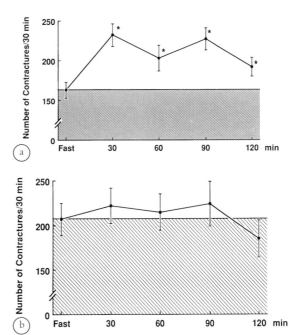

Figure 7.4 — Motor responses to feeding in infants who received small enteral feedings with formula (top panel) and water (bottom panel). Overall motor activity during fasting is shown by the hatched area with feeding. Motor activity increases briskly with feeding and is sustained for 12 minutes. In contrast, when infants who have been fed water are given a formula feeding there is little change in motor activity. From Berseth & Nordyke (1993), with permission.

infants who received sterile water (Figs. 7.3 and 7.4) (Berseth 1993). Infants who had received minimal enteral feedings established full EN and full nipple feedings sooner than those fed water. Thus, both of these studies show that the early administration of EN optimizes the maturation of intestinal muscular function in pre-term infants.

Vascular effects

In adults, the provision of enteral nutrients results in the post-prandial hyperaemic response, which is described as a decrease in splanchnic-bed resistance, an increase in intestinal blood flow, and an increase in oxygen uptake. Splanchnic-vascular resistance fails to drop in response

to feeding in the newborn pig on the first day of life; however, a brisk reduction is present by the third day (Crissenger 1989). Thereafter, splanchnic-bed resistance decreases and oxygen consumption increases in neonates following the ingestion of protein or lipid but not glucose. Hence, ingestion of glucose appears to induce less metabolic stress than does the ingestion of protein or lipid. In the human infant, post-prandial vascular responses to feeding are present in the human pre-term and term infant by the third post-natal day (Martinussen et al 1994, 1996). Unlike the term infant, however, the splanchnic hyperaemic response in the pre-term infant results in compensatory systemic haemodynamic changes, especially increases in cardiac output. Whether the volume or nutrient load of the eternal feeding alters these vascular responses has not been tested yet, and one could speculate that the use of minimal volumes of enteral feeding may cause less stress on cardiac output. The dual effects of feeding and hypoxia in the neonatal animal result in diminished oxygen uptake and mucosal damage. (Crissenger 1989, Szabo et al 1987). Although hyperaemic responses to specific nutrients or hypoxic challenge have been tested in human pre-term infants, these two studies in animals suggest that the pre-term infant who is marginally oxygenated is more vulnerable to the metabolic stress caused by enteral feedings.

Endocrine and metabolic effects

Fasting plasma concentrations of many gastrointestinal peptides are similar in pre-term and term infants (Berseth 1992, Lucas 1982) Pre-term infants also demonstrate the ability to release peptides in response to feeding. Fasting plasma concentrations of peptides increase post-natally if babies receive full enteral feedings for a week (Berseth 1992). Recent studies show that fasting plasma concentrations of gastro-intestinal peptides are lower and that the post-prandial release of peptides is blunted in infants who do not receive enteral feedings (Berseth 1992, Lucas, Meetze 1992).

Several investigators have compared fasting plasma concentrations of various gastrointestinal peptides in infants who have received EN and those who have received only PN. The plasma concentrations of the following peptides were found to be significantly elevated in enterally-fed infants: gastrin, enteroglucagon, motilin, neurotensin, gastric inhibitory peptide, pancreatic polypeptide and peptide YY (Lucas 1982, 1983, Berseth 1992, Meetze 1992). Gastrin and enteroglucagon are potent trophic agents for intestinal mucosa, and gastric inhibitory peptide regulates the release of insulin, which is another potent growth factor in the newborn. In addition, all of these peptides regulate a variety of gastrointestinal and endocrine functions that maintain the integrity of the intestine and contribute to the digestion and absorption of nutrients.

The enteral administration of nutrients induces the post-prandial release of plasma peptides. Babies who have received full enteral feedings show a greater post-prandial release of peptides than those who have received only parenteral nutrition. Indeed, infants who have received exclusive PN may fail to show any post-prandial release of some peptides and a blunted release of others when compared to that seen in enterally-fed infants (Lucas 1983). Two recent studies have demonstrated that fasting concentrations of peptides are also increased significantly in infants who received minimal enteral feedings at volumes of 0.1–4 ml/kg (Fig. 7.5) (Berseth 1992, Meetze 1992) and that a significant post-prandial release of peptides occurs in

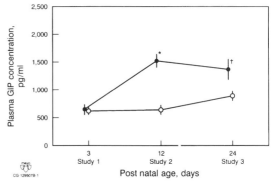

Figure 7.5 — Plasma gastric intestinal polypeptide concentrations in babies who received small enteral feedings (solid circles) and babies who received no enteral feedings (open circles) on post-natal days 3–12. Babies had higher plasma concentrations of peptide on post-natal days 12 and 24 (see Berseth 1992 for full data).

response to feeding volumes of 4 cm^3/kg (Berseth 1992). In older infants, Hyman et al (1983) showed that gastric acid secretion was significantly reduced in patients who were TPN dependent compared to those who were receiving enteral feedings to supplement their TPN. This reduction in gastric acid secretion was reversed within 6–8 weeks of the institution of small enteral feedings, and gastric acid output was similar between infants receiving small feedings compared to those receiving full feedings. Thus, it appears that the administration of either full or minimal EN results in comparable metabolic responses.

Other metabolic differences are seen among infants who receive early EN. In Dunn et al (1988), babies fed minimal enteral nutrients demonstrated lower serum concentrations of bilirubin and bone alkaline phosphatase than infants who were maintained solely on PN, although the clinical outcome of the two groups after hospital discharge did not differ.

Effects on intestinal flora

Although the gut is sterile *in utero*, it becomes colonized rapidly after birth with *E. coli*, streptococci and anaerobes. A complex flora has been established by the fourth post-natal day in term infants receiving routine enteral feedings. Bacteria are introduced to the neonatal gut as they are present in ingested milk. Infants who are breast-fed have a predominance of lactobacilli and bifidobacteria, which are commonly found in freshly-expressed breast milk. In contrast, infants who are formula-fed become colonized with a predominance of *Enterobacteriaceae*, *Bacteroides* and *Colstridium* species (Meinssen-Verhage 1987).

Although the gut flora has not been evaluated in infants who have not been fed, animal studies suggest that normal colonization is delayed until EN is given.

Another concern now emerging with the routine use of TPN is that of bacterial translocation, or the presence of bacteria in mesenteric lymph nodes due to reduced barrier function. It has been shown previously in a variety of animal models that the use of small enteral feedings reduces significantly the rate of bacterial translocation. Pierro et al (1996) have recently shown that a small number of infants (about 6%) developed sepsis due to microbial translocation of enteric micro-organisms after receiving TPN for approximately 58 days (range 32–286 days). Infants with short-gut bowel syndrome who received enteral feedings were more likely to develop bacterial translocation than age-matched control infants who did not receive feedings (Weber 1995). On the other hand, Sax (1996) has shown that there is a dose-response reduction in bacterial translocation in TPN-fed rats given 0–25% of their total caloric intake enterally. In neonatal animals, it has been noted that animals fed conventional formula have a greater incidence of translocation than do animals fed species-specific breast milk (Steinwender et al 1996). However, Ford (1996) has shown that bacterial translocation can be eliminated if animals are fed pasteurized formula and are maintained in a meticulously-clean environment.

Efficacy of early enteral nutrition

The use of early nutrition for the very-low-birth-weight infant was introduced over a decade ago. In early descriptive trials, babies with birth weights < 1250 g gained weight normally when they received enteral feedings (Moyer-Mileur & Chan 1986, Brosirs et al 1994). After two randomized controlled trials demonstrated that the introduction of enteral feedings early in the post-natal period did not increase the incidence of NEC, several randomized trials were instituted to evaluate the efficacy of minimal enteral feedings. In the study by Dunn et al 1988, 39 infants who had birth weights <1500 g were given parenteral nutrition. Of the 39 infants, 19 received small amounts of enteral feeds for the first 9 post-natal days and 20 were used as controls. The infants who received minimal enteral feedings established full enteral feedings. In the study by Slagle & Gross (1988), 46 infants with birth weights < 1500 g received parental nutrients. Half of the infants were randomly assigned to begin early feedings on the seventh post-natal day at rates of 12 ml/kg/d; the other half began feedings late on the

seventeenth day of life. Infants whose enteral feedings were initiated later experienced more frequent gastric residuals and had their feedings withheld twice as often as infants who had been fed earlier. Moreover, late-fed infants required a longer course of PN. In the study by Berseth (1992), 27 infants born at 32 weeks gestation or less were randomly assigned to begin enteral feedings at the age of 3 days (early) or at the age of 10 days (late). Infants who received early enteral feedings had fewer days of feeding intolerance and gained weight faster than did infants who were fed late. These studies, as well as others, have shown that there are benefits in providing early EN that directly accrue to the gastrointestinal tissue and indirectly enhance overall metabolic function.

Discussion

A variety of enteral feeding volumes have been used to provide minimal EN ranging from 1.3–24 ml/kg/d. Although clinical studies have shown that use of these small volumes for 7–14 days results in improvement of gastrointestinal function, it is not known if these volumes promote intestinal growth. Because the promotion of intestinal growth is a major concern in the treatment of short gut, there is a need to identify the feeding volume that is needed to achieve growth as well as functional maturation. When chronically-parenterally-fed dogs were given enteral feeding volumes that provided 2.5–5% of their daily caloric intake, no difference in gut growth or function was seen compared to pups given no enteral feedings (Owens et al 1997). When pups were given 7.5, 10, 30 or 100% of their caloric intake enterally, improvement in motor function occurred in a dose-response fashion; however intestinal growth did not occur until enteral feeding volumes provided 30% or more of daily caloric intake. Enteral feeding volumes that exceed 20% of total caloric intake result in the reduction of bacterial translocation (Sax 1996). Enteral feeding volumes that provide approximately 10% of total caloric intake result in a significant increase in plasma concentrations of gastrointestinal hormones and peptides. Thus, it appears that minimal enteral feeding volumes provide the greatest benefit and the least risk when volumes range from 10–30% of full caloric intake, if gut mucosal growth is sought.

Enteral feeding volumes must be selected based upon the goal to be achieved. Enteral feeding can be used to maintain mucosal integrity, promote gut growth or provide caloric intake. Neonatologists and gastroenterologists often attempt to maintain mucosal integrity in premature infants or those who have chronic lung disease for whom fluid balance is a major concern. For these smaller infants, enteral feeding volumes may be adequate. For infants with short gut, promotion of gut growth may be more important and larger feeding volumes may be necessary. The achievement of this goal should be tempered with caution as larger feeding volumes can increase the risk for NEC in pre-term infants. Retrospective studies have shown that the use of feeding volumes that exceed 60% of caloric intake or provide daily incremental increases that exceed 24 cc/kg/d may increase the risk for NEC (McKeown et al 1992, Owens & Berseth 1995). It would seem prudent, then, to give high-risk populations of pre-term infants enteral feedings that provide < 60% of caloric intake or less than 25 cc/kg/d in daily increments until prospective trials confirm that volumes beyond this range are safe.

Feedings can be given orally or by tube into the stomach or pylorus. Because many pre-term infants lack an intact sucking mechanism they are fed by tube. Although feedings using sterile water may be used to assess whether the gastrointestinal tract is patent and, as such, may be used for initial feedings, water does not stimulate mucosal growth, the release of hormones or the maturation of motor function. Solutions containing glucose or diluted nutrients may stimulate mucosal growth and modest hormone release, but full strength formula or breast milk provide the best stimulus for motor function. Thus, when feeding the intact gastro-intestinal tract, the physician may wish to use undiluted formula or breast milk. The use of diluted and/or specialized modular formulas may be warranted in the treatment of short-gut syndrome, whereas formulas that are calorically denser may be used to feed infants who have chronic lung disease.

Infants fed by transpyloric tube are often fed by continuous infusion in order to avoid a dumping syndrome. However, a continuous infusion may stimulate the continuous release of gastrointestinal hormones or, alternatively, cause only a modest release of hormones because the small volume is insufficient to stimulate optimal hormone release. There are also concerns that continuous infusions do not allow complete emptying of intraluminal contents. Some researchers have used regimens that provide intermittent interruptions in the continuous feeding, such as 3 h of continuous infusion followed by 1 h of no infusion or 2 h of infusion followed by 2 h of no infusion. Such a regimen permits more physiological cycling of

hormone release as well as permits motor function to cycle between feeding and fasting states.

References

Bauman, W.A. (1960) Early feedings of dextrose and saline solutions to premature infants. *Pediatrics*, 26, 756–761.

Benda, G.I.M. (1979) Modes of feeding low-birth weight infants. *Sem Perinatol*, 3, 407–415.

Berseth, C.L. (1987) Enhancement of intestinal growth in neonatal rats by epidermal growth factor in milk. *Am J Physiol*, 253, G662–665.

Berseth, C.L. (1990) Neonatal small intestinal motility: The motor responses to feeding in term and preterm infants. *J Pediatr*, 117, 777–782.

Berseth, C.L. (1992) Early feeding enhances maturation of the preterm small Intestine. *J Pediatr*, 120, 947–953.

Berseth, C.L., Lichtenberger, L.M., Morriss, F.H., Jr. (1983) Comparison of the gastrointestinal growth-promoting effects of rat colostrum and mature milk in newborn rats in vitro. *Am J Clin Nutr*, 37, 52–60.

Berseth, C.L., Nordyke, C. (1993) Enteral nutrients promote postnatal maturation of intestinal motor activity in preterm infants. *Am J Physiol*, 27, G1046–1051.

Berseth, C.L., Nordyke, C.K., Valdes, M.G. (1992) Responses of gastrointestinal peptides and motor activity to milk and water feedings in preterm and term infants. *Pediatr Res*, 31, 587–590.

Brosirs, K.K., Ritter, D.A., Kenney, J.D. (1994) Postnatal growth curve of the infant with extremely low birth weight who was fed enterally. *Pediatrics*, 74, 778–782.

Brown, H.O., Levine, M.L., Lipkin, M. (1963) Inhibition of intestinal epithelial cell renewal and migration induced by starvation. *Am J Physiol*, 205, 868–872.

Carver, J.D., Barness, L.A. (1996) Trophic factors for the gastrointestinal tract. *Clinics Perinatal* 23, 265–285.

Churella, H.R., Backhuber, W.L., Machean, W.C., Jr. et al (1985) Survey-Methods of feeding low-birth-weight infants. *Pediatrics*, 76, 342–349.

Cobin, R.M., Weintraub, A., DiMarino, A., Jr. (1994) Gastroesophageal reflux during gastrostomy feeding. *Gastroenteroloy*, 106, 13–18.

Crissinger, K.D., Burney, D.L. (1992) Influence of luminal nutrient composition on hemodynamics and oxygenation in developing piglet intestine. *Pediatr Res*, 31, 106A.

Crissinger, K.D., Granger, D.N. (1989) Mucosal injury induced by ischemia and re-perfusion in the piglet intestines: Influence of age and feeding. *Gastroenterology*, 97, 920–926.

Dembinski, A.B., Yamaguchi, T., Johnson, L.R. (1984) Stimulation of mucosal growth by a dietary amine. *Am J Physiol*, 247, G352–356.

Dunn, L., Hulman, S., Weiner, J. (1988) Beneficial effects of early hypocaloric enteral feeding on neonatal gastrointestinal function: Preliminary report of a randomized trial. *J Pediatr*, 112, 622–629.

Ford, H.R., Avanoglue, A., Boechar, P.R. et al (1996) The microenvironment influences the pattern of bacterial translocation in formula-fed neonates. *J Pediatr Surg*, 31, 486–489.

Greene, H.L., McCabe, D.R., Merenstein, G.B. (1974) Protracted diarrhea and malnutrition in infancy: Changes in intestinal morphology and disaccharidase activity. *Gastroenterology*, 67, 975–982.

Heird, W.C., Schwarz, S.M., Hansen, T.H. (1984) Colostrum induces enteric mucosal growth in beagle puppies. *Pediatr Res*, 18, 512–515.

Hyman, P.E., Feldman, E.J., Ament, M.E., Byrne, W.J., Euler, A.R. (1983) Effect of enteral feeding on the maintenance of gastric acid secretory function. *Gastroenterol*, 84, 341–345.

Jahnke, G.D., Lazarus, L.H. (1984) A bombesin immuno-reactive peptide in milk. *Proc Natl Acad Sci USA*, 81, 578–580.

Klagsbrun, M. (1978) Human milk stimulates DNA synthesis and cellular proliferation in cultured fibroblasts. *Proc Natl Acad Sci USA*, 75, 5057–5061.

Koldovsky, O., Thornburg, W. (1987) Hormones in milk. *J Pediatr Gastroenterol Nutr*, 6, 172–196.

LaGamma, E.F., Ostertag, S.G., Birenbaum, H. (1985) Failure of delayed oral feedings to prevent necrotizing enterocolitis. *Am J Dis Child*, 139; 385–389.

Lucas, A., Bloom, S.R., Anysley-Green, A. (1982) Postnatal surges in plasma gut hormones in term and preterm infants. *Biol Neonate*, 41, 63–67.

Lucas, A., Bloom, S.R., Anysley-Green, A. (1983) Metabolic and endocrine consequences of depriving preterm infants of enteral nutrition. *Acta Paediatr*, 72, 245–249.

McKeown, R.E., Marsh, T.D., Amarnath, V. (1992) Role of delayed feedings and of feeding increments in necrotizing enterocolitis. *Pediatr*, 12, 764–770.

Martinussen, M., Brubakk, A., Lunker, D.T., Vik, T., Yao, A.C. (1994) Mesenteric blood flow and its relation to circulatory adaptation during the first week of life in healthy term infants. *Pediatr Res*, 36, 334–339.

Martinussen, M., Brubakk, A., Vik, T., Yao, A.C. (1996) Mesenteric blood flow velocity and its relation to transitional circulatory adaptation in appropriate for gestational age preterm infants. *Pediatr Res*, 39, 275–278.

Meetze, W.H., Valentine, C., McGuigan, J.E. (1992) Gastrointestinal priming prior to full enteral nutrition in very low birth weight infants. *J Pediatr Gastroenterol Nutr*, 15, 163–170.

Meinssen-Verhage, E.A., Marcelis, J.H., de Vos, M.N. (1987) Bifido bacterium, Bacterordis and Clostridium ssp in fecal samples from breast-fed and bottle-fed infants with and without iron supplement. *J Clin Microbiol*, 25, 285–289.

Morin, C.L., Ling, V., Bovrassa, D. (1980) Small intestinal and colonic changes induced by a chemically defined diet. *Dig Dis Sci*, 25, 123–128.

Moyer-Mileur, L., Chan, G.M. (1986) Nutritional support of very-low-birth-weight infants requiring prolonged assisted ventilation. *Am J Dis Child*, 140, 929–932.

Orenstein, S.R. (1986) Enteral vs. parenteral therapy for intractable diarrhea of infancy. *J Pediatr*, 109, 277–286.

Ostertag, S.H., LaGamma, E.F., Reisen, C.E. (1986) Early enteral feeding does not affect the incidence of necrotizing enterocolitis. *Pediatrics*, 77, 275–280.

Owens, L., Berseth, C.L. (1995) Is there a volume threshold for enteral feeding and necrotizing enterocolitis? *Pediatr Res*, 37, 315A.

Owens, L., Burn, D., Berseth, C.L. (1997) Intestinal growth and function increase in a dose-response fashion to enteral feeding in the parenterally fed neonatal dog. *Pediatr Res*, 41, 237A.

Pierro, A., Van Saene, H.K., Donell, S.C., Hughes, J., Ewan, C., Nunn, A.J., Lloyd, D.A. (1996) Microbial translocation in neonates and infants receiving long term parenteral nutrition. *Archives of Surgery*, 131, 176–179.

Read, L.C., Upton, F.M., Francis, G.L. (1984) Changes in the growth promoting activity of human milk during lactation. *Pediatr Res*, 18, 133–139.

Sax, H.C. (1996) Low-dose enteral feeding is beneficial during total parenteral nutrition. *Amer J Surgery*, 171, 587–590.

Slagle, T.A., Gross, S.J. (1988) Effect of early low-volume enteral substrate on subsequent feeding tolerance in very low birth weight infants. *J Pediatr*, 113, 526–531.

Smallpiece, V., Davies, P.A. (1964) Immediate feeding of premature infants with undiluted breast milk. *Lancet*, 2, 1349–1352.

Steinwender, G., Schimpl, G., Sixl, B., Siegfried, K., Ranschek, M., Kilzer, S., Höllwarth, M.E., Wenzl, H. (1996) Effect of early nutritional deprivation and diet on translocation of bacteria from the gastrointestinal tract in the newborn rat. *Pediatr Res*, 39, 415–420.

Stoll, B.J. (1994) Epidemiology of necrotozing enterocolitis. *Clin Perinatol*, 21, 205–218.

Szabo, J.S., Mayfield, S.R., Oh. W. (1987) Postprandial

gastrointestinal blood flow and oxygen consumption: Effects of hypoxia in neonatal piglet. *Pediatr Res*, 21, 93–98.

Weber, T.R. (1995) Enteral feeding increases sepsis in infants with short bowel syndrome. *J Pediatr Surgery*, 30, 1086–1088.

Widdowson, E.M., Columbo, V.E., Artavanis, C.A. (1976) Changes in the organs of pigs in response to feeding for the first 24 hours after birth: II The digestive tract. *Biol Neonate*, 28, 272–281.

Wilmore, D.W., Dudrick, S.J. (1968) Growth and development of an infant receiving all nutrients exclusively by vein. *JAMA*, 203, 140–144.

Young, E.A., Cioletti, L.A., Traylor, J.B. (1982) Gastrointestinal response to oral versus gastric feeding of defined formula diets. *Am J Clin Nutr*, 36, 715–726.

8

Home enteral nutrition in infants and children

Alexandra Papadopoulou and Ian W. Booth

Introduction

Malnutrition is common in chronically-ill children and has adverse effects on the course of chronic disease (Table 8.1) (Meritt & Suskind 1979, Parsons et al 1980, Donaldson et al 1981, van Eys 1985, Chantler C 1988, Moy et al 1990, Taj et al 1993) and on well being (Broude-Heller et al 1979). Furthermore, malnourished patients have more complications and consume more resources (Twomey & Patchings 1985, Jendteg et al 1987, Reilly et al 1987, Robinson et al 1987). Managing malnutrition is therefore a primary clinical target in the treatment of chronically-ill children.

Enteral nutrition (EN) is safer, cheaper and simpler to provide than parenteral nutrition (PN) (Mughal & Irving 1986, Elia 1990, Payne-James et al 1990), and it has been used increasingly in children over the last years (Fig. 8.1). The role of EN in children with chronic disorders has been studied extensively. EN has been associated with: 1) an arrest in the deterioration of lung function in children with cystic fibrosis (CF) (Levy et al 1985, Boland et al 1986, Shepherd et al 1986); 2) reduced spasticity in children with cerebral palsy (CP) (Patrick et al 1986); 3) avoidance of surgery in infants with gastro-oesophageal reflux (Ferry et al

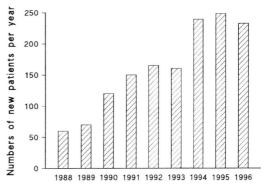

Figure 8.1 — The frequency of home enteral nutrition (HEN) at the Children's Hospital, Birmingham.

1983); 4) induction of remission in Crohn's disease and better growth in children with Crohn's disease compared with treatment with steroids (Belli et al 1988, Papadopoulou et al 1995a); and 5) weight gain in children with congenital heart disease (Bougle et al 1986 Vanderhoof et al 1982) and with chronic renal failure (Rees et al 1989).

The provision of nutritional support at home has a number of attractions such as return to a comfortable environment, avoidance of the negative emotional effects of hospitalization, reduction of the risk of infection and reduction in costs (Raymond 1990, Smith & Smith 1992). Home enteral nutrition (HEN) has been shown to be safe with acceptably few side effects, tolerated well by most patients and acceptable by patients' parents despite the effort (Holden et al 1991, Papadopoulou et al 1995b).

Table 8.1 — The multi-system implications of protein-energy malnutrition

Impaired gastrointestinal function
    hypochlorhydria
    reduced mucosal function
    pancreatic exocrine insufficiency

Immunodeficiency
    impaired cell-mediated immunity
    anergy

Respiratory dysfunction
    reduced inspiratory force and minute volume

Myocardial dysfunction

Reduced muscle mass

Increased operative mortality/morbidity

Delayed wound healing

Possible delay in intellectual development

Altered behaviour
    apathy
    depression

Growth failure

Practice and procedures

Indications for home enteral nutrition

Home enteral nutrition (HEN) is an invasive, time consuming procedure, and although it has been shown that the benefits are worth the cost and discomfort (Holden et al 1991, Papadopoulou et al 1995b), strict criteria for patient selection are required. The patients who require HEN often are a diverse group with different primary disorders (Table 8.2).

Nutritional targets of HEN

The major indications for providing HEN are threefold: 1) reversal of stunting; 2) correction of wasting; and 3) maintenance of nutritional status during nutritional insult. The nutritional criteria for providing

Table 8.2 — Disorders that are potential indications for home enteral nutrition

Gastrointestinal disorders
gastro-oesophageal reflux
Crohn's disease
cystic fibrosis
short bowel syndrome
intestinal pseudo-obstruction
Malignant disorders
during chemotherapy
Renal disorders
chronic renal failure
Liver disorders
chronic liver failure
Neurological disorders
cerebral palsy
Cardiology disorders
congenital heart disease awaiting surgery

Table 8.3 — Nutritional criteria for the provision of enteral nutrition

Impaired energy consumption: usually 50–60% of recommended daily amount despite high-energy supplements
plus
Severe and deteriorating wasting: weight-for-height > 2 SD below the mean plus skinfold thickness below the third centile
and/or
Depressed linear growth: fall in height of > 0.3 SD/year or height velocity < 5 cm/year or decrease in height velocity of at least 2 cm from the preceding year during early to mid-puberty

HEN are shown in Table 8.3. Recent work has showed that improvements in nutritional status depend directly on the duration of feeds, and the longer the duration of feeding the better the impact on nutritional status (Papadopoulou et al 1997). However, correction of wasting is easier than correcting stunting, which usually requires for at least several months HEN (Papadopoulou et al 1995b) (Fig. 8.2).

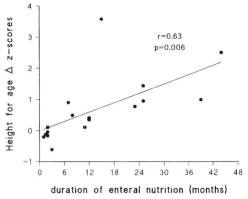

Figure 8.2 — Correlations between the duration of HEN and changes in height for age Z-scores (Papadopoulou et al 1995a). The longer the feeds the better the changes in height (r = 0.63; p = 0.006).

Methods of providing HEN

Nasogastric feeding

Nasogastric feeding via a nasogastric tube is the most preferable way for providing HEN as by the time the feeds reach the duodenum they have become iso-osmolar. This is possible due to the ability of the stomach to regulate its motility in relation to the osmolality of the feeds. This process continues until gastric contents become iso-osmolar and only then does their transfer across the pylorus start. The disadvantages of nasogastric feeding are the risk for reflux and aspiration pneumonia.

Gastrostomy feeding

Anatomical abnormalities or injury of the upper gastrointestinal tract are indications for providing gastrostomy feeds. Contraindications are severe gastro-oesophageal reflux or delayed gastric emptying. Gastrostomy tubes may be inserted using a percutaneous endoscopic technique (Larson et al 1987), and button gastrostomies flush with the skin are available (Gauderer et al 1988).

Nasojejunal feeding

In order to avoid gastric retention and therefore the risk of pulmonary aspiration, the provision of feeding directly to the jejunum is indicated when nasogastric feeding is not tolerated due to impaired gastric emptying. The administration of feeds intrajejunally bypasses the pyloric sphincter and duodenal osmoreceptors, which normally delay gastric emptying until isotonicity is achieved. Therefore, the administered feeds should be isotonic and infused continuously, via a pump, in order to avoid symptoms related to dumping syndrome, which occurs when bolus feeds are given directly into the jejunum, and to osmotic diarrhoea, which is usually associated with the use of hyperosmolar feeds. Similarly, sterile feeds and sterile water for flushing should be used as the stomach's anti-infective functions are bypassed. When long-term feeds are needed, then a jejunostomy is required. A *jejunostomy* is defined as an incision into the jejunum to make an opening through which feed can be administered. They are usually placed surgically under a general anaesthesia.

Equipment used for HEN

Continuous feeding is safe and increasingly used (Puntis & Holden 1991) as it has certain advantages over bolus feeding such as more positive nitrogen balance and less stool output in patients with diarrhoea (Parker et al 1981). Overnight feeding allows the child to be fed during the day.

Nasogastric-nasojejunal tubes

Polyurethane or silicone are the recommended tubes for long-term EN as they cause minimal local irritation and do not require replacement more often than monthly. Polyethylene and polyvinylchloride (PVC) tubes are stiffer and have the advantage that they do not become easily displaced. However, they are not recommended for long-term HEN as they require weekly replacement because otherwise they become rigid (Moor & Green 1985). Polyurethane and silicone tubes are soft and easily inserted. As well, they are particularly popular with parents. Their disadvantages are that they block easily, need regular flushing and may be displaced during vomiting. The choice of the external diameter also matters as smaller diameters are more comfortable for the patients. In general, 6-French gauge are used in infants and 8-French gauge in older children (Moore and Green 1985).

Enteral pumps (Table 8.4)

The most suitable pumps for the provision of HEN should combine a number of characteristics. They should be simple to use, accurate, friendly, quiet and have incorporated safety alarms indicating disconnection, blockage or running out of feeds (Torrance & Harrison 1988). Portable pumps are particularly useful for older children who need the feeding during the day as well as overnight. Alarms on these are usually limited but portability is their advantage.

Formulas recommended for HEN
(Table 8.5)

A wide range of feeds are currently available in the

Table 8.4 — Pumps and nasogastric tubes used for home enteral nutrition

PUMPS	Flow rate (ml/h)	Battery (hrs)	Weight (Kg)
Flexiflo II (Abbott)	29–250	8	1.2
Enteroport (Braun)	20–240	48	0.5
Frenta II (Fresenius)	25–250	10	0.4
Flocare (Nutricia)	1–400	30	0.7
Kangaroo K 324 (Sherwood)	1–295	24	1.8
NASOGASTRIC TUBES	Material	Length (cm)	Gauge (FG)
Flexiflo (Abbott)	PVC	110	8–12
Freka (Fresenius)	Polyurethane	60–120	8
Flocare (Nutricia)	PVC Polyurethane	50–110	6–8
Indwell (Sherwood)	Polyurethane	110	12
Vygon (Vygon)	Polyurethane	125	10–14

Table 8.5 — Diets indicated for home enteral nutrition

Diets	Clinical indications	Commercially-available products
Polymeric diets	normal gastrointestinal function	Fresubin, Fresubin 750 (Fresenius); Nutrison paediatric, Nutrison high energy (Nutricia); Osmolite, Paediasure, Advera, Ensure HN, Ensure plus (Abbott)
Oligomeric diets	drug/irradiation-induced enteropathy cow's milk protein intolerance post-gastroenteritis diarrhoea	Fresenius OPD (Fresenius); Pepti-2000 (Nutricia); Peptide$^{0-2}$ (SHS); Pepdite^{2+} (SHS)
Modular feed	short gut post-gastroenteritis glucose-galactose malabsorption advanced liver disease	Chix (Cow & Gate)
Elemental diets	Crohn's disease short gut	Alitraque (Abbott); Elemental 028 (SHS); Neocate (SHS); Nutri-2000 (Nutricia)
MCT-diets	cholestasis intestinal lymphangiectasia Anderson's disease pancreatic insufficiency Abeta-lipoproteinaemia	Osmolite (Abbott); Fresubin 750 MCT (Fresenius); MCT-Pepdite$^{0-2}$ (SHS); MCT- Pepdite^{2+} (SHS)

market. Formula selection for HEN is usually dictated by a number of factors such as the underlying disorder, the availability and the cost. Ready-to-use formulas are preferable to powdered as the cost of powdered formulas is higher due to the bigger amount of labour involved in preparation.

Volume of the feeds and energy intake

The total intake depends on the nutritional targets of the clinician, the estimated average requirements for energy taking into account the patient's clinical condition and physical activity (COMA 1987) and the oral intake that is tolerated during the day time. When the target is to reverse stunting and/or wasting, the total daily intake should provide 120% of the estimated average requirements for energy. Nasogastric or nasojejunal feeding usually provides part (50–70%) of the daily requirements, depending on the oral intake of the patient during the daytime. As mentioned before, continuous, overnight feeding is preferable as it does not suppress the oral intake during the daytime and does not interfere with the child's normal daytime activity.

The volume of the feeds is usually individualized. Feeding is introduced at a rate of 10 ml/h, increasing by 10 ml/h/day if tolerated. The total volume should be reached within 5–7 days from the start of EN. The infusion rate is then increased in order to provide the same volume during 10–14 hours overnight. Oral intake is encouraged in almost all cases during the day, with the exception of Crohn's disease, and energy supplements are recommended.

Training patients and parents

The initiation of the feeds should always be carried out by a well-trained, nutritional-care nurse (Holden 1990). However, it is important to prepare the child well before admission to hospital so that he/she looks at HEN positively and not as a punishment. The support of a play specialist where available is welcomed (Holden et al 1997). Alternatively, the nutritional-care nurse may cope with this important issue. Booklets with information on the feeds, photograph albums, diagrams showing the relevant anatomy, video-tapes, dolls, bravery awards and stickers are all used depending on the age of the patients (Holden et al 1987).

Training usually takes 2–3 days in hospital and depends mainly on the level of understanding of the parents and the patients (Park et al 1988). Other clinicians find home teaching to be an effective alternative to hospitalization because it requires less time (average 3.2 h) without being associated with any particular complication (Berezin et al 1988). People whose first language is other than that spoken by the medical and nursing staff usually require more time, and their training is extremely difficult without the help of an interpreter service in the base hospital (Holden 1994). Recently, Sexton et al suggested the development of pictorial teaching tools in order to assist such people to learn the procedure of feeding step-by-step (Sexton et al 1996).

Follow-up: monitoring nutritional status

An important element of HEN is continuous parental support and regular follow-up of the patients by both the nutritional care team of the base hospital and the community medical and nursing staff. The outpatient follow-up routine consists of regular assessment of the anthropometric indices of nutritional status (i.e., weight, height, mid-arm circumference, skin folds) together with regular review of the clinicians' nutritional targets.

Indications for discontinuing HEN

The criteria for discontinuing HEN are: 1) achievement of nutritional targets; 2) achievement of an oral intake covering at least 90% of the estimated average requirements for energy (COMA 1987) during the daytime; and 3) no existence of the clinical condition that caused the nutritional insult (e.g., chemotherapy).

Discussion

Complications of HEN

Gastrointestinal disturbances during HEN

HEN is a relatively safe procedure with no major side effects (Park et al 1988). However, all patients should be aware of the potential complications of the feeds, including pulmonary aspiration, gastro-oesophageal reflux, delayed gastric emptying and diarrhoea. Nausea and vomiting have been reported in 10% of adults

receiving EN and have been attributed mainly to high osmolality of the feeds (Keohane et al 1984). However, Papadopoulou et al found in a study in 44 children receiving HEN that vomiting was only transient and associated mainly with the initiation of feeds; it gradually settled in most patients (Papadopoulou et al 1995b). Diarrhoea occurs during HEN and has been associated either with bacterial contamination of the feeds or the use of hyper-osmolar feeds (Casewell et al 1981).

Mechanical complications

Mechanical complications are usually related to the insertion of the tubes (nasogastric/nasojejunal, gastrostomy/jejunostomy) or the presence of the tubes in situ. Perforation of the upper respiratory tract or pneumothorax may occur rarely, particularly in unconscious patients during the insertion of the nasogastric tubes. Peritonitis may occur during the insertion of gastrostomy tubes. Complications related to the presence of nasogastric tubes in situ are usually caused by excessive mucous production due to the irritation of the upper respiratory tract, particularly in infants undergoing an upper respiratory tract infection. One general rule to prevent this kind of problem is to insert the smallest tube to the smallest nosdre (Stocks 1980). Certainly, in cases of bronchiolitis in such infants, it may be safer to interrupt the nasogastric feeding for a short time and admit the patient to hospital in order to provide intravenous fluids if necessary (Berman et al 1991). Aspiration pneumonia has been reported in adult patients receiving enteral feeding (Olivares et al 1974), but it does not appear to be a problem in children. However, it is always advisable to feed the patient at an angle of approximately 30 degrees in order to avoid this complication and to switch neurological patients with gastro-oesophageal reflux to nasojejunal feeds. Leaking of the gastrostomy buttons and inflammation of the skin around the buttons are some of the complications of gastrostomy feeds.

Metabolic complications

The authors are not aware of any serious metabolic complications having been reported in children receiving HEN, such as hypoglycaemia when interrupting the feeds. However, magnesium depletion has been reported in patients with Crohn's disease receiving HEN and it has been attributed to the impaired absorption of the inflamed intestinal mucosa of the administered nutrients (Motil et al 1985, Park et al 1990).

Bacterial contamination of the feeds

It is well recognized from previous studies that 'home brew' diets are often associated with diarrhoea (Keighley et al 1982) and infections (Casewell 1979). Therefore, these should be avoided when commercial formulas are available. Furthermore, ready-to-use liquids are preferable to powdered formulas as the reconstitution and blending that are required with powdered formulas have been reported to predispose to contamination with bacteria (Hostetler et al 1982). Recently, Sami et al suggested the safety and efficiency of 'all-in-one' sterile and modular formulas consisting of carbohydrate, protein and lipid sterilized separately (Sami et al 1990). Regarding the tubes used for HEN, it is preferred to avoid wide-bore feeding tubes, which are often used in jejunostomies, as they have been reported to facilitate retrograde contamination with bacteria (van Alsenoy et al 1985).

Other unpleasant side effects of HEN

Sleep disturbance is a common side effect of the overnight feeds due to the noise or nicturia (Park et al 1988, Holden et al 1991). Distress due to aesthetic problems as well as unwelcome public interest for the presence of the nasogastric tube are both common problems particularly in older children. These problems can be solved by teaching the older patients to insert their own tubes at night and remove them before going out to school.

The role of the nutritional care team

Despite the wide use of HEN, many hospitals and community health teams still do not have the appropriate organization to guarantee that nutritional support is provided in the best manner for the patients. A number of studies have agreed that the presence of a multi-disciplinary nutritional care team in regional hospitals can improve the quality of the nutritional support and reduce the cost (Brown et al 1987, Puntis & Booth 1990). The nutritional care team comprises a clinician with special experience in nutrition, a nurse specialist and a dietician. The responsibilities of the team and of the clinician in nutritional support are shown in Tables 8.6 and 8.7, respectively. The nutritional care team should be in a close contact with the community health teams. The community medical and nursing staff should always be aware of the potential complications of the feeds so that they can provide first-line help to the patients when necessary. Certainly, contact phone numbers

Table 8.6 — The role of the nutritional care team

identification of 'at risk' patients
nutritional assessment
provision of specialized nutritional support
clinical and biochemical monitoring
audit
teaching
research

Table 8.7 — The clinican's role in nutritional care

lobbying for staff appointments
advertising cost benefits
liaison with clinical colleagues
clinical admission
enteral access
prescription of feeds
overall responsibility for nutritional care

with a member of the nutritional care team of the hospital should be available 24 h/day for the more complicated cases.

Budgets and organization of HEN

HEN is one of the most rapidly growing sectors of home care (Rucker & Holmstedt 1984, Sexton et al 1996). However, the level of budgeting arrangements for HEN is still unsatisfactory. General practitioners are still asked to decide on prescribing the feeds, and still carry the legal responsibility for HEN. In practice, general practitioners are easily convinced to prescribe the feeds but not the equipment required for HEN (McFadzean 1988), and this is clearly an irregularity. Therefore, guidelines relating to funding and supply of the equipment for HEN are needed (Scott 1988). A possible solution might be the availability of a reserve stock of pumps and disposables brought with a community budget so that patients may borrow them. Furthermore, increased public awareness (via relevant articles in journals, radio/television programmes, etc.) would be associated with an increased consumer pressure on hospital catering as well as on budgeting arrangements and home supply services.

Conclusions

HEN has been shown to be safe and effective in reversing wasting and stunting and in maintaining nutritional status during insult. Its major economic benefits are based on the well-recognized reduction in costs and the shorter duration of hospital stays for well-nourished patients compared with malnourished ones.

References

Belli, D.C., Seidman, E., Bouthillier, L. et al (1988) Chronic intermittent elemental diet improves growth failure in children with Crohn's disease. *Gastroenterology*, 94, 603–610.

Berezin, S., Medow, M.S., Bernarducci, J. et al (1988) Home teaching of nocturnal nasogastric feeding. *J Parent Ent Nutr*, 12, 392–393.

Berman, S., Simoes, E.A.F., Lanata, C. et al (1991) Respiratory rate and pneumonia in infancy. *Arch Dis Child*, 66, 81–84.

Boland, M.P., McDonald, N.E., Stoski, D.S. et al (1986) Chronic jejunostomy feeding with a non-elemental formula in undernourished patients with cystic fibrosis. *Lancet*, i, 232–234.

Bougle, D., Iselin, M., Kahyat, A. et al (1986) Nutritional treatment of congenital heart disease. *Arch Dis Child*, 61, 799–801.

Broude-Heller, A., Rotbalsam, I., Elbinger, R. (1979) Clinical Aspects of Hunger Disease in Children. In: Winick, M. (ed.) *Hunger Disease. Studies by Jewish Physicians in the Warsaw Ghetto*, pp. 45–57. John Wiley: New York.

Brown, R.O., Carlson, S.D., Cowan, G.S.M. et al (1987) Enteral nutritional support management in a university teaching hospital : Team vs no team. *J Parent Ent Nutr*, 11, 52–56.

Casewell, M.W., (1979) Nasogastric feeds as a source of Klebsiella infection for intensive care patients. 1, 101–105.

Casewell, M.W., Cooper, J.E., Webster, M. (1981) Enteral feeds contaminated with Enterobacter cloacae as a cause of septicaemia. *BMJ*, 282, 973.

Chantler, C. (1988) Growth and metabolism in renal failure. *J R Coll Physicians Lond*, 22, 69–73.

COMA. (1987) *Department of Health Dietary Reference Values for Food Energy and Nutrients for the United Kingdom*. London.

Donaldson, S.S., Welsey, M.N., Dewys, W.D. et al (1981) A study of the nutritional status of pediatric cancer patients. *Amer J Dis Child*, 135, 1107–1112.

Elia, M. (1990) Artificial nutritional support. *Med Intern*, 82, 3392–3396.

Gauderer, M.W.L., Olsen, M.M., Stellato, T.A., Dokter, M.L.

(1988) Feeding gastrostomy button: Experience and recommendation. *J Pediatr Surg*, 23, 24–28.

Holden, C.E. (1987) *Feeding Time with Roo And Joe*. Crawley: Sherwood Medical Industries Ltd.

Holden, C.E. (1990) *Tube Feeding at Home: A Parents' Guide*. Sussex: Sherwood Medical Industries Ltd.

Holden, C.E., Puntis, J.W., Charlton, C.P., Booth, I.W. (1991) Nasogastric feeding at home acceptability and safety. *Arch Dis Child*, 61, 148–151.

Holden, C.E. (1994) *Enteral and Parenteral Nutrition. Feeding at Home: Impact on Family Life And The Implications for Home Care*. Unpublished MSc dissertation. The Birmingham Children's Hospital NHS Trust.

Holden, C.E., MacDonald, A., Handy, D. et al (1997) Psychological preparation for nasogastric feeding in children. *Br J Nursing*, 6, 34–37.

Hostetler, C., Lipman, T.O., Geraghty, M. et al (1982) Bacterial safety of reconstituted continuous drip tube feeding. *JPEN*, 6, 232–235.

Ferry, G.D., Selby, M., Peitro, T.J. (1983) Clinical response to short-term nasogastic feeding in infants with gastro-esophageal reflux and growth failure. *J Pediatr Gastroenterol Nutr*, 2, 57–61.

Jendteg, S., Larsson, J., Lindgren, B. (1987) Clinical and economic aspects on nutritional supply. *Clin Nutr*, 6, 185–190.

Keighley, M.R.B., Mogg, B., Beatley, S., Allan, C. (1982) "Home brew" compared with commercial preparations for enteral feeding. *BMJ*, 284, 163.

Keohane, P.P., Attrill, H., Love, M. et al (1984) Relation between osmolality of diet and gastrointestinal side effects in enteral nutrition. *BMJ*, 288, 678–681.

Larson, D.E., Burton, D.B., Schroeder, A.W., Di Magno, E.P. (1987) Percutaneous endoscopic gastrostomy. Indications, success, complications and mortality in 314 consecutive patients. *Gastroenterology*, 93, 48–52.

Levy, L.D., Durie, P.R., Pencharz, P.B. et al (1985) Effects of long-term nutritional rehabilitation on body composition and clinical status in malnourished children and adolescents with cystic fibrosis. *J Pediatr*, 107, 225–230.

McFadzean, W. (1988) Support for BDA bid for prescrible plastics. *Clin Nutr Update*, 1, 5.

Merritt, R.J., Suskind, R.M. (1979) Nutiritional survey of hospitalised paediatric patients. *Am J Clin Nutr*, 32, 1320–1325.

Moore, M.C., Green, H.L. (1985) Tube feeding of infants and children. *Pediatr Clin N Amer*, 32, 401–417.

Motil, K.J., Altchuler, S.I., Grand, R.J. (1985) Mineral balance during nutritional supplementation in adolescents with Crohn disease and growth failure. *J Pediatr*, 107, 473–479.

Moy, R.J.D., Smallman, S., Booth, I.W. (1990) Malnutrition in a UK children's hospital. *J Hum Nutr Dietet*, 3, 93–100.

Mughal, M., Irving, M. (1986) Home parenteral nutrition in the United Kingdom and Ireland. *Lancet*, ii, 383–387.

Olivares, L., Segovia, A., Revuelta, R. (1974) Tube feeding and lethal aspiration in neurological patients: A review of 720 autopsy cases. *Stroke*, 5, 654–657.

Papadopoulou, A., Rawashdeh, M.O., Brown, G.A. et al (1995a) Remission following an elemental diet or prednisolone. *Acta Paediatr*, 84, 79–83.

Papadopoulou, A., Holden, C.E., Paul, L. et al (1995b) The nutritional response to home enteral nutrition in childhood. *Acta Paediatr*, 84, 528–531.

Papadopoulou, A., MacDonald, A., Williams, M.D. et al (1997) Enteral nutrition in children following bone marrow transplantation. *Arch Dis Child*. 77, 131–160.

Park, R.H.R., Galloway, A., Russell, R.I. (1988) Practical aspects of home enteral nutrition. *Gut*, 29, A1470–1471.

Park, R.H.R., Galloway, R.H.R., Shenkin, A. et al (1990) Magnesium deficiency in patients on home enteral nutrition. *Clin Nutr*, 9, 147–149.

Parker, P., Stroop, S., Greene, H.L. (1981) A controlled comparison of continuous versus intermittent feeding in the treatment of infants with intestinal disease. *J Pediatr*, 99, 360–364.

Parsons, H.G., Francoeur, T.E., Howland, P. et al (1980) The nutritional status of hospitalized children. *Am J Clin Nutr*, 33, 1140–1146.

Patrick, J., Boland, M., Stoski, D., Murray, G.E. (1986) Rapid correction of wasting in children with cerebral palsy. *Dev Med Child Neurol*; 28, 734–739.

Payne-James, J., deGara, C., Grimble, G. et al (1990) Nutritional support in hospitals in the United Kingdom: National survey 1988. *Health Trends*, 22, 9–13.

Puntis, J.W.E., Holden, C.E. (1991) Home enteral nutrition in paediatric practice. *Brit J Hosp Med*, 45, 104–107.

Puntis, J.W.L., Booth, I.W. (1990) The place of a nutritional care team in paediatric practice. *J Parent Ent Nutr*, 7, 132–135.

Raymond, J.L. (1990) State and federal reimbursement for home nutrition support. *Caring*, Oct, 16–18.

Rees, L., Rigden, S.P.A., Ward, G.M. (1989) Chronic renal failure and growth. *Arch Dis Child*, 64, 573–577.

Reilly, J.J., Hull, S.F., Albert, N. et al (1987) Economic impact of malnutrition: A Model System for Hospitalised patients *JPEN*, 12, 372–376.

Rucker, B.B., Holmstedt, K.A. (1984) Trends in the home infusion therapy market. *Caring* 3, 65–70.

Robinson, G., Goldstein, M., Levine, G.M. (1987) Impact of nutritional status on DRG length of stay. *J Parent Ent Nutr* 11, 49–51.

Sami, H., Saint-Aubert, B., Szawlowski, A.W. et al (1990) Home Enteral Nutrition System: One patient, one daily ration of an "all-in-one" sterile and modular formula in a single container. *J Parent Ent Nutr*, 14, 173–176.

Scott, C. (1988) Home to home: Important issues to be resolved. *Clin Nutr Update*, 1, 8.

Sexton, E., Paul, L., Holden, C. (1996) A pictorial assisted teaching tool for families. *Paediatr Nurs*, 8, 24–26.

Shepherd, R.W., Holt, T.L., Thomas, B.J.K. et al (1986) Nutritional rehabilitation in cystic fibrosis: controlled studies of effect on nutritional and growth retardation, body protein turnover and cause of pulmonary disease. *J Pediatr*, 109, 788–794.

Smith, A.E., Smith, P.E. (1992) Reimbursement for clinical nutrition services: A 10-year experience. *J Am Diet Assoc*, 92, 1385–1388.

Stocks, J. (1980) Effect of nasogastric tubes on nasal resistance during infancy. *Arch Dis Child*, 55, 17–21.

Taj, M.M., Pearson, A.D., Mumford, D.B., Price, L. (1993) Effect of nutritional status on the incidence of infection in childhood cancer. *Pediatr Heamatol Oncol*, 10, 283–287.

Torrance, A., Harrison, C. (1988) A controlled study of the performance of five enteral feeding pumps. *J Hum Nutr Dietet*, 1, 1–7.

Twomey, P.L., Patchings, S.C. (1985) Cost effectiveness of nutritional support. *J Parent Ent Nutr*, 9, 3–10.

van Alsenoy, J., De Leeuw, I., Delvigne, C., Vandewoude, M. (1985) Ascending contamination of a jejunostomy feeding reservoir. *Clinical Nutrition*, 4, 95–98.

van Eys, J. (1985) Nutrition and cancer: Physiological interrelationships. *Annual Rev Nutr*, 5, 435–461.

Vanderhoof, J.A., Hofschire, P.J., Baluff, M.A. et al (1982) Continuous enteral feedings. An important adjunct to the management of complex congenital heart disease. *Am J Dis Child*, 136, 825–827.

9

Parenteral nutrition
in infants

John W.L. Puntis

Introduction

The premature newborn and the term infant under-going surgery for congenital or acquired gastrointestinal disease comprise the two largest groups of children receiving parenteral nutrition (PN). Although the premature infant may have a functional gastrointestinal tract, a rapid build-up of enteral nutrition (EN) to full requirements is frequently precluded by immature gastrointestinal motility. Because reserves of energy are limited (Heird et al 1972) whilst demands are high, PN is often given as a matter of routine when birth weight is < 1500 g. Conventionally (Herid 1992), PN has been commenced after some days of clinical stabilization. More recently, there has been a move towards earlier introduction and faster incrementation of feeds (Forsyth et al 1995). In addition, minimal enteral feeding (MEF) to stimulate bowel growth and development is often used as an adjunct to PN, even in ventilated infants with neuromuscular blockade (McClure et al 1996). The potential benefits of MEF include protection against sepsis, a decreased risk of cholestasis, faster growth and less time to establish full enteral feeding (Troche et al 1995).

Many infants receive PN for no more than 2–3 weeks (Puntis & Booth 1987). In a minority of surgical new-born, however, PN extends beyond the post-operative phase of gut failure, for example when there is short bowel (Stringer & Puntis 1995) or severe dysmotility. These indications together with protracted diarrhoea (Walker-Smith 1994) are the commonest diagnoses amongst children on long-term home PN (Bisset et al 1992). Although PN has undoubtedly led to greater survival in such patients, its contribution to improved survival in pre-term infants is uncertain given the many other advances in neonatal intensive care and the lack of prospective studies.

Historical background

Physicians were first stimulated to use intravenous fluid therapy in the early part of the last century following insights gained into the pathophysiology of cholera (O'Shaughnessy 1831). One of those involved predicted that 'this.... astonishing method of medication.... will lead to wonderful improvements in the practice of medicine' (Cosnett 1989). However, not until over 100 years later was it possible to provide the complete nutritional requirements of a child using the intravenous route (Helfrick & Abelson 1944). This was in a 5-month-old infant with vomiting,

constipation and severe failure to thrive secondary to Hirschsprung's disease. Feeds delivered from a peripheral vein consisted of 50% glucose, 10% amino acid solution, and a fat emulsion made from olive oil and lecithin. Over a 5-day period, nutritional and general clinical status improved, followed by successful re-establishment of enteral feeding. The widespread use of PN in the newborn infant is an even more recent phenomenon dating from a landmark case report published in 1968 (Wilmore & Dudrick 1968). This was a child with ileal atresia who received total PN via a central venous catheter and who maintained normal growth and development over a 44-day period.

Practice and procedures

Who to feed

The most common indications for PN are shown in Table 9.1. PN is mandatory when there is a contra-dication to enteral feeding. There is a good deal of agreement amongst neonatologists that PN is an important therapeutic intervention in the pre-term infant, even though there are virtually no prospective studies comparing PN with enteral feeding (Heird 1992). In practice, however, there is considerable variation in PN usage between units. This often reflects clinicians' perceptions of the relative merits of

Table 9.1 — Common indications for parenteral nutrition in infants

Newborn	
Unequivocal:	intestinal failure
	functional immaturity
	necrotizing enterocolitis
	short bowel
Equivocal:	respiratory failure requiring IPPV
	promotion of growth in pre-term infants
	prevention of necrotizing enterocolitis
Infants	
Intestinal failure:	post-operative gastrointestinal surgery
	short bowel
	protracted diarrhoea
	chronic pseudo-obstruction
Intensive care / multi-organ failure:	hyper-catabolism (e.g., extensive burns; severe trauma)
	severe fluid restriction required (e.g., renal impairment; inappropriate ADH)

Abbreviations: IPPV = Intermittent Positive Pressure Ventilation
ADH = Antidiuretic Hormone

PN and enteral feeding, as well as the sophistication of local pharmacy services. Despite such variation, a birth weight of < 1500 g is often used as an arbitrary indication for PN in this group in the expectation that meeting full nutritional requirements with enteral feeding will be a slow process. In addition, rapid incrementation of milk feeds is recognized as a risk factor for *necrotizing enterocolitis* (NEC) (Anderson & Kliegman 1991), a serious condition affecting up to 8% of very-low-birth-weight infants and associated with a mortality of around 25–40%.

Whether or not PN or EN is most effective in promoting growth in the pre-term newborn is unclear. By *in utero* standards, parenterally-fed premature infants often show growth failure and even at 1 year corrected age may have significantly impaired head circumference (Georgieff et al 1985). The rarity of NEC in infants who have never been given enteral feeds suggests that total PN for several weeks might be used as a prophylactic measure. However, there is little objective evidence to support this viewpoint, even in infants thought to be at especially-high risk of the disease (McDonnell et al 1994). Although PN is universally used in the management of NEC once it has developed, its role as a preventive measure cannot be regarded as firmly established. Severe fluid restriction, as is sometimes necessary during multi-system failure,

is another indication for PN in sick infants because nutritional goals are more achievable if concentrated PN fluids are given in conjunction with MEF rather than using all the limited fluid space available for enteral feeding which can only partially meet requirements.

What to feed

Suggested feeding regimens suitable for infants are shown in Table 9.2. These are based on Fresenius Kabi Ltd nutritional products; more information is available from the relevant data sheets. Vaminolact should be used as the amino acid source in infants under 6 months of age, and Vamin 9 for those above.

Amino acids

Requirements are supplied using a solution of crystalline L-amino acids. The pre-term newborn infant with an average energy intake of 80 kcal/kg/day needs approximately 3 g/kg/day of amino acids to produce nitrogen retention similar to that found *in utero* (Zlotkin et al 1981). In term infants, 2.5 g/kg/day amino acids (equivalent to 300–360 mg of nitrogen/kg/day) is adequate for growth. The growth demands of infants require a higher proportion of essential amino acids to be given than in adult patients. Because metabolic pathways are not fully developed,

Table 9.2 — Parenteral nutrition for infants

Regimen number:	/Kg/day	1	2	3	4	5	6	7	8
amino acid	g	0.8	1.5	2.0	2.5	1	1.5	2.0	2.5
carbohydrate	g	10	12	13	14	10	12	13	14
fat	g	1	2	3	3.5	1	2	2	3
sodium	mmol	3	3	3	3	3	3	3	3
potassium	mmol	2.5	2.5	2.5	2.5	2.5	2.5	2.5	2.5
calcium	mmol	1	1	1	1	0.6	0.6	0.6	0.6
magnesium	mmol	0.2	0.2	0.2	0.2	0.1	0.1	0.1	0.1
phosphate	mmol	0.4★	0.4★	0.4★	0.4★	0.4★	0.4★	0.4★	0.4★
iron	µg	100	100	100	100	100	100	100	100
Solivito N	ml	1	1	1	1	1	1	1	1
Vitlipid N Infant	ml	4	4	4	4	4	4	4	4
Peditrace	ml	0.5	1	1	1	1	1	1	1

Regimens 1 to 3 are used in the newborn for the first 3 days of PN; regimen 4 is used for day 4 and beyond; regimens 5 to 7 are used in patients over 1 month but under 10 kg bodyweight for the first 3 days of PN; regimen 8 is used for day 4 and beyond. The phosphate should be increased to 1 mmol/kg/day if the infant is pre-term

★When phosphate is added using Addiphos, the sodium and potassium content of this product should be included in calculations; if using sodium glycerophosphate injection, the sodium content should be included. Solivito N may be reconstituted with Vitlipid N Infant and 1 ml of mixture used. [Addiphos, Peditrace, Solivito N and Vitlipid N are manufactured by Fresenius Kabi Ltd, Hampton Court, Tudor Road, Manor Park, Runcorn, Cheshire, WA7 1UE.]

Table 9.3 — Amino acid composition (mg/g) of some commercially-available amino acid solutions and of breast milk

Amino Acid	Vaminolact (Fresenius Kabi Ltd)	Primène (Cernep Synthelabo)	Aminoplasmal ped (Braun)	Milk (mother's)
Isoleucine	47	67	28	48
Leucine	107	99	50	104
Lysine	86	109	90	81
Methionine	20	24	16	19
Phenylalanine	41	42	38	41
Threonine	55	37	60	53
Tryptophan	21	20	12	20
Valine	55	76	32	54
Histidine	32	38	60	30
Cystine/cysteine	15	19	29★	16
Tyrosine	8	9	23★★	39
Taurine	5	6	0	3
Alanine	96	79	116	47
Aspartate	63	60	38	101
Glutamate	109	99	196	181
Glycine	32	40	0	30
Proline	86	30	54	85
Serine	58	40	20	55
Arginine	63	84	44	46

★cysteine; ★★tyrosine 6 mg, n-acetyl-tyrosine 17 mg

several amino acids regarded as non-essential in adults are essential in the newborn. These include histidine, taurine, cystine/cysteine, tyrosine, proline and glycine. There are a number of different nitrogen sources available, some of which are shown in Table 9.3 together with the composition of breast milk for comparison. Solutions have been designed on the basis of various different premises with regard to optimal composition, constrained by such factors as solubility or stability of individual amino acids. For example, tyrosine is poorly soluble and cystine unstable. Increasing the intake of these amino acids by using the more soluble and stable acetylated forms appears to result in increased urinary losses (Van Goudoever et al 1994), and delivery using dipeptides may be the solution to this problem in the future.

Vaminolact (Fresenius Kabi Ltd) is based on the amino acid profile of egg protein, modified in certain respects to make it more similar to breast milk. The content of phenylalanine was considerably reduced and led to a significant reduction in plasma phenylalanine concentration (Puntis et al 1989) during PN. Although elevated plasma phenylalanine concentrations reported in infants given amino acid solutions designed for adults were a cause for concern, subsequent follow-up studies did not demonstrate any adverse effect on neuro-development (Lucas 1993). Recent investigation in piglets has suggested that the intake of aromatic amino acids with Vaminolact may now be so low as to limit growth and nitrogen retention (Wykes et al 1994).

Primène (Cernep Synthelabo) was formulated to mimic the umbilical cord plasma amino acid concentrations of pre- and full-term infants. The composition of Aminoplasmal ped (Braun) reflects amino acid utilization data from pharmacokinetic studies in the premature infant and newborn. It can be seen from Table 9.3 that solutions are broadly similar, and whether one represents a particular advance over another is not yet established. Further evaluation, including measures of protein turnover and nitrogen balance, are required. Such studies have already suggested that there is a resistance to suppression of proteolysis during PN in the premature infant compared with the term infant (Denne et al 1996). Given the unique metabolism of pre-term infants, their wide variation in developmental and nutritional status at birth, and the effects of illness and medication on nutrient requirements, it is unlikely there will be one amino acid solution that perfectly suits the needs of all infants at all times.

Carbohydrate

Glucose is the carbohydrate of choice for PN as it is metabolized by all cells, and is an essential nutrient for central nervous tissues, erythrocytes and renal cortex. High infusion rates may lead to hyperglycaemia, glycosuria and osmotic diuresis. Tolerance can usually be achieved by increasing intake over a number of days (see Table 9.2). Insulin infusion has been used to increase carbohydrate intake in the very-low-birth-weight infant and may be helpful in those usually very immature infants who develop hyperglycaemia even at low dextrose intakes (Binder et al 1989).

Fat

Lipid emulsions are non-irritant to veins, calorie dense and provide essential fatty acids. Increasing energy intake by adding fat to carbohydrate-based regimens improves nitrogen retention (Van Aerde et al 1994). Intralipid (Fresenius Kabi Ltd) is available as a 10%, 20% or 30% emulsion, and is made from soybean oil emulsified with egg yolk phospholipid. It is composed entirely of long-chain triglycerides (LCTs) and infusion gives rise to an increase in plasma cholesterol and phospholipid concentration (less evident with 20% than 10% emulsion). Lipofundin (Braun) in addition to LCTs contains medium-chain triglycerides (MCTs), which have the theoretical advantage of more rapid clearance from the blood and more complete oxidation. There is relatively little experience with MCT emulsions in infants and their advantages over LCT preparations remain unclear.

Tolerance of lipid may be reduced in the pre-term infant, particularly in those who are growth retarded, and plasma triglyceride concentration should be monitored in such patients. Lipid emulsions do not contain L-carnitine which enhances transfer of fatty acids across the inner mitochondrial membrane before oxidation. Although low-plasma carnitine concentrations have been reported during PN there is no compelling evidence to support routine supplementation. Free fatty acids from metabolism of lipid emulsion in the newborn might theoretically displace bilirubin from albumin binding sites and increase the risk of kernicterus in a jaundiced baby. Recent evidence indicates the risk is probably very low, particularly if lipid is withheld when unconjugated

plasma bilirubin is above 180 μmol/L. In the pre-term infant with respiratory distress, lipid infusion can lead to a reduction in arterial oxygen tension, possibly through vasoactive metabolites unblocking hypoxic vasoconstriction in the lung and thereby effectively increasing ventilation perfusion mismatch. A number of different studies have implicated lipid emulsion in pulmonary function abnormalities (Stahl et al 1992), and the development of chronic lung disease in the pre-term. Prospective randomized trials have not substantiated any link between early use of Intralipid and subsequent lung disease (Alwaidh et al 1996). However, continuous infusion of lipid has been shown to cause a significant dose and time-dependent increase in pulmonary vascular resistance in the pre-term infant (Prasertsom et al 1996) and should therefore be used with caution in the infant with pulmonary hypertension.

Much has been written regarding the potential for lipid emulsion to compromise host defence against infection. Few studies have demonstrated a clinically-significant effect, although lipid emulsion does appear to increase the risk of coagulase-negative *staphylococci* septicaemia in pre-term infants with in-dwelling central venous catheters. Unless there is overwhelming sepsis, the nutritional advantages of continuing lipid infusion almost certainly outweigh the theoretical disadvantages (Palmblad 1991).

Calcium and phosphate

Bone mineralization is dependent upon an adequate supply of calcium and phosphate. Metabolic bone disease in the pre-term infant receiving PN appears to be related to insufficient mineral intake. The limited solubilities of calcium and phosphate in PN solutions make it difficult to satisfy the relatively-high requirements of these infants. In the pre-term infant a calcium:phosphate ratio of 1.7:1 (the ratio of retention in the fetus) in PN solution has been suggested as the ideal. The use of calcium glycerophosphate rather than the usual combination of calcium gluconate with monobasic and dibasic potassium phosphate allows a higher concentration of calcium and phosphate to be held in solution. Plasma phosphate should generally be kept above 2.0 mmol/L in the very-low-birth-weight infants (Holland et al 1990).

Vitamins and trace elements

Based on a review of the available evidence, the American Society for Clinical Nutrition (ASCN)

Table 9.4 — Vitamin and trace element intakes recommended by the American Society of Clinical Nutrition

Vitamin	Infants dose/day	Pre-term infants dose/Kg/day	Intake/Kg/day as provided in Table 9.2
Water Soluble:			
Ascorbic acid (mg)	80	25	10
Thiamin (mg)	1.2	0.35	0.32
Riboflavin (mg)	1.4	0.45	0.36
Niacin (mg)	17	5	4
Pyridoxine (mg)	1	0.3	0.4
Folate (μg)	140	40	40
Cyanocobalamin (μg)	5	1.5	1.5
Pantothenate (mg)	20	6	6
Biotin (μg)	20	6	6
Lipid soluble:			
A (μg) ★	700	500 (max. 700/day)	276
D (μg) ★	10	4 (max. 10/day)	4
K (μg)	200	80 (max. 200/day)	80
E (mg) ★	7	2.8 (max. 7/day)	2.56

Element	Pre-term infant μg/Kg/day	Term infant μg/Kg/day	Intake μg/Kg/day as provided in Table 9.2
Zn	400	250 < 3 months	250
		100 > 3 months	250
Cu	20	20	20
Se	2	2	2
Cr	0.2	0.2	0
Mn	1	1	1
Mo	0.25	0.25	0
I	1	1	1
Fe	200	200	100

★700 μg retinol = 2300 international units (IU); 10 μg vitamin D = 400 IU;
7 mg α-tocopherol = 7 IU; Intakes as per regimens in Table 9.2 shown in column four. From Greene et al (1988) with permission.

published guidelines for intake of vitamins and trace elements during PN (Table 9.4) as well as calcium, magnesium and phosphorus (Greene et al 1988); optimal intakes continue to be debated.

Novel substrates

A number of novel supplements to PN have undergone evaluation in recent years, although none has yet become incorporated into standard infant regimens. Inositol is a component of membrane phospholipids and is found in breast milk. The administration of inositol increases levels of pulmonary surfactant in immature animals and it is therefore of particular

interest in pre-term infants who are at high risk of developing surfactant-deficient respiratory distress syndrome. A 5-day trial of intravenous inositol supplementation significantly reduced the risk of chronic lung disease in infants who had not received exogenous surfactant therapy (Hallman et al 1992). Glutamine is a specific energy source for cells of the gut and immune system. Efflux of glutamine from muscle provides a carbon source for oxidative metabolism in these tissues. Suggested potential benefits of glutamine include provision of a specific fuel for the gastro-intestinal tract, repletion of the intracellular muscle glutamine pool, and maintenance of gut barrier function. Free glutamine is unstable in solution and a new infusion solution (Fresenius Kabi Ltd) supplies 20 g of glutamine per litre in the form of glycine-L-glutamine. This solution is not designed for use in infants. In one study of glutamine supplementation in the pre-term newborn (Lacey et al 1996), conventional PN was compared with glutamine supplemented PN. In the group of infants who were < 800 g birth weight, there appeared to be a decreased number of ventilator days and total PN days required by those receiving glutamine. Ornithine α-ketoglutarate (OKG) is the ornithine salt of α-ketoglutaric acid, has the same carbon skeleton as glutamine and has been shown to reduce nitrogen loss post-operatively. Enteral supplementation with OKG accelerates growth velocity in rats and stimulates insulin and human growth hormone secretion. OKG added to PN fluids has been shown to increase linear height velocity and growth factor (IGF1) concentrations in parenterally-fed children with growth failure, although the mechanism of action remains uncertain (Moukarzel et al 1994). Randomized trials of sufficient size will be required to determine whether such novel substrates have an important role in clinical practice.

When to feed

How soon feeding is instituted depends on the age and nutritional status of the patient (Heird 1972) as well as the anticipated course of the illness. Clearly, there must be more urgency in the growth-retarded 800 g pre-term infant than the acutely-ill 9-month-old who is on the fiftieth centile for weight. Until recently, it has been customary to delay introduction of amino acids and lipids in the premature infant until clinically stable, and then to build up feeds over a week or more. This practice was influenced by past concerns regarding metabolic complications of PN such as acidosis, hyperammonaemia and coma, which are now very uncommon. Serial 24 h balance studies in pre-term infants given parenteral amino acids within 24 h of birth or from 72 h of age showed that positive nitrogen balance could be achieved from day 1 with early feeds but not until day 4 with later feeds (Saini et al 1989). In another study comparing introduction of amino acids from day 2 or after day 4, early introduction of amino acids was shown to have a positive effect on protein balance by increasing protein synthesis (Van Lingen et al 1992). Administration of amino acids to pre-term infants from birth seems safe and prevents loss of protein mass (Van Goudoever et al 1995). Murdock et al (1995) studied the tolerance of different feeding regimens given during the first 48 h of life; these comprised glucose, glucose/amino acids, or amino

acid/glucose/lipid. Plasma amino acid concentrations declined only in those infants not given intravenous amino acids. Plasma triglyceride and cholesterol concentrations were similar in each group, as was plasma bilirubin; hypoglycaemia was least common in the group given fat. Whether or not maintaining positive nitrogen and energy balance has long-term clinical benefits is unknown, but it seems reasonable for nutritional support to aim to bring about nutrient accretion and growth rates seen in the foetus of comparable post-conceptional age. These recent studies suggest that such a policy is practical and safe; however, some caution should be exercised when there is sepsis, marked acidosis, extreme prematurity and severe respiratory disease.

How to deliver parenteral nutrition

Prescribing and compounding

Where possible, provision of PN should be centralized through a multi-disciplinary nutritional care team (Puntis 1997). Recognized benefits include a reduction in metabolic and catheter-related complications as well as a reduction in unnecessary courses of PN. Parenteral feeds can be made up using standard solutions combined to give an appropriate fluid volume or with the aid of a computer program containing details of regimens appropriate to weight and age (Ball et al 1985). The latter allows the nutritional contribution of partial enteral feeds and additional intravascular fluids to be 'balanced' against the PN prescription. Such flexibility is most useful in those children with abnormal fluid and electrolyte requirements (Cade et al 1997) when feed components can be varied independently of one another. The prescription can be relayed directly via the ward computer to the computer in the pharmacy compounding unit or printed out in hard copy and sent to pharmacy. Grams of fat, glucose, amino acids, et cetera are 'translated' by the pharmacy computer into volumes of stock solution. A work sheet is produced for the pharmacist and printed labels are made for the feed bags. Feeds are made up in an aseptic unit, automatic titration devices speeding up the process.

Although most PN for adults is now given as a mixture of dextrose, amino acids and fat (an all-in-one mix), a two-bag system comprising separate infusion of lipid emulsion is generally used in infants. This is because of problems of stability of solutions (Barnett & Cosslett 1995), particularly given the high volume of divalent cations required in paediatric PN. What happens when the two infusions mix immediately prior to entering the circulation has until recently received little attention. It seems likely that coalescence of lipid droplets is quite common, particularly if heparin is being routinely added to solutions (Murphy et al 1996). The clinical significance of this observation remains uncertain.

Venous access

PN fluids may be delivered via a peripheral venous cannula or a central venous catheter. Solutions are irritant to veins and may cause tissue necrosis if extravasation occurs. When a peripheral vein is used overall dextrose concentration should not normally exceed 12.5%. In infants, 2FG (0.6 mm) Silastic catheters are widely used for central venous access. They also perform well as peripheral cannulae when advancement into a central vein is impossible. If reliable peripheral venous access cannot be maintained, feeds contain a high dextrose concentration, or when giving cyclical PN (all fluids infused overnight) a larger diameter Broviac-type catheter should be inserted surgically under a general anaesthetic (Stringer 1995). The tip of the catheter is usually placed just within the right atrium and the correct positioning should be confirmed radiologically.

Filters and pumps

Amino acid and dextrose solution is commonly filtered through a 0.22 μ pore size filter in order to remove bacteria. Because bacterial contamination of feeds made up in an aseptic compounding unit is rare, the role of the filter in removing particulate matter is probably more important. Recently an in-line filter suitable for use with lipid emulsion has also been developed. Filtration may be of greater consequence in infants than adults due to the high fluid requirements and relatively large particulate load, although the additional cost of a lipid filter is difficult to justify for short-term feeding. Particulate contamination is known to be associated not only with phlebitis but with more severe clinical consequences such as granulomatous pulmonary arteritis and cor pulmonale (Puntis et al 1992). Particulate matter is derived from chemical interactions in the feed solution as well as from the administration system itself. Filtration also offers protection against unstable solutions resulting from potentially-fatal compounding errors (Hill et al 1996). A volumetric pump should be used to deliver PN fluids; these are usually calibrated in ml/h and use a peristaltic pumping mechanism which delivers volumes within an accuracy of ±5%. For flow rates below 5 ml/h either a syringe pump or a neonatal volumetric pump can be used.

What to look out for

Metabolic complications

Many metabolic complications of PN have been reported in the literature, although few serious abnormalities arise unexpectedly directly as a consequence of short-term PN. A suggested protocol for routine monitoring of stable patients is shown in Table 9.5. Whilst increasing carbohydrate intake, blood glucose should be monitored several times each day in order to identify intolerance and avoid glycosuria and osmotic diuresis. In more long-term patients, urine testing for glucose is sufficient. Fat tolerance should be monitored by measuring plasma triglycerides with a view to keeping concentrations below 2.5 mmol/L. With PN extending over months, other metabolic derangements may be encountered. The most common of these is cholestasis, which can ultimately lead to cirrhosis and liver failure. Although multifactorial in origin, lack of pancreatico-biliary stimulation when enteral feeds are withheld is an important contributor, emphasizing the need to avoid complete enteral starvation whenever possible. Prematurity and sepsis are additional key factors and infants with short bowel or severe dysmotility (e.g., gastroschisis) are most at risk from severe liver disease. When liver function is deteriorating with no prospect of establishing full enteral feeding, treatment may be given with ceruletide, an analogue of cholecystokinin. A single daily dose of 300 μg/kg by subcutaneous or intramuscular injection is given in order to stimulate gallbladder contraction and biliary flow. In addition, ursodeoxycholic acid (10 mg/kg t.d.s.) has been shown to reverse cholestasis in long-term PN (Spagnuolo et al 1996). Recent evidence points to a possible role for plant sterols found in lipid emulsions in PN-associated liver disease (Clayton et al 1993); jaundice may improve when lipid intake is reduced.

Selenium is now included in Peditrace but prior to routine supplementation selenium deficiency presenting as a skeletal myopathy was described as a complication of long-term PN. Zinc requirements in the pre-term infant are high, and zinc deficiency sometimes occurs despite supplementation with Peditrace, particularly in infants with gastrointestinal fluid losses. A low plasma alkaline phosphatase (a zinc-dependent enzyme) activity may be seen before the typical skin lesions of

Table 9.5 — Monitoring protocol for parenteral nutrition (for clinically-stable patients)

	Before PN	Daily	Twice weekly	Once weekly	Monthly	Six monthly
Plasma						
Na	✓		✓			
K	✓		✓			
PO$_4$				✓		
bilirubin	✓			✓		
Ca				✓		
ALP				✓		
BM stix (glucose)		✓ week 1		✓		
Cu, Zn, Se, Mn					✓	
cholesterol, triglycerides				if fat ↑ > 3g/Kg		✓
FBC, PT/PTT						✓
ferritin						
Al, Cr						✓
folate; vitamins A, E, D, B1, B2 B6, B12						✓
Urine						
Na	✓		✓			
K	✓		✓			
glucose		✓				
Other						
CXR						✓
cardiac echo						✓
ECG						✓

PN = parenteral nutrition, Na = sodium, K = potassium, PO$_4$ = phosphate, Ca= calcium, ALP = alkaline phosphatase, BM = Boehringer-Monnheim, Cu = copper, Zn = zinc, Se = selenium, Mn = monganese, FBC = full blood count, PT = prothrombin time, PTT = partial thromboplastine time, Al = aluminium, Cr = chromium, CXR = chest X-ray, ECG = electrocardiogram

zinc deficiency manifest. Chromium added to long-term PN regimens has been associated with hepatic and renal impairment. There is probably sufficient chromium contaminating PN solutions for it to be unnecessary to make any specific addition; it is not included in Peditrace. Recently, manganese intake has been greatly reduced (along the lines of the ASCN proposals) following reports of accumulation in children with cholestasis associated with basal ganglia damage (Fell et al 1996). Trace element concentrations should be monitored periodically as described in Table 9.5 because requirements are variable. Aluminium contaminates PN solutions and has also been associated with cholestasis, central nervous system abnormality, anaemia and bone disease. Both pre-term and term infants are susceptible to accumulation of aluminium in tissue during PN (Moreno et al 1994). Further refinements in manufacture of feed products are needed to reduce aluminium load.

Catheter sepsis

The most common catheter related complication is sepsis, although mechanical problems also occur. Infection may occur with coagulase-negative *staphylococci* from the skin of the patient or carers following contamination of the hub of the catheter during disconnection or reconnection of the infusion. Gram-negative bacteria and yeasts also cause catheter sepsis. Presentation is usually with fever, but may be non-specific with instability of temperature or blood glucose or diarrhoea. Blood cultures from the catheter and a peripheral vein should be taken on first suspicion of sepsis; the possibility of infection elsewhere (e.g., urinary tract, chest, cerebrospinal fluid) must be considered. A tenfold excess of colony forming units in the through-catheter blood specimen helps distinguish between catheter sepsis and bacteraemia or contamination. Examination of the through-catheter specimen for bacteria following red cell lysis using acridine orange stain is a rapid test (1 h) that has proved useful for diagnosing catheter sepsis and has an accuracy of 92% (Rushforth et al 1993). Following blood sampling, broad-spectrum antibiotic treatment should be commenced with a combination of vancomycin and gentamicin. Ten-days treatment is given via the catheter with an antibiotic to which the cultured organism is sensitive. Sometimes there is only suppression of growth of organisms and clinical sepsis recurs soon after stopping antibiotic treatment. In the child who appears to be septicaemic and ill, the catheter may need to be removed at the outset, although most episodes of suspected catheter sepsis are disproved. The decision whether or not to remove a catheter is also influenced by small size and low gestational age (low threshold), anticipated difficulties in maintaining venous access and the likely duration of PN. Shock, septic emboli, yeast infection, continuing bacteraemia despite antibiotic treatment, or persistent thrombocytopenia are indications for catheter removal. Prevention of catheter sepsis requires adherence to strict aseptic technique when disconnecting and reconnecting the infusion, standardization of care protocols and staff training.

Mechanical catheter complications

These include blockage, fracture, and occasionally knotting, as well as injuries caused at insertion. Catheters can sometimes be unblocked by injecting saline, urokinase, 1M hydrochloric acid or 90% ethanol into the catheter lumen. It is possible to repair a fracture of the external part of a Broviac-type catheter using a kit supplied by the manufacturer. A fragment of catheter left behind after removal can be removed by the cardiologist using myocardial biopsy forceps or a venous catheter with a loop snare. Cardiac tamponade following erosion of the atrial wall by the catheter tip is well described even with Silastic neonatal catheters and may cause sudden collapse. PN leaking into the pleural space, lung, cranium or abdomen have all been described in catheters that have been mal-positioned. The risk of mechanical complications is reduced by limiting insertion to a small number of skilled operators and by always checking the position of the catheter radiologically. A worryingly-high prevalence of major thromboembolic complications has

recently been described in children dependent upon long-term PN (Dollery 1996). Further studies are required to establish the precise incidence of this complication and the role of anti-coagulation in prevention.

Delayed psycho-social development

Delayed psycho-social development is an inevitable consequence of long-term hospitalization for PN. Oral stimulation programmes should be encouraged from an early stage under the expert supervision of a speech therapist in order to prevent feeding difficulties once the time has come to establish full EN. Occupational, physio- and play therapists can provide additional stimulation for the child, and infusion of nutrients overnight leaves the child free of pumps during the day so that mobility can be increased. Care of the infant should be delegated to a small number of nursing staff, and visits from parents or trips home for the day encouraged. In children dependent on PN for longer than 3 months, home therapy should be considered (Bisset et al 1992).

Discussion

There have been few randomized clinical trials of PN in infancy. Despite this, PN is used successfully to promote growth in a wide range of disorders in early life. Although immature gastrointestinal function in the pre-term infant represents one of the commonest indications for PN, there is little evidence that its use has contributed to decreased mortality. For children with congenital gastrointestinal abnormalities, protracted diarrhoea, and severe dysmotility, however, PN represents a life-saving intervention. Developments in nutrient formulation and understanding of nutritional requirements have led to a reduction in metabolic complications, although these may still occur with long-term feeding. Metabolic and catheter related complications can be minimized if PN is supervised by a nutritional care team, strict protocols are followed and practical procedures are limited to a minimum number of operators. Home parenteral nutrition is an important option for the minority of infants who are dependent on long-term PN (see Chapter 10); advantages include a reduction in catheter sepsis and improved psycho-social development. Further refinements of PN require large scale prospective studies; these should include assessment of a number of novel energy substrates, a re-examination of specific nutrient needs, and investigation of the effects of disease states on nutritional requirements.

References

Alwaidh, M.H., Bowden, L., Shaw, B., Ryan, S.W. (1996) Randomised trial of effect of delayed intravenous lipid administration on chronic lung disease in preterm neonates. *J Pediat Gastroent Nutr*, 22, 303–306.

Anderson, D.M., Kliegman, R.M. (1991) The relationship of neonatal alimentation practices to the occurrence of endemic necrotizing enterocolitis. *Am J Perinatol*, 8, 62–67.

Ball, P.A., Candy, D.C.A., Puntis, J.W.L., McNeish, A.S. (1985) Portable bedside microcomputer system for management of parenteral nutrition in all age groups. *Arch Dis Child*, 60, 435–439.

Barnett, M.I., Cosslett, A.G. (1995) *Parenteral Nutrition Formulation*. In: Payne-James, J., Grimble, G., Silk, D. (eds.) *Artificial Nutrition Support in Clinical Practice*, pp. 321–332. London: Edward Arnold.

Binder, N.D., Raschko, P.K., Benda, G.I., Reynolds, J.W. (1989) Insulin infusion with parenteral nutrition in extremely low birth weight infants with hyperglycaemia. *J Pediatrics*, 114, 272–280.

Bisset, W.M., Stapleford, P., Long. S., Chamberlain, A., Sokel, B., Milla, P.J. (1992) Home parenteral nutrition in chronic intestinal failure. *Arch Dis Child*, 67, 109–114.

Cade, A., Thorp, H., Puntis, J.W.L. (1997) Does the computer improve the nutritional support of the newborn? *Clin Nutr*, 16, 19–23.

Clayton, P.T., Bowron, A., Mills, K.A., Massoud, A., Casteels, M., Milla, P.J. (1993) Phytosterolemia in children with parenteral nutrition-associated cholestatic liver disease. *Gastroenterology*, 105, 1806–1813.

Cosnett, J.E. (1989) The origins of intravenous fluid therapy. *Lancet*, 1, 768–771.

Denne, S.C., Karn, C.A., Ahlrichs, J.A., Dorotheo, A.R., Wang, J., Liechty, E. (1996) Proteolysis and phenylalanine hydroxylation in response to parenteral nutrition in extremely premature and normal newborns. *J Clin Invest*, 97, 746–754.

Dollery, C.M. (1996) Pulmonary embolism in parenteral nutrition. *Arch Dis Child*, 74, 95–98.

Fell, J.M.E., Reynnolds, A.P., Meadows, N., Khan, K., Long, S.G., Quaghebeur, G., Taylor, W.J., Milla, P.J. (1996) Manganese toxicity in children receiving long-term parenteral nutrition. *Lancet*, 347, 1218–1221.

Forsyth, J.S., Murdock, N., Crighton, A. (1995) Low birth weight infants and total parenteral nutrition immediately after birth. III. Randomised study of energy substrate utilisation, nitrogen balance, and carbon dioxide production. *Arch Dis Child*, 73, F13–F16.

Georgieff, M.K., Hoffman, J.S., Pereira, G.R., Bernbaum, J., Hoffman-Williamson, M. (1985) Effect of neonatal caloric deprivation on head growth and 1-year developmental status in preterm infants. *J Pediat*, 107, 581–587.

Greene, H.L., Hambidge, K.M., Schanler, R., Tsang, R.C. (1988) Guidelines for the use of vitamins, trace elements, calcium, magnesium, and phosphorus in infants and children receiving total parenteral nutrition: Report of the Subcommittee on Pediatric Parenteral Nutrition Requirements from the Committee on Clinical Practice Issues of the American Society for Clinical Nutrition. *Am J Clin Nutr*, 48, 1324–1342.

Hallman, M., Bry, K., Hoppu, K., Lappi, M., Pohjavuori, M. (1992) Inositol supplementation in premature infants with respiratory distress syndrome. *N Engl J Med*, 326, 1233–1239.

Heird, W.C. (1992) Parenteral Feeding. In: Sinclair, J.C., Bracken, M.B. (eds.) *Effective Care of The Newborn Infant*, pp. 141–160. Oxford: Oxford University Press.

Heird, W.C., Driscoll, J.M., Schullinger, J.N., Grebin, B., Winters, R.W. (1972) IV alimentation in pediatric patients. *J Pediatrics*, 80; 351–372.

Helfrick, F.W., Abelson, N.M. (1944) Intravenous feeding of a complete diet in a child. *J Pediatrics*, 25, 400–403.

Hill, S.E., Heldman, L.S., Goo, E.D.H., Whippo, P.E., Perkinson, J.C. (1996) Fatal microvascular pulmonary emboli from precipitation of a total nutrient admixture. *J Parent Ent Nutr*, 20, 81–87.

Holland, P.C., Wilkinson, A.R., Diez, J., Lindsell, D.R.M. (1990) Prenatal deficiency of phosphate, phosphate supplementation, and rickets in very-low-birthweight infants. *Lancet*, 335, 697–701.

Lacey, J., Crouch, J., Benefell, K., Ringer, S., Wilmore, C., Maguire, D., Wilmore, D. (1996) The effects of glutamine-supplemented parenteral nutrition in premature infants. *J Parent Enter Nutr*, 20, 74–80.

Lucas, A., Baker, B.A., Morley, R.M. (1993) Hyperphenylalaninaemia and outcome in intravenously fed neonates. *Arch Dis Child*, 68, 579–583.

McClure, R., Chatrath, M.K., Newell, S.J. (1996) Changing trends in feeding policies for ventilated preterm infants. *Acta Paediatr*, 85, 1123–1125.

McDonnell, M., Serra-Serra, V., Gaffney, G., Redman, C.W.G., Hope, P.L. (1994) Neonatal outcome after pregnancy complicated by abnormal velocity waveforms in the umbilical artery. *Arch Dis Child*, 70, F84–F89.

Moreno, A., Dominguez, C., Ballabriga, A. (1994) Aluminium in the neonate related to parenteral nutrition. *Acta Paediatr*, 83, 25–29.

Moukarzel, A.A., Goulet, O., Salas, J.S., Marti-Henneberg, C., Buchman, A.L., Cynober, L., Rappaport, R., Ricour, C. (1994) Growth retardation in children receiving long-term total parenteral nutrition: Effects of ornithine α-ketoglutarate. *Am J Clin Nutr*, 60, 408–413.

Murdock, N., Crighton, A., Nelson, L.M., Forsyth, J.S. (1995) Low birth weight infants and total parenteral nutrition immediately after birth. II. Randomised study of biochemical tolerance of intravenous glucose, amino acids, and lipid. *Arch Dis Child*, 73, F8–F12.

Murphy, S., Craig, D.Q.M., Murphy, A. (1996) An investigation into the physical stability of a neonatal parenteral nutrition formulation. *Acta Paediatr*, 85, 1483–1486.

O'Shaughnessy, W.B. (1831/2) Experiments on the blood in cholera. *Lancet*, 1, 490.

Palmblad, J. (1991) Intravenous lipid emulsions and host defence – a critical review. *Clin Nutr*, 10, 303–308.

Prasertsom, W., Phillipos, E.Z., Van Aerde, J.E., Robertson, M. (1996) Pulmonary vascular resistance during lipid infusion in neonates. *Arch Dis Child*, 74, F95–F98.

Puntis, J.W.L. (1997) Establishing a nutrition support team. *Baillières Clinical Paediatrics*, 5, 177–178.

Puntis, J.W.L., Ball, P.A., Preece, M.A., Green, A., Brown, G.A., Booth, I.W. (1989) Egg and breast milk based nitrogen sources compared. *Arch Dis Child*, 64, 1472–1477.

Puntis, J.W.L., Booth, I.W. (1987) Complications of neonatal parenteral nutrition. *Intensive Therapy and Clinical Monitoring*, 8, 48–56.

Puntis, J.W.L., Wilkins, K.M., Ball, P.A., Rushton, D.I., Booth, I.W. (1992) Hazards of parenteral nutrition: Do particles count? *Arch Dis Child*, 67, 1475–1477.

Rushforth, J.A., Hoy, C.M., Kite, P., Puntis, J.W.L (1993) Rapid diagnosis of central venous catheter sepsis. *Lancet*, 342, 402–403.

Saini, J., Macmahon, P., Morgan, J.B., Kovar, I.Z. Early parenteral feeding of amino acids. *Arch Dis Child*, 64, 1362–1366.

Spagnuolo, M.I., Iorio, R., Vegnente, A., Guarino, A. (1996) Ursodeoxycholic acid for treatment of cholestasis in children on long-term parenteral nutrition: A pilot study. *Gastroenterology*, 111, 716–719.

Stahl, G.E., Spear, M.L., Hamosh, M. (1992) *Lipid Infusions and Pulmonary Function Abnormalities*. In: Polin, R.A., Fox, W.W. (eds.) *Fetal and Neonatal Physiology*, pp. 346–353. Philadelphia: WB Saunders Company.

Stringer, M.D. (1995) Vascular Access. In: Spitz, L., Coran, A.G. (eds.) *Pediatric Surgery*, pp. 25–37, 5th edn. London: Chapman and Hall Medical.

Stringer, M.D., Puntis, J.W.L. (1995) Short bowel syndrome. *Arch Dis Child*, 73, 170–173.

Troche, B., Harvey-Wilkes, K., Engle, W.D., Nielsen, H.C., Frantz, I.D., Mitchell, M.L., Hermos, R.J. (1995) Early minimal feedings promote growth in critically ill premature infants. *Biol Neonate*, 67, 172–181.

Van Aerde, J.E., Sauer, P.J., Pencharz, P.B., Smith, J.M., Heim, T., Swyer, P.R. (1994) Metabolic consequences of increasing energy intake by adding lipid to parenteral nutrition in full term infants. *Am J Clin Nutr*, 59, 659–662.

Van Goudoever, J.B., Sulkers, E.J., Timmerman, M., Huijmans, J.G.M., Langer, K., Carnielli, V.P., Sauer, P.J.J. (1994) Amino acid solutions for premature neonates during the first week of life: The role of n-acetyl-L-cysteine and n-acetyl-L-tyrosine. *J Parent Ent Nutr*, 18, 404–408.

Van Goudoever, J.B., Colen, T., Wattimena, J.L.D., Huijmans, J.G.M., Carnielli, V.P., Sauer, P.J.J. (1995) Immediate commencement of amino acid supplementtion in preterm infants: Effect on serum amino acid concentrations and protein kinetics on the first day of life. *J Pediatr*, 127, 458–465.

Van Lingen, R.A., Van Goudoever, J.B., Luijendijk, I.H.T., Wattimena, J.L.D., Sauer, P.J.J. (1992) Effects of early amino acid administration during total parenteral nutrition on protein metabolism in pre-term infants. *Clin Sci*, 82, 199–203.

Walker-Smith, J.A. (1994) Intractable diarrhoea in infancy: continuing challenge for the paediatric gastroenterologist *Acta Paediatr*, Suppl 395, 6–9.

Wilmore, D.M., Dudrick, S.J. (1968) Growth and development of an infant receiving all nutrients by vein. *JAMA*, 203, 860–864.

Wykes, L.J., House, J.D., Ball, R.O., Pencharz, P.B. (1994) Amino acid profile and aromatic amino acid concentation in total parenteral nutrition: Effect on growth, protein metabolism and aromatic amino acid metabolism in the neonatal piglet. *Clin Sci*, 87, 75–84.

Zlotkin, S.H., Bryan, M.H., Anderson, G.H. (1981) Intravenous nitrogen and energy intakes required to duplicate in utero nitrogen accretion in prematurely born human infants. *J Pediat*, 99, 115–120.

10

Home parenteral nutrition

John W.L. Puntis

Introduction

A description of *home parenteral nutrition* (HPN) in an adult patient (Shils et al 1970) appeared just 2 years after the first report of prolonged parenteral nutrition (PN) in an infant (Wilmore & Dudrick 1968). HPN for children developed a decade later, although progress in the United Kingdom (Bisset et al 1992) was slower than in the United States (Cannon et al 1980) and France (Gorski et al 1989). The main factors that favoured the development of HPN in the United States have been summarized as pressures from insurers to reduce costs of treatment, the availability of equipment (e.g., ambulatory infusion pumps), competition between private providers and patient preference (Payne-James 1991). In the United Kingdom, the need for long-term PN should now no longer be the sole reason for keeping a child in hospital, even though this may still happen (British Paediatric Surveillance Unit 1992). Although the development of both the nutritional support industry and hospital outreach services have simplified the provision of HPN, the necessary organization and supervision remain complex and time consuming. For this reason it is desirable that HPN be restricted to regional centres providing both gastroenterology and surgical services. A nutrition-nurse specialist working within the framework of a multi-disciplinary nutritional care team (Puntis 1997a) is a further essential requirement.

Historical background

Home care

Home care has been defined as 'the provision of equipment and services to the patient in the home for the purpose of maintaining his/her maximal level of comfort, function and health' (Anonymous 1990). HPN is one of an increasing number of home-care services available as alternatives to treatment in hospital. Despite recent evidence for an increase in home care of children, there is considerable scope for further expansion (Tatman & Woodroffe 1993). The possible cost saving advantage of caring for patients at home holds obvious attractions for budget holders. For HPN, as well as other home-care services however, there are few data available on cost effectiveness (Anonymous 1991). Because the definition of home care given by the Council on Scientific Affairs of the American Medical Association (Anonymous 1990) includes reference to 'comfort, function and health' it is clear that 'quality' aspects are important. Savings to

be made from provision of high-quality home care, whilst considerable, have probably been overestimated (Cade and Puntis 1997).

With resource implications in mind, the British Association of Parenteral and Enteral Nutrition (BAPEN) has called for the establishment of local and national registers of patients in order to provide data on numbers and likely future trends in home nutritional support (BAPEN 1993). Subsequently, the British Artificial Nutrition Survey was instituted, encompassing both children and adult patients. Acknowledging the importance of experience and 'critical mass,' BAPEN recommended that HPN be concentrated in a limited number of centres, with one adult and one paediatric unit per region (BAPEN 1993). A more centralized model has been adopted in France where from 1984 HPN has been managed through just five recognized centres (Colomb 1995).

Practice and procedures

Which children should be considered for HPN?

One unique aspect of HPN for children is that it offers not only a good quality of life but the possibility of fully realizing growth and developmental potential (Loras Duclaux et al 1993, Carlsson et al 1997). Most children can expect to attend school and take part in normal social life, including sporting activities and holidays (Ricour et al 1990, Bisset et al 1992). Another benefit is reduced risk of central venous catheter sepsis, a major complication of PN (O'Connor et al 1988, Melville et al 1997). All children with chronic intestinal failure, therefore, should be considered potential candidates for HPN, other factors permitting. However, initiating PN in the child with little or no prospect of eventually adapting to full EN (such as a child with a congenital enteropathy or who has had massive gut resection in the newborn period) presents a major ethical dilemma requiring careful consideration (Hancock & Wiseman 1990; Paris et al 1994).

Long-term PN makes it possible to sustain growth and has considerably improved the prognosis of children with intestinal failure. In short-bowel syndrome, for example, Goulet et al (1991) were able to report an increase in survival of children with < 40 cm of small intestine from 42% before 1980 to a figure approaching 94%; for those with 40–80 cm of small bowel, survival improved to 97%. Such outcomes reflect an aggressive and meticulous approach to nutritional support. In addition to children with short bowel, similar numbers of patients with both congenital enteropathy and severe motility disorders (pseudo-obstruction) figure among HPN patients in one UK centre (Bisset et al 1992). In a larger series from France, short bowel was the most common condition (44 out of 112 children), followed by motility disorders, Crohn's disease, protracted diarrhoea and immune deficiency (Ricour et al 1990). During an 8-year period, 49 of these children progressed to full EN, and 18 died. Failure to achieve full EN after 4 years in short bowel syndrome was generally indicative of the need for life-long PN.

It is reasonable to consider HPN when the need for PN extends (or is likely to extend) beyond 3 months. Severity of underlying gastrointestinal disease must be taken into account, and fluid losses and tolerance of partial enteral feeding have important practical implications as does the presence of associated medical conditions. For example, care may be simplified if there is sufficient enteral intake to obviate the need for a separate intravenous lipid infusion and daily addition of vitamins to the parenteral nutrition bag. The overall clinical state must be relatively stable.

Parents need to be highly motivated to take responsibility for their child's day-to-day medical care. They must be able to cope not only with the emotional demands of HPN but also master technical aspects. Suitable housing and a supportive partner, relation, or friend who can share all aspects of care are both necessary prerequisites. In some conditions such as short bowel syndrome, specialized enteral support may also be needed (Booth 1994), imposing additional demands for carers (Puntis & Holden 1991). A survey undertaken by the British Paediatric Surveillance Unit (1992) identified 34 children receiving HPN in the United Kingdom. More recently, this figure had increased to 64 (British Artificial Nutrition Support Survey, 1999).

The role of the nurse specialist in nutritional support

A nurse specialist in nutritional support is central to the success of HPN and essential for assessing the suitability of the family, providing structured teaching, organizing community support, providing the link with hospital after discharge and co-ordinating the input of other professionals. In addition to facilitating home care, the nutrition nurse working within the paediatric unit can help reduce the incidence of

central venous catheter sepsis as well as play a key role within the multi-disciplinary care team (Puntis et al 1991, Lennard-Jones 1992, Puntis 1997a).

Assessment and teaching of parents

Family assessment can be undertaken in conjunction with ward staff and members of the primary health care team. This should include a home visit during which practical details such as availability of storage space, power points, lighting and hand-washing facilities are reviewed. If the family is suitable and the home circumstances adequate, detailed preparation can begin. A teaching programme should be formulated to make sure that the parents are confident and competent in all aspects of their child's care. This would include: hand washing and aseptic technique; knowledge of central venous catheters; catheter care and dressing changes; care of the infusion pump; running feed solutions through and connecting to the central venous catheter; setting up the infusion and making the necessary connections; urine testing; temperature taking; problem solving; and what to do in an emergency.

The teaching programme can be completed within a few weeks if both parents are able to be resident in hospital, but because this is often not the case, teaching may need to be extended over a longer period of time. Each session is focused on one particular skill, allowing time for practice; a written record is made of progress. Only when competence is achieved in one area is a new subject introduced. Before discharge home, the family and nutritional nurse draw up a care plan to fit in with the family's routine (Bilodeau 1995).

Family-held records

Children receiving HPN may be seen by a large number of different health care professionals in various locations (e.g., home, general practice, district hospital, HPN centre). The family is provided with a set of medical records both for their reference and for the benefit of any professionals unfamiliar with the child, such as new junior staff. A folder is compiled for the family that includes a medical summary and a list of contact names and telephone numbers for the ward and nutritional care team. Written information to back up the teaching sessions in hospital, instruction manuals for equipment, problem solving advice, growth charts, and flow charts recording the results of biochemical monitoring should also be included. Much of this information is available in the form of a

Table 10.1 — Equipment required for an HPN patient with short-bowel syndrome

Chlorhexidine 1/200 with alcohol 70%, 500 ml
Aquasept, 500 ml; 5 ml dispenser
Manusept, 500 ml; 3 ml dispenser

Parenteral nutrition feed bags, 2 weeks' supply
Refrigerator
IVAC 597 intravenous (IV) infusion pump
IV stand
IVAC IV administration sets with Y site and luer lock
IBEX-HP 0.22 micron high-pressure vented filter set

Enteral feed (Chix, Maxijul, Calogen, Liquigen, Aminogram, pectin)
Kangaroo 500 ml easy cap pump set (box 36)
Kangaroo 2100 enteral feeding pump
Vygon nasogastric tubes
Blue litmus paper
Stoma-hesive
Zinc oxide adhesive tape

NHS supplies wound care pack
Latex gloves (50 pairs)
Paper towels
5 ml syringes
5 micron filter needles
Hepflush 100 units heparin/ml, 2 ml ampoules
normal saline, 5 ml plastic ampoules
Durapore tape
Mediwipes
Absorbent dressings
Gauze swabs
Urine ketodiastix
Emla cream with Tegaderm dressings
Sterilizing solution (Milton)
Disposal bin for 'sharps'
Yellow plastic waste bags

well-illustrated and parent-friendly booklet (Holden 1993).

Supply of equipment

Equipment supply can be arranged through the hospital or by contracting with one of a number of commercial home-care companies (see appendix). A stock list of necessary equipment and disposables (Table 10.1) should be compiled by the nutrition nurse. By the time of discharge the PN formulation should require infrequent modification. It is relayed to the compounding unit by the nutrition team pharmacist.

Standard nutritional regimens (Puntis 1997b) modified to take into account both intake of enteral nutrients and fluid and electrolyte losses can be used. Fluid bags and disposables are usually delivered every 2 weeks; adequate storage space at home is essential. The home-care company provides a folding trolley and a refrigerator large enough for a 2-weeks' supply of PN. Disposal of sharps and clinical waste needs special arrangements with the local authority. In the United Kingdom, the council cleansing department must be contacted to ensure that yellow bags for clinical waste are collected once a week for incineration; the appropriate form is obtainable from district nurses. The electricity company should be made aware of the importance of maintaining supply.

Costs and funding

Bisset et al (1992) estimated the annual cost of HPN solutions to be between £20,000–25,000, with the infusion pump and disposable equipment a further £3000–5000. This was contrasted with the cost of 1 year in hospital of around £100,000. Current annual costs for HPN when contracted with a home-care company are in the order of £22,000 for PN solutions, £10,000 for disposables, and £3600 for pump rental (Cade and Puntis 1997). The home-care company charge 15% of this total as a service charge, covering 2-week stock holding; free loan of trolley, refrigerator and drip stand; help with arranging holidays; fast response to change in regimen; and quarterly financial reports.

Difficulty agreeing funding arrangements in the absence of a universally-accepted system often resulted in delay of discharge from hospital (Bisset et al 1992), with both community and hospital care budget holders arguing inadequate funding for long-term home care. January 1995 saw the launch of a new strategy for the supply of complex home care treatments, including PN. This policy was described in the Department of Health Executive Letter EL(95)5 titled 'Purchasing high-tech health-care for patients at home'. Subsequently, there have been formal contracts for providing HPN between purchasers and providers that have simplified the process of sending a child home. Unfortunately, the costs of nutritional-care-team time and effort expended in order to manage children at home go unrecognized.

Liaison with primary health care team

The primary health care team should be contacted at

an early stage of discharge planning, beginning with the general practitioner. A full medical summary is provided at the time it is decided that HPN is going to be pursued. The nutrition nurse then visits the general practitioner surgery to explain the implications and discuss prescribing and funding with the primary health care team. The health visitor and district nurse are invited to the ward for a case discussion and explanation of HPN, and joint home visits arranged after discharge. Where available, the active involvement of a paediatric community nurse facilitates discharge and provides excellent local support for parents.

Venous access

In hospital and at home venous access is maintained by a central venous catheter. While in hospital the amount of time PN is infused gradually decreases, the aim being to give solutions over 12 h at night so that the child is free of the infusion pumps during the day (Francois et al 1997). This pattern is associated with a regular rhythm of growth hormone secretion and normal growth (Yokoyama et al 1997). Central venous catheters are usually of the Broviac or Hickman type, the catheter being positioned with its tip just within the right atrium and exiting from a skin tunnel below the nipple. There is less experience of long-term PN using totally implantable devices, which must be accessed using a Huber needle. Catheters are filled with heparin solution during the day but may block acutely with blood or slowly with a gradual build-up of a hard waxy deposit, which seems to be a mixture of both lipid, fibrin and particulate plastic debris. If the central venous catheter is to be saved, blockage of either type requires prompt action, which may involve a urokinase lock or infusion, hydrochloric acid, ethanol, passage of a guide wire (Ball 1993), or sodium hydroxide (Sando et al 1997).

Catheter sepsis appears to be more common in children than adults receiving HPN, with around two-thirds of infections being due to gram-negative organisms (Buchman et al 1994). Parents must be taught about the signs of catheter sepsis and the need for prompt review by medical staff. After clinical assessment, peripheral and central venous blood samples are taken for quantitative bacterial culture (Ruderman et al 1988) and Acridine Orange Leucocyte Cytospin test (Rushforth et al 1993); alternative sites of primary infection must be excluded. When catheter sepsis is suspected, treatment with intravenous gentamicin and vancomycin via the catheter should be started while awaiting the results of blood culture and sensitivity

testing. Every effort must be made to salvage blocked, infected or damaged catheters in children requiring long-term intravenous therapy. If the catheter has to be removed, it may be possible for the surgeon to place a new catheter at the same time through the existing track in order to preserve the vein.

Support

Continuing practical and psychological support for parents/home carers is essential. The hospital social worker can provide support to families as well as information regarding sources of financial assistance such as the disability living allowance. Help with disposable nappies may also be available. The support group for Patients on Intravenous and Nasogastric Nutrition Therapy (PINNT) share helpful advice, produce a newsletter, and organize meetings for patients and their families. An introduction to another family who have experience of HPN can be invaluable. A member of the nutritional care team should be contactable 24 h a day to discuss any acute problems once the child has gone home

Monitoring and follow-up

Once discharged from hospital, regular outpatient follow-up is arranged initially at monthly intervals. PN is generally safe, and although many different metabolic complications are described, sudden unexpected and serious biochemical disturbances seem relatively rare in stable patients both in hospital (Puntis et al 1993) and at home (Bisset 1992). Trace element and vitamin requirements are, however, uncertain and status should be monitored. Blood can be taken from the central venous catheter by the nutrition nurse at the time of clinic visit. In addition to anthropometry, a range of haematological and biochemical parameters (Table 10.2) should be checked periodically. Thromboembolism (Dollery et al 1994) and granulomatous pulmonary arteritis (Puntis et al 1992) have been reported in children on long-term PN. For this reason electrocardiography twice a year and annual echocardiography are advocated. The risk of cholestatic liver disease and gallstones are increased both by short-bowel syndrome and long-term PN and can be monitored by abdominal ultra-sound every 6 months. A yearly developmental assessment for children receiving HPN has also been suggested as part of clinical follow-up and audit.

Long-term complications

Although almost half of those children starting HPN

Table 9.2 — Recommended monitoring during long-term parenteral nutrition

---

Monthly

full blood count; clotting studies

sodium, potassium; chloride; calcium; magnesium; phosphate; alkaline phosphatase; albumin; aspartate transaminase; bilirubin (conjugated/unconjugated); ferritin; copper; zinc; selenium; cholesterol; triglycerides

Every 6 months

aluminium; chromium; manganese; folate; vitamins A, E, D, B1, B2, B6, B12

Annual

echocardiography and ECG; MRI brain; developmental assessment; abdominal ultrasound

---

Abbreviations: ECG, electrocardiogram; MRI, magnetic resonance imaging.

may eventually achieve full enteral feeding (Vargas et al 1987, Ricour et al 1990), the remainder are committed to long-term intravenous support. Although in many respects their quality of life may be excellent, there are a number of important, and sometimes life-threatening, complications that may occur. Despite adequate provision of protein and energy, some children fail to grow. One study has indicated that provision of ornithine α-ketoglutarate may reverse this growth failure, possibly by stimulating production of growth hormone or insulin-like growth factor-1 (Moukarzel et al 1994). Standard iron intakes of around 100 μg/kg/day have been associated with iron overload, a possible factor in PN-associated liver disease (Ben Hariz et al 1993). Iron status improves if parenteral iron is withdrawn (Ban Hariz et al 1997). Plant sterols in lipid emulsions are implicated in PN cholestasis; liver function may improve if a sustained reduction in lipid intake is possible (Clayton et al 1993). Manganese toxicity causing damage to the basal ganglia has been reported in children receiving PN (Fell et al 1996) and prompted modification of the trace element preparation by the manufacturers, resulting in a fifty-fold reduction in manganese intake. Patients with liver disease and impaired biliary excretion of manganese may still be at risk of toxicity even at the lower intake, and they require monitoring.

Aluminium contaminating PN solutions may also be a contributory factor to liver disease, in addition to metabolic bone disease (Klein 1995). A further major concern related to long-term PN is the risk of thromboembolic events. A paper from the largest UK children's HPN centre identified thrombosis or embolism in 12 of 32 patients on long-term PN (Dollery et al 1994); there were four deaths. How far these might be preventable by routine use of anti-coagulants as well as the risks of this treatment remain unclear at the present time.

Discussion

HPN requires a remarkable commitment from parents, who in return must be adequately supported. The practical difficulties remain considerable and, as the number of suitable children is likely to remain small, a restricted number of HPN centres should develop expertise in this area. Major advantages of HPN over hospital care include an improved quality of life, the opportunity for normal psycho-social development, decreased risk of catheter sepsis, and cost savings to the health service. The alternative to long-term PN for some children is small-bowel transplantation. Initial experience proved disappointing (Schroeder et al 1990) but technical advances now mean that surgery has progressed well beyond the experimental stage. Transplantation (at present not readily available) will probably be seen as a solution when, for whatever reason, HPN fails. In the meantime, for the child committed to long-term PN it seems reasonable to conclude that 'if the home works—use it'!

Appendix

The following home-care companies undertake HPN in the UK:

1. Baxter, Wallingford Road, Compton, Newbury, Berks RG20 7QW.

2. B Braun, B Braun House, Aylesbury Vale Industrial Park, Stocklake, Aylesbury, Bucks HP20 1DQ.

3. Central Home Care Ltd, HRH House, Mill Lane, Alton, Hampshire GU34 2QG.

4. Health Care at Home, 15 Brentford Business Centre, Commerce Road, Brentford, Middlesex TW8 8LG.

5. Fresenius Kabi Ltd, Hampton Court, Tudor Road, Manor park, Runcorn, Cheshire, WA7 1UF.

Half PINNT is the childrens' section of PINNT (i.e., Patients on Intravenous and Nasogastric Nutrition Therapy), 258 Wennington Road, Rainham, Essex RM13 9UU.

References

Anonymous. (1990) Council on Scientific Affairs. Home care in the 1990s. *JAMA*, 263, 1241–1244.

Anonymous. (1991) Who cares about home care? *Lancet*, 338, 1303–1304.

Ball, P.A., Booth, I.W., Holden, C.E., Puntis, J.W.L. (1993) *Paediatric Parenteral Nutrition*, pp. 69–74. Milton Keynes: Pharmacia Limited.

British Association of Parenteral and Enteral Nutrition. (1993) Progress report of the British Association of Parenteral and Enteral Nutrition sub-committee on home artificial nutritional support. London: BAPEN.

Ben Hariz, M., Goulet, O., De Potter, S. et al. (1993) Iron overload in children receiving prolonged parenteral nutrition. *J Pediatr*, 123, 238–241.

Ben Hariz, M., Goulet, O., Colomb, V. et al. (1997) Inappropriate iron intake in children on long-term parenteral nutrition: Outcome after iron withdrawal. *Clin Nutr*, 16, 109–112.

Bilodeau, J.A. (1995) A home parenteral nutrition program for infants. *J Obstet, Gynecol Neonat Nurs*, 24, 72–76.

Bisset, W.M., Stapleford, P., Long, S., Chamberlain, A., Sokel, B., Milla, P.J. (1992) Home parenteral nutrition in chronic intestinal failure. *Arch Dis Child*, 67, 109–114.

Booth, I.W. (1994) Enteral nutrition as primary therapy in short bowel syndrome. *Gut*, suppl 1, S69–S72.

British Artificial Nutrition Survey (BANS) (August 1999). British Association of Parenteral and Enteral Nutrition, Maidenhead.

British Paediatric Surveillance Unit. (1992) *7th Annual Report*, pp. 16–17. London: BPSU.

Buchman, A.L., Moukarzel, A., Goodson, B., Herzog, F., Pollack, P., Reyen, L., Alvarez, M., Ament, M.E., Gornbein, J. (1994) Catheter-related infections associated with home parenteral nutrition and predictive factors for the need for catheter removal in their treatment. *J Parent Enter Nutr*, 18, 297–302.

Cade, A., Puntis, J.W.L. (1997) Economics of home parenteral nutrition. *Pharmacoeconomics*, 12, 327–338.

Cannon, R.A., Byrne, M.J., Ament, M.E., Gates, B. (1980) Home parenteral nutrition in infants. *J Pediatr*, 96, 1098–1104.

Carlsson, G., Håkansson, A., Rubensson, A., Finkel, Y. (1997) Home parenteral nutrition (HPN) in Sweden. *Pediatric Nursing*, 23, 272–274.

Clayton, P.T., Bowron, A., Mills, K.A., Massoud, A., Casteels, M., Milla, P.J. (1993) Phytosteroloemia in children with parenteral nutrition-associated cholestatic liver disease. *Gastroenterology*, 105, 1806–1813.

Colomb, V., Goulet, O., de Potter, S., Ricour, C. (1995) Nutrition parentérale à domicile chez l'enfant. *Méd et Nut*, 31, 193–197.

Department of Health (1995). Purchasing high-tech health care for patients at home. Executive Letter EL(95)5; London, Department of Health.

Dollery, C.M., Sullivan, I.D., Bauraind, O. et al. (1994) Pulmonary embolism and long term central venous access for parenteral nutrition. *Lancet*, 344, 1043–1045.

Fell, J.M.E., Reynolds, A.P., Meadows, N. et al. (1996) Manganese toxicity in children receiving long-term parenteral nutrition. *Lancet*, 347, 1218–1221.

François, B., Colomb, V., Bonnefont, J.P., Goulet, O., Benhariz, M., Vassault, A., Rabier, D., Ricour, C. (1997) Tolerance to starvation in children on long-term total parenteral nutrition. *Clin Nutr*, 16, 113–117.

Gorski, A.M., Goulet, O., Lamor, M. (1989) Nutrition parentérale à domicile chez l'enfant. Bilan de 8 ans d'activité chez 88 malades. *Arch Fr Pediatr*, 46, 323–329.

Goulet, O., Revillon, Y., Jan, D. et al. (1991) Neonatal short bowel syndrome. *J Pediat*, 119, 18–23.

Hancock, B.J., Wiseman, N.E. (1990) Lethal short bowel syndrome. *J Pediat Surg*, 25, 1131–1135.

Holden, C.E. (1993) *Home Parenteral Nutrition for Your Child*. Yorkshire: Blackwell Masters.

Klein, G.L. (1995) Aluminum in parenteral solutions revisited - Again. *Am J Clin Nutr*, 61, 449–456.

Lennard-Jones, J.E. (1992) A positive approach to nutrition as treatment. Report of a working party on the role of enteral and parenteral feeding in hospital and at home. London: King's Fund.

Loras Duclaux, I., De Potter, S., Pharaon, I., Olives, J.P., Hermier, M. (1993) Qualité de view des enfants en nutrition parentérale à domicile et de leurs parents. *Pédiatrie*, 7/8, 555–560.

Melville, C.A., Bisset, W.M., Long, S., Milla, P.J. (1997) Counting the cost: Hospital versus home central venous catheter survival. *J Hosp Infect*, 35, 197–205.

Moukarzel, A.A., Goulet, O., Salas, J.S. et al. (1994) Growth retardation in children receiving long-term total parenteral nutrition: Effects of ornithine α-ketoglutarate. *Am J Clin Nutr*, 60, 408–413.

O'Connor, M.L., Ralston, C.W., Ament, M.E. (1988) Intellectual and perceptual-motor performance of children receiving prolonged home total parenteral nutrition. *Pediatrics*, 81, 231–236.

Paris, J.J., Bell, A.J., Morley, C. (1994) Lethal short-bowel syndrome: More than a medical challenge. *J Perinatol*, 14, 226–229.

Payne-James, J. (1991) Home care in the 1990s. *Brit J Hosp Med*, 45, 355.

Puntis, J.W.L, Holden, C.E. (1991) Home enteral nutrition in paediatric practice. *Br J Hosp Med*, 45, 104–107.

Puntis, J.W.L., Holden, C.E., Smallman, S., Finkel, Y., George, R.H., Booth, I.W. (1991) Staff training: A key factor in reducing intravascular catheter sepsis. *Arch Dis Child*, 66, 335–337.

Puntis, J.W.L., Wilkins, K.M., Ball, P.A., Rushton, D.I., Booth, I.W. (1992) Hazards of parenteral treatment: Do particles count? *Arch Dis Child*, 67, 1475–1477.

Puntis, J.W.L., Hall, S.K., Green, A., Smith, D.E., Ball, P.A., Booth, I.W. (1993) Biochemical stability during parenteral nutrition in children. *Clin Nutr*, 12, 153–159.

Puntis, J.W.L. (1997a) Establishing a nutrition support team. *Baillières Clinical Paediatrics*, 5, 177–188.

Puntis, J.W.L. (1997b) Parenteral Nutrition. In: Campbell, A.G.M., McIntosh, N. (eds.) *Forfar and Arneil's Textbook of Paediatrics*, pp. 1219–1230, 5th edn. Edinburgh: Churchill Livingstone.

Ricour, C., Gorski, A., Goulet, O. et al. (1990) Home parenteral nutrition in children: 8 years of experience with 112 patients. *Clin Nutr*, 9, 65–71.

Ruderman, J.W., Morgan, M.A., Klein, A.H. (1988) Quantitative blood cultures and the diagnosis of catheter sepsis in infants with umbilical and Broviac catheters. *J Pediatr*, 112, 748–751.

Rushforth, J.A., Hoy, C.M., Kite, P., Puntis, J.W.L. (1993) Rapid diagnosis of central venous catheter sepsis. *Lancet*, 342, 402–403.

Sando, K., Fujii, M., Tanaka, K., Chen, K., Yoshida, H., Iiboshi, Y., Nezu, R., Konishi, K., Takagi, Y., Okada, A. (1997) Lock method using sodium hydroxide solution to clear occluded central venous access devices. *Clin Nutr*, 16, 185–188.

Schroeder, P., Goulet, O., Lear, P.A. (1990) Small bowel transplantation: European experience. *Lancet*, 336, 110–111.

Shils, M.E., Wright, W.L., Turnbull, A. (1970) Long-term parenteral nutrition through external arteriovenous shunt. *N Engl J Med*, 283, 341–344.

Tatman, M.A., Woodroffe, C. (1993) Paediatric care in the UK. *Arch Dis Child*, 69, 677–680.

Vargas, J.H., Ament, M.A., Berquist, W.E. (1987) Long term home parenteral nutrition in paediatrics: Ten years of experience in 102 patients. *J Pediatr Gastroenterol Nutr*, 6, 24–32.

Wilmore, D.W., Dudrick, S.J. (1968) Growth and development of an infant receiving all nutrients exclusively by vein. *JAMA*, 203, 860–864.

Yokoyama, S., Hirakawa, H., Soeda, J., Ueno, S., Mitomi, T. (1997) Twenty-four-hour profile of growth hormone in cyclic nocturnal total parenteral nutrition. *Pediatrics*, 100, 973–976.

11

Percutaneous endoscopic gastrostomy

Patricia Davidson

Introduction

Children who cannot maintain adequate oral nutrition either because they cannot swallow properly or because they have increased nutritional requirements require enteral feeding (Moore & Greene 1985, Goulet 1991, Amundson et al 1994, Heine et al 1995). In this situation, a clinical judgment is made between either nasogastric feeds or gastrostomy. The decision hinges on the benefits of a permanent gastrostomy versus the risks of the procedure (Rabeneck et al 1997). Often the parent or child has found difficulties with maintenance of the nasogastric tube and decides to proceed to gastrostomy. *Percutaneous endoscopic gastrostomy* (PEG) was initially described as a method of gastrostomy placement for children who were unsuitable for laparotomy (Gauderer et al 1980). Subsequent experience has confirmed that this is a suitable method for insertion of a gastrostomy (Coughlin et al 1991, Gauderer 1991, Davidson et al 1994, Marin et al 1994). It is the method of choice if no other intra-abdominal procedure is required. Careful attention to detail ensures the risks of the procedure are minimized (Beasley et al 1995). Common indications for insertion are: 1) loss of the ability to swallow (e.g., patients with cerebral palsy or severe head injuries); 2) anatomical abnormalities precluding swallowing (e.g., oesophageal stricture and dysmotility following oesophageal atresia repair), and 3) inability to maintain nutrition (e.g., patients with cystic fibrosis or congenital cardiac disease). A PEG is contraindicated if the child requires a surgical anti-reflux procedure for gastro-oesophageal reflux, as a gastrostomy is ideally placed at the same time. Previous surgery may be a contraindication to insertion of a PEG because of the risks of interposition of an organ (usually liver) or viscus (usually colon) between the abdominal wall and the stomach. This complication can still occur without any previous surgery (Coughlin et al 1991).

This Chapter details the principles of insertion and emphasizes the common problems that may be encountered.

Practice and procedures

Pre-operative preparation

Patient information

The risks and benefits of the technique are discussed so that the child and parent understand and are able to give informed consent (Huddleston & Ferraro 1991). A video of the procedure and/or written information is useful. The parent should discuss the details of the feeding regimen with the dietitian and/or nurse to ensure that all additional equipment is available prior to insertion of the PEG. An opportunity to meet with other parents and children who have a gastrostomy is beneficial.

Nutritional requirements

The feeding regimen should be chosen beforehand so that this can be implemented once the PEG is *in situ*. Alternatives include infant formula, liquid enteral feeds and ordinary food processed in a blender. This decision influences the size of the PEG inserted. If a child is to receive continuous feeds a feeding pump is needed.

Fasting and wound site preparation

The children should be fasted for the time consistent with local hospital practice. Antibiotic prophylaxis is given to prevent post-operative wound infection (options include a broad-spectrum cyclosporin or flucloxacillin). The site for insertion of the PEG is selected pre-operatively and marked on the anterior abdominal wall. This position is normally mid-way between the umbilicus and the costal margin in the mid-clavicular line (Fig. 11.1). Preparation of the skin with an iodine-containing solution just prior to departure for the operating suite may minimize the risks of wound infection.

Operating room procedure

Instruments required

There are a large number of PEG kits available that include all the instruments necessary for insertion. The contents include: a PEG feeding tube with internal bumper and external bolsters, a trocar with removable stylet, a flexible-tipped guide wire, syringe, needle, and scalpel. The PEG kit that is used depends on the size of the child, the dimension requirements for the gastrostomy and the choice of the operator. A PEG catheter can be made from a modified latex catheter (e.g., a foley type). The selected PEG catheter should be immersed in an iodine-containing solution prior to insertion to minimize post-operative wound infections. A paediatric endoscope with accompanying snare or forceps is necessary as is an a-septic trolley with equipment for skin preparation and draping.

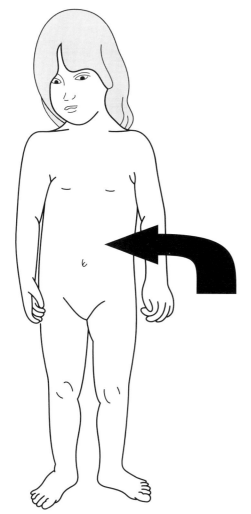

Figure 11.1 — Insertion site of the PEG.

Method of anaesthesia

Opinions regarding the most appropriate technique by which a patient can achieve both adequate pain relief and a lack of awareness of the procedure are divided. Options include intravenous sedation or general anaesthetic. Either method should include local anaesthetic at the site of the PEG to provide post-operative pain relief. The patient's needs and experience of the staff involved determine which method is chosen.

Operative technique (Fig. 11.2)

Insertion of a PEG requires two operators. One to perform the endoscopy (the endoscopist) and one

gloved in an a-septic manner (surgeon) to prepare the abdominal wall and insert tile trocar. The procedure can be performed by one operator but is more time-consuming and difficult. Once in the operating room, place the child in the supine position. Perform a routine upper gastrointestinal endoscopy with biopsies of oesophagus, stomach and duodenum to confirm the presence of normal anatomy and to identify any additional abnormalities (e.g., oesophagitis).

Inflate the stomach with air to ensure that it approximates to the anterior abdominal wall. At the same time, prepare the abdominal wall with an iodine-containing solution. The surgeon identifies the anticipated site for the PEG by pressing down with an index finger at the site for insertion. This produces an indentation on the anterior aspect of the stomach that is clearly visible to the endoscopist. The endoscopist then directs the tip of the flexible endoscope towards this site. The bright light from the endoscope should be clearly visible transilluminating the abdominal wall maximal at the prospective site of insertion. If not, dim the operating room lights to allow the light to be seen more easily. If the indentation caused by the index finger of the surgeon is not visible and/or if transillumination suggests an interposed viscus or organ, then a different site should be chosen for insertion or the gastrostomy should be inserted by the open technique.

Infiltrate the PEG site with local anaesthetic. Make a small incision in the skin and introduce the trocar into the stomach. This is accompanied by a 'pop' as the trocar enters the stomach. The tip of the trocar should be visible through the endoscope. If it is not, it may be lying within the peritoneal cavity. The trocar should then be removed and a second attempt made to introduce it into the stomach. Multiple tries should not be attempted because of the risks of leakage of gastric contents or pneumoperitoneum. Once successful, the stylet is removed and a flexible-tipped guide wire is passed into the stomach and retrieved, either with an endoscopic snare or forceps and then withdrawn through the oesophagus and mouth. The trocar is removed from the anterior abdominal wall. The tip of the PEG catheter is pushed over, or attached to, the guide wire and pulled down into the stomach and out through the abdominal wall.

The endoscope is returned to the stomach and the internal bumper of the PEG catheter is visualized. It should lie comfortably against the gastric mucosa. The external bolster should be placed against the skin to ensure the PEG catheter is retained in position. The bolster should not be too tightly applied as this leads

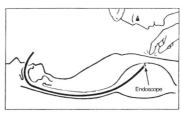

1. Prepare insertion site.

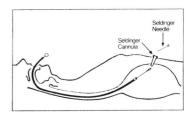

2. Make incision. Insert Seldinger Needle. Remove inner stylet, leaving outer cannula in place. Loop endoscopic snare loosely over end of cannula.

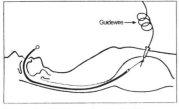

3. Insert guidewire and grasp it with snare. Remove endoscope to bring guidewire out through mouth.

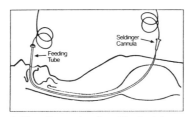

4. Thread tapered portion of feeding tube over guidewire, pass into oropharynx, then out through abdominal wall, pushing cannula out.

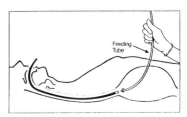

5. As tapered end of feeding tube emerges through abdominal wall, bumper is delivered through oropharynx by endoscopist.

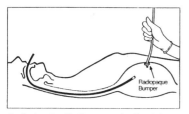

6. Under visualization, snug feeding-tube bumper gently up against gastric mucosa. Remove guidewire through abdominal site.

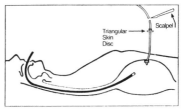

7. Pass external bolster over tapered end of feeding tube and secure close to skin. Cut off tapered dilator portion of tube and confirm bumper position by endoscopy.

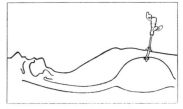

8. Insert adapter into tube and close caps.

Figure 11.2 — Overview of operative technique.

to skin and gastric mucosal ischaemia predisposing to infection at the site of insertion. The endoscope is removed at completion of the procedure.

Post-operative care

The PEG catheter can be used immediately after the procedure. A crystalloid solution is commenced at a rate appropriate for age and weight. This enables adequate fluid balance to be maintained in the immediate post-operative period. The patient should avoid oral intake in the early post-operative period until the PEG is functioning without complication.

Despite the smaller incision required for insertion of a PEG, the wound is often painful post-operatively. After the local anaesthetic has ceased to provide pain relief, provision should be made for administration of adequate analgesia. Opiates, as an intravenous infusion, may be required during the first 24 h.

Once the patient is stable and recovered from the anaesthetic, a regime of gastrostomy feeds can be commenced. Parents need instruction on use of the catheter and how to vent the catheter in the event of gastric dilatation. Parents and or the patient should also be given instructions on meticulous cleaning of the PEG feeding catheter around the insertion site. This helps prevent wound infection and subsequent granuloma formation. The feeding catheter requires to be rotated at regular intervals (daily for two weeks) to maintain mobility within the gastrostomy. This

Table 11.1 — Common problems and possible solutions with the percutaneous gastrostomy technique

Problem	Action
Identifying correct site for PEG	Check for interposed viscus or organ Position endoscope in 'j' shape and rotate endoscope Avoid inserting too much endoscope
Failure to introduce trocar into stomach	Fully inflate stomach Angle trocar towards xiphisternum Push trocar firmly into stomach
Post-operative wound infection	Antibiotic prophylaxis Soak catheter in iodine-containing solution Avoid tension under the external bolster
Granulation tissue at PEG site	Frequent local cleaning with iodine-containing solution Topical application of paw-paw ointment or 1% hydrocortisone cream Cautery to granulation tissue
Leakage around PEG	Treat granulation tissue Decrease feeding rate
PEG catheter submucosal migration	Rotate catheter daily for 2 weeks
PEG catheter migration with gastric outlet obstruction	Withdraw and reposition PEG catheter comfortably adjacent to stomach wall (1–2 cm)
PEG catheter extrusion	Treat wound infection if necessary; remove PEG catheter and replace with another

helps prevent submucosal migration of the internal bumper.

Discussion

Common problems and possible solutions

(Table 11.1)

Operative and early post-operative problems (within 6 h)

- **Difficulty in manipulating the tip of the endoscope directly underneath the site selected for insertion of the PEG**: once a 'j' shape has been obtained with the endoscope, rotation of the endoscope may bring the tip around to the position required. Insertion of too great a length of the endoscope adversely affects the position.

- **Failure to introduce the cannula into the stomach**: this results in a false passage into the peritoneum. Make sure the stomach is fully inflated against the abdominal wall. Ensure that the trocar is introduced at an angle pointing slightly upwards and towards the xiphisternum. A firm push ensures puncture of the stomach rather than allowing the tip of the trocar to deflect off the external stomach wall.

- **Difficulty passing the PEG feeding catheter through the oesophagus**: this occurs particularly in smaller children. Ensure that the guidewire runs freely and that the external diameter of the PEG catheter selected is not too great for the oesophagus.

- **Interposed viscus or organ**: this can be avoided by ensuring that the indentation caused by an index finger is clearly visible and that no tissue is visible on transillumination of the abdomen.

- **Post-operative bleeding**: the superior epigastric

artery can be visualized by transillumination of the abdomen and should be avoided; multiple passes with the trocar should not be performed.

- **Surgical emphysema or pneumoperitoneum**: persistent surgical emphysema or pneumo-peritoneum suggests perforation of a viscus. If the distance between the internal bumper and the external bolster is greater than the anticipated depth of the abdominal wall this supports interposition of a viscus.

- **Post-operative pain**: local anaesthetic should be instilled in the wound pre-operatively and adequate post-operative analgesia should be prescribed.

Post-operative problems (1 week)

- **Post-operative wound infection**: antibiotic prophylaxis should be administered routinely; the abdominal skin should be prepared in an a-septic manner; the PEG catheter may be coated with an iodine-containing solution; and excessive pressure between the internal bumper and external bolster should be avoided.

- **Submucosal migration of the internal bumper**: the PEG catheter should be rotated daily for 2 weeks after insertion to avoid the internal bolster migrating under the gastric mucosa.

Late post-operative problems (weeks or months later)

- **Granulation tissue at the site of the PEG**: the parents and child should clean around the external PEG site twice daily with mild soap and water, particularly under the external bolster. An iodine solution may be useful to help keep the site clean. Applications of paw-paw ointment are useful in minimizing granulation tissue. If this becomes a severe problem, application of 1% hydrocortisone cream (usually 3 times/day) or, if this fails, cautery (e.g., silver nitrate pencil) to the granulation tissue may be necessary.

- **Leakage around the PEG catheter**: this is unusual with a PEG and the main cause is granulation tissue (see above), but the integrity of the catheter should be confirmed. If necessary, decrease the rate of intragastric feeds until the leakage ceases, then slowly increase to meet requirements.

- **PEG catheter extrusion**: this most often happens in association with a wound infection (see above), which should be treated. Occasionally, the catheter can be accidently removed. Provided the stomach remains adherent to the abdominal wall no consequences occur.

- **PEG catheter migration**: the catheter can migrate inwards into the pylorus if the external bolster slips. This can cause gastric-outlet obstruction. The catheter should be pulled comfortably back against the stomach wall and the bolster re-positioned.

- **Gastro-oesophageal reflux**: gastrostomies can produce gastro-oesophageal reflux for reasons that are not fully apparent (Jolley et al 1986). However a PEG may be less likely to do so (Launay et al 1996). If gastro-oesophageal reflux develops following insertion of a PEG, it is possible to perform an anti-reflux procedure at laparotomy without taking the PEG down.

Conclusion

PEG is a simple and effective method of gastrostomy insertion. Careful preventative measures minimize complications. The PEG catheter can be replaced with a low-profile device after 3 months.

References

Amundson, J.A. et al. (1994) Early identification and treatment necessary to prevent malnutrition in children and adolescents with severe disabilities. *J Am Diet Assoc*, 94, 880–883.

Beasley, S.W., Davidson, P.M., Catto-Smith, A.G. (1995) How to avoid complications during percutaneous endoscopic gastrostomy. *J Paediatr Surg*, 3, 671–673.

Coughlin, J.P., Gauderer, M.W.L., Stellato, T.A. (1991) Percutaneous gastrostomy in children under 1 year of age: Indications, complications and outcome. *Pediatric Surg Int*, 6, 88–91.

Davidson, P.M., Catto-Smith, A.G., Beasley, S.W. (1994) Technique and complications of percutaneous endoscopic gastrostomy in children. *ANZ J Surg*, 65, 194–196.

Gaskin, K.J. et al. (1990) Nutritional status, growth and development in children undergoing intensive treatment for cystic fibrosis. *Acta Paediatr*, 6, S106–S110.

Gauderer, M.W.L., Ponsky, J.L., lzant, R.J. (1980) Gastrostomy without laparatomy: A percutaneous endoscopic technique. *J Paediatr Surg*, 15, 872–875.

Gauderer, M.W.L. (1991) Percutaneous endoscopic gastrostomy: A 10 year experience with children. *J Pediatr Surg*, 26, 288–292.

Goulet, O. (1991) Enteral feeding in children. *Rev-Prat*, 41, 703–709.

Heine, R.G., Reddihough, D.S., Catto-Smith, A.G. (1995)

Gastro-oesophageal reflux and feeding problems after gastrostomy in children with severe neurological impairment. *Dev Med Child Neurol*, 37, 320–329.

Huddleston, K.C., Ferraro, A.R. (1991) Preparing families of children with gastrostomies. *Pediatr Nurs*, 17, 153–158.

Jolley, S.G. et al. (1986) Lower esophageal pressure changes with tube gastrostomy: A causative factor of gastro-esophageal reflux in children? *J Pediatr Surg*, 21, 624–627.

Launay, V. et al. (1996) Percutaneous endoscopic gastrostomy in children: Influence on gastroesophageal reflux. *Pediatr*, 97, 726–728.

Marin, O.E. et al. (1994) Safety and efficacy of percutaneous endoscopic gastrostomy in children. *Am J Gastroenterol*, 89, 357–361.

Moore, M.C., Greene, H.L. (1985) Tube feeding of infants and children. *Pediatr Clin North Am*, 32, 401–417.

Rabeneck, L., McCullough, L.B., Wray, N.P. (1997) Ethically justified, clinically comprehensive guidelines for percutaneous endoscopic gastrostomy tube placement. *Lancet*, 349, 496–498.

12

Trace element requirements in artificial support

Kinya Sando and Akira Okada

Introduction

Trace element

Twenty-seven of the 95 naturally occurring elements are known to be essential for life. In general, the term, *trace element*, is used to indicate an element for which the requirement is measured in quantities of < 1 mg. Iron, zinc, copper, manganese, nickel, cobalt, molybdenum, selenium, chromium, iodine, fluorine, tin, silicon, vanadium, and arsenic are generally recognized as trace elements (Underwood 1977). This chapter is limited primarily to iron, zinc, copper, selenium, manganese, molybdenum, chromium, iodine, fluoride and cobalt.

With the development and widespread use of artificial nutritional support such as total parenteral nutrition (TPN) and enteral nutrition (EN), abnormalities of trace elements related to their metabolism and pharmacokinetics have received much attention. It would appear that they have an essential role in a large number of enzyme activities, usually as an integral part of the enzyme where these are metallo-proteins. The trace element deficiencies occur in only a limited proportion of nutritionally-compromised patients. Generally, insufficiency of intestinal absorption due to malabsorption, increased excretion, increased demand, and altered distribution in tissues are precipitating factors. Each trace element deficiency displays a specific clinical feature.

Infancy

Infancy is probably the most demanding period of life for meeting the body's nutritional requirements. Weight typically doubles during the first 4–6 months of life and triples by the end of the first year. In general, during this period, infants receive a single source of nourishment, either human milk or a product formulated to resemble human milk. The problem of trace-element deficiency is especially important in infants and children because normal growth and development are dependent on sufficient amounts in the diet.

Practice and procedures

Requirements in artificial support

There are a certain number of essential trace elements for which essentiality in humans is not established. The dietary intake of trace elements is greatly influenced by the choice of foods and by their materials. The dietary needs for them are known with varying degrees of certainty, especially during infancy. In addition to the rate of growth, tissue reserves as well as the content and bioavailability of the element are major issues that need to be considered in evaluating the adequacy of a diet. The estimates of dietary needs during infancy are frequently based on the extrapolation of data from animal studies, from studies of adult human beings, or on typical nutrient intakes of apparently healthy infants.

The World Health Organisation (WHO) Expert Committee on Trace Elements in Human Nutrition (1973, 1996) and the National Research Council (1980, 1989) published recommended intakes of trace elements to cover normal physiological needs. Allowances for increased needs during illness have not been considered. Table 12.1 shows the recommended dietary allowances (RDAs) in the United States for nine important trace elements, which was revised in 1989.

RDAs are expressed as average daily intakes over time and are intended to provide variations amongst most normal persons living in the United States under usual environmental stresses. Diets should be based on a variety of common foods in order to provide other nutrients for which human requirements have been less well defined. *Estimated safe and adequate daily intakes* (ESADIs) are defined as follows: there is less information on which to base allowances, [so] these figures are provided in the form of ranges of recommended intakes. Because the toxic levels for many trace elements may be only several times the usual intakes, the upper levels for the trace elements given in this table should not be exceeded habitually.

Enteral nutrition

There are at most five trace elements (iron, zinc, copper, manganese, and iodine) whose contents in EN solutions currently on the market or under development in Japan are explicitly stated (Table 12.2) (Okada et al 1993). Ample heed must be paid also to selenium, chromium, and molybdenum, which are not contained in any of the nutritional formulas on the market in Japan. On the other hand, many of the products available in the United States document iron, zinc, copper, manganese, and iodine. In addition, in the United Kingdom, all products to be used on a long-term basis contain adequate amounts of selenium, chromium, and molybdenum (see Table 12.2) Okada et al 1993). Moreover, in the United Kingdom amounts of trace elements are smaller than the RDA, which are

Table 12.1 — Recommended dietary allowances (RDAs) and estimated safe and adequate daily intakes (ESADIs)★ of trace elements

Age range (years)	Iron (mg)	Zinc (mg)	Copper★ (mg)	Selenium (µg)	Manganese★ (mg)	Molybdenum★ (µg)	Chromium★ (µg)	Iodine (µg)	Fluoride★ (mg)
Infants									
0–0.5	6	5	0.4–0.6	10	0.3–0.6	15–30	10–40	40	0.1–0.5
0.5–1	10	5	0.6–0.7	15	0.6–1	20–40	20–60	50	0.2–1
Children									
1–3	10	10	0.7–1	20	1–1.5	25–50	20–80	70	0.5–1.5
4–6	10	10	1–1.5	20	1.5–2	30–75	30–120	90	1–2.5
7–10	10	10	1–2.0	30	2–3	50–150	50–200	120	1.5–2.5
Males									
11–14	12	15	1.5–2.5	40	2–5	75–250	50–200	150	1.5–2.5
Fmales									
11–14	15	12	1.5–2.5	45	2–5	75–250	50–200	150	1.5–2.5

Table 12.2 — Trace elements in various enteral nutrition solutions (per 100 kcal)

Products in Japan		Elental Elemental Diet (Ajinomoto)	Enterud (Terumo)	Sastagen (Bristol Myers)	Hinex (Otsuka)	Low-Residue Diet Clinimeal (Eizai)	Besvion (Fujisawa)	Ensure (Dinabbot)
Iron	(mg)	6	7	10	6.5	9.0	11	9
Zinc	(mg)	6	3.7	11.2	2	1.5	3.4	15
Copper	(mg)	0.7	0.5	1.1	0.07	1	not detected	1
Manganese	(mg)	1	1.5	2.8	0.07	0.5	not detected	2
Iodine	(µg)	50	not detected	85	85	not detected	not detected	75

Products in the United Kingdom and United States		Ensure (Abbott)	Enrich (Abbott)	Nutrison (Cow&Gate)	Nutrison Fibre (Cow&Gate)	Fresubin (Fresenius)	Liquisorb (Merck)	Elemental 028 (Fresenius)
Iron	(mg)	2.3	2.4	1.7	1.8	1.7	1.3	1.9
Zinc	(mg)	3	3.2	1.7	1.8	1.3	1.1	1.9
Copper	(mg)	0.28	0.3	0.25	0.28	0.17	0.22	0.18
Selenium	(µg)	10.8	11.7	6.2	6.7	8.3	5	6.8
Manganese	(mg)	0.63	0.67	0.5	0.55	0.25	0.22	0.27
Molybdenum	(µg)	20	20.8	8.3	9.2	12.5	16.7	15.2
Chromium	(µg)	10.8	11.7	5.5	6.2	12.5	16.7	6.8
Iodine	(µg)	16.7	18.3	16.7	18.3	12.5	10	15.2
Fluoride	(mg)	2.25	2.42	1.67	1.83	1.67	1.25	1.92

Table 12.3 — Representative values of some trace elements in human milk and in infant formula

		Mature human milk	Infant formulas
Iron	(mg/L)	0.3–0.5	
Zinc	(mg/L)	0.14–4	3.7–12
Copper	(µg/L)	90–630	500–2000
Selenium	(µg/L)	8–50	5–10
Manganese	(µg/L)	1.9–27.5	70–530
Molybdenum	(µg/L)	0.1–1.7	30–70
Chromium	(µg/L)	40–80	10–20
Iodine	(µg/L)	5–50	
Fluoride	(µg/L)	5–50	30–100

designed for maintenance of good health in the United States. Long-term nutritional support with such commercial EN solutions alone would probably result in the manifestation of signs and symptoms of deficiencies of those elements.

Table 12.3 shows representative values of some of the trace elements found in human milk and infant formulas (Milner 1990).

Parenteral nutrition

The actual parenteral requirements of each trace element are uncertain because their appropriate dosages in TPN vary depending on disease or deficiency. The American Medical Association (AMA) (1979, 1984) developed guidelines for essential trace element preparations for parenteral use. Provisional recommendations for trace elements in infants and children from a number of sources, including Japan, are summarized in Table 12.4 (Jeejeebhoy 1990,

Okada et al 1993) and are expressed per kg/day in Table 12.5 (Greene et al 1988, Chan 1995).

Trace-element deficiency may occur in children receiving long-term parenteral nutrition (PN). It may be thought that essential trace elements (copper, zinc, chromium, manganese, selenium, iodine, and iron) need not be supplied for patients receiving TPN for < 2 weeks. The authors are of the opinion that trace elements must be provided immediately on instituting nutritional support because the immediate supplementation from day one of therapy may be in the best interest of the patient.

Prematurity

There is particular difficulty in recommendations for premature infants (weighing < 1500 g). Their requirements may be more than the RDA because of their low body reserves and increased requirements for rapid growth. The premature infant is at increased risk for all nutrient deficiencies.

The Nutrition Committee of the Canadian Paediatric Society (1995) suggested a different method to establish nutrition recommendations (Table 12.6) and defined new categories on the basis of the infant's birth weight and age after birth as follows:

1. **Birth-weight categories**: either below 1000 g or 1000 g or more.

2. **Age categories**: 'transition' period from birth to 7 days; 'stable-growing' period form stabilization to discharge from the neonatal intensive care unit (NICU); and 'post-discharge' period from 1 year following discharge from the NICU.

The birth-weight categories reflect the difference in accretion of nutrients before birth, and the post-natal

Table 12.4 — Recommended paediatric TPN dose (µg/kg/day)

	Wilmore (1969)	Wretlind (1972)	Ricour (1976)	James & McMahon (1976)	Shenkin & Wretlind (1978)	AMA (1979, 1984)	Jeejeebhoy (1990)
Iron	20	112		200	112–224		20
Zinc	40	39	50–60	200	39–100	100–300	50–100
Copper	22	19	20	50	19	20	20
Selenium			4		4		30
Manganese	40	55	20	10	20–55	2–10	10–20
Chromium			0.14–0.2	0.7	0.8	0.14–0.2	0.2–0.5
Iodine	15	5.8			5.8		5
Fluoride		57			57		1
Cobalt	14						

Table 12.5 — RDA for components of maintenance parenteral nutrition in infants and children

	Zinc (µg/kg)	Copper (µg/kg)	Selenium (µg/kg)	Manganese (µg/kg)	Molybdenum (µg/kg)	Chromium (µg/kg)	Iodine (µg/kg)
Pre-term Infants	300 or 400	20 or 40	1–2	1★, 5 or 10	0.25	0.2 or 0.4	1★
Infants/Toddlers	200–300 250 < 3 mo, 100 > 3 mo★	20–30	1–2	1★, 5–7.5	0.25	0.2–0.3	1★
Children (≥ 2–11 years of age)	50★, 100–200	10–20	1–2	1★, 2.5–5	0.25	0.1–0.2	1★
Adolescents (≥ 11 years of age)	100	10	1–2	2.5	0.25	0.1	
Maximum	[5000]	[500]	[30]	[5]	[50]★, [125]	[5]	[1]★

★Data from Chan (1995): Pre-term infants = premature infants; Infant = full term infants appropriate for gestational age (AGA) or small for gestational age (SGA) to 3 months of age; Infants/Toddlers = full term AGA or SGA infants to 2 years of age; If patient is on TPN for > 30 days with no significant enteral intake the addition of these elements is advisable; Copper, Manganese: Omit in patients with obstructive jaundice; Selenium, Chromium, Molybdenum: Omit in patients with renal dysfunction. Other data from Greene et al (1988): When TPN is only supplemental or limited to < 4 weeks, only zinc needs to be added. Thereafter, addition of the remaining elements is advisable; Pre-term: Available concentrations of manganese and molybdenum are such that dilution of the manufacturer's product may be necessary.

Table 12.6 — Recommended nutrient intakes for premature infants

Period after birth	Iron (mg/kg)	Zinc (mg/kg)	Copper[1] (µg/kg)	Selenium[1] (µg/kg)	Manganese[1] (µg/kg)	Molybdenum[1] (µg/kg)	Chromium[1] (µg/kg)	Iodine (µg/kg)
Transition (birth to 7 days)	0	0.43	70–120	3.2–4.7	0.55–1.1	0.19–0.38	0.05–0.1	25
Stable-growing (stabilization to discharge from NICU[2])	3–4[3,4] 2–3[5]	0.5–0.8	70–120[6]	3.2–4.7	0.55–1.1	0.19–0.38	0.05–0.1	32–63
Post-discharge (1 year following discharge from NICU)	3–4[4] 2–3[5]	0.98[7]	70–120[6]	3.2–4.7	0.55–1.1	0.19–0.38	0.05–0.1	32–63

[1]amount required if the infant is fed parenterally differs. May be omitted from parenteral nutrition during the transition period; [2]neonatal intensive care unit; [3]starting 6–8 weeks after birth; [4]birth weight < 1000 g; [5]birth weight ≥ 1000 g; [6]for infants fed formula this amount may differ; [7]estimate.

periods reflect the changing growth and nutrient metabolism that accompany post-natal maturation. During the 'transition' period, the minimum achievable goal is the provision of sufficient nutrients to prevent deficiencies and substrate catabolism. During the 'stable-growing' period the primary nutritional goal is growth and nutrient retention rates similar to those that would have been achieved *in utero*. During the 'post-discharge' period, the goal is a nutrient intake that is adequate to achieve catch-up growth.

Iron

Dietary iron intake in Western diets is usually about 5–6 mg/100 kcal/day. The RDA in the United States for iron is 6–10 mg for infants and 10–15 mg for children (see Table 12.1). Although breast milk contains only a small amount of iron, 0.3–0.5 mg/L, about 50% of it is absorbed. This is in contrast with low-birth-weight (LBW) infants. LBW infants fed human milk almost invariably develop iron deficiency anaemia unless they are given iron supplements (Siimes 1984). LBW infants are born with inadequate iron stores.

The Committee on Nutrition of the American Academy of Paediatrics (1969) recommends 2 mg/kg/day to a maximum of 15 mg iron/day for LBW infants. The Nutrition Committee of Canadian Paediatric Society (1995) recommends 3–4 mg/kg/day for infants with below 1000 g of body weight and 2–3 mg/kg/day for those with more than 1000 g of body weight (see Table 12.6). Approximately 2.5 mg/kg of elemental iron raises the haemoglobin concentration by 1 g/100 ml. However, target-site delivery and incorporation into the erythrocyte takes at least 3 weeks. The duration of administration in most instances is 3 months from any indication of improvement of anaemia.

Controversies still exist concerning parenteral administration of iron (Weinberg et al 1978). Parenteral iron may not need to be repleted during short periods of parenteral therapy if iron stores are adequate prior to the initiation of parenteral feeding (Cook 1984). Patients hospitalized and receiving PN for < 30 days may not need iron added to their solutions.

Zinc

The RDA for zinc in the United States is 5 mg for infants and 10–15 mg for children (see Table 12.1). Infants require even larger amounts of zinc on a mg/kg basis because of their growth. Zinc requirements are in the region of 1 mg/kg/day in infancy (Lentner 1981). At least 100 μgrams/kg/day should be given to infants beyond the first 6 months of life (Widdowson et al 1974, Arakawa et al 1976, James & MacMahan 1976, Shaw 1979). To maintain a positive zinc balance, 300 (James & MacMahan 1976) or 300–500 μgrams/kg/day (Widdowson et al 1974) are recommended. In older children (James & MacMahan 1976, Ricour et al 1977) and after adolescence (Widdowson et al 1974, James & MacMahan 1976, Shaw 1979) 50 μgrams/kg/day maintains normal serum levels and 100 μgrams/kg/day is a safe intake for growth. Zinc requirements are 10 mg/day between 1–10 years of age (Lentner 1981). Zinc bio-availability from human milk is considerably greater than that from bovine milk (Lonnerdal et al 1981). Zinc requirements of infants fed cow-milk-based formula appear to be higher than in those fed human milk.

In immature infants at the time of birth, there is a greater need for zinc in those who require parenteral nutrition (Widdowson et al 1974). Premature babies should be given greater amounts, 430–980 μgrams/kg/day of zinc (see Table 12.6).

Copper

In infants, the requirements based on balance are 50 μgrams/kg/day (James & MacMahan 1976). The RDA for copper in the United States is settled at 80 μgrams/kg/day for infants and children, and 40 μgrams/kg/day for older children. However, the range is very wide, varying from 10–50 μgrams/kg/day. Malnourished infants require 40–135 μgrams/kg/day. It was reported that children receiving 100 μgrams/kg/day show serum copper levels in the normal range (Ament 1991). For the pre-term infant, no consensus has been obtained about the minimal daily requirements for copper (Salim et al 1986, Anon 1987, Wharton 1987). The Canadian Paediatric Society (1995) presented 70–120 μg/kg/day as a minimal requirement.

Human milk contains about 390 (90–630) μgrams/L of copper but levels fall in prolonged lactation. Cow's milk contains only about 90 μg/L. Copper deficiency has been reported in term infants fed unprocessed cow's milk, which is a poor source of copper in early infancy (Levy et al 1985). In the United States, the Food and Nutrition Board has recommended infant formulas supplemented with a minimum of 60 μgrams/100 kcal (and higher concentrations in premature baby formulas).

In infants, the recommended dosage of copper during PN ranges between 10–50 μgrams/kg/day (see Table 12.5) (Mertz et al 1961). Deficiency symptoms can become evident within 7 weeks in pre-term infants receiving TPN with no oral supplements. Copper should be omitted in infants with obstructive biliary disease, because it is excreted primarily through the biliary tract.

Selenium

The infant's requirement for selenium has not been defined. A range of safe and adequate dietary intakes of selenium has been estimated (see Table 12.1), primarily by extrapolation from the selenium requirement of mammalian animal species. The daily oral intake of selenium varies between 20–200 mg, depending on geographical district. The selenium content of enteral feeds used in the United Kingdom range from 60–140 mg/2000 kcal (see Table 12.4). Because commercially-available EN solutions in Japan contain virtually no selenium (< 20 mg/L), long-term nutritional support with such preparations alone is likely to result in selenium deficiency.

Human milk contains about 15–20 or 8–50 µgrams/L selenium (see Table 12.3). It may represent the minimum needs of human infants for selenium. The selenium content of cow's milk is lower than that of human milk. There are no recommendations for the minimum selenium content of cow-milk-derived formulas. The content of selenium infant formulas in the United States has been reported to be approximately half or lower than that of human milk from US women (see Table 12.3)(Smith et al 1982).

The recommended TPN dose for paediatrics are replete with 1–2 or 4 µgrams/kg/day.

Manganese

The RDA of manganese in the United States is 0.5–3 mg for children and 5 mg for adolescents. An ordinary Japanese diet is said to provide 3–9 mg manganese, which is enough to prevent deficiency. The manganese content of human milk was reported during the early 1970s to be 15 µgrams/L and 1.9–27.5 µgrams/L in 1990 (see Table 12.3). Recent data indicate lower amounts, with the concentration declining from approximately 7 µgrams/L in the first month to 4 µgrams/L in later months (Vouri et al 1980). The quantity of manganese in cows milk is about 35 µgrams/L, whereas US formulas provide between 70–530 µgrams/L.

Daily TPN doses vary widely among different reported series, ranging from 10–55 mg/kg for children. In Europe (Shenkin et al 1986) an intravenous dose of 1 mg/kg has been shown to be adequate to sustain serum manganese concentrations in infants. The natural concentration of manganese in TPN solutions is sufficient to meet the needs of paediatrics.

In the presence of biliary obstruction, excretion of manganese is impaired (Hambidge et al 1989) as is that of copper. Under such circumstances, care should be exercised to avoid administration of manganese in excessive amounts.

Molybdenum

The normal diet appears to contain sufficient molybdenum to meet the need for this element. The preliminary balance studies indicates RDA for molybdenum is 15–250 mg for paediatrics. Minimum requirements for molybdenum are unknown. The safe and adequate range of intakes for infants was derived by extrapolation

from these balance studies. Recommended dose of TPN is 0.25 µgrams/kg/day (see Table 12.5)(Greene et al 1988).

Chromium

In a study of infants (James & MacMahan 1976), a requirement of 0.14–0.2 µgrams/kg/day was determined. Recommendations for infants are extrapolated from expected food intake. The RDA in the United States is 10–200 µgrams/kg/day and 0.05–0.1 µgrams/kg/day for premature infants in Canada. Cow's milk is reported to contain less chromium than human milk, and the element is present in cow's milk in a form that is not biologically available. The recommended dose of TPN is 0.1–0.4 µgrams/kg/day (see Tables 12.4 and 12.5). Chromium concentration of standard PN fluid may meet the requirements in infants (Kien et al 1986, Moukarzel et al 1992).

Iodine

The iodine content of foods varies with that of the soil from which the food has originated. Precise recommendations are not yet available. The minimum requirement of adults has been estimated as 50–75 µgrams/day; children and pregnant women have a higher requirement. The RDA of paediatrics for this element is 40–150 mg. In Japan, because an ordinary diet provides more than the daily allowance, ingestion of excess iodine should be avoided.

The requirement for this element during TPN is nearly equal to its daily dietary intake of 1 or 5.8–15 µgrams/kg/day in children (see Tables 12.4 and 12.5). However, because iodine is present in many ointments, cutaneous absorption should allow adequate levels to meet a child's needs. Iodine overdosage should be avoided, especially in newborns and immature infants.

Short-term TPN without iodine supplementations did not cause iodine deficiency in immature babies (Gough et al 1982). Iodine is not added to ordinary TPN solutions; however, the routine administration of parenteral sodium iodide is recommended for long-term patients who are receiving solely parenteral support or are not absorbing enterally ingested nutrients.

Fluoride

The American Academy of Pediatrics Committee on

Nutrition (1979) recently revised its recommendation for fluoride supplementation during infancy. For this group, the RDA was 0.25 mg/day. 0.1–2.5 mg/day has been proposed by the Food and Nutrition Board of the National Research Council (see Table 12.1).

The concentration of fluoride in human milk ranges from approximately 5–50 µgrams/L. This is similar for women drinking water. Cow's milk normally contains greater amounts of fluoride. Fluoride supplementation for infants is advised only when the water supply contains fluoride at concentrations < 0.3 ppm and human milk provides TPN for more than 6 months. In areas where the fluoride content of natural water is low, fluoridation (1 part per 1 million) of drinking water is recommended by the Food and Nutrition Board, although the desirability of this measure is still internationally debated.

Cobalt

Because cobalt is a component of vitamin B12, which is not used by the human body in any other way when supplied from this vitamin, cobalt deficiency of dietary origin has never been observed in humans. Estimates of daily oral intake of 140–580 mg have been reported. Recommended TPN dose is 14 µgrams/kg/day (see Table 12.4).

Discussion

With an increasing number of patients receiving artificial nutrition (i.e., TPN and EN) deficiencies of various essential trace elements have appeared. Because symptomatic deficiencies may be only a small part of an abnormality, we should recognize the much wider background of abnormal metabolism and physiology of such elements and examine their possible participation in most diseases. Measurements of biochemical indices of trace elements in these patients frequently reveal decreased levels. To prevent marginal deficiencies and maintain good balance in the body, routine administration of trace elements is therefore essential.

The discussion has focused on daily requirements, including the recommended doses of each trace element in TPN and EN formulas. The range of different recommended doses in different countries as well as the content and completeness of trace element mixtures available in these countries is a matter of concern. A consensus based on better data from patients with different clinical states is urgently required.

References

Ament, M. (1991) Trace Metals in Parenteral Nutrition. In: Chandra, R.K. (ed.) *Trace Elements in Nutrition of Children*, pp. 181–199. New York: Vevey/Raven Press.

American Academy of Pediatrics Committee on Nutrition. (1969) Iron balance and requirements in infancy. *Pediatrics*, 43, 134–142.

American Academy of Pediatrics Committee on Nutrition. (1979) Fluoride supple-mentation: Revised dosage schedule. *Pediatrics*, 63, 150–152.

American Medical Association, Department of Foods and Nutrition. (1979) Guidelines for essential trace element preparations for parenteral use. *JAMA*, 241, 2051–2054.

American Medical Association, Department of Foods and Nutrition. (1984) Working conference on parenteral trace elements. *Bull NY Acad of Med*, 60, 115–209.

Anon, (1987) Copper and the infant. *Lancet*, 1, 900–901.

Arakawa, T., Tamura, T., Igarashi, Y., et al. (1976). Zinc deficiency in two infants during total parenteral alimentation for diarrhea. *Am J Clin Nutr*, 29, 197–204.

Canadian Paediatric Society Nutrition Committee. (1995) Nutrient needs and feeding of premature infants. *Can Med Assoc J*, 152, 1765–1785.

Cook, J.D. (1984) Parenteral trace elements: Iron. *Bull NY Acad Med*, 60, 156–162.

Gough, D.C., Laing, I., Astley, P. (1982) Thyroid function on short-term total parenteral nutrition without iodine supplements. *JPEN*, 6, 439–440.

Greene, H.L., Hambidge, K.M., Schanler, R. et al. (1988) Guidelines for use of vitamins, trace elements, calcium, magnesium and phosphorous in infants and children receiving total parenteral nutrition. *Am J Clin Nutr*, 48, 1324–1342.

Hambidge, M.K., Sokol, R.J., Fidanza, S.J. et al. (1989) Plasma manganese concentrations in infants and children receiving parenteral nutrition. *JPEN*, 13, 168–171.

James, B.E., MacMahon, R.A. (1976) Balance studies of 9 elements during complete intravenous feeding of small premature infants. *Aust Pediatr J*, 12, 154–162.

Jeejeebhoy, K.N. (1990) Trace Elements in Total Parenteral Nutrition. In: Tomita, H. (ed.) *Trace Elements in Clinical Medicine*, pp. 203–225. Tokyo: Springer-Verlag.

Kien, C.L., Veillon, C., Patterson, K.Y. et al. (1986) Mild, peripheral neuropathy but biochemical chromium deficiency during 16 months of "chromium-free" total parenteral nutrition. *JPEN*, 10, 662–664.

Lentner, C. (1981) Nutritional Standards. In: *Geigy Scientific Tables, Volume 1. Units of Measurement, Composition of the Body, Nutrition*, pp. 232–240. Basle: Ciba-Geigy.

Levy, Y., Zaharia, A., Grunebaum, M. et al. (1985) Copper deficiency in infants fed cow milk. *J Pediatr*, 786–788.

Lonnerdal, B., Keen, C.L., Hurley, L.S. (1981) Iron, copper, zinc, and manganese in milk. *Ann Rev Nutr*, 1, 149–174.

Mertz, W., Roginski, E.E., Schwartz, K. (1961) Effects of trivalent chromium complexes on glucose uptake by epididymal fat tissue of rats. *J Biol Chem*, 236, 318–322.

Milner, J.A. (1990) Trace minerals in the nutrition of children. *J Pediatr*, 117, S147–S155.

Moukarzel, A.A., Song, M.K., Buchman, A.L. et al. (1992) Excessive chromium intake in children receiving total parenteral nutrition. *Lancet*, 339, 385–388.

National Research Council. (1980) *Food and Nutrition Board Recommended Dietary Allowances*, 9th edn. Washington DC: National Academy of Sciences.

National Research Council. (1989) *Food and Nutrition Board Subcommittee on the Tenth Edition of the RDAs. Recommended Dietary Allowances*. Washington DC: National Academy of Sciences.

Okada, A., Takagi, Y., Nezu, R. et al. (1993) Trace elements metabolism in parenteral and enteral nutrition. *Nutr*, 11, 106–113.

Ricour, C., Gros, J., Maiere, B. et al. (1976) Trace elements in children on total parenteral Nutrition (TPN). *Acta Chir Scand*, 466, 22.

Ricour, C., Duhamel, J.F., Gros, J. et al. (1977) Estimates of trace element requirements of children receiving total parenteral nutrition. *Arch Fr Pediatr*, 34, 92–100.

Salim, S., Farquharson, J., Arneil, G. et al. (1986) Dietary copper in artificially fed infants. *Arch Dis Child*, 61, 1068–1075.

Shaw, J.C.L. (1979) Trace elements in the fetus and young infant. I. Zinc. *Am J Dis Child*, 133, 1260–1268.

Shenkin, A., Fell, GS., Halls, D.J. et al. (1986) Essential trace element provision to patients receiving home intravenous nutrition in the United Kingdom. *Clin Nutr*, 5, 91–97.

Shenkin, A, Wretlind, A. (1978) Parenteral nutrition. *World Rev Nutr Diet*, 28, 1–111.

Siimes, M.A. (1984) Iron Nutrition in Low-Birth-Weight Infants. In: Stekel, A. (ed.) *Iron Nutrition in Infancy And Childhood*, pp. 75–91. New York: Raven Press.

Smith, A.M., Picciano, M.F., Milner, J.A. (1982) Selenium intake and status of human milk and formula fed infants *Am J Clin Nutr*, 35, 521–562.

Underwood, E.J. (1977) *Trace Elements in Human and Animal Nutrition*, 4th edn. New York: Academic Press.

Vouri, E., Makinen, S.M., Kara, R. et al. (1980) The effect on dietary intake of copper, iron, manganese and zinc on the trace element content of human milk. *Am J Clin Nutr*, 33, 227–231.

Weinberg, E.D. (1978) Iron and infection. *Microbiol Rev*, 42, 45–66.

Wharton, B.A. (1987) *Nutrition and Feeding of Preterm Infants*. Oxford: Blackwell Scientific.

Widdowson, E.M., Dauncey, J., Shaw, J.C.L. (1974) Trace elements in foetal and early postnatal development. *Proc Nutr Soc*, 33, 275–284.

Wilmore, D.W., Groff, D.B., Bishop, H.C. et al. (1969) Total parenteral nutrition in infants with catastrophic gastro-intestinal anomalies. *J Pediatr Surg*, 4, 181–189.

World Health Organisation. (1973) *Trace Elements in Human Nutrition. Report of a WHO Expert Committee. Technical Report Series No. 532*. Geneva: WHO.

World Health Organisation. (1996) *Trace Elements in Human Nutrition and Health*. Geneva: WHO.

Wretlind, A. (1972) Complete intravenous nutrition. Theoretical and experimental background. *Nutr Metab*, 14, 1–57.

13

Protein requirements and the use of parenteral amino acids in the pre-term neonate

David Adamkin

Introduction

Protein is the building block of lean body tissue and is the nutrient that receives primary attention with respect to neonatal requirements. The consensus from various international organizations (Food and Nutrition Board 1980, WHO/FAO 1973, 1985, ESPGAN 1977, 1981, 1987, Committee on Nutrition 1976) is that neonatal protein requirements for the term infant are ~2–2.2 g/kg of body weight/day (g/kg/day) during the first 4 months of life, declining by about 0.2 g/kg/day after 4 months. Pre-term infant needs are about 1 g/kg/day higher than term neonates. All these recommendations assume that a complete protein is being used, which is one that contains sufficient amounts of the classically-defined essential amino acids. Interestingly, although all these groups recommend breastfeeding as the first choice for the healthy term neonate, they do not address the paradox that human milk does not fall within their own recommended guidelines for protein intake, based on the fact that human milk contains about 1 g/dL and would have to be fed at a rate of approximately 200 mL/kg/day to meet their recommendation.

Using the factorial approach, Fomon (1991) also estimates that the protein requirement of the normal male infant is about 2 g/kg/day during the first month of life, decreasing to about 1.2 g/kg/day by 4–5 months of age, and remaining relatively constant for the first year of life. This estimate assumes a 90% conversion of dietary protein to body protein and that obligatory losses from urine, stool and skin remain constant through the first post-natal year. Protein accretion in female infants is similar to that in males after the first 2 months of age, so the requirement for both is nearly identical.

Historical background

The original classification of amino acids as essential or non-essential was based upon the requirement for maintenance of growth and/or nitrogen balance. These categories have been modified as new understandings of the functions and biochemistry of amino acids have developed and are as follows (Irwin & Hegsted 1971, Jackson et al 1981, Laidlaw & Kopple 1987):

1. non-essential amino acids such as glutamate and aspartate that can be completely synthesized;

2. essential carbon skeleton amino acids such as valine and leucine that have a carbon skeleton that can be aminated, but not synthesized;

3. semi-essential amino acids such as glycine and serine that can undergo carbon skeleton synthesis, but cannot be aminated;

4. essential amino acids such as lysine that have a carbon skeleton that cannot be synthesized or aminated.

Additional categories have included: 1) genetically-required amino acids such as tyrosine and phenylalanine that cannot be synthesized due to an inherited metabolic defect; 2) disease-induced essential amino acids such as the branched-chain amino acids that cannot be synthesized due to a disease not specifically related to amino acid metabolism (such as hepatic dysfunction); 3) nutritionally-induced requirements such as arginine that appear to be required due to special nutritional circumstances, including total parenteral nutrition (TPN); and 4) developmentally-required amino acids such as cysteine in the premature infant that cannot be synthesized in sufficient quantities due to the biochemical immaturity of the neonate.

As a result of this increased understanding of neonatal amino acid requirements, it is generally accepted that most amino acids ought to be provided in the diet during this period to support optimal growth and development, including amino acids that are not considered essential or semi-essential. Some amino acids may still be classified as non-essential because all of their functions are not yet completely understood. When non-essential amino acids are omitted from the diet of neonates, it is generally because of concerns regarding toxicity. For example, the exclusion of glutamate from TPN solutions is generally due to its potential neurotoxicity (Olney et al 1972). Potential effects of amino acid intake, from deficiency to sufficiency to excess, must be considered particularly in the vulnerable, developing human being. The experience with the use of parenteral protein solutions in pre-term neonates illustrates all of these effects.

The current widespread use of TPN in low-birth-weight (LBW) infants can be attributed to a general increase in awareness of the importance of nutritional support. In addition, several changes in its composition and delivery have enhanced its overall safety and efficacy: 1) crystalline amino acid mixtures have replaced protein hydrolysates; 2) safe parenteral lipid emulsions have become available; 3) knowledge of parenteral requirements of trace minerals and vitamins has improved; 4) some of the metabolic complications reported during the early days of parenteral nutrition therapy have been solved; and 5) the types of catheters and the precision of infusion pumps available for use have improved and medical personnel are generally much more familiar with the details of their use.

In this chapter, emphasis is on the role of amino acids in the parenteral delivery of nutrients, especially to LBW infants who form the largest group of patients using TPN and who have relatively high total amino acid requirements to support their maintenance, growth, and developmental needs.

Practice and procedures

Protein quantity

Estimating the protein or amino acid requirements of the typical infant requiring TPN is more difficult than estimating requirements for the well, enterally-fed infant. Suboptimal nutrition in the period prior to the initiation of TPN can lead to catabolism of body protein. Amino acids are required for catch-up and normal growth. Furthermore, obligatory nitrogen losses are likely to be quite variable, reflecting primarily the degree of ongoing stress (e.g., illness, infection, or surgery), which may increase such losses by two- or threefold.

The parenteral amino acid requirement of the pre-term infant is greater than that of the term infant, due primarily to more rapid growth. For example, the rate of weight gain during the last trimester of gestation averages 15 g/kg/day and nitrogen retention averages 300 mg/kg/day (about 1.9 g/kg/day of protein) (Zlotkin et al 1981a). Several studies (Shore et al 1953, Pencharz et al 1977, Saini et al 1989, Rivera et al 1989, 1993, Heird & Kashyap 1994) have shown that pre-term infants who are not receiving exogenous nitrogen excrete 150–180 mg/kg/day of nitrogen (equivalent to about 1 g/kg/day of protein) during the first week of life. Using this value and assuming that parenterally-administered amino acids are converted to body protein with an efficiency of 75%, the estimated parenteral amino acid requirement for normal growth amounts to 3.7 g/kg/day, which is about 20% above that generally accepted as necessary for achieving intrauterine rates of nitrogen retention (i.e., 3 g/kg/day) (Zlotkin et al 1981a). The differences in these numbers may be due to a variety of factors: overestimates of body protein accretion, greater efficiency of conversion of parenteral amino acids to body protein (> 75%), or lower obligatory nitrogen losses beyond the first week than previously assumed. Clearly, the amino acid needs of the growing pre-term infant are greater than those of

the older term infant, especially when catch-up growth is also required (Heird 1995).

Energy

There must be an equilibrium between energy and nitrogen intakes to promote positive nitrogen balance. In pre-term infants, if the total energy intake is < 50 kcal/kg/day (maintenance), nitrogen is not retained effectively (Hanning & Zlotkin 1989, Anderson et al 1979). However, energy intakes approaching maintenance levels combined with parenteral amino acid intakes above 2 g/kg/day, promote positive nitrogen balance (Anderson et al 1979, Rivera et al 1989, Saini et al 1989). For pre-term infants receiving adequate non-protein energy calories, > 70 kcal/kg/day, the level of nitrogen intake is the primary influence on nitrogen retention (Zlotkin et al 1981a, Hanning & Zlotkin 1997) (Fig. 13.1). Amino acid intakes of 2–2.5 g/kg/ day result in nitrogen retention comparable to that in the healthy, enterally-fed term infant (Heird & Gomez 1994), whereas intakes of up to 4 g/kg/day may be required to mimic the rate of nitrogen retention that occurs in the reference foetus *in utero* (approximately 3 g/kg/day) (Widdowson 1979, Zlotkin et al 1981a, Heird & Kashyap 1994).

Protein quality

Twenty amino acids are required for protein synthesis and each must be present in sufficient concentration to meet the metabolic need for that amino acid. Protein synthesis is limited by the amino acid present in the lowest quantity in relation to its requirement. Other amino acids, which are present in amounts

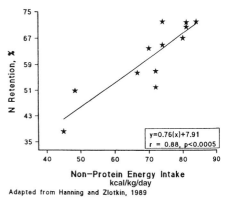

Figure 13.1 — Nitrogen retention in relation to non-protein energy intake. From Hanning, R.H., Zlotkin, S.H. (1997) with permission.

above this limit, cannot participate in protein synthesis and are oxidized. The goal in protein nutrition, then, is to provide a balanced amino acid source that maximizes protein synthesis and minimizes the degradation of amino acids.

Formerly, amino acid sources for parenteral nutrition consisted of protein hydrolysates of casein and fibrin. Metabolic complications (hyperammonaemia and azotaemia) with these solutions were not uncommon (Johnson et al 1972). Technological advances have made the production of crystalline amino acids economically feasible in recent years, and a number of different formulations have been introduced (Table 13.1). In general, the ratio of essential: non-essential amino acids, as well as the pattern of essential amino acids, in the early mixtures resembled that of high-quality dietary proteins. Concentrations of non-essential amino acids varied from mixture to mixture, but the glycine content was quite high in most adult (general purpose) solutions. In addition, none of these adult solutions contained glutamic or aspartic acid and some lacked one or more of the other non-essential amino acids. Of greatest concern with respect to use of these mixtures in infants was that because of the relative insolubility of tyrosine and cysteine none contained appreciable amounts of these two amino acids, both of which are considered to be conditionally essential for the infant (Atkinson & Hanning 1989) and particularly for the LBW infant. Special functions in the neonate could be compromised by insufficient substrate, such as catecholamine production from tyrosine.

A number of special-purpose crystalline amino acid mixtures have become available over the past few years, including some designed specifically for infants. Amino acid profiles influence nitrogen retention, even when the amounts of energy and nitrogen used are comparable (Hanning & Zlotkin 1989). The amino acid mix of one of these infant solutions is based on that of human milk (Vaminolact). Another is designed from a mathematic model to result in a plasma amino acid pattern similar to that of a normally-growing, breastfed term infant (TrophAmine). The pattern of a third solution appears to have been chosen arbitrarily to result in a more 'normal' plasma amino acid pattern than with other mixtures (Aminosyn PF). Although these newer solutions contain a higher ratio of essential:non-essential amino acids, none contain appreciable amounts of tyrosine or cysteine, although one Trophamine contains N-acetyl-L-tyrosine, a soluble tyrosine derivative. The bioavailability of this form of tyrosine appears to be questionable, whereas cysteine-

hydrochloride is now available as an additive. Both of these amino acids are discussed in more detail in the next section.

A number of randomized studies have compared the different formulations (Bell et al 1983, Burger et al 1983, Chase & Nixt 1983, Ogata et al 1983, Zlotkin 1984, Chessex et al 1985, Coran and Drongowski 1987, Helms et al 1987, Rosenthal et al 1987, Puntis et al 1989, Adamkin et al 1991). In general, these trials showed that plasma amino acid concentrations are reflections of the pattern of the specific amino acid mixture infused. The adult solutions, FreAmine II, Vamin, Travasol, and Aminosyn have resulted in abnormal plasma amino acid profiles in infants. Despite differences in individual plasma amino acids, few clinical benefits of one mixture versus another have been demonstrated. The standards against which plasma amino acid concentrations are evaluated are variable and no single standard has been accepted to define 'normal' (Atkinson & Hanning 1989). One study did show a beneficial effect of one crystalline amino acid mixture over another (Helms et al 1987). In this study, infants who received a parenteral amino acid mixture that was designed for infants gained weight more rapidly and retained nitrogen more efficiently than historical controls who had received a TPN regimen that was similar in energy and amino acid content but which used egg protein as the model. A multi-centre trial comparing two parenteral amino acid mixtures designed for infants demonstrated similar nitrogen balance and weight gain in the two groups (Adamkin et al 1991). Both formulas contained supplemental taurine, based on data showing a potentially deleterious effect of taurine deficiency on the developing brain and retina (Zelikovic et al 1990). Large scale randomized trials will be required for a valid assessment of the impact of nitrogen quality on nitrogen retention, growth, and neurodevelopment. Developmental outcome is relevant in light of old and new reports that parenterally-administered amino acid formulations can result in abnormalities in plasma amino acid concentrations (e.g., hyperphenylalaninaemia, hyperglycinaemia), which may have an impact on a vulnerable central nervous system.

Specific amino acids

In addition to the nine amino acids that are essential for infants, some amino acids are considered conditionally essential because of metabolic immaturity, heightened needs, or special functions in the infants. These amino acids include cysteine, tyrosine, glycine,

Table 13.1 Amino Acid Solutions

Product Manufacturer	Paediatric		General Purpose				
	Trophamine 6% (McGaw)	Aminosyn-PF 7% (Abbott)	Aminosyn 10% (Abbott)	Aminosyn II 10% (Abbott)	Travasol 10% (Baxter)	FreAmine III 10% (McGaw)	Vamin 7%[+] (Clintec)
Amino acid concentration	6%	7%	10%	10%	10%	10%	7%
Nitrogen (g/100 mL)	0.93	1.07	1.57	1.53	1.65	1.53	1.32
Essential amino acids (mg/100 mL)							
Histidine	290	220	300	300	480	280	240
Isoleucine	490	534	720	660	600	690	390
Leucine	840	831	940	1000	730	910	530
Lysine	490	475	720	1050	580	730	390
Methionine	200	125	400	172	400	530	190
Phenylalanine	290	300	440	298	560	560	550
Threonine	250	360	520	400	420	400	300
Tryptophan	120	125	160	200	180	150	100
Valine	470	452	800	500	580	660	425
Non-essential amino acids (mg/100 mL)							
Alanine	320	490	1280	993	2070	710	300
Arginine	730	861	980	1018	1150	950	330
Proline	410	570	860	722	680	1120	810
Serine	230	347	420	530	500	590	750
Taurine[a]	15	50	–	–	–	–	–
Tyrosine	140★	44	44	–	40	–	50
N–Acetyl-L-Tyrosine	–	–	–	270	–	–	–
Glycine	220	270	1280	500	1030	1400	210
Cysteine[a]	< 14	–	–	–	–	< 20	140
Glutamic Acid	300	576	–	738	–	–	900
Aspartic Acid	190	370	–	700	–	–	410
Electrolytes (mEq/L)							
Calcium	–	–	–	–	–	–	5
Sodium	5	3.4	–	45.3	–	10	50
Potassium	–	–	5.4	–	–	–	20
Magnesium	–	–	–	–	–	–	3
Chloride	< 3	–	–	–	40	< 3	55
Acetate	56	32.5	148	71.8	87	89	–
Phosphate (mMol/L)	–	–	–	–	–	10	–
mOsmol/L	525	586	1000	873	1000	950	690
pH	5–6	5.4	5.3	5–6.5	6	6–7	5.2

Source: 1996 product information. [a]These amino acids are considered essential in infants and young children; [+]MicroMedex, Inc. 1997; ★Mixture of tyrosine and N–Acetyl-L-Tyrosine.

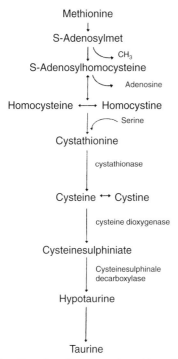

Methionine
↓
S-Adenosylmet
↓ ↘ CH₃
S-Adenosylhomocysteine
↑ ↘ Adenosine
Homocysteine ⟷ Homocystine
↓ ↘ Serine
Cystathionine
cystathionase
↓
Cysteine ⟷ Cystine
cysteine dioxygenase
↓
Cysteinesulphiniate
Cysteinesulphinale
decarboxylase
↓
Hypotaurine
↓
Taurine

Figure 13.2 — Overview of sulphur amino acid metabolism.

arginine, taurine, and glutamine. Hepatic cystathionase activity is reduced in the foetus and during the early post-natal period; therefore, plasma cysteine concentrations are low in pre-term compared to term infants (Fig. 13.2) (Zlotkin et al 1981b, Zlotkin & Anderson 1982). Whether adequate amounts of cysteine can be synthesized in the absence of an exogenous source is debatable. Infants with hyaline membrane disease and newborns with persistent pulmonary hypertension may have low plasma cysteine levels due more to oxidative stress than nutritional factors (White et al 1994). Cysteine is unstable in parenteral solutions and is rapidly oxidized to cystine, which is insoluble. Although some of the adult TPN products contain high methionine levels to permit the endogenous synthesis of cysteine and taurine, these solutions have resulted in hypermethioninaemia in infants (Wong & Pildes 1974, Adamkin et al 1995). The manufacturers of many solutions such as Aminosyn-PF, Primene, and TrophAmine, recommend using a cysteine-HCl additive, which is soluble and relatively stable for a short time. Although cysteine-HCl supports improved plasma cysteine levels, improvements in nitrogen retention have not been shown (Malloy et al 1984, Van Goudoever et al 1994). Additionally, there is the potential for the low pH of

the additive to aggravate metabolic acidosis in immature infants (Heird et al 1988, Laine et al 1991).

Taurine

Some of the newer parenteral amino acid solutions designed for infants do contain taurine (see Table 13.1). Although this sulphur-containing amino acid is not used in protein synthesis, it is found in large concentrations in the free amino acid pool of breast milk and in the retinal and nervous tissue of the newborn. Observations during taurine-free or taurine-supplemented nutrition have included abnormal electroretinograms in paediatric patients receiving taurine-free parenteral nutrition (Geggel et al 1985) and enhancement of auditory brainstem-evoked responses in infants < 1300 g birth weight receiving taurine-supplemented formula (Tyson et al 1989). Taurine may also be important in cellular osmoregulation (Jackson et al 1994).

Phenylalanine and tyrosine

The limited ability of the premature or young infant to metabolize phenylalanine prompted some researchers in the 1970s to consider tyrosine a conditionally-essential amino acid for the neonate (Hanning & Zlotkin 1989). In referenced proteins such as egg albumin or that in human milk, as well as foetal tissue (Widdowson 1979), phenylalanine and tyrosine are found in similar concentrations. Thus, it seems reasonable to design feedings with a balance of these aromatic amino acids. The makers of parenteral solutions have attempted to compensate for a lack of tyrosine by providing additional phenylalanine with the expectation that infants will convert it to tyrosine. This does not happen to any significant degree (Radmacher et al 1993). Infants receiving one of the commercially-available solutions with this added phenylalanine have been reported to have elevated plasma phenylalanine levels and to excrete organic acids recognized as alternative catabolites of phenylalanine (Chessex et al 1985, Evans et al 1986, Puntis et al 1986, Walker et al 1986, Bjorkman and Lindholm 1987, Puntis et al 1989, McIntosh & Mitchell 1990, Thornton & Griffin 1991, Lucas et al 1993, Radmacher et al 1993). The clinical significance of elevated plasma phenylalanine is of concern because patients with phenylketonuria, exhibiting mild hyperphenylalaninaemia, have levels similar to those of some pre-term infants receiving this solution (Lucas et al 1993). This elevated phenylalanine was seen even when the ratio of energy:protein was low (< 26 kcal/g protein). However, at 18-month follow-up in these patients, there were no differences in Bayley scales of mental or psycho-motor development based on early peak phenylalanine concentration.

Hypertyrosinaemia does occur in infants, especially premature infants who are enterally fed with high protein or high phenylalanine-containing diets (McIntosh & Mitchell 1990). Tyrosine degradation is limited by immaturity of tyrosine aminotransferase during the perinatal period (Delvalle & Greengard 1977). Transient neonatal hypertyrosinaemia has been associated with intellectual impairment (Mammunes et al 1976), therefore it is desirable to maintain normal plasma tyrosine levels. Newer parenteral amino acid formulations have lower phenylalanine concentrations and do not produce hyperphenylalaninaemia (Evans et al 1986, Puntis et al 1986, Walker et al 1986, Bjorkman & Lindholm 1987, Mitton & Garlick 1992). However, the tyrosine content of these solutions remains low, resulting in sub-normal plasma tyrosine concentrations (Mitton & Garlick 1992).

To address tyrosine insolubility, tyrosine precursors, and dipeptides containing tyrosine have been tested. N-acetyl-L-tyrosine, a stable and more soluble form of tyrosine, has been incorporated in some currently available commercial parenteral amino acid formulations such as TrophAmine and Aminosyn-II. Initial studies in rats suggest that deacylation occurred and that N-acetyl-L-tyrosine supported protein production (Neuhauser et al 1985, Im & Rennie 1988). Studies in humans have not borne this out. In parenterally-fed LBW infants, the use of N-acetyl-tyrosine resulted in elevated plasma and urinary N-acetyl-L-tyrosine levels (Heird et al 1987, Hanning et al 1990, Van Goudoever et al 1994), but there was no improvement in nitrogen retention. Thus the bioavailability of tyrosine from this source, at least for the neonate, is questionable probably because of limited acylase activity.

Peptides have been used experimentally to deliver amino acids in solution in a more stable or soluble form. A number of animal studies investigated tyrosine-based peptides. Using alanyl-tyrosine in rats receiving TPN, investigators observed an increase in plasma tyrosine without an increase in plasma or urinary levels of the dipeptide (Daabees & Steglink 1978). From our studies in mice we have shown that the stable peptide, gamma-glutamyl-tyrosine, given in a single intravenous dose, resulted in a rise in plasma tyrosine concentrations without excretion of peptide in the urine (Hilton et al 1991). In a subsequent experiment, parenterally-fed rats received either a commercial amino acid solution

(a solution in which glutamyl-tyrosine was substituted for half of the phenylalanine in the commercial amino acid solution) or saline infusion and chow. Rats receiving the peptide-containing solution showed normalized plasma phenylalanine and tyrosine levels compared with rats receiving the standard amino acid solution, as well as improved brain tyrosine concentrations (Radmacher et al 1993). Tyrosine peptides appear to be rapidly hydrolysed and may provide a soluble source of tyrosine without the potential risks associated with accumulation of the precursor. More investigation and investment need to be made in their development.

Glutamine

Glutamine is not present in prepared amino acid solutions because it is unstable following heat sterilization (Furst et al 1990). Glutamine supplementation of TPN solutions has drawn attention because of its potential for reducing intestinal atrophy, its role in energy metabolism, and its immune function in states of trauma or stress (Abumrad et al 1989, Furst et al 1989, Heyman 1990). Some newer formulations have increased glutamic acid content in an effort to promote glutamine synthesis. Other solutions have incorporated peptides containing glutamine such as alanylglutamine and glycylglutamine, which are stable (Jiang et al 1993). Animal studies (Kweon et al 1991, Okuma et al 1994) and adult human studies (Lowe et al 1991, Scheltinga et al 1991) have been promising.

There are limited data on the benefits of glutamine in the neonate. In a recent randomized double-blind trial, glutamine (15–25%) was added to amino acid solutions infused in infants weighing < 1300 g (Lacey et al 1996). No elevations of blood glutamate, ammonia, or urea were observed. In infants < 800 g, those receiving glutamine-supplemented TPN required fewer days of TPN until full feeds were established and less time on the ventilator than those who did not. Because similar observations were not seen in infants between 800–1300 g, one must wonder if glutamine is conditionally essential in the very, very LBW infant. Further investigation into this question is certainly warranted.

Glycine

Glycine was proposed as a conditionally-essential amino acid for infants based on altered turnover in enterally-fed infants (Jackson et al 1981). However, the high levels of glycine in some parenteral formulations have resulted in blood concentrations in infants similar to those observed in non-ketotic hyperglycinaemia (Adamkin et al 1991). The more moderate glycine levels in the newer solutions designed for infants appear to be well-tolerated.

Early post-natal amino acid administration

It is common practice in neonatal intensive care units to start intravenous nutrition with a simple glucose solution on admission and to refrain from adding amino acids during the first post-natal day, or even longer if the infant is unstable. Withholding amino acids is accompanied by a loss of body protein, from 0.5–1 g/kg/day as the infant catabolizes muscle for energy. A frequently cited reason for withholding protein or amino acids is concern for the premature infant's ability to metabolize them. Such concern is probably unwarranted. Despite the fact that the hepatic activity of enzymes involved in catabolism of a number of amino acids is low in LBW infants, the plasma concentrations of most amino acids fall precipitously within hours after birth in infants who receive no exogenous protein (Renee et al 1989). A number of studies (Zlotkin et al 1981a, Renee et al 1989, Saini et al 1989, Van Lingen et al 1992, Rivera et al 1993, Heird & Kashyap 1994) have documented the apparent efficacy of early amino acid intake in LBW infants. These studies show that provision of amino acids reverses the net nitrogen loss characteristic of infants who receive amino acid-free intravenous fluids (equivalent to a daily loss of at least 1% of endogenous protein stores). Even an intake of 1.15 g/kg/day of amino acids with an energy intake of < 30 kcal/kg/day from birth onward resulted in improved nitrogen retention (Van Lingen 1992). The studies of early amino acid initiation (Van Lingen et al 1992, Rivera et al 1993, Heird & Kashyap 1994, Van Goudoever et al 1995) showed improved plasma aminograms without evidence of hyperaminoacidaemia or azotaemia. Other studies in LBW infants (Zlotkin et al 1981a, Duffy & Pencharz 1981, Pineault et al 1988) showed minimal effects of energy intake on retention of amino acids at a dose of < 2.5 g/kg/day but more marked effects on retention at higher amino acid intakes. Most infants will tolerate ~2 g/kg/day of amino acids to initiate TPN, but in the most immature and critically-ill infants a lower starting dose is still helpful, even with modest energy intake. Finally, administering amino acids as soon as possible after birth may stimulate endogenous insulin secretion and prevent, in many cases, the need for intravenous insulin infusion to control hyperglycaemia.

Discussion

Human milk should be the standard for determining amino acid needs in the healthy term infant. Formulas and parenteral solutions used to nourish term and pre-term infants must take into account the route of administration as well as the developmental status of the infant because these can have both short- and long-term influence on behaviour and neurological development of the neonate. Amino acid solutions administered to neonates should reflect a content and composition based on human milk until the consequences of deviating from this standard are fully understood. Long-term evaluation of neonatal amino acid requirements must consider growth, nitrogen balance, biochemical response and behavioural development to ensure optimal outcome. It is clear that parenteral amino acid solutions in LBW infants can support nitrogen retention equivalent to the reference foetus if adequate non-protein energy is supplied. Newer solutions designed for infants have resulted in more normal plasma amino acid profiles in infants, although there have not been appreciable gains in nitrogen retention. The problem of delivering poorly-soluble or unstable nutrients in parenteral formulations has not been effectively addressed. However, peptides show promise. Finally, the early initiation of amino acids appears to have particular benefit for the very LBW infant.

References

Abumrad, N.N., Morse, E.L., Lochs, H. et al. (1989) Possible sources of glutamine for parenteral nutrition: Impact on glutamine metabolism. *Am J Physiol*, 257, E228–E234.

Adamkin, D.H., McClead, R.E. Jr., Desai, N.S. et al. (1991) Comparison of two neonatal intravenous amino acid formulations in preterm infants: A multicenter study. *J Perinatol*, 11, 375–382.

Adamkin, D.H., Radmacher, P., Rosen, P. (1995) Comparison of a neonatal versus general purpose amino acid formulation in preterm neonates. *J Perinatol*, 15, 108–113.

Anderson, T.L., Muttart, C., Bierber, M.A. et al. (1979) A controlled trial of glucose versus glucose and amino acids in premature infants. *J Pediatr*, 94, 947–951.

Atkinson, S.A., Hanning, R.M. (1989) Amino Acid Metabolism And Requirements Of The Premature Infant: Is Human Milk The 'Gold Standard'? In: Atkinson, S.A., Lonnerdal, B. (eds.) *Protein And Non-Protein Nitrogen in Human Milk*, p. 187. Boca Raton: CRC Press. 14, 187–209.

Bell, E.F., Filder, L.J. Jr., Wong, A.P., Stegink, L.D. (1983) Effects of a parenteral nutrition regimen containing dicarboxylic amino acids on plasma, erythrocyte, and urinary amino acid concentrations of young infants. *Am J Clin Nutr*, 37, 99–107.

Bjorkman, O., Lindholm, M. (1987) Phenylalanine content and parenteral nutrition. *Lancet*, 1, 1311.

Burger, U., Wolf, H., Fritsch, U., Bauer, M. (1983) Parenteral nutrition in preterm infants: Influence of respiratory treatment and effect of different amino acid compositions. *J Pediatr Gastroenterol Nutr*, 2, 644–652.

Chase, H.P., Nixt, T.L.A. (1983) A double-blind study comparing Neopham with Freamine III in infants receiving parenteral nutrition. *Acta Chir Scand*, 517(Suppl), 49–55.

Chessex, P., Zebiche, H., Pineault, M., Lepage, D., Dallaire, L. (1985) Effect of amino acid composition of parenteral solutions on nitrogen retention and metabolic response in very-low-birth-weight infants. *J Pediatr*, 106, 111–117.

Committee on Nutrition, American Academy of Pediatrics. (1976) Commentary on breast-feeding and infant formulas including proposed standards for formulas. *Pediatr*, 57, 278–285.

Coran, A.G., Drongowski, R.A. (1987) Studies on the toxicity and efficacy of a new amino acid solution in pediatric parenteral nutrition. *J Parent Enter Nutr*, 11, 368–377.

Daabees, T.T., Stegink, L.D. (1978) L-alanyl-L-tyrosine as a tyrosine source during intravenous nutrition of the rat. *J Nutr*, 108, 1104–1113.

Delvalle, J.A., Greengard, O. (1977) Phenylalanine hydroxylase and tyrosine amino transferase in human fetal and adult liver. *Pediatr Res*, 11, 2–5.

Duffy, B., Pencharz, P. (1981) The effect of varying protein quality and energy intake on the nitrogen metabolism of parenterally fed very low birth weight (< 1600 g) infants. *Pediatr Res*, 15, 1040–1044.

European Society for Paediatric Gastroenterology Committee on Nutrition. (1977) Guidelines on infant nutrition: I. Recommendations for the composition of an adapted formula. *Acta Paediatr Scand*, 262(Suppl), 5–8.

European Society for Paediatric Gastroenterology Committee on Nutrition. (1981) Guidelines on infant nutrition: II. Recommendations for the composition of a follow-up formula and beikost. *Acta Paediatr Scand*, 287(Suppl), 1–25.

European Society for Paediatric Gastroenterology Committee on Nutrition. 1987. Nutrition and feeding of preterm infants. *Acta Paediatr Scand*, 336(Suppl), 1–14.

Evans, S.J., Wynne-Williams, T.C.J.E., Russell, D.A. et al. (1986) Hyperphenylalaninaemia in parenterally fed new-born infants. *Lancet*, 2, 1404–1405.

Fomon, S.J. (1991) Requirements and recommended dietary intake of protein during infancy. *Pediatr Res*, 30, 391–395.

Food and Nutrition Board. (1980) *Recommended Dietary Allowances*, 9th edn. Washington DC: National Academy of Sciences–National Research Council.

Furst, P., Albers, S., Stehle, P. (1989) Evidence for nutritional needs for glutamine in catabolic patients. *Kidney Int*, 36, S287–S292.

Furst, P., Albers, S., Stehle, P. (1990) Glutamine-containing dipeptides in parenteral nutrition. *JPEN*, 14, 118S–124S.

Geggel, H.S., Ament, M.E., Heckenlively, H.R., Martin, D.A., Kopple, J.D. (1985) Nutritional requirement for taurine in patients receiving long-term parenteral nutrition. *N Engl J Med*, 312, 142–146.

Hanning, R.M., Moss, L.A., Flanagan, J. (1990) N-acetyltyrosine: A source of tyrosine for total parenteral nutrition in premature infants. *J Can Diet Assoc*, 51, 416.

Hanning, R.M., Zlotkin, S.H. (1989) Amino acid and protein needs of the neonate: Effects of excess and deficiency. *Sem in Perinat*, 13, 131–141.

Hanning, R.M., Zlotkin, S.H. (1992) Nitrogen Needs of The Parenterally Fed Neonate. In: Yu, V., McMahon, B. (eds.) *Intravenous Feeding of The Neonate*, p. 32. Kent: Hodder and Stoughton. 47, 32–41.

Hanning, R.H., Zlotkin, S.H. (1997) Parenteral Proteins. In: Baker, R.D., Baker, S.S., Davis, A.M. (eds.) *Pediatric Parenteral Nutrition*, p. 130. New York: Chapman and Hall. 10, 128–148.

Heird, W.C. (1995) Amino acid and energy needs of pediatric patients receiving parenteral nutrition. *Pediat Clin N Am*, 42, 765–789.

Heird, W.C., Dell, R.B., Helms, R.A., Greene, H.L., Ament, M.E., Karna, P., Storm, M.C. (1987) Amino acid mixture designed to maintain normal plasma amino acid patterns in infants and children requiring parenteral nutrition. *Pediatr*, 80, 401–408.

Heird, W.C., Hay, W., Helms, R.A., Storm, M.C., Kashyap, S., Dell, R.B. (1988) Pediatric parenteral amino acid mixture in low birth weight infants. *Pediatr*, 81, 41–50.

Heird, W.C., Gomez, M.R. (1994) Total parenteral nutrition in necrotizing enterocolitis. *Clin Perinato*, 21, 389–409.

Heird, W.C., Kashyap, S. (1994) Protein Requirements of Low Birth Weight, Very Low Birth Weight And Small for Gestational Age Infants. In: Raiha, N.C.R. (ed.) *Protein Metabolism During Infancy. Nestle Nutrition Workshop*, Vol. 33. New York: Raven Press.

Helms, R.A., Christensen, M.L., Mauer, E.C., Storm, M.C. (1987) Comparison of a pediatric versus standard amino acid formulation in preterm neonates requiring parenteral nutrition. *J Pediatr*, 110, 466–469.

Heyman, M.B. (1990) General and specialized parenteral amino acid formulations for nutrition support. *J Am Diet Assoc*, 90, 401–408.

Hilton, M., Hilton, F., Montgomery, W. et al. (1991) Use of the stable peptide, gamma-L-glutamyl-L-tyrosine as an intravenous source of tyrosine in mice. *Metabolism*, 10, 634–638.

Im, H.A., Rennie, M.J. (1988) Skeletal muscle contains extracellular aminopeptidase against ala-gln but no peptide transporter. *Eur J Clin Invest*, 18, A34.

Irwin, M.I., Hegsted, D.M. (1971) A conspectus of research on amino acid requirements of man. *J Nutr*, 101, 539–566.

Jackson, A.A., Shaw, J.C., Barber, A., Golden, M.H.N. (1981) Nitrogen metabolism in preterm infants fed donor breast milk: The possible essentiality of glycine. *Pediatr Res*, 15, 1454–1461.

Jackson, P.S., Morrison, R., Stange, K. (1994) The volume-sensitive organic osmolyte-anion channel VSOAC is regulated by nonhydrolytic ATP binding. *Am J Physiol*, 267, C1203–C1209.

Jiang, Z.M., Wang, L.J., Qi, Y. et al. (1993) Comparison of parenteral nutrition supplemented with L-glutamine or glutamine dipeptides. *J Parent Enter Nutr*, 17, 134–141.

Johnson, J.D., Albritton, W.L., Sunshine, P. (1972) Hyperammonemia accompanying parenteral nutrition in newborn infants. *J Pediatr*, 81, 154–161.

Kweon, M.N., Moriguchi, S., Mukai, K. et al. (1991) Effect of alanylglutamine enriched infusion on tumor growth and cellular immune function in rats. *Amino Acids*, 1, 7–16.

Lacey, J.M., Crouch, J.B., Benfell, K. et al. (1996) The effects of glutamine-supplemented parenteral nutrition in premature infants. *JPEN*, 20, 74–80.

Laidlaw, S.A., Kopple, J.D. (1987) Newer concepts of the indispensable amino acids. *Am J Clin Nutr*, 46, 593–605.

Laine, L., Shulman, R.J., Pitre, D., Lifschitz, C.H., Adams, J. (1991) Cysteine usage increases the need for acetate in neonates who receive total parenteral nutrition. *Am J Clin Nutr*, 54, 565–567.

Lowe, D.K., Benfell, K., Smith, R.J. et al. (1991) Safety of glutamine-enriched parenteral nutrient solutions in humans. *Am J Clin Nutr*, 52, 1101–1106.

Lucas, A., Baker, B.A., Morley, R.M. (1993) Hyper-phenylalaninaemia and outcome in intravenously fed preterm neonates. *Arch Dis Child*, 68, 579–583.

McIntosh, N., Mitchell, V. (1990) A clinical trial of two parenteral nutrition solutions in neonates. *Arch Dis Child*, 65, 692–699.

Malloy, M.H., Rassin, D.K., Richardson, C.J. (1984) Total parenteral nutrition in sick preterm infants: Effects of cysteine supplementation with nitrogen intakes of 240 and 400 mg/kg/day. *J Pediatr Gastroenterol Nutr*, 3, 239–244.

Mammunes, P., Prince, P.E., Thornton, N.H., Hunt, P.A., Hitchcock, E.S. (1976) Intellectual deficits after transient tyrosinaemia of the newborn. *Pediatr*, 57, 675–680.

Mitton, S.G., Garlick, P.J. (1992) Changes in protein turnover after the introduction of parenteral nutrition in premature infants: Comparison of breast milk and egg protein-based amino acid solutions. *Pediatr Res*, 32, 447–454.

Neuhauser, M., Wandira, J.A., Gottman, U., Bassier, K.H., Langer, K. (1985) Utilization of N-acetyltyrosine and glycyltyrosine during long term parenteral nutrition in the growing rat. *Am J Clin Nutr*, 42, 585–596.

Ogata, E.S., Boehm, J.J., Deddish, R.B., Wiringa, K.S., Yanagi, R.B., Bussey, M.E. (1983) Clinical trial of a 6.5 percent amino acid infusion in appropriate-for-gestational-age premature neonates. *Acta Chir Scand*, 517(Suppl), 39–47.

Okuma, T., Kaneko, H., Chen, K. et al. (1994) Total parenteral nutrition supplemented with L-alanyl-L-glutamine and gut structure and protein metabolism in septic rats. *Nutrition*, 10, 241–245.

Olney, J.W., Sharpe, L.G., Feigin, R.D. (1972) Glutamate-induced brain damage in infant primates. *J Neuropathol Exp Neurol*, 31, 464–488.

Pencharz, P.B., Stefee, W.P., Cochran, W. et al. (1977) Protein metabolism in human neonates: Nitrogen-balance studies, estimated obligatory losses of nitrogen and whole-body turnover of nitrogen. *Clin Sci Mol Med*, 52, 485–498.

Pineault, M., Chessex, P., Bisaillon, S., Bresson, G. (1988) Total parenteral nutrition in the newborn: Impact of the quality of infused energy on nitrogen metabolism. *Am J Clin Nutr*, 47, 298–304.

Puntis, J.W.L., Ball, P.A., Preece, M.A., Green, A., Brown, G.A., Booth, I.W. (1989) Egg and breast milk based nitrogen sources compared. *Arch Dis Child*, 64, 1472–1477.

Puntis, J.W.L., Edwards, M.A., Green, A. (1986) Hyper-phenylalaninaemia in parenterally fed newborn babies. *Lancet*, 2, 1105–1106.

Radmacher, P.G., Hilton, M.A., Hilton, F.K. et al. (1993) Use of the soluble L-glutamyl-L-tyrosine to provide tyrosine in total parenteral nutrition in rats. *JPEN*, 17, 337–344.

Renee, J., Goldberg, A., Rementeria, J.L. et al. (1989) Amino acid patterns of infants of very low birth weight. I. Characterization and clinical significance of change over time. *Nutrition*, 5, 101–106.

Rivera, A. Jr., Bell, E.F., Bier, D.M. (1993) Effect of intravenous amino acids on protein metabolism of preterm infants during the first three days of life. *Pediatr Res*, 33, 106–111.

Rivera, A. Jr., Bell, E.F., Steginy, L.D., Ziegler, E.E. (1989) Plasma amino acid profiles during the first three days of life in infants with respiratory distress syndrome: Effect of parenteral amino acid supplementation. *J Pediatr*, 115, 465–468.

Rosenthal, M., Sinha, S., Laywood, E., Levene, M. (1987) A double-blind comparison of a new paediatric amino acid solution in neonatal total parenteral nutrition. *Early Hum Dev*, 15, 137–146.

Saini, J., MacMahon, P., Morgan, J.B. et al. (1989) Early parenteral feeding of amino acids. *Arch Dis Child*, 64, 1362–1366.

Scheltinga, M.R., Young, L.S., Benfell, K. et al. (1991) Glutamine enriched intravenous feedings attenuate extra-cellular fluid expansion after a standard stress. *Ann Surg*, 214, 385–393.

Shore, B., Nichols, A., Freeman, N. (1953) Evidence for lipolytic action by human plasma obtained after intravenous administration of heparin. *Proc Soc Exp Biol Med*, 83, 216–220.

Thorton, L., Griffin, E. (1991) Evaluation of a taurine containing amino acid solution in parenteral nutrition. *Arch Dis Child*, 66, 21–25.

Tyson, J.E., Lasky, R., Flood, D. et al. (1989) Randomized trial of taurine supplementation for infants < 1300 g birth weight: Effect on auditory brainstem-evoked responses. *Pediatr*, 83, 406–415.

Van Goudoever, J.B., Colen, T., Wattimens, J.L.D., Juigmans J.G.M., Carnielli, V.P., Sauer, P.J. (1995) Immediate commencement of amino acid supplementation in preterm infants: Effect on serum amino acid concentrations and protein kinetics on the first day of life. *J Pediatr*, 127, 458–465.

Van Goudoever, J.B., Sulkers, E.J., Timmerman, M., Huijmans, J.G.M., Langer, K., Carnielli, V.P., Sauer, P.J.J. (1994) Amino acid solutions for premature neonates during the first week of life: The role of N-acetyl-L-cysteine and N-acetyl-L-tyrosine. *J Parent Enter Nutr*, 18, 404–408.

Van Lingen, R.A., Van Goudoever, J.B., Luijendijk, H.T. et al. (1992) Effects of early amino acid administration during total parenteral nutrition on protein metabolism in pre-term infants. *Clin Sci*, 82, 199–203.

Walker, V., Hall, M.A., Bulusu, S. et al. (1986) Hyper-phenylalaninaemia in parenterally fed newborn infants. *Lancet*, 2, 1284.

White, C.W., Stabler, S.P., Allen, R.H., Moreland, S., Rosenberg, A.A. (1994) Plasma cysteine concentrations in infants with respiratory distress. *J Pediatr*, 125, 769–777.

Widdowson, E.M. (1979) Body Composition of The Fetus and Infant. In: Visser, H.K.A. (ed.) *Nutrition And Metabolism of The Fetus And Infant. Fifth Nutricia Symposium*, p. 147. The Hague: Martinus Nijhoff Session III, 169–177.

Wong, P.W.K., Pildes, R.S. (1974) Plasma amino acids in low birth weight infants treated with intravenous infusions. *Biol Neonate*, 25, 300–306.

World Health Organization/Food Agricultural Organization. (1973) *Energy And Protein Requirements. WHO Technical Report Series No. 522*. Geneva: World Health Organization.

World Health Organization/Food Agricultural Organization. (1985) *Energy And Protein Requirements. Technical Report Series No. 724*. Geneva: World Health Organization.

Zelikovic, I., Chesney, R.W., Friedman, A.L. et al. (1990) Taurine depletion in very-low-birth weight infants receiving prolonged total parenteral nutrition: Role of renal immaturity. *J Pediatr*, 116, 301–306.

Zlotkin, S.H. (1984) Intravenous nitrogen intake requirements in full-term newborns undergoing surgery. *Pediatr*, 73, 493–496.

Zlotkin, S.H., Anderson, G.D. (1982) The development of cystathionase activity during the first year of life. *Pediatr Res*, 16, 65–68.

Zlotkin, S.H., Bryan, M.H., Anderson, G.H. (1981a) Intravenous nitrogen and energy intakes required to duplicate in utero nitrogen accretion in prematurely born human infants. *J Pediatr*, 99, 115–120.

Zlotkin, S.H., Bryan, M.H., Anderson, G.H. (1981b) Cysteine supplementation to cysteine free intravenous feeding regimens in newborn infants. *Am J Clin Nutr*, 34, 914–923.

14

Essential fatty acid requirements: Implication for neural development

Jitka S. Vobecky and J.R. Iglesias

Abbreviations

AA   arachidonic acid (20:4n-6)
DHA   docosahexaenoic acid (22:6n-3)
EFA   essential fatty acids
SFA   saturated fatty acids

Introduction

Amongst the polyunsaturated fatty acids, (omega-6) linoleic (18:2n-6) acid and (omega-3) alpha-linolenic (18:3n-3) acid are considered essential because they are necessary for optimal health. However, the organism is not able to produce a sufficient quantity of these (Spector 1999).

In this short chapter on the role of the essential fatty acids (EFA), the focus is limited to the available studies about EFA status during pregnancy, lactation and early infancy. The omega-3 fatty acids have a very important role during pregnancy and for the growth and development of young infants. The n-3 fatty acids, especially 22:6n-3 (docosahexaenoic acid) are deposited in the baby's brain during the third trimester of pregnancy and it is then that myelin formation starts and continues to increase (Crawford et al 1997) until the eighteenth month after birth.

There are two series of EFAs. One is derived from linoleic acid (n-6) and the second one from alpha-linolenic acid (n-3). Both are supplied by foods of plant origin. The deficiency of linoleic acid results in a failure of several physiological systems and is characterized by scaly dermatitis, increased susceptibility to infection and poor growth (British Nutrition Foundation 1992).

Historical background

The polyunsaturated fatty acids belonging to the n-6 and n-3 families are not interconvertible. Plants can synthesize EFAs but animals can not because of their inability to form double bonds of carbon at positions n-6 and n-3. Linoleic fatty acid (18:2n-6) is present in vegetable oils and can be converted in organisms to other n-6 fatty acids for example arachidonic acid (AA) (20:4n-6). Some vegetable oils, namely canola and soy bean oil, contain an important quantity of alpha-linolenic fatty acid (18:3n-3). This fatty acid can be converted to long-chain polyunsaturated fatty acids of the n-3 family such as eicosapentanoic (20:3n-3) and DHA (22:6n-3).

Maternal malnutrition, whether primary or secondary to illness, and placental malfunction can result in intrauterine malnutrition. In early pregnancy, the formation of the placenta and its development can be disrupted by inadequate nutrition, resulting in insufficient foetal growth even if later in the pregnancy nutrition is adequate. In this situation, the maternal malnutrition affecting the omega-3 AA and DHA supply influence vascular development (Crawford et al 1997).

As yet, the available evidence supporting the causal links between DHA deficiency and neurological symptoms is not very solid. Nevertheless, Salem & Ward (1993) reported that the levels of DHA correlate with various diseases. On the contrary, diets containing a high level of omega-3 fatty acids are associated with a much lower incidence of multiple sclerosis when compared to diets containing low levels.

Pre-term infants

Inadequate maternal diet before conception is often associated with low birth weight (LBW) and also with deficiencies of vitamins, namely B vitamins, magnesium and many other nutrients. According to Uauy et al (1990), Carlson et al (1996) and others, pre-term infants cannot sufficiently synthesize DHA nor possibly AA from precursors. Consequently, both of these fatty acids should be added to their diets. Because DHA and AA are also found in breast milk, it is important to be sure that the substitutes of maternal milk for formula-fed pre-term infants have a comparable concentration of long-chain polyunsaturated fatty acids. The immaturity and the rapid brain growth of premature infants influence the complexity of essential fatty acid requirements. Sanders (1999) underlines that some controversy still exists about whether full-term infants require any dietary supply of long-chain polyunsaturated fatty acids. Some authors (Makrides et al 1995, Carlson et al 1996) found improvement of visual function in full-term infants fed with fortified formulas. However, other authors (Innis et al 1996, Auestad et al 1997) have not found any difference between full-term infants fed formulas either with or without DHA and AA in comparison with breastfed infants. Recently, Bakker et al (1999) investigated the influence of fatty acid status and early nutrition on the visual acuity of term infants at 7 months of age. No influence of EFA status, infant diet or potential confounders on visual acuity was found.

Pre-term lipid nutrition should be revised to be more in line with placental lipid transfer to the foetus.

Central nervous system development

Pregnancy and the first post-natal months are the critical time for growth and development of the nervous system (Koletzko et al 1998). Therefore, it is essential to supply adequate nutrients that have long-term effects on sensory and cognitive abilities during this period.

The role of fatty acids on brain function beyond the period of rapid brain growth is not quite understood. It seems that EFA deficiency is not as important for the alternations of these functions as is SFA deficiency (Kaplan & Greenwood 1998).

The polyunsaturated fatty acids, especially those derived from the linoleic and alpha-linolenic acids, are necessary for normal development of the central nervous system and the retinae. It should be emphasized that these are not present in plant foods.

The possibility that intrauterine nutrition may play a part in the aetiology of developmental central nervous system and visual disorders is frequently discussed. DHA is mobilized from tissue stores during the early weeks of pregnancy, but in the third trimester its concentration is decreased.

Retinal development

A large quantity of DHA is present in the membranes of the retinae. This acid is also present in cerebral lipids. According to Neuringer et al (1988) and Connor et al (1984), the insufficiency of this fatty acid can produce a decrease in visual acuity. DHA increases during the third trimester of pregnancy up to the eighth month after the birth.

The level of DHA in the red cells of newborns that are fed formulas that are poor in alpha-linolenic fatty acid is lower than in the red cells of breastfed newborns. Crawford et al (1997) reviewed the available studies concerning the pre-natal or post-natal deficits of AA and DHA as well as those concerned with underdeveloped antioxidant protection. These deficits contributed to nervous and visual developmental disorders and other premature birth complications.

The most important polyunsaturated fatty acids belonging to the n–6 and n–3 families and their derivatives are incorporated into membrane phospho-lipids of cells. The polyunsaturated fatty acids are an important nutrient in early human development for neural tissues such as the brain and the retinae. The food supply of pregnant women and neonates should be adequate (Antal & Gaal 1998).

Growth and development

According to Koletzko et al (1998), the evaluation of dietary effects on infant growth requires epidemiological studies. Growth factors and some essential nutrients such as amino acids and polyunsaturated fatty acids may be potentially useful as ingredients in functional foods. Early diet seems to have long-term effects on sensory and cognitive abilities as well as on behaviour (Koletzko et al 1998). The potential beneficial effects of a balanced supply of nutrients such as iodine, iron, zinc and polyunsaturated fatty acids should be further evaluated.

Risk of vegetarian nutrition

It is not quite clear if and how the required essential fatty acids are supplied by a vegetarian diet. In his instructive review of this problem, Sanders (1991) concluded that there are differences in the EFA status of vegetarians and omnivores. The most important is the higher intake of linoleic acid by vegetarians and, to a lesser degree, the different intakes of long-chain polyunsaturated fatty acids.

However, in the breast milk of lactating vegetarian women, long-chain polyunsaturated fatty acids are present.

Practice and procedures

Modern biotechnology offers the possibility to include in special dietary products the necessary bioactive substances that have adequate physiological effects. Individual growth patterns, as well as the different developmental needs of children, exist and differ greatly according to age. Because of the rapid growth during the first 2 years of life, infants at this age are nutritionally vulnerable. Therefore, it seems that in infancy a high-fat diet is fully recommended. The consumption of approximately 50% energy from fat can ensure an adequate intake of energy and fatty acids needed for growth and development (Nutrition Recommendations Update. Dietary Fat and Children 1993).

Recommendations for infants

Based on the reviewed evidence, Crawford et al (1997)suggested that parenteral and enteral nutrition for pre-term babies should correspond with placental lipid transfer to the foetus. Even if full-term milk composition is the basis for pre-term foods, the placenta is richer in AA and DHA than milk. Some authors suggest that supplementation with DHA is important during pregnancy and lactation for the needs of pregnant women and growing infants (Connor et al 1996). Al et al (1995) studied the effect of maternal linoleic acid supplementation during pregnancy on neonatal essential fatty acid status. The results indicate that maternal linoleic acid supplementation can affect some aspects of neonatal essential fatty acid status. A significant negative correlation has been observed between EFA deficiency in the umbilical artery and birth weight. Because a low birth weight may have negative consequences later in life, the increase of foetal EFA status by maternal supplementation during pregnancy is recommended.

Discussion

The Workshop on the Essentiality of and Recommended Dietary Intakes for Omega-6 and Omega-3 Fatty Acids held in 1999 (Simopoulos et al 1999) discussed thespecific recommendations for:

1. healthy adults;

2. pregnant and lactating women; and

3. the composition of infant formula that will support the growth and development of the formula-fed infant to the same extent as the breastfed infant.

The workshop did not determine dietary reference intakes because of insufficient data. It was, however, possible to recommend adequate intakes for adults. The similar recommendations for pregnant and lactating women were accepted as for adults with an additional recommendation that a DHA intake of 300 mg/day must be ensured.

The supply of linoleic acid equal to 1% of the total energy intake is enough to prevent deficiency symptoms. The FAO (1977) recommended supply of EFAs is 3% of total energy intake. The fatty acid n-6 should represent at least 3% of the total energy intake and the fatty acid n-3 at least 0.5% of this energy intake. The ratio of fatty acids n-6:n-3 should be between 4:1 and 10:1. For infants whose diets do not cover the fatty acids n-3 with 20 and 22 atoms of carbon, the intake of linolenic fatty acid (n-3) should correspond to 1% of total energy intake. The formula diet for premature infants merits special attention. Its composition should be similar to breast milk in order to support growth and neural development in

Table 14.1 — Adequate intake for infant formula diet★

Fatty acids	Percentage of fatty acids
Linoleic acid	10
Alpha-linolenic acid	1.5
Arachidonic acid	0.5
Docosahexaenoic acid	0.35
Eicosapentaenoic acid	
Upper limit	< 0.1

★ According to Simopoulos et al (1999).

the same manner as breastfeeding. The workshop's proposal for adequate intakes are shown in Table 14.1.

The recommended intake of EFAs is based on values found in maternal milk. They are very low, even if 6 times higher than in cow's milk. Because the supply of omega-3 unsaturated fatty acids is almost absent, the recommended value is expressed by alpha-linolenic acid and represents 1% of total energy intake.

References

Al, M.D., van Houwelingen, A.C., Badart-Smook, A., Hornstra, G. (1995) Some aspects of neonatal essential fatty acid status are altered by linoleic acid supplementation of women during pregnancy. *J Nutr*, 125, 2822–2830.

Antal, M., Gaal, O. (1998) Nutritional value of polyunsaturated fatty acids. *Otv Hetil*, 139, 1153–1158.

Auestad, N., Montalto, M.B., Hall, R.T. et al. (1997) Visual acuity, erythrocyte fatty acid composition and growth in term infants fed formulas with long chain polyunsaturated fatty acids for one year. *Pediatr Res*, 41, 1–10.

Bakker, E.C., van Houwelingen, A.C., Hornstra, G. (1999) Early nutrition, essential fatty acid status and visual acuity of term infants at 7 months of age. *Eur J Clin Nutr*, 53, 872–879.

British Nutrition Foundation. (1992) *Task Force on Unsaturated Fatty Acids*. London: Chapman and Hall.

Carlson, S.E., Ford, A.J., Werkman, S.H., Peeples, J.M., Koo, W.W.K. (1996) Visual acuity and fatty acid status of term infants fed human milk and formulas with and without docosahexaenoic and arachidonate from egg yolk lecithin. *Pediatr Res*, 39, 882–888.

Connor, W.E., Lowensohn, R., Hatcher, L. (1996) Increased docosaheaenoic acid levels in human new born infants by administration of sardines and fish oil during pregnancy. *Lipids*, 31, S183–S187.

Crawford, M.A., Costeloe, K., Ghebremeskel, K., Phylactos, A., Skirvin, L., Stacey, F. (1997) Are deficits of arachidonic and docosahexaenoic acids responsible for the neural and vascular complications of preterm babies? *Am J Clin Nutr*, 66(Suppl), S1032–S1041.

Innis, S.M., Nelson, C.M., Lwanga, D., Rioux, F.M., Waslen, P. (1996) Feeding formula without arachidonic acid and docosahexaenoic acid has no effect on preferential looking acuity or recognition memory in healthy full-term infants at 9 mo of age. *Am J Clin Nutr*, 64, 40–46.

Kaplan, R.R., Greenwood, C.E. (1998) Dietary saturated fatty acids and brain function. *Neurochem Res*, 23, 615–626.

Koletzko, B., Aggett, P.J., Bindels, J.G., Bung, P., Ferre, P., Gill, A., Lentze, M.J., Roberfroid, M., Strobel, S. (1998) Growth, development and differentiation: A functional food science approach. *Br J Nutr*, 80(Suppl), S5–S45.

Koletzko, B., Demmelmair, H., Socha, P. (1998) Nutritional support of infants and children: Supply and metabolism of lipids. *Baillières Clin Gastroenterol*, 12, 671–696.

Makrides, M., Neumann, M.A., Simmer, K., Pater, J., Gibson, R.A. (1995) Are long-chain polyunsaturated fatty acids essential nutrients in infancy? *Lancet*, 345, 1463–1468.

Neuringer, M., Anderson, G.J., Connor, W.E. (1988) The essentiality of n-3 fatty acids for the development and function of the retina and brain. *Ann Rev Nutr*, 8, 517–541.

Nutrition Recommendations Update. Dietary Fat and Children. (1993) Report of the Joint Working Group of the Canadian Paediatric Society and Health Canada.

Ratnayake, W.M., Chardigny, J.M., Wolff, R.L., Bayard, C.C., Sebedio, J.L., Martin, L. (1997) Essential fatty acids and their transgeometrical isomers in powdered and liquid infant formulas sold in Canada. *J Pediatr Gastroenterol Nutr*, 25, 400–407.

Reece, M.S., McGregor, J.A., Allen, K.G., Harris, M.A. (1997) Maternal and perinatal long-chain fatty acids: Possible roles in preterm birth. *Am J Obstet Gynecol*, 176, 907–914.

Salem, N.Jr, Ward, G.R. (1993) Are Omega 3 fatty acids essential nutients for mammals? *Rev Nutr Diet*, 72, 128–147.

Sanders, T.A.B. (1999) Essential fatty acid requirements of vegetarians in pregnancy, lactation, and infancy. *Am J Clin Nutr*, 70(Suppl), S555–S559.

Simopoulos, A.P., Leaf, A., Salem, N. Jr. (1999) Workshop on the Essentiality of and Recommended Dietary Intakes for Omega-6 and Omega-3 Fatty Acids. *Asia Pacific J Clin Nutr*, 8, 300–301.

Spector, A.A. (1999) Essentiality of fatty acids. *Lipids*, 34(Suppl), S1–S3.

Stevens, L., Zentall, S., Abate, M., Kucsek, T., Burgess, J. (1996) Omega-3 fatty acids in boys with behaviour, learning and health problems. *Physiology & Behaviour*, 59, 915–920.

Uauy, R.D., Birch, D.G., Birch, E.E., Tyson, J.E., Hoffman, D.R. (1990) Effect of dietary omega-3 fatty acids on retinal function of very low birth weight neonates. *Pediatr Res*, 28, 485–492.

Uauy, R., Mena, P. (1999) Requirements for long-chain polyunsaturated fatty acids in the preterm infant. *Curr Opin Pediatr*, 11, 115–120.

15

Prevention of iron deficiency in infants: issues and approaches

Martin Bloem, Rainer Gross, Werner Schultink, Roger Shrimpton and Ray Yip

Introduction

Iron deficiency is the most prevalent nutritional disorder worldwide, when anaemia is used as an indicator (ACC/SCN 1992). Although anaemia can also be caused by other factors, such as folic acid deficiency or genetic disorders, iron deficiency is the most common cause. Young children and pregnant women are at highest risk of suffering from iron deficiency because they have relatively-high requirements related to the rapid increase in cell mass. A selection of data on the prevalence of low haemoglobin and low ferritin amongst young children is shown in Table 15.1. These data have to be interpreted with some caution because they are not representative of the respective countries, and low values for haemoglobin or ferritin per se are not always indicative of iron deficiency in infants. However, the percentage of infants with anaemia is still quite high in developed countries, and even up to half of the infants in the developing world have anaemia. In spite of being an unrepresentative as well as a possible inaccurate indicator for iron deficiency, the data indicate a high likelihood that iron deficiency amongst infants is a public health problem in many countries, especially in developing ones. Figure 15.1 shows the prevalence of anaemia (Hb < 110 g/L) in a randomized sample of Indonesian infants (total n=1352) from 118 villages in Central Java, Indonesia. The high prevalence of anaemia starts from 1 month of age onwards.

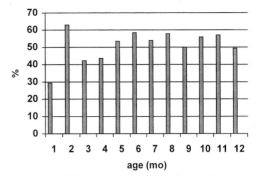

Figure 15.1 — The prevalence of anaemia according to age as indicated by haemoglobin concentration < 110 g/L amongst a sample of 1352 Indonesian infants randomly selected from 118 villages in Central Java. From Survey Helen Keller International (1997), with permission.

Historical background

Iron deficiency anaemia amongst infants has long been recognized as a significant problem in Western Europe (Stevens 1991). The major risk factors were low stores of iron in low-birth-weight infants, feeding of foods that were based on cow's milk without added iron, and the type of weaning foods used (MacKay & Goodfellow 1931). In spite of the early identification of the causal factors, it appears to be difficult to alleviate iron deficiency amongst infants as indicated by the current prevalence rates. Reasons for this prolonged

Table 15.1 — Prevalence of iron deficiency among infants

Age (months)	Ethnicity/Country	Indicator	Prevalence (%)	Reference
3–12	Asian/United Kingdom	Hb < 110 g/L	11	(4)
6	Asian/United Kingdom	Hb < 110 g/L	12	(5)
6	Non-asian/United Kingdom	Ferritin < 10 ug/L	36	(5)
6	Asian/United Kingdom	Ferritin < 10 ug/L	40	(5)
12–24	United States of America	Iron deficient★	9	(6)
4–36	Brazil	Hb < 110 g/L	20–50	(7)
12	Brazil	Hb < 110 g/L	40–44	(8)
0–6	Brazil, Sao Paolo	Hb < 110 g/L	35	(9)
6–18	Vietnam	Hb < 110 g/L	45	(10)
0–6	Indonesia	Hb < 110 g/L	46	(11)
6–12	Indonesia	Hb < 110 g/L	51	(11)
6–24	Vietnam	Hb < 110 g/L	56	(12)

★Considered iron deficient when two or more of the iron-status tests of serum ferritin (< 10 g/L), transferrin saturation (< 10%), and erythrocyte protoporphyrin (> 1.42 umol/L RBC) were inadequate.

unsatisfactory situation probably include a lack of awareness about the negative impact of iron deficiency on infant development and health, causing inadequate or total absence of interventions by parents and/or authorities. In developing countries, additional reasons such as a lack of resources to achieve improvement and a lack of adequate intervention possibilities also play an important role in the prolongation of the widespread presence of iron deficiency.

The influence of maternal iron status on infant iron status

A healthy full-term baby is born with about 75 mg iron/kg bodyweight endowed by the mother (Dallman et al 1980), and most of this is deposited during the last trimester of pregnancy. During the first weeks after birth, iron is re-distributed in the body. In the period between birth and 4 weeks post-partum the haemoglobin concentration of healthy infants decreases from about 170 g/L to 110–120 g/L, and there is a decrease in erythropoiesis (Dallman et al 1980). Between 2–4 months of age, the mean haemoglobin concentration increases again to about 125 g/L. Ferritin concentrations in the first 2 months of life were reported to be 200–240 µg/L in healthy infants from Finland, thereafter the concentration dropped to about 30 µg/L in infants older than 6 months (Saarinen & Simes 1978).

The influence of maternal iron status on the iron status of infants continues to be under investigation, and available studies show conflicting results. Iron status (both haemoglobin and ferritin) at birth of a full-term infant has been reported not to be associated with maternal iron status (Dallman et al 1980) unless mothers are severely anaemic (Singla et al 1978). A lack of association between iron status of mothers and their newborns has also been reported by other studies (Rios et al 1975, Gebre-Madhin & Birgegard 1981). However, some studies have reported an association. A correlation between maternal and newborn iron indicators has been reported for Nigerian (Daouda et al 1991) and Ecuadorian (Yepez et al 1987) women. Iron-supplemented women with a ferritin level at delivery of 22 µg/L had infants with higher cord-blood ferritin (15 µg/L) compared with infants from unsupplemented women who had ferritin levels at delivery of 118 µg/L and infants with cord-blood ferritin of 14 µg/L (Milman et al 1994). Discrepancies between studies may be explained partially by the fact that most studies were cross-sectional and only investigated iron status of mothers and newborns at the time of delivery. The association between maternal and infant iron status may be confounded by practices during delivery. At birth, the bulk of an infant's iron is present in circulating haemoglobin and the amount of iron in the body at the time of birth depends on the blood volume and haemoglobin concentration. Therefore, factors that influence the blood volume of the newborn, such as the timing of the clamping of the umbilical cord, influence the infant's iron stores (Wilson et al 1941, Kinmond et al 1993).

Most studies on the relationship between infants and maternal iron status were limited to the moment of birth or to the period shortly afterwards. Few studies were longitudinal and investigated the maternal iron status during pregnancy in relation to the iron status of older infants. Iron status of English infants at 6 months and 1 year showed to be correlated positively with cord ferritin levels and with maternal ferritin levels at 37 weeks of gestation (Morton et al 1988). A Spanish study indicated that infants born from a mother with iron deficiency anaemia at delivery had a 6.6 times higher chance of becoming iron deficit during the first year of life compared to infants from non-anaemic mothers (Colomer et al 1990). The impact of iron supplementation was investigated amongst pregnant women from Niger (Preziosi et al 1997) of whom 67% were anaemic. Women who received 100 mg iron/day throughout the third trimester of pregnancy had significantly higher ferritin levels at delivery and 3 months post-partum compared to women who did not receive iron-supplements. The infants from the iron-supplemented women did not have better iron status immediately after delivery, but had significantly higher ferritin concentration at 3 and 6 months. These three longitudinal studies clearly demonstrate the importance of an adequate maternal iron status during pregnancy for the iron status of infants, especially in developing countries.

Iron requirements in infancy

Rapid increase in body size is the major reason for the usually high requirement of iron during infancy. During the first 6 months of life, body weight should increase from about 3 kg at birth to 7–8 kg at 6 months of age. The natural food of infants during this period of life is breast milk, which contains 0.6–0.9 mg iron/L depending on the period of lactation. Although iron from breast milk is absorbed well, the requirement needed for rapid growth can not be covered by the milk intake and the endowed iron stores are used up to satisfy the requirements. After the stores are finished, the infant becomes completely dependent upon external iron sources. Iron stores of healthy, full-term infants last until 4–6 months of age.

Pre-term and low-birth-weight babies have extra-high iron requirements during infancy because they experience a greater rate of growth compared to term infants (Dallman et al 1980). Pre-term and low-birth-weight babies are also born with lesser iron stores. Therefore, their iron stores often are already depleted by 2–3 months of age and they require additional iron much earlier than full-term infants.

The same situation is valid for many full-term infants from developing countries. For example, 73% of a group of children from Niger, whose mothers were anaemic in 69% of cases during pregnancy, were already iron deficient at 6 months of age (Preziosi et al 1997). Whether physiological iron requirements can be satisfied by the daily diet depends on the iron content of the food as well as the bioavailability. Generally only a small part of the iron in the diet can be absorbed (10% or less).

A child aged between 6–12 months should on average absorb about 0.1–0.2 mg iron/kg body weight (totally 0.8–1.2 mg), which almost equals the daily dietary requirements of an adult man (Hallberg et al 1993) at 8–10 mg iron/day (necessary to absorb 1 mg). After a child has become 1 year of age, the requirements for growth decrease by about half and the total requirements are lower than during infancy.

Consequences of deficiency

The most well known consequence of iron deficiency is anaemia. However, unless severe (Hb < 80 g/L when reduced oxygen-carrying capacity becomes significant), anaemia in itself does not constitute a major health threat. Rather, it is an indicator of the severity of iron deficiency. Amongst the major consequences of iron deficiency that have been studied, the evidence that it adversely affects child development and behaviour is of greatest concern. Several studies show that iron deficiency is associated with impaired cognitive performance and motor development (Soemantri et al 1985, Aukett et al 1986, Soewondo et al 1989). The causal relationship between iron deficiency and mental development was demonstrated by a study amongst Indonesian children aged 1–2 years (Idjradinata & Pollitt 1993). Anaemic children who received iron treatment had higher mental test scale scores than a placebo group and had similar scores compared to

an iron replete control group at the end of the supplementation. This study demonstrated that the developmental delays were reversible (Lozoff et al 1991). However, a study amongst Costa Rican children who had been treated for iron deficiency anaemia during infancy and who were followed up at 5 years of age indicated that the delay was not reversible. Another study amongst 12–23-month-old iron-deficient anaemic children who were treated for 6 months with orally-administered iron, also indicated that delays in mental development persisted in spite of improved haematological status (Lozoff et al 1996). The evidence that prolonged iron deficiency during early childhood leads to irreversible impaired development is therefore not conclusive, and the effects may vary depending on age and severity. However, the possibility of an irreversible effect must be considered and therefore the prevention of iron deficiency is important to avoid negative developmental consequences.

It was demonstrated that when iron-deficient pre-schoolers with growth retardation were treated with iron their linear growth rate increased (Aukett et al 1986, Soewando et al 1989, Angeles et al 1993, Lawless et al 1994). However, the evidence is not conclusive because other studies do not report a positive impact of iron on growth (Palupi et al 1997, Rosado et al 1997). Iron deficiency also negatively influences the normal defence systems against infection (Srikantia et al 1976, Brock 1993). Clinical evidence of increased infection associated with iron deficiency was provided by a study amongst African children: incidence of upper respiratory and gastrointestinal infections increased in iron-deficient infants with depressed levels of T-helper cells (Berger et al 1992).

Another health consequence of iron deficiency that is of particular concern for children, especially those living in an urban environment, is enhanced lead absorption. Animal and human studies have demonstrated that gastrointestinal absorption of lead increases with the severity of iron deficiency (Watson et al 1980). Both clinical and epidemiological studies demonstrate an association between elevated blood levels of lead and iron deficiency (Centre for Disease Control 1985). Given that childhood lead poisoning is a well documented cause of neurological and developmental deficits, iron deficiency appears to contribute to this problem.

Causes of iron deficiency

Iron in the diet is present as heme-iron from meat,

poultry or fish, or as non-heme iron from vegetable foods. Heme-iron is present only in a small amount in the diet (maximally 10–15% of total iron intake) but it has a high absorption rate of 20–30%. The absorption rate of non-heme iron is generally much lower (1–5%) and is influenced by dietary factors and physiological status. Important dietary factors are absorption inhibitors such as phytate, polyphenols, and calcium, and absorption enhancers such as vitamin C and heme-iron (Hallberg 1981). Phytate is present, for example, in the outer layers of cereals, and green leafy vegetables contain polyphenols.

A typical infant in a developing country is still breastfed at 6 months of age. Assuming that breast milk provides about 400 kcal/day for an infant of 6–8 months, about 300 kcal/day and 0.5–0.7 mg iron needs to be absorbed from the complementary food. With an average dietary iron absorption of 10%, the daily diet needs to contain 5–7 mg of iron. This requires a high bioavailable diet, containing ample amounts of animal products and vitamin C and low amounts of iron absorption inhibitors such as phytate. However, the typical diet in developing countries is low in iron bioavailability and can be characterized by a small amount of heme-iron and a large quantity of absorption inhibitors. Even in industrialized countries when infants are fed non-fortified diets without sufficient amounts of meat, a risk for deficiency is induced. The major cause of iron deficiency in infants is therefore the low content as well as the low absorption of iron from the diet.

A specific dietary factor associated with anaemia amongst infants is the consumption of unfortified cow's milk. A high prevalence of anaemia amongst 9–24-month-old children in Argentina (Calvo & Gnazzo 1990) and 9-month-old children in Chile (Pizarro et al 1991) was associated with the early introduction of cow's milk. The study from Chile indicated that children consuming non-fortified cow's milk have a 30–40% risk of becoming iron deficient by 9 months of age. Factors leading to anaemia with consumption of larger amounts of cow's milk are the low content and bioavailability of iron in milk, the inhibitory effect of milk on the absorption of iron from other foods (Hallberg et al 1991), and the possible effect on gastrointestinal bleeding (Wharton 1990, Ziegler et al 1990).

A nutrient that has been shown to influence iron metabolism is vitamin A. Vitamin A deficiency may lead to a decrease in haemoglobin concentration, even when sufficient iron is stored in the liver (Bloem 1995). A main source of vitamin A for many infants is breast milk. However, the vitamin A content of breast milk is influenced by the vitamin A status of the mother (Stolzfus et al 1993). Although no information is available about the influence of breast milk vitamin-A concentration on infant iron status, it may be a determinant factor in developing countries.

Practice and procedures

Options for improvement

Dietary approach

Given the high iron requirement and low iron bioavailability of most infant diets, the dietary approach is a challenge. The possibility of satisfying the iron needs from natural unfortified foods seems to be limited especially considering the limited gastric capacity of infants. Considering the protective effect of breastfeeding on the iron status of healthy infants, it is recommended to breastfeed for 4–6 months without giving additional food because it may influence the bioavailability of iron from the breast milk and, especially in developing countries, introduce the risk of food-borne infections. If breastfeeding is not possible, it is essential to feed young infants an adequately fortified formula. When breastfeeding is continued until 1 year of age a part of the iron requirements would be covered by the breast milk. Complementary foods providing highly-bioavailable iron are meat (2–4.3 mg/100 g) and liver (6–14 mg/100 g). The best possibility of maintaining or improving an infant's iron status is to include generous amounts (30–50 g) of these foods in the daily diet. Vegetable foods such as pulses and green leafy vegetables are also rich in iron but the bioavailability is low, especially when eaten in combination with cereals that contain phytate. The negative impact of phytate on iron absorption can be overcome by improved milling techniques (taking away the outer layer) or by adding vitamin C rich foods to a meal (Tuntawiroon et al 1990). Preparing a small volume meal with a small amount of cereal fibre with high phytate content but with adequate amounts of meat and vitamin C is possible for parents in industrialized countries. Unfortunately, it is not possible for many parents in developing countries. For example, many households in rural Indonesia do consume fish as the most important animal food source, but only do so 2–3 times per week in small amounts (Gross et al 1994). Vitamin C rich foods such as fruits are only consumed seasonally.

Achieving adequate iron absorption from the diet is ideal, but in developing countries this is difficult to achieve in the near future.

Food fortification

Considering the difficulty of providing enough iron for infants through the normal diet, fortification of infant foods has long been recognized as an efficient way to guarantee adequate iron uptake. This appears to be the most effective option in industrialized countries where infants often consume industrially-produced foods such as formulas and cereals. In industrialized countries, almost all infant formulas are fortified with iron at a level of 5–12 mg/L; the formulas from Europe contain less than the formulas from the United States. The importance of these industrially-prepared foods in industrialized countries is indicated by a survey in the United Kingdom that shows that about 80% of infants are fed some commercial infant food rather than family foods (Mills & Tyler 1990). Epidemiological studies suggest that the iron status of children can improve through fortification of infant foods. In the United States, the use of infant formulas and cereals has been identified as an important factor in reducing the prevalence of anaemia amongst infants from low and middle-income families (Vasquez-Soanne et al 1985, Dallman 1990). In most developing countries, the use of fortified infant foods is limited due to the unavailability in smaller villages and towns and the relatively-high prices that make these foods unattainable for a large part of the population. Furthermore, in developing countries, formula feeding is associated with an increased risk of diarrhoea and under-nutrition due to incorrect usage and polluted water. The use of infant formula as a way to improve iron nutrition in developing countries is therefore very limited.

A factor of concern in developed countries is the level of iron fortification. An excess of iron may have adverse effects, and may negatively influence zinc and copper absorption (Lönnerdal 1989). The results of a recent study suggest that under the conditions of industrialized countries, formulas for infants younger than 6 months do not need to be fortified with more than 10 mg iron/L (Fomon et al 1997). The adequate level of fortification of infant formulas for children from developing countries may be higher, but no studies have been undertaken to investigate the most appropriate level for these countries.

Another micro-nutrient of special concern during infancy is zinc. Zinc deficiency may be common in developing countries, and iron influences its absorption (Solomons 1986). The effect of fortification on zinc absorption from a vegetable-based weaning food was tested in 9-month-old infants (Fairweather-Tait et al 1995). The absorption of 1-mg-enriched stable isotope was measured comparing unfortified and iron-fortified (5 mg iron/portion) product. No differences in zinc absorption were observed, and it was concluded that iron fortification of the vegetable-weaning food did not reduce zinc absorption, which was about 28–30%. The type of cereal is probably of little importance in the preparation of infant foods when considering iron absorption. The absorption from a rice, wheat, maize, oats, millet, or quinoa based cereal product was reported to be similar. Methods to reduce the phytate content are therefore of greater importance in improving iron absorption than the choice of a certain cereal (Cook et al 1997).

Supplementation

Iron status of an individual can be improved in a short period of time through supplementation with iron. Iron status of infants can be improved by giving 2 mg iron/kg body weight/day (DeMaeyer 1989). The World Health Organization (WHO) recommends that countries provide iron supplements to all members of at-risk groups when the prevalence of iron deficiency is high. When, for example, the prevalence of anaemia is 40% in a population group and iron deficiency is the main cause of the anaemia, then it can be expected that virtually all members of this population group are iron deficient and therefore all should receive additional iron. In line with these recommendations, pregnant women in many countries are supplemented with iron during the second half of pregnancy. These supplementation programmes are usually organized through the public health sector. However, the effectiveness of these programmes is disappointing mainly because of a low coverage of the target population, inadequate tablet supply, and low compliance with tablet intake (ACC/SCN 1991, Schultink & Gross 1996, Yip 1996). It also is recommended to provide iron supplements on a large scale to infants from developing countries considering the high prevalence of iron deficiency and the absence of other effective dietary-based interventions. The WHO-recommended dose for infants is 3 mg/kg body weight/day, and no adverse side effects have been reported by parents of infants when this was given on a daily basis for 3 months (Reeves & Yip 1985). However up-to-date, most countries have not started such a large-scale supplementation programme for infants. Reasons for this absence include the costs of the programme and problems related to the distribution mechanism. A pilot study in Brazil reported on compliance problems when supplementing infants on a daily basis with iron supplements (Szarfarc et al 1996). More than half of the mothers who were provided with iron supplements for their infants did not continue with the supplementation for more than 1 month. An alternative for the traditional form of supplementation can be supplementation on a weekly basis.

Supplementation on a weekly instead of a daily basis may possibly improve compliance and reduce the amount of supplements needed. Studies amongst Indonesian (Schultink et al 1995) and Chinese (Liu et al 1995) pre-school children indicate that the impact of daily versus intermittent supplementation is similar. A study amongst Indonesian pre-school children who were supplemented under programme conditions showed that the compliance with supplement intake during a 10-week period was quite high at about 70% and that prevalence of anaemia was reduced from 37% to 16% (Palupi et al 1997). Until now, no studies have been published on the comparison of weekly versus daily supplementation in infants. However, preliminary data are available of a study amongst Vietnamese infants. This study compared a daily supplementation of 8 mg iron, 5 mg zinc and 330 μg retinol with a weekly supplementation of 20 mg iron, 17 mg zinc and 1700 μg retinol under double-blind, placebo controlled conditions. The two intervention groups had similar haemoglobin values at the start of the study (110–112 g/L). After 3 months of supplementation, the increase in haemoglobin concentration was similar (6–7 g/L higher compared to placebo) in both treatment groups (Thu 1997). Before making decisions on the initiation of large scale programmes, the effectiveness of supplementation on a weekly or daily basis needs to be investigated further.

Discussion

To prevent early iron deficiency, breastfeeding should possibly continue for 4–6 months because it is a source of highly-bioavailable iron. If possible, complementary foods for infants should contain meat, fish or liver to assure uptake of iron with a high bioavailability. If meat/fish are not available or too expensive, other locally-available and acceptable foods that are rich in iron should be identified for the promotion of complementary feeding. Furthermore, fortified foods should be fed on a daily basis. Optimal levels of

fortification should be investigated, both for usage in industrialized as well as in developing countries. Research is also needed to develop acceptable and affordable high-quality complementary foods for developing countries.

In countries where iron deficiency anaemia amongst infants is common (prevalence > 20%) iron supplementation programmes should be initiated. For any implementation of iron supplementation during infancy other nutrients such as vitamin A and zinc should be considered because of the generally poor quality diet. The impact of weekly and daily supplementation was shown to be similar in one study. More information from additional studies is needed before considering application in supplementation schemes.

The high prevalence of anaemia amongst infants younger than 6 months of age in Indonesia (see Fig. 15.1) suggests that there are factors other than low iron dietary content and availability causing iron deficiency. In developing countries, the influence of factors such as early additional feeding, quality and quantity of breast milk, maternal iron status and infectious diseases should be further investigated.

Iron deficiency amongst infants cannot be seen in isolation. Attention has to be given to pregnant mothers to assure adequate iron status of both mothers and their infants.

References

ACC/SCN. (1991) Controlling iron deficiency (Nutrition policy paper no.9). Geneva: United Nations Administrative Committee on Coordination: Subcommittee on Nutrition.

ACC/SCN. (1992) Second report on the world nutrition situation. Vol 1. Global and regional results. Geneva: United Nations Administrative Committee on Coordination: Subcommittee on Nutrition.

Angeles, I.T., Schultink, J.W., Matulessi, P., Gross, R., Sastroamidjojo, S. (1993) Decreased rate of stunting among anemic Indonesian preschool children through iron supplementation. *Am J Clin Nutr*, 58, 339–342.

Aukett, M.A., Parks, Y.A., Scott, P.H., Warburton, B.A. (1986) Treatment with iron increases weight gain and psychomotor development. *Arch Dis Childh*, 61, 849.

Berger, J., Schneider, D., Dyck, J.L. et al. (1992) Iron deficiency, cell mediated immunity and infection among 6–36 month old children living in rural Togo. *Nutr Res*, 12, 39–49.

Bloem, M.W. (1995) Interdependence of vitamin A and

iron: An important association for programmes of anaemia control. *Proceedings of the Nutrition Society*, 54, 501–508.

Brock, J.H. (1993) Iron and imunity. *J Nutr Immunol*, 2, 47–106.

Calvo, E.B, Gnazzo, N. (1990) Prevalence of iron deficiency in children aged 9–24 months from a large urban area from Argentina. *Am J Clin Nutr*, 52, 534–540.

Centre for Disease Control. (1985) Prevention of lead poisoning in young children: A statement by the Centre for Disease Control. report no 99–2230. Atlanta: CDC.

Colomer, J., Colomer, C., Gutierrez, D., Jubert, A., Nolasco, A., Donat, J., Fernandez-Delgado, R., Donat, F., Alvarez-Dardet, C. (1990) Anemia during pregnancy as a risk factor for infant iron deficiency: Report from the Valencia Infant Anemia Cohort (VIAC) study. *Paediatr Perinat Epidemiol*, 4, 196–204.

Cook, J.D., Reddy, M.B., Burri, J., Juillerat, M.A., Hurrell, R.F. (1997) The influence of different cereal grains on iron absorption from infant cereal foods. *Am J Clin Nutr*, 65, 964–969.

Dallman, P.R. (1990) Progress in the prevalence of iron deficiency in infants. *Acta Paediatr Scan*, 365, 28–37.

Dallman, P.R., Simes, M.A., Stekel, A. (1980) Iron deficiency in infancy and childhood. *Am J Clin Nutr*, 33, 86–118.

Daouda, H., Galan, P., Prual, A., Sekou, H., Hercberg, S. (1991) Iron status in Nigerian mothers and their newborns. *Int J Vitam Nutr Res*, 61, 46–50.

DeMaeyer, E.M. (1989) Preventing and controlling iron deficiency anaemia through primary health care. Geneva: World Health Organization.

Duggan, M.B., Steel, G., Elwys, G., Harbottle, L., Noble, C. (1991) Iron status, energy intake, and nutritional status of healthy young Asian children. *Arch Dis Childh*; 66, 1386–1389.

Fairweather-Tait, S.J., Wharf, S.G., Fox, T.E. (1995) Zinc absorption in infants fed iron-fortified weaning food. *Am J Clin Nutr*, 62, 785–789.

Fomon, S.J., Ziegler, E.E., Serfass, R.E., Nelson, S.E., Frantz, J.A. (1997) Erythrocyte incorporation of iron is similar in infants fed formulas fortified with 12 mg/L or 8 mg/L of iron. *J Nutr*, 127, 83–88.

Gebre-Madhin, M., Birgegard, G. (1981) Serum ferritin in Ethiopian mothers and their newborn infants. *Scan J Haematol*, 27, 247–252.

Gross, R., Schultink, W., Sastroamidjojo, S. (1994) Trends in food consumption and basic needs coverage in rural India. Changes in food consumption in Asia: Effects on production and use of upland crops. CGPRT no.28. Proceedings of a workshop held in Kandy, Sri Lanka October 6–9, 1992.

Hallberg, L. (1981) Bioavailability of dietary iron in man. *Annu Rev Nutr*, 1, 123–148.

Hallberg, L., Brune, M., Erlandson, M. et al. (1991) Calcium effect of different amounts on non-heme iron and heme-iron absorption in humans. *Am J Clin Nutr*, 53, 112–119.

Hallberg, L., Sandström, B., Aggett, P.J. (1993) Iron, Zinc and Other Trace Elements. In: Garrow, J.S., James, W.P.T. (eds.) *Human Nutrition and Dietetics*, 9th edn. Edinburgh: Churchill Livingstone.

Helen Keller International. (1997) Central Java Project: Maternal post-partum vitamin A supplementation: Increased intake of vitamin A rich foods and early childhood survival in Central Java. Special Report. Jakarta: Helen International.

Idjradinata, P., Pollitt, E. (1993) Reversal of developmental delays in iron deficient anaemic infants treated with iron. *Lancet*, 341, 1–4.

Kinmond, S., Aitchison, T.C., Holland, B.M., Jones, J.G., Turner, T.L., Wardrop, C.A.J. (1993) Umbilical cord clamping and preterm infants: A randomized trial. *BMJ*, 306, 172–175.

Lawless, J.W., Latham, M.C., Stephenson, L.S., Kinoti, S.N., Pertet, A.M. (1994) Iron supplementation improves appetite and growth in anemic Kenyan primary school children. *J Nutr*, 124, 645–654.

Liu, X.N., Khang, J., Zhao, L., Viteri, F.E. (1995) Intermittant iron supplementation is efficient and safe in controlling iron deficiency and anemia in preschool children. *Food and Nutrition Bulletin*, 16, 139–146.

Lönnerdal, B. (1989) Trace element absorption in infants as a foundation to setting upper limits for trace elements in infant formulas. *J Nutr*, 119, 1839–1845.

Lozoff, B., Jimenez, E., Wolf, W. (1991) Long-term developmental outcome of infants with iron deficiency. *NEJM*, 325, 687.

Lozoff, B., Wolf, A. W., Jimenez, E. (1996) Iron deficiency anemia and infant development: Effects of extended oral therapy. *J Pediatr*, 129, 382–389.

Mackay, H.M.M, Goodfellow, L. (1931) Nutritional anaemia in infancy, with particular reference to iron deficiency. Medical Research Council Special Report Series 252.

Mills, A.M.E, Tyler, H.A. (1990) Infant feeding practices in Britain. *Health Visitor*, 63, 346–349.

Milman, N., Agger, A.O., Nielsen, O.J. (1994) Iron status markers and serum erythopoietin in 120 mothers and newborn infants. Effect of iron supplementation in normal pregnancy. *Acta Obstet Gunecol Scand*, 73, 200–204.

Morton, R.E., Nysenbaum, A., Price, K. (1988) Iron status in the first year of life. *J Pediatr Gastoenterol Nutr*, 7, 707–712.

Palupi, L., Schultink, W., Achadi, E., Gross, R. (1997) Effective community intervention to improve haemoglobin status in preschoolers receiving once-weekly iron supplementation. *Am J Clin Nutr*, 65, 1057–1061.

Pizarro, F., Yip, R., Dallman, P.R., Olivares, M., Hertrampf, E., Walter, T. (1991) Iron status with different infant feeding regimens: Relevance of screening and prevention of iron deficiency. *J Pediatr*, 118, 687.

Preziosi, P., Prual, P., Galan, P., Daouda, H., Boureima, H., Hercberg, S. (1997) Effect of iron supplementation on the iron status of pregnant women: Consequences for new-borns. *Am J Clin Nutr*, 66, 1178–1182.

Reeves, J.D., Yip, R. (1985) Lack of adverse side-effects of oral ferrous sulphate therapy in 1 year old infants. *Paediatr*, 75, 353–355.

Rios, E., Lipschitz, D.A., Cook, J.D., Smith, N.J. (1975) Relationship of maternal and infants iron stores as assessed by the determination of plasma ferritin. *Pediatrics*, 55, 694–699.

Rosado, J.L., Lopez, P., Munoz, E., Martinez, H., Allen, L.H. (1997) Zinc supplementation reduced morbidity, but neither zinc nor iron supplementation affected growth or body composition of Mexican preschoolers. *Am J Clin Nutr*, 65, 13–19.

Saarinen, U.M., Simes, M.A. (1978) Serum ferritin in the assessment of iron nutrition in healthy infants. *Acta Paediatr Scand*, 67, 741–751.

Schultink, W., Gross, R. (1996) Iron deficiency alleviation in developing countries. *Nutrition Research Reviews*, 9, 281–293.

Schultink, W., Gross, R., Gliwitzki, M., Karyadi, D., Matulessi, P. (1995) Effect of daily vs twice weekly iron supplementation in Indonesian preschool children with low iron status. *Am J Clin Nutr*, 61, 111–115.

Singla, P.N., Chand, S., Khanna, S., Agarwal, K.N. (1978) Effect of maternal anemia on the placenta and the newborn infant. *Acta Paed Scand*, 67, 645–648.

Soemantri, A.G., Pollitt, E., Kim, I. (1985) Iron deficiency anemia and educational achievement. *Am J Clin Nutr*, 42, 1221.

Soewondo, S., Husaini, Pollitt, E. (1989) Effects of iron deficiency on attention and learning processes in preschool children. Bandung, Indonesia. *Am J Clin Nutr*, 50, 667.

Solomons, N.W. (1986) Competitive interaction of iron and zinc in the diet: Consequences for human nutrition. *J Nutr*, 116, 927–935.

Srikantia, S.G., Bhaskaram, C., Prasad, J.S., Krishnachari, K.A.V.R. (1976) Anaemia and the immune response. *Lancet*, I, 1307–1309.

Stevens, D. (1991) Helen Mackay and anaemia in infancy – then and now. *Arch Dis Childh*, 66, 1451–1453.

Stolzfus, R., Hakimi, M., Miller, K.W., Rasmussen, K.M., Dawiesah, S., Habicht, J.P., Dibley, M.J. (1993) High dose vitamin A supplementation of breast-feeding Indonesian mothers: Effects on the vitamin A status of mother and infant. *J Nutr*, 123, 666–675.

Szarfarc, S.C., Berg, G., Santos, A.L.S., de Souza, S.B., Monteiro, C.A. (1996) Prevencao de anemia no primerio ano de vida em centros de saude do municipio de Santo Andre, Sao Paolo. *Jornal de Pediatria*, 72, 329–334.

Tuntawiroon, M., Sritongkul, N., Rossander-Hulten, L., Pleehachinda, R., Suwanik, R., Brune, M., Hallberg, L. (1990) Rice and iron absorption in man, *Eur J Clin Nutr*, 44, 489–497.

Vasquez-Soanne, P., Windom, R., Pearson, H. (1985) Disappearance of iron-deficiency anemia in a high-risk infant population given supplemental iron. *N Eng J Med*, 313, 1239–1240.

Watson, W.S., Hume, R., Moore, M.R. (1980) Oral absorption of lead and iron. *Lancet*, 2, 236–237.

Wharton, B.A. (1990) Milk for babies and children. *BMJ*, 301, 774–775.

Wilson, E.E., Windle, W.F., Alt, H.L. (1941) Deprivation of placental blood as a cause for iron deficiency in infants. *Am J Dis Child*, 62, 320–327.

Yepez, R., Calle, A., Galan, P., Estevez, E., Davila, M., Estrella, R,, Masse-Raimbault, A.M., Hercberg, S. (1987) Iron status in Ecuadorian pregnant women living at 2800 m altitude: Relationship with infant iron status. *Int J Vitam Nutr Res*, 57, 327–332.

Yip, R. (1996) Prevention and control of iron deficiency in developing countries. *Current Issues in Public Health*, 2, 253–263.

Ziegler, E.E., Fomon, S.J., Nelson, S.E. et al. (1990) Cow milk feeding in infancy: Further observations on blood loss from the gastrointestinal tract. *J Pediatr*, 116, 11–18.

16

Magnesium

Gema Ariceta and Juan Rodríguez-Soriano

Introduction

Biological function

Magnesium (MG) is a divalent cation characterized by an atomic number of 12 and an atomic mass of 24.3 daltons (12.3 mg are equivalent to 0.5 mmol or 1 mEq) (Elin 1987). It is widely distributed in nature (Alfrey 1985). In humans, it is mainly present in the intracellular space where it represents the second-most abundant cation after Potassium (K) (Reinhart 1988). The biological significance of Mg is its condition as a co-factor of adenosine triphosphate (ATP) synthesis, which takes place in the mitochondria (Quamme & Dirks 1987). Thus, Mg participates as an activator of as many as 300 enzymes (Gums 1987), including phosphokinases, phosphatases and ATPases (Monserrat et al 1979).

The biological function of Mg is expressed fundamentally in the nervous system (participating in axonal conductivity, synaptic activity and physiology of the motor plate) and in the cardiovascular system (participating in cardiac rhythm and in peripheral resistance) (Gums 1987). Mg is also important in many other organs and systems and, especially, in the modulation of both the secretion and the peripheral action of parathyroid hormone (Anast et al 1976, Freitag et al 1979). Mg metabolism is closely linked to K metabolism, not only because both cations are intracellular and have common regulatory mechanisms (Solomon 1987), but also because Mg regulates the intracellular content of K through its action on Na-K-ATPase (Whang et al 1981).

There is indirect evidence that Mg may play a physiological role in the development of the foetus and maintenance of normal gestation (Husain & Sibley 1993). In animals, but not in humans, Mg deficiency is followed by an increased rate of abortions and malformations (Hurley et al 1976). Also, the possible role of Mg deficiency in the development of neonatal apnoeas, bronchopulmonary dysplasia and sudden infant death syndrome has been speculated (Miller et al 1990).

Body distribution of Mg

Total content of Mg in adult subject of about 70 kg oscilates between 21 and 28 g (875–1200 mmol or 1750–2400 mEq). This represents, approximately, 45 mg of Mg/kg of lean body mass (Quamme & Dirks 1987). Total content of Mg in a newborn infant of 3.5 kg is about 5 g (30 mmol or 60 mEq) (Jukarainen 1971).

Intracellular Mg

More than 99% of body Mg is present inside the cells (Shafik & Dirks 1992). Intracellular Mg is present in bone (68%), skeletal muscle (20%) and other soft tissues (11%). It is not uniformily distributed: a small portion is free and may potentially interchange with plasma Mg. However, the most intracellular Mg is not diffusible and is attached to cellular ligandins (Quamme & Dirks 1987). Intracellular Mg is difficult to measure. It is accepted that measurement of erythrocyte Mg concentration (about three times higher than plasma Mg concentration) is an acceptable indicator of Mg content in other tissues (Elin 1987).

Extracellular Mg

Less than 1% of body Mg is present in the extracellular space, and its concentration is maintained within narrow limits. In an adults, values of 0.85 mmol/L (0.7–1.05 mmol/L) (Reinhart 1988), 1.55 mEq/L (1.4–1.9 mEq/L) (Ducanson & Worth 1990) and 2 mg/dl (1.7–2.4 mg/dl) (González-Revalderría et al 1990) have been reported.

Plasma concentration of Mg is elevated in term newborn infants, and especially in pre-term newborn infants (1.97 ± 0.4 mg/dl) (Ariceta et al 1995). There is an inverse relationship between plasma Mg and either gestational age or birth weight (Tsang & Oh 1970, Nelson et al 1989, Ariceta et al 1955). Plasma Mg is still comparatively higher during the first year of life (1.86 ± 0.2 mg/dl), but soon after infancy it reaches values comparable to those present in adult life (1.7–2.4 mg/dl) (Venkataram et al 1987, Ariceta et al 1995).

Plasma Mg circulates in three separate fractions: about 55–60% is present in ionized form; 20–25% is bound to different salts such as citrate, phosphate, oxalate and sulphate; and the remaining 20–30% is bound to proteins (Alfrey 1985). Of the latter part, about 75% is bound to albumin and the rest is bound to globulins (Kroll & Elin 1985). The sum of ionized and complexed Mg constitutes the diffusible or ultra-filterable form of Mg (UfMg), which is the one that is freely filtered at the glomerulus. Although UfMg concentration in plasma remains almost constant, the proportion of this diffusible form in relation to total Mg increases progressively with age (pre-term newborn infants: 1.08 ± 0.21 mg/dl and 52%, respectively; term newborn infants: 1.07 ± 0.23 mg/dl and 62%, respectively; infants: 1.24 ± 0.17 mg/dl and 66%, respectively; children: 1.18 ± 0.1 mg/dl and 70%, recpectively) (Ariceta et al 1995).

Perinatal Mg metabolism

Mg concentration in amniotic fluid is about 1.7 mg/dl or 0.7 mmol/L. It is known that Mg freely crosses the placental barrier and mainly accumulates in the foetus during the first trimester of pregnancy (Jukarainen 1971). Placental transfer continues during the whole gestation with a daily accumulation of Mg of about 6 mg (Mimouni & Tsang 1991). Transfer of Mg across the placenta depends upon an active transport mechanism, which is necessary to maintain higher foetal than maternal concentrations (Shaw et al 1990). Mg concentration in cord blood oscilates between 1.89 ± 0.36 mg/dl and 2.09 ± 0.2 mg/dl (Jukarainen 1971). Obviously, situations of Mg excess or Mg deficiency in the mother are also reflected in the foetus (Mimouni & Tsang 1991).

Body balance of Mg

Body Mg content depends upon the balance between the amount ingested and the amount excreted, mainly through the kidneys. The Mg filtered through the glomerulus is almost completely re-absorbed along the renal tubules, and this re-absorption is almost complete under circumstances of poor intake. However, Mg concentration in plasma not only depends upon the mentioned balance between intake and excretion but also upon the dynamic equilibrium of diffusible Mg between intracellular and extracellular spaces (Shafik & Dirks 1992).

Intake of Mg

The standard diet in Western countries provides enough Mg to fulfil normal daily requirements. Foods richer in Mg are bran, peanuts, soy beans, wheats, rice, chocolate and seafood (Gums 1987). Mg content in human milk is about 25–35 mg/dl and in cow's-milk-adapted formula is about 40–50 mg/dl (Lönnerdal 1997). However, significant differences in plasma Mg concentration do not exist between the two types of infant feeding (Lönnerdal 1997).

The daily requirements of Mg increase with age and are depicted in Table 16.1.

Table 16.1 — Daily requirements of magnesium

Age	Daily requirements
Very pre-term newborn infant	20 mg/kg (Giles et al 1990)
Pre-term newborn infant	10 mg/kg (Koo & Tsang 1991)
Term newborn infant – Infant 4 months	30 mg (Fomon & Nelson 1993)
Infant 4–12 months	40 mg (Fomon & Nelson 1993)
Child 1–18 years	6 mg/kg (National Research Council 1989)
Adult	300 mg (National Research Council 1989)

Intestinal absorption of Mg

About 40% of ingested Mg is absorbed along the gut, mainly in proximal parts of the small intestine (Alfrey 1985, Elin 1987). Newborn infants, and especially pre-term infants, have a high capacity for intestinal absoption of Mg (Lönnerdal 1997).

The mechanisms governing intestinal absorption of Mg are still scarcely known (Elin 1987). It is accepted that there are two distinct systems of intestinal transport. The one system appears to depend on a saturable carrier present in the luminal membrane, which probably is altered genetically in congenital chronic hypomagnesaemia (Salet et al 1966, Paunier et al 1968). The second system is not saturable and may transport Mg through the paracellular spaces by gradient-mediated diffusion. A third transport system may be operative in humans, because as Shafik & Dirks (1992) showed in experimental animals, Mg may also follow water absorption passively through the paracellular channels.

The factor regulating intestinal absorption of Mg are largely unknown. Mg absorption is influenced by the food content not only of Mg but also of calcium, K proteins and carbohydrates (Norman et al 1981). In this sense, the absorption of Mg may be altered by the formation of intraluminal complexes containing fitate (Reinhart 1988). Several hormones (parathyroid hormone, 1.25 $(OH)_2$ & vitamin D_3, aldosterone, growth hormone, calciotionin) may also play a regulatory role (Ferment & Touitou 1988).

Renal homeostasis of Mg

Mg filtered through the glomerulus is almost completely re-absorbed along the renal tubules. Of approximately 2500 mg of Mg filtered each day in the adult, only about 3% is excreted in the urine. The tubular handling of Mg has been characterized by micro-puncture and micro-perfusion experiments (Quamme & Dirks 1987). The proximal convoluted tubule reclaims 5–15%, which is considerably less than fractional re-absorption of sodium or calcium. Re-absorption takes place trans-cellularly, following the favourable trans-epithelial Mg concentration gradient resulting from water absorption. The thick ascending limb of the loop of Henle has a major role in the re-absorption of Mg, and it absorbs 70–80% of the filtered Mg. This re-absorption is mainly passive and depends upon the favourable trans-epithelial electric gradient. Recently a paracellular protein called paracellin 1 has been proposed to be involved in controlling Mg permeability at this level. The distal convoluted tubule only re-absorbs the remaining 10–15%, but this re-absorption is especially important because it determines the final amount of Mg present in the urine. In this part of the nephron, Mg is trans-celullarly re-absorbed by an active mechanism (Cole & Quamme 2000). Overall, tubular re-absorption of Mg is a process that is quantitatively limited: maximal rate of tubular re-absorption or MgTm (magnesium thulium) is estimated to be about 1.4 mg/dl of glomerular filtrate (Rude et al 1980).

Renal homeostasis of Mg is regulated by many hormonal and non-hormonal factors. The hormonal factors interact to modify either the trans-epithelial electric gradient or the tubular permeability at the level of the loop of Henle or the mechanism of active transport at the level of the distal convoluted tubule (Ferment & Touitou 1988). Parathyroid hormone, calciotonin, glucagons, vasopressin and insulin increase tubular re-absorption of Mg. The role of aldosterone is misunderstood, but Mg re-absorption follows sodium reabsorption: it increases under conditions of volume depletion and decreases under conditions of volume expansion.

The non-hormonal factors include concentration of Mg in the tubular lumen, acid-base equilibrium and plasma concentrations of K and inorganic phosphate. Tubular re-absorption of Mg is closely linked to that of calcium. It has been shown recently that epithelial cells of Henle's loop and distal convoluted tubule have receptors that sense the extracellular concentration of both Mg^{2+} and Ca^{2+} (Quamme 1997).

Daily excretion is about 120–140 mg in adults (Quamme & Dirks 1987). In healthy individuals, the urine excretion of Mg closely reflects the body content of Mg and becomes almost nil under conditions of Mg deficiency (Shafik & Dirks 1992). Urinary excretion in normal children oscillates between 1.6–2.8 mg/kg body weight (Paunier et al 1970, Ghazali & Barratt 1974, Hernández Macro et al 1988, Rodríguez Soriano et al 1987). Normal values for the U_{Mg}:U_{Cr} ratio (mg/mg) change with age and vary between 0.13 ± 0.8 in infants and 0.08 ± 0.4 in children (Ariceta et al 1996). The raised value observed during infancy does not represent a higher excretion of Mg, but is related to diminished excretion of creatinine per unit of lean body mass in this age period. In fact, fractional excretion of Mg remains quite constant during infancy and childhood: 1.7 (0.38–8.2%) in neonates, 3.8 ± 2.1% in infants, and 3.9 ± 1.7% in children (Ariceta et al 1996).

Practice and procedures

Hypomagnesaemia

Definition

The term *hypomagnesaemia* should be applied to situations in which plasma Mg concentration is situated below 2 standard deviations (SD) of normal values for age. Therefore, the authors define hypomagnesaemia in infants and children above 3 months of age when plasma Mg concentration is situated below 1.4 mg/dl, and in infants below 3 months of age when plasma Mg concentration is situated below 1.6 mg/dl (Ariceta et al 1995, 1996). Hypomagnesaemia may result from insufficient intake or from excessive losses of Mg (Table 16.2). the following syndromes are especially relevant during infancy and childhood.

Transient neonatal hypomagnesaemia

Transient neonatal hypomagnesaemia is often observed in infants born to diabetic mothers (Jukärainen 1971) and in low-birth-weight infants (Tsang & Oh 1970), as well it often coexists with hyperphosphataemia (Mimouni & Tsang 1991). Generally, the disorder corrects itself spontaneously but on occasion it may require the therapeutic administration of Mg (Fomon & Nelson 1993).

Congenital chronic hypomagnesaemia

Congenital chronic hypomagnesaemia, also called *familial hypomagnesaemia with secondary hypocalcaemia*, constitutes

Table 16.2 — Aetiology of hypomagnesaemia

Nutritional deficiency
Alcoholism
Protein-calorie malnutrition
Prolonged fluid or total parenteral therapy
Insufficient Mg intake during pregnancy or
lactation
Bulimia and anorexia nervosa

Digestive
Prolonged gastric suction
Malabsorption syndromes (celiac disease,
pancreatic insufficiency, Crohn's disease, ulcerative
colitis, etc.)
Short-bowell syndrome
Abuse of laxatives
Colon neoplasias
Congenital chronic hypomagnesaemia

Renal
Congenital 'Mg-losing' tubulopathies (isolated
renal hypomagnesaemia, Bartter's syndrome,
Gitelmans syndrome, familial hypomagnesaemia-
hypercalciuria syndrome)
Post-tubular necrosis
Post-obstructive uropathy
Distal renal tubular acidosis

Endocrine
Hyperaldosteronism
Hyperparathyroidism
Hyperthyroidism

Drugs
Diuretics
Aminoglycosides
Amphotericin B
Cysplatinum
Cyclosporin A

Associated to other electrolyte disorders
Hypercalcaemia
Hypervolaemia
Uremia
Hyperglycaemia
Phosphate depletion
Alcohol administration

Miscellaneous causes
Transient neonatal hypomagnesaemia
Chronic renal insufficiency during infancy
Porfiria associated with the syndrome of
inappropriate ADH secretion
Exchange-transfusion or repeat transfusions with
citrated blood
Burns

Adapted from Whang (1987), with permission.
ADH = Anti Diuretic Hormone

a rare entity that is characterized by an inherited defect in intestinal absorption of Mg (Salet et al 1966, Paunier et al 1968). Although an X-linked transmission has been suggested (Dudin & Teebi 1987), recent linkage studies have established that the disorder is autosomal recessive with the responsible gene mapping to the long arm of chromosome 9 (9q12–9q22.2) (Walder et al 1997). Identification of gene mutations or deletions will probably confirm the current hypothesis that this disease represents an inherited defect of the saturable Mg carrier present in the luminal membrane of the small intestine. Both histology and enzymatic components of the intestinal mucosa have been found strictly normal.

Clinically it presents in early infancy with generalized, convulsions hypocalcaemia and hypomagnesaemia, although occasionally it may have more delayed onset (Romero et al 1996). Convulsions are refractory to administration of calcium salts, and their correction requires the simultaneous administrations of Mg salts. Oral administration of Mg salts must be maintained long-life to prevent symptoms. Prognosis is favourable if diagnosis is made early enough. There is an exceptional case reported associating this entity with a defect in renal transport of Mg (Matzkin et al 1989).

Hypomagnesaemia of renal origin
A renal origin must be suspected when Mg is present in the urine despite the coexistence of significant hypomagnesaemia. This situation may have an intrinsic renal origin or be secondary to metabolic and endocrine causes or administrations of drugs and toxins (Rodríguez Soriano et al 1987).

Clinical findings

Clinical findings of hypomagnesaemia generally appear when plasma Mg concentration drops below 1.2 mg/dl. Many symptoms are not directly related to hypo-magnesaemia but are secondary to associated hypo-kalaemia or hypocalcaemia. Table 16.3 summarizes the clinical signs and symptoms and its possible pathogenic mechanism. It must be recognized that states of severe Mg deficiency may remain completely asymptomatic (Quamme & Dirks 1987).

Diagnosis

Mg deficiency remains an undiagnosed disorder. Mg determination in plasma is not a routine determination in many centres so clinical findings may be mistakenly attributed to associated hypokalaemia or hypocalcaemia (Elin 1987). Also, plasma Mg determination only partly

Table 16.3 — Clinical and biochemical findings in hypomagnesaemia

	Symptom	Mechanism
Biochemical	Hypocalcaemia	Impaired PTH secretion
		PTH resistance of end organs
		Resistance to vitamin D
	Hypokalaemia	Renal K wasting
Neuromuscular	Muscular irritability	Hypocalcaemia
	Hyper-reflexia	Hypomagnesaemia
	Tetany	
	Muscle weakness	
	Nystagmus, dizziness, ataxia	
	Depression, psychosis	
Cardiovascular	Arrythmias	Hypocalcaemia
	Increased sensitivity to digitalis	Hypomagnesaemia
	Arterial hypertension	
Digestive	Dysphagia	Muscular irritability
Endocrine	Bone resistance to PTH	
	Hyper-reninism	
	Hyperaldosteronism	
	Reduced lipolysis	
Haematological	Anaemia	Diminished erythrocyte half-life

Adapted from Quamme & Dirks (1987), with permission. PTH = Parathyroid Hormone, K = Potassium.

reflects the intracellular content of Mg, and many subclinical deficiencies may remain unapparent. Techniques designed to determine intracellular Mg content (i.e., selective microelectrodes, isotopic markers, nuclear magnetic resonance) are not yet applicable to patients (Shafik & Dirks 1992).

In clinical practice, a state of Mg deficiency is always diagnosed by the presence of hypomagnesaemia. The simultaneous determination of urinary Mg permits suspicion of its pathogenesis. If urinary Mg excretion is low or nil, a carencial or digestive origin is probably the cause. If Mg present in the urine in appreciable quantities, the hypomagnesaemia is probably of renal origin (Rodríguez Soriano & Vallo 1986). In situations of hypomagnesaemia of carencial or digestive origin, the intracellular content of Mg may be estimated by a parenteral loading test: the lower the proportional amount of Mg excreted in the urine the higher the intracellular deficit of that cation (Thoren 1963, Caddell 1975). In situations of hypomagnesaemia of renal origin, the rate of tubular Mg re-absorption may be estimated by standard clearance techniques during an infusion of Mg sulphate (Rude et al 1980).

This study permits a functional classifications of the different Mg-losing tubulopathies (Rodríguez Soriano et al 1987, Scheiman et al 1999).

Therapy

Replenishment of intracellular Mg stores remains largely empirical. The amount of Mg to be administered is usually based on an estimated deficit of 1–2 mEq/kg body weight. In many circumstances oral administration of 10–20 mg/kg/day of a Mg salt (hydroxide, lactate, chloride, citrate, glycerophosphate, etc.) may be sufficient. It must be taken into account that only about 50% of administered Mg is being absorbed and that large doses have a noxious cathartic effect. In cases of symptomatic severe hypomagnesaemia, it may be necessary to give Mg parenterally in the form of Mg sulphate. About half of the calculated deficit must be given during 24 h and the remaining amount during the following 2–4 days (Rodríguez Soriano & Vallo 1986). In patients with chronic deficiency of digestive origin, parenteral Mg supplements should be given repeatedly to avoid states of symptomatic hypomagnesaemia (Gums 1987).

Table 16.4 — Aetiology of hypermagnesaemia

Renal insufficiency
    Acute (oliguric)
    Chronic

Acute metabolic acidosis
    Ketoacidosis
    Addison's disease
    Hypothyroidism
    Pheochromocytoma

Exogenous Mg administration
    Laxatives
    Antacids
    Enemas
    Solutions for irrigation of urinary bladder
    As parenteral Mg therapy (myocardial ischaemia, arrythmias, eclampsia, placental insufficiency, neonatal pulmonary hypertension, etc.)

Hypermagnesaemia

Definition

The term *hypermagnesaemia* should be applied to situations in which plasma Mg concentration is situated above 2 SD of normal values for age. Therefore, the authors define hypermagnesaemia in infants below 1 year of age when plasma Mg concentration is situated above 2.5 mg/dl and in infants and children above 1 year of age when plasma Mg concentration is situated above 2.0 mg/dl (Ariceta et al 1995, 1996).

Aetiology

Hypermagnesaemia usually follows the administration of large doses of Mg in patients with diminished renal function (Table 16.4). in neonates, the authors have observed this situation following Mg sulphate administration given as therapy for neonatal pulmonary hypertension. It may also be observed transiently following perinatal asphyxia (Caddell & Reed 1989), as the consequence of transcellular Mg exit (Whong et al 1986).

Clinical findings

Moderate elevation of plasma concentration is accompanied by only a few signs such as nausea and vomiting, but marked hypermagnesaemia is followed by severe neurological and cardiovascular impairment (Table 16.5).

Therapy

In situations of moderate hypermagnesaemia it may be sufficient to stop the administration of the offending Mg salt and to increase diuresis by administering a loop diuretic such as furosemide. However, in cases of severe hypermagnesaemia the patient is in risk of immediate death and therapy must include intravenous administration of calcium gluconate and urgent initiation of peritoneal dialysis if there is

Table 16.5 — Clinical and biochemical findings in hypermagnesaemia

	Symptom	**Mechanism**
Biochemical	Hypocalcaemia	Impaired PTH secretion Renal Ca loss
Neuromuscular	Neuromuscular depression Muscular weakness Hypo-reflexia Cephalalgia Dizziness Depression Lethargy	Impaired nerve transmission Hypermagnesaemia Altered post-synaptic response
Cardiovascular	Facial redness Arrhythmias	Hypermagnesaemia Hypocalcaemia
Digestive	Nausea Vomiting	

Adapted from Quamme & Dirks (1987), with permission.

evidence of impaired renal function (Shafik & Dirks 1992).

Reference

Alfrey, A.C. (1985) Disorders of Magnesium Metabolism. In: Seldin D.W., Giebisch, G. (eds.) *The Kidney: Physiology and Pathophysiology*, pp. 1281–1295. New York: Raven Press.

Anast, C.S., Winnacker, J.L., Forte, L.R., Burns, T.W. (1976) Impaired released of the Parathyroid hormone in Magnesium deficiency. *J Clin Endocrinol Metabol*, 42, 707–717.

Ariceta, G., Rodríguez Soriano, J., Vallo, A. (1995) Magnesium homeostasis in premature and full-term neonates. *Pediatr Nephrol*, 9, 423–427.

Ariceta, G., Rodríguez Soriano, J., Vallo, A. (1996) Renal magnesium handling in infants and children. *Acta Paediatr*, 85, 1019–1023.

Caddell, J.L. (1975) The Magnesium load test: A design for infants. *Clin Pediatr*, 14, 449–452.

Caddell, J.L., Reed, G.F. (1989) Unrealiability of plasma magnesium values in axphysiated neonates. *Magnesium*, 8, 11–16.

Cole, D.C., Quamme, G.A. (2000) Inherited disorders of renal magnesium handling. *J Am Soc Nephrol*, 11, 1937–1947.

Ducanson, G.O., Worth, H.G.J. (1990) Determination of reference intervals for serum Magnesium. *Clin Chem*, 36, 756–758.

Dudin, K.L., Teebi, A.S. (1987) Primary hypomagnesaemia. *Eur J Pediatr*, 146, 303–305.

Elin, R.J. (1987) Assesment of Magnesium status. *Clin Chem*, 33, 1965–1970.

Ferment, O., Touitou, Y. (1988) Régulation hormonale et interrelations métaboliques du magnésium. *Presse Méd*, 17, 584–587.

Fomon, S.J., Nelson, S.E. (1993) Calcium, Phosphorus, Magnesium and Sulfur. In: Fomon, S.J. (eds.) *Nutrition of Normal infants*, 11, pp. 192–218. St Louis: Mosby Year Book.

Freitag, J.J., Martin, K.J., Conrades, M.B., Balanin-Font, E., Teitelbaum, S., Khahr, S., et al. (1979) Evidence for squeletal resistance to Parathyroid hormone in Magnesium deficiency. *J Clin Invest*, 64, 1238–1244.

Ghazali, S., Barratt, T.M. (1974) Urinary excretion of Calcium and Magnesium iin children. *Arch Dis Child*, 49, 97–101.

Giles, M.M., Laing, I.A., Elton, R.A., Robins, J.B., Sanderson, M., Hume, R. (1990) Magnesium metabolism in preterm infants: Effects of Calcium, Magnesium and Phosphorus and of postanal and gestational age. *J Pediatr*, 117, 147–154.

González-Revalderría, J., García Bermejo, A., Menchén, A., Fernández Rodríguez, E. (1990) Biologycal variation of Zn, Cu and Mg in serum of healthy subjects. *Clin Chem*, 36, 2140–2141.

Gums, J.G. (1987) Clinical significance of Magnesium: A review. *Drug Int Clin Phat*, 21, 240–246.

Hernández-Macro, R., Nuñez, F., Martínez, C., Fons, J., Peris, A., Brines, J. (1988) Excreción urinaria de Calcio, Magnesio, ácido úrico y ácido oxálico en niños normales. *An Esp Pediatr*, 29, 99–104.

Hurley, L.S., Cosens C., Theriault, L.L. (1976) Terratogenic effects of magnesium deficiency in rats. *J Nutr*, 106, 1254–1260.

Husain, S.M., Sibley, C.P. (1993) Magnesium and pregnancy. *Miner Electrolyte Metab*, 19, 296–307.

Jukärainen, E. (1971) Plasma Magnesium levels during the first five days of life. *Acta Paediatr Scand*, 222(Suppl), 1–58.

Koo, W.W., Tsang, R.C. (1991) Mineral requirements of low-birth-weight infants. *J Am Coll Nutr*, 10, 474–486.

Kroll, M.H., Elin, R.J. (1985) Relationships between Magnesium and protein concentrations in serum. *Clin Chem*, 31, 244–246.

Lönnerdal, B. (1997) Effects of milk and milk components on Calcium, Magnesium and trace element absorption during infancy. *Physiol Rev*, 77, 643–669.

Lönnerdal, B., Yuen, M., Glazier, C., Litov, R.E. (1993) Magnesium bioavailability from human milk, cow milk and infant formula in suckling rat pups. *Am J Clin Nutr*, 58, 392–397.

Matzkin, H., Lotan, D., Boichis, H. (1989) Primary hypomagnesemia with a probable double magnesium transport defect. *Nephron*, 52, 83–86.

Miller, J.K., Schneider, M.D., Ramsey, N., White, P.K., Bell, M.C. (1990) Effects of hypomagnesemia on reactivity of bovine and ovine platelets: Possible relevance to infantile apnea and sudden infant death syndrome. *J Am Coll Nutr*, 9, 58–64.

Mimouni, F., Tsang, R.C. (1991) Perinatal magnesium metabolism: personal data and challenges for the 1990s. *Magnesium Res*, 4(2), 109–117.

Monserrat, J.L., Rapado, A., Castrillo, J.M. et al (1979) Nephrocalcinosis as a clinical syndrome. Study of 77 cases. *Med Clin* (Barc), 73(8), 305–311.

National Research Council. (1989) *Recommended Dietary Allowances*, 10th edn. Washington DC: National Academy Press.

Nelson, N., Finnström, O., Larsson, L. (1989) Plasma ionized Calcium, Phosphate and Magnesium in preterm and small for gestational age infants. *Acta Paediatr Scand*, 78, 351–357.

Norman, D.A., Fordtran, J.S., Brinkley, R.J. (1981) Jejunal and ileal adaptation to alterations in dietary Calcium. Changes in Calcium and Magnesium absorption and pathogenetic role of Parathyroid hormone and 1,25-dihydroxyvitamin D. *J Clin Invest*, 67, 1599–1603.

Paunier, L., Borgeaud, M., Wyss, M. (1970) Urinary excretion of Magnesium and Calcium in normal children. *Helv Acta Paediatr*, 25, 577–584.

Paunier, L., Radde, I.C., Koch, S.W., Conen, P.E., Fraser, D. (1968) Primary hypomagnesemia with secondary hypocalcemia in an infant. *Pediatr*, 41, 385–402.

Quamme, G.A., Dirks, J.H. (1987) Magnesium Metabolism. In: Maxwell, M.H., Kleeman, C.R., Naims, R.G. (eds.) *Clinical Disorders of Fluid and Electrolyte metabolism*, 13, pp. 297–316, 4th edn. New York: McGraw-Hill.

Reinhart, R.A. (1988) Magnesium metabolism. *Arch Int Med*, 148, 2415–2420.

Rodríguez Soriano, J., Vallo, A. (1987) Hypomagnesemia. *An Esp Pediatr*, 24, 27–35.

Rodríguez Soriano, J., Vallo, A., García-Fuentes, M. (1987) Hypomagnesaemia of hereditary renal origin. *Pediatr Nephrol*, 1, 465–472.

Romero, R., Meacham, L.R., Winn, K.T. (1996) Isolated Magnesium malabsorption in a 10-year boy. *AJG*, 91, 611–613.

Rude, R.K., Bethune, J.E., Singer, F.R. (1980) Renal tubular maximum for Magnesium in normal, hyperparathyroid and hypoparathyroid man. *J Clin Endocrinol Metab*, 51, 1425–1431.

Salet, J., Polonovsky, C., de Gouyou, F., Peau, G., Melekian, B., Fournet, J.P. et al. (1966) Tétanie hypocalcémique récidivante par hypomagnésémie congénitale. *Arch Franc Péd*, 23, 749–768.

Scheinman, S.J., Guay-Woodford, L.M., Thakker, R.V. et al (1999) Genetic disorders of renal electrolyte transport. *N Eng J Med* 340(15), 1177–1187.

Shafik, I.M., Dirks, J.H. (1992) Hypo- and Hyper-magnesaemia. In: Cameron, S., Davidson, A.M., Grünfeld, J.P., Kerr, D., Ritz, E. (eds.) *Oxford Textbook of Clinical Nephrology*. Oxford: Oxford University Press. 143, pp. 1802–1821.

Shaw, A.J., Mughal, M.Z., Mohammed, T., Maresh, M.J.A, Sibley, C.P. (1990) Evidence for active maternofetal transfer of Magnesium across the in situ perfussed rat placenta. *Pediatr Res*, 27, 622–625.

Solomon, R. (1987) The relationships between disorders of K and Mg homeostasis. *Seminars Nephrol*, 7, 253–262.

Thoren, L. (1963) Magnesium deficiency in gastrointestinal fluid loss. *Acta Chir Scand*, 306(suppl), 1–65.

Tsang, R.C., Oh, W. (1970) Serum Magnesium levels in low birth weight infants. *AJDC*, 120, 44–48.

Venkataraman, P.S., Kirk, M.S., Tsang, R.C., Wen-Chen, I. (1987) Calcium, Phosphorus, Magnesium and Calcitonin concentrations in the serum and cerebrospinal fluid of children. *AJDC*, 141, 751–753.

Walder, R.Y., Shalev, H., Brennan, T.M., Carmi, R., Elbedour, K., Scott, D.A. et al. (1997) Familial hypomagnesemia maps to chromosome 9q, not to the X chromosome: Genetic linkage mapping and analysis of a balanced translocation breakpoint. *Hum Mol Genet*, 6, 1491–1497.

Whang, R. (1987) Magnesium deficiency: Pathogenesis, prevalence and clinical implications. *Am J Med*, 82(3A suppl), 24–29.

Whang, R., Oei, T.O., Aikawa, J.K. (1981). Magnesium and Potassium interrelationships experimental and clinical. *Acta Med Scand*, 647(Suppl), 139–144.

Whong, N.L.M., Quamme, G.A., Dirks, J.H. (1986) Effects of acid-bases disturbances on renal handling of Magnesium in the dog. *Clin Sci*, 70, 277–284.

17

Nutritional antioxidants: Modulation in malnutrition and requirements

Katja Becker, Stephan Gromer and R. Heiner Schirmer

Abbreviations

EGRAC	erythrocyte glutathione reductase activation coefficient
FAD	flavin adenine dinucleotide
FMN	fllavin mononucleotide
G6PDH	glucose-6-phosphate dehydrogenase
GPX	glutathione peroxidase
GR	glutathione reductase
GSSG	glutathione disulphide
NADPH	nicotinomide adenine dinucleotide phosphate
PEM	protein energy malnutrition
ROS	reactive oxygen species
PUFAs	polyun-staturated fatty acids
SOD	superoxide dismutase

Introduction

Protein energy malnutrition (PEM) represents one of the most severe socio-economic and health problems in the world. Clinically, it manifests in various forms. One of them, *marasmus*, is characterized by a severe deficit of body mass—according to the Wellcome classification (Wellcome Trust Working Party 1970) the deficit is < 60% of the corresponding weight-for-age standards. A second form of PEM is *kwashiorkor*, which is defined as 60–80% of weight-for-age standards in combination with generalized oedema. The full clinical picture of kwashiorkor includes skin lesions, red hair colouring and partial loss of hair, a fatty liver, apathy and irritability. Kwashiorkor is typically precipitated by infections. A third form of PEM, namely *marasmic kwashiorkor*, is characterized by a mixed clinical picture: the children are below 60% weight-for-age *and* have oedema (Suskind et al 1990).

Marasmus seems to quite clearly result from a quantitative lack of nutrients; once the clinical problems of the acute phase, often dehydration and infection, are under control, the prognosis is rather good. This is different, however, for kwashiorkor and marasmic kwashiorkor. The clinical management of these conditions is still highly insufficient; the lethality of kwashiorkor ranges between 10–50%, and is even higher for marasmic kwashiorkor (Golden 1994). During the last 40 years this situation has not significantly improved. As indicated in a study done by Erinoso et al (1993), the lethality of mal-nourished children in Nigeria was 47% for kwash-iorkor, 60% for marasmic kwashiorkor, and still as high as 35% for marasmus. These worrying numbers are certainly due to socio-economic problems but also to the fact that we do not know enough about aetiology, pathogenesis and pathophysiology of kwashiorkor.

Historical background

Kwashiorkor was described for the first time by Cicely Williams working in the Gold Coast Area. Williams identified a relationship between the low-protein maize diet of the children and the occurrence of the syndrome (Williams 1935). Since then, kwashiorkor has been considered to be due to protein deficiency and relative carbohydrate excess. However, as shown by Golden et al (1980), the clinical picture of kwashiorkor, especially oedema formation, does not correlate with plasma protein concentrations; hypoproteinosis can therefore not be the only causative factor.

Consecutive results of Hendrickse (1988) suggested that the hepatotoxic effects of aflatoxins might be involved in the pathogenesis of kwashiorkor. In humid and moist climates, aflatoxins are generated by extensive fungal growth on stored grain or crops. However, the pathological changes of acute aflatoxinosis involve scattered areas of hepatic necrosis and not, as expected, fatty liver development; in addition, a number of studies have shown that aflatoxin contamination of food or urinary aflatoxin excretion do not correlate with the frequency of kwashiorkor (Househam & Hundt 1991).

Because of this, another hypothesis by Golden & Ramdath (1987) has attracted interest. They ask whether an imbalance between oxidative stress and antioxidant capacity could be responsible for the development of kwashiorkor. Toxic derivatives of oxygen and nitrogen, like hydrogen peroxide, nitric oxide, superoxide radicals and hydroxyl radicals, are continuously generated in the human body (Table 17.1). These so called 'reactive oxygen species' (ROS) or 'reactive nitrogen species' (RNS) are, for example, produced as a by-product in cell respiration, as defence agents against infections, during detoxification of xenobiotics, and by UV-radiation. These compounds can directly or indirectly oxidize biological macromolecules. Oxidation of proteins can impair enzyme function and induce false crosslinking. Lipid peroxidation disturbs membrane integrity, and oxidative DNA-damage (El Ghazali et al 1990) can impair protein synthesis and cell division. Against this oxidative stress as a whole but

Table 17.1 — Reactive oxygen and nitrogen species

Reactive Oxygen Species (ROS)

Radicals	Non-Radicals
Superoxide, O_2^{-}	Hydrogen peroxide, H_2O_2
Hydroxyl, $OH\cdot$	Hypochlorous acid, HOCl
Peroxyl, $RO_2\cdot$	Ozone, O_3
Alkoxyl, $RO\cdot$	Singlet oxygen, $^1\Delta g$
Hydroperoxyl, $HO_2\cdot$	

Reactive Nitrogen Species (RNS)

Radicals	Non-Radicals
	Nitrosyl, NO^{-}
Nitric oxide, $NO\cdot$	Nitrous acid, HNO_2
	Nitroxide, NO
Nitrogen dioxide, $NO_2\cdot$	Dinitrogen tetroxide, N_2O_4
	Dinitrogen trioxide, N_2O_3
	Peroxynitrite, $ONOO^{-}$
	Peroxynitrous acid, ONOOH
	Nitronium cation, (Nitryl), NO_2^{+}
	Alkyl peroxynitrites, ROONO

Data from Halliwell (1996).

also against individual ROS a number of biochemical defence systems have evolved that include anti-oxidant enzymes and low molecular weight anti-oxidants. It should be kept in mind that the definition of a compound as an antioxidant is not very precise and is sometimes arbitrary. Antioxidants are redox active compounds, precursors, or parts of redox-active systems. This implies that a given 'antioxidant' can become a pro-oxidant in a given metabolic constellation (Sies 1991).

An imbalance between ROS generated and the available antioxidant capacity might play a significant role in the pathophysiology of PEM, particularly in kwashiorkor (Ashôur et al 1999, Fechner et al 2001). The syndrome was, for example, found to be associated with low concentrations of vitamin E, carotene, zinc, selenium, or glutathione. It was reported further to be associated with a reduced $NADPH: NADP^{+}$ ratio, low glutathione peroxidase and elevated glutathione-S-transferase activities. High concentrations of circulating iron as a possible source of oxidative stress has been reported as well (Golden & Ramdath 1987, Becker et al 1995b, Dempster et al 1995).

Supplying PEM patients adequately with nutritional antioxidants and the avoidance of additional oxidant intake is likely to support recovery from PEM as well as have preventive effects (Halliwell et al 1992, Aruoma 1994).

Practice and procedures

Antioxidants in the blood

The blood is rich in antioxidants and because it is an easily-accessible organ it is possible to determine numerous blood antioxidants in PEM. Well-studied examples are: the copper- and zinc-dependent super-oxide dismutase (SOD); the selenium-containing glutathione peroxidase (GPX) and other erythrocyte enzymes; the cysteine peptide glutathione of red blood cells; and ascorbic acid (vitamin C). The albumin/bilirubin system and selenoprotein P are important antioxidants of the blood plasma. The presence of high antioxidant concentrations and activities reflects the fact that blood is exposed to high oxygen tensions not encountered by other organs. A complementary aspect is that blood as a fluid organ can assist other tissues in the detoxification of ROS (Sies 1991).

Alterations of antioxidant concentrations in plasma, serum or erythrocytes of PEM patients as well as recommended daily intakes should be judged with great caution. This is underlined for the following reasons: 1) the concentrations of many blood parameters are often not well regulated; they reflect current nutritional intake and excretion, both of which depend on a variety of other parameters; 2) in mal-nutrition, the onset of muscular wasting can lead to overloading of other tissues and physiological fluids with metabolites and co-factors released from the wasting cells. Thus, although 'normal' values might be measured in acute PEM, deficiency could develop during recovery; 3) oedema formation and resolution can derange the level of blood plasma antioxidants by dilution or concentration; 4) the interpretation of data remains difficult. For example, is reduced enzyme activity due to a co-factor deficiency, to a protein deficiency leading to impaired enzyme synthesis, to protein inactivation by ROS, or to adaptive transcription control?- and 5) depending on the surrounding milieu and the relative concentrations of compounds in reductive pathways, many antioxidants can become pro-oxidants. This list indicates that our practical knowledge vis-à-vis the complex metabolic constellation in PEM is most limited. Ideally one should therefore estimate the deficit of a given nutritional antioxidant and, under regular control of the parameter, slowly make up for this deficit.

In this chapter we summarize how the nutritional antioxidants, which are recognized so far, are altered in malnutrition. The currently accepted treatment of PEM, particularly of marasmus, with fluids, electrolytes, glucose and various drugs is discussed in other chapters of this book.

Antioxidant enzymes and trace elements

Superoxide dismutase (SOD) is responsible for the scavenging of superoxide radicals ($2 O_2^- + 2 H^+ \rightarrow O_2 + H_2O_2$; H_2O_2 is then detoxified by catalase and glutathione peroxidase). Reduction in hepatic levels of copper as well as in erythrocyte SOD, a copper-zinc-dependent enzyme, have been described in PEM patients. The mitochondrial manganese-dependent SOD has not yet been measured in PEM but a marked reduction in hepatic manganese was reported. Zinc concentrations in plasma are reduced in kwashiorkor and marasmic kwashiorkor down to approximately 60% of control values (Golden & Ramdath 1987). In the form of zinc-metallothionein and copper-zinc SOD, zinc is likely to contribute to free radical scavenging *in vivo* (Hemalatha et al 1993).

Cytosolic glutathione peroxidase (GPX) is a selenium-containing enzyme, reducing peroxides at the expense of glutathione. Erythrocyte GPX-activity was found to be reduced in PEM, particularly in kwashiorkor (Golden & Ramdath 1987, Sive et al 1993). In the blood of PEM patients, reduction in activity was also observed for *catalase* — a heme–iron–enzyme which, in addition, needs bound NADPH to be functional. However, the activity of *glutathione-S-transferase* (an enzyme detoxifying peroxides, epoxides and other oxidizing agents using glutathione as a second substrate) was described to be elevated in erythrocytes of kwashiorkor patients (Ramdath & Golden 1993). *Selenium*, a component of the antioxidant enzymes glutathione peroxidase and thioredoxin reductase (Thomas et al 1994, Becker et al 2000), plays a critical role in oxygen metabolism, particularly in the breakdown of H_2O_2 and other peroxides. Selenium is required for the growth of human fibroblasts and other cells in tissue culture; furthermore, it protects from carcinogenic agents and prevents or cures Keshan disease, a condition characterized by myocardial necrosis (Levander & Beck 1999). Blood selenium concentrations are reduced in PEM as reported in a number of studies (Golden & Ramdath 1987, Salih et al 1994). It will be of interest to study if the concentration of selenoprotein P (Persson-Moschos et al 1995)—which contains more than 10 selenocysteine residues and which appears to function as an antioxidant in blood plasma—is also decreased in PEM.

Data on the trace elements zinc and selenium are

Table 17.2 — Reference values and recommended daily intake of (nutritional) antioxidants for healthy children aged 1–3 years

Antioxidant	Reference value	Recommended daily intake
Total protein	60–80 g/L (S)	3–5 g protein/kg[1]
Albumin	40–50 g/L (S)	[see total protein]
Glutathione	2–2.5 mM (E)	[see total protein]
Retinol	200–400 µg/L (P)	250–400 µg retinol equivalent)[2]
β-Carotene	300–800 µg/L (P)	[see retinol]
Ascorbate	4–10 mg/L (P)	20–45 mg
α-Tocopherol	5–9 mg/L (P)	3–5 mg
Riboflavin	100–200 µg/L (P)	0.6–0.8 mg
Ubiquinone-10	0.75 ± 0.26 µg/mL (P)	additional intake not proven to be beneficial
Selenium	0.07–0.14 mg/L (P)	10–60 µg
Zinc	0.6–1.2 mg/L (P)	3–8 mg[3]

Values given in the table represent a synopsis of data taken from various sources (Avery & Lewis 1994, Geigy Scientific Tables 1985 [including recommendations of FAO/WHO; the Food and Nutrition Board, USA; and the Department of Health and Security, UK], van Dusseldorp et al 1996). It should be noted that methodological differences are not accounted for in this table. 1. Protein intake in PEM-patients should gradually be increased from 1.5 g/kg/day upwards. 2. The immediate injection of 100.000–200.000 IU vitamin A or the oral application of 200.000 IU vitamin A for 2 days in PEM patients protects from keratomalacia and blindness. 3. Zinc can be applied as zinc acetate (2 mg/kg/day). P = plasma, S = serum, E = erythrocyte

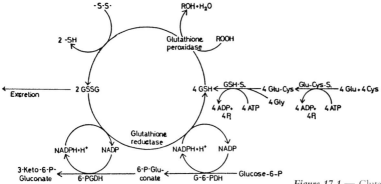

6-PGDH	=	6-Phosphogluconatdehydrogenase
G-6-PDH	=	Glucose-6-Phosphatdehydrogenase
GSH-S	=	Glutathionsynthetase
Glu-Cys-S	=	γ-Glutamyl-Cysteinsynthetase

Figure 17.1 — Glutathione redox cycle in red blood cells. The cycle that utilizes glutathione peroxidase and glutathione reductase provides reducing equivalents for H_2O_2 and organic peroxide detoxification. The small cycles indicate that the reduction of glutathione disulphide is based on the NADPH-regenerating enzymes glucose-6-phosphate dehydrogenase and 6-phosphogluconate dehydrogenase.

given in Table 17.2. Nutritional application of copper and iron should, according to the authors' current knowledge, be avoided in PEM-patients. Although both ions are essential co-factors of antioxidant enzymes, they can act as strong oxidants when not bound to proteins (Zhang et al 1996).

Glutathione reductase (GR) is a homodimeric FAD-dependent enzyme that keeps glutathione to more than 95% in its reduced state using NADPH as the source of reducing equivalents. An overview over the glutathione redox cycle is given in Figure 17.1; Figure 17.2 shows the active site of glutathione reductase. In one study, GR-activity was found to be increased in malnourished patients (Fondu et al 1978). In another study GR-activity per g haemoglobin was similar in controls, marasmic and kwashiorkor patients indicating that GR-protein synthesis was neither significantly impaired nor induced in PEM (Becker et al 1995b). *Glucose-6-phosphate dehydrogenase* (G6PDH) is the key enzyme of the pentose phosphate shunt and, in many cells, the main source for NADPH. This co-enzyme is essential for maintainance of a reducing milieu in the cytosol and for stabilizing the enzyme catalase. The activity of G6PDH was found to be increased or not significantly altered in PEM, indicating that G6PDH deficiency is not correlated with the oxidative disturbances observed (Macdougall et al 1982, Golden & Ramdath 1987, Becker et al 1995b).

Antioxidant proteins do of course not really represent 'nutritional antioxidants'; however, an adequate, slowly-increasing intake of amino acids is important to ensure sufficient protein synthesis.

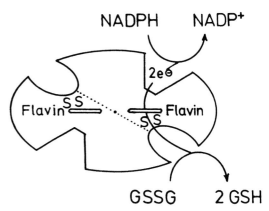

Figure 17.2 — The molecular focus of the antioxidant defence. Shown is the dimeric flavoenzyme glutathione reductase where electrons are transferred from NADPH via FAD and a protein disulphide to glutathione disulphide, which is reduced to give two molecules of glutathione.

Glutathione

The tripeptide glutathione (γ-glutamyl-cysteinyl-glycine) represents the major non-enzymatic intracellular antioxidant (see Fig. 17.1). Glutathione protects cells from oxidizing agents and electrophilic xenobiotics and is involved in a wide range of other metabolic functions like neutrophil locomotion and neuronal receptor modulation (Beutler & Dale 1988, Dringen et al 2000). In kwashiorkor, intraerythrocytic glutathione concentrations have been found to be reduced to 30% of the reference range of 2–2.5 mM (Golden & Ramdath 1987, Becker et al 1995b). These values are close to glutathione concentrations measured in children with inherited glutathione synthetase deficiency. The drastic glutathione depletion strongly supports the hypothesis that a lack in antioxidant capacity might be involved in the pathophysiology of kwashiorkor. Marasmic children have been described to either have normal values (Golden & Ramdath 1987) or to exhibit glutathione deficiency that is milder than in kwashiorkor (Becker et al 1995b). The percentage of oxidized glutathione in total glutathione was normal in all patient groups studied by different authors. Only desperately-ill kwashiorkor children exhibited an increased proportion of glutathione disulphide. However, a decreased $NADPH:NADP^+$ ratio observed in many kwashiorkor patients indicates disturbances in the intracellular redox milieu (Golden & Ramdath 1987).

For glutathione synthesis in PEM, availability of the three amino acids required (glutamate, cysteine, glycine) should be guaranteed by sufficient protein intake; particularly the sulphur containing amino acid cysteine might become rate limiting for glutathione synthesis. As recently shown, the application of glutathione and other cysteine donors like N-acetylcysteine do (Baker 1987, Roediger 1995) support the recovery of the cellular glutathione pool in kwashiorkor has to be investigated in systematic clinical studies (Bray & Taylor 1993, Becker et al unpublished.

Vitamin B₂ (Riboflavin)

Riboflavin is mainly contained in food of high quality like eggs, liver, nuts or grains. Therefore, riboflavin status—estimated, for example, on the basis of the erythrocyte glutathione reductase activation coefficient (EGRAC) (Becker et al 1991, Bates 1992)—has often been used as a parameter to quantify malnutrition biochemically. Riboflavin is needed in the human body for the synthesis of flavin mononucleotide (FMN) and flavin adenine dinucleotide (FAD) both representing essential co-factors for a number of redox reactions. The riboflavin deficiency syndrome in children is characterized by sore throat, cheilosis, angular stomatitis, glossitis, seborrhoeic dermatitis, and anaemia.

Surprisingly, in severely-malnourished patients, normal or even slightly elevated FAD levels were determined in erythrocytes (Becker et al 1995b). These high concentrations are unlikely to indicate an adequate riboflavin intake. Rather, they might reflect muscular wasting in severe malnutrition: riboflavin released

from muscle tissue can normalize the FAD status of other cells including erythrocytes. Concerning riboflavin supplementation, two aspects should be taken into account: 1) The activity of the FAD-dependent enzyme glutathione reductase—a marker for FAD status—is not impaired in severe PEM; and 2) free FAD might even contribute to the production of reactive oxygen species (Becker & Wilkinson 1993). Therefore, riboflavin supplementation in PEM should not exceed the daily intakes recommended for healthy children. Only in children with intact kidney function, excess riboflavin is readily excreted.

Albumin

The concentrations of albumin (approximately 30% of reference values) and consequently of total serum protein (approximately 60% of reference values) are drastically decreased in kwashiorkor and to a lesser degree in marasmus (Golden & Ramdath 1987, Becker et al 1995b). In a study carried out in Nigeria, it was detected that the molar ratio of whole blood glutathione over plasma albumin was approximately 1.5 for control children as well as for marasmic and kwashiorkor patients (Becker et al 1995b). This indicates a parallel decrease of glutathione and albumin in PEM patients. *Albumin*, a large plasma transport protein, represents by itself an important antioxidant. For example, it guarantees the bilirubin-protected transport of unsaturated fatty acids in blood, that is in a medium of high oxygen tension. In addition, albumin appears to be a self-sacrificing scavenger of reactive oxygen species (Halliwell 1988). Indeed, albumin deficiency was shown to increase lipid peroxidation in an animal model (Huang & Fwu 1992). In PEM, a vicious cycle can develop if oxidized albumin cannot be replaced by an adequate rate of synthesis—a likely situation precipitated by amino acid deficiency and/or impaired liver function. As discussed by Phadke et al (1995) disturbances in amino acid metabolism of PEM patients might also be related to altered transaminase functions of genetic origin. This interesting hypothesis has to be proven in further studies.

Vitamin E (tocopherol)

Vitamin E is the generic name for a group of closely-related, naturally-occurring, fat-soluble compounds, the *tocopherols*. Of these, α-tocopherol is biologically the most potent (1 IU = 1 mg α-tocopherol). Vitamin E acts as an antioxidant in food and in animal tissues by inhibiting the peroxidation of unsaturated fatty acids and of such labile compounds as vitamin A. In the absence of vitamin E, rabbits develop muscular dystrophy, chickens exhibit exudative diathesis and encephalomalacia, and rodents show defective reproduction. Erythrocytes from tocopherol-deficient humans show an increased susceptibility to haemolysis.

Tocopherol concentrations (both absolute and relative to plasma lipid concentrations) have been found to be low in PEM (Golden & Ramdath 1987). Although different studies on that topic do not provide a completely uniform picture, vitamin E deficiency can be stated to be a major feature of PEM. Vitamin E concentrations might furthermore be specifically related to the prognosis of malnutrition. In a recent study, plasma α-tocopherol, total tocopherol and the tocopherol:lipid ratio were found to be decreased in PEM, and again, kwashiorkor patients who had approximately 50% of control values were more seriously affected than marasmic children; β- and γ-tocopherol concentrations did not deviate significantly from normal values (Becker et al 1994). Tocopherol supplementation in therapy and possibly also prevention of PEM might therefore be considered (Beau & Sy 1996). In this context, however, it should be pointed out that tocopherol applied in high concentrations might also act as a pro-oxidant if it is not accompanied by sufficient amounts of water-soluble antioxidants like ascorbate, which are able to export radicals from the hydrophobic to the aqueous phase. The potential pro-oxidant effect was demonstrated for tocopherol and low-density lipoproteins by Bowry & Stocker (1993) (Fig. 17.3).

Vitamin A (retinol)

Retinol can either be ingested or synthesized within

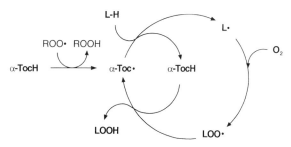

Figure 17.3 — Tocopherol-mediated peroxidation (after Bowry & Stocker 1993). The pro-oxidant effect of vitamin E on the radical-initiated oxidation of human low-density lipoprotein. Tocopherol is usually classified as an antioxidant. However, vitamin E radicals forming, for example, under the influence of peroxyl radicals can promote lipid peroxidation.

the body from plant carotenoids. Preformed vitamin A is present in animal tissues, and the best sources are liver, milk and kidney. β-Carotene can either be absorbed intact or cleaved in the intestinal tract to form two molecules of retinal, which are then reduced to retinol. Retinol from whatever source is stored as retinyl ester in the cells of the liver. Prior to release from the liver, retinyl esters are hydrolyzed, and the free alcohol is bound to a specific plasma protein, the retinol-binding protein, for transport to peripheral tissues.

The best-defined function of vitamin A is related to the role of retinol as a prosthetic group in visual proteins. In addition, vitamin A is required for growth and reproduction. Clinical manifestations of vitamin A deficiency are night blindness, followed by reversible degenerative changes in the conjunctiva and cornea (xerosis and Bitot's spots) and then by irreversible keratomalacia and blindness. Dryness and hyperkeratosis of the skin are also observed.

In developing countries, vitamin A deficiency is a major cause of blindness in the young due to inadequate food intake. Deficiency in vitamin A often accompanies PEM; defective synthesis or defective release of retinol-binding protein from the liver may aggravate the condition (Smith et al 1973, Golden & Ramdath 1987, Mayatepek et al 1991). In many hospitals, the immediate injection of 100,000–200,000 IU vitamin A or the oral application of 200,000 IU for 2 days in malnourished children has proven to restore retinol levels and to prevent keratomalacia.

Vitamin C (ascorbate)

Ascorbate is a water-soluble vitamin that is widely distributed in fruits and vegetables but also in milk and some meats. L-Ascorbic acid readily undergoes reversible oxidation and is thus a co factor for physiological redox reactions. Ascorbic acid and glutathione furthermore are likely to represent a redox system *in vivo* (Winkler et al 1994). The best understood function of ascorbate is its role in collagen synthesis; absence of the vitamin leads to impairment of post-translational hydroxylation of procollagen with ensuing reduction in collagen stability. Ascorbate deficiency causes scurvy, the peak age incidence in children being 8 months. The most prominent sign on physical examination is painful tenderness of the lower extremities, which are also usually swollen. Also observed are enlargement of costochondral junctions, subcutaneous haemorrhages, swollen and haemorrhagic gums. Many of these features can be explained by defective collagen synthesis.

Although few data are available on vitamin C status in PEM, the importance of ascorbate in detoxification of reactive oxygen species is obvious. Ascorbate is an essential water-soluble 'co-antioxidant' of tocopherol and glutathione. However, as reviewed by Halliwell (1996), ascorbate can also exert pro-oxidant properties. Systematic studies have to show whether increasing the ascorbate intake in malnourished patients over the established recommended intakes is beneficial.

Ubiquinone-10

Ubiquinone-10 (co enzyme Q) represents not only an essential constituent of the respiratory chain electron transport system but is also an important blood plasma antioxidant. The reduced form of co enzyme Q, ubiquinol-10, was shown to protect low-density lipoproteins against lipid peroxidation (Beyer 1990, Stocker et al 1991). In the only study carried out on co enzyme Q in PEM, no decreased plasma concentrations were detected in malnourished children (Becker et al 1994). Marasmic patients had co enzyme Q levels very similar to local and European controls (Becker et al 1995a), whereas children with kwashiorkor exhibited slightly increased values. This increase is likely to reflect a compensatory mechanism (Navarro et al 1998).

Ubiquinone-10 is produced in humans in a biochemical pathway closely linked to cholesterol synthesis. Additional oral intake of co-enzyme Q might enhance the overall antioxidant capacity and is recommended in the context of other diseases (Folkers et al 1993). However, there is still no evidence that application of co-enzyme Q in PEM is beneficial.

Fatty acids

Analysis of plasma and erythrocyte fatty acid composition showed a significant reduction of polyunsaturated fatty acids (PUFAs) like docosahexaenoic acid, arachidonic acid, and linoleic acid in PEM, particularly in kwashiorkor (Wolff et al 1984, Leichsenring et al 1995). These findings are likely to indicate increased oxidative stress inducing lipid peroxidation (Lenhartz et al 1999), although it is difficult to exclude completely a nutritional deficit. Lipid peroxidation of membrane lipids can impair membrane integrity and function. Leaky cell membranes have been observed in leukocytes

(Patrick & Golden 1977) and in erythrocytes (Kaplay 1978) of kwashiorkor patients. These changes are accompanied by an increased activity of the adenosine triphosphate (ATP) consuming sodium pumps and a raised intracellular sodium concentration. Alterations in fatty acid and/or glutathione metabolism might also contribute to the changes in leukotriene metabolism observed in kwashiorkor. Taken together, these changes are likely to be relevant for oedema formation and susceptibility to infections (Mayatepek et al 1993). Food enrichment with polyunsaturated fatty acids cannot be recommended in PEM because PUFAs promote lipid peroxidation and therefore enhance oxidative stress.

Discussion

New strategies for improving the clinical situation of severely-malnourished patients, especially kwashiorkor patients, are urgently required. A therapy directed to the restoration of the antioxidant capacity is likely to be beneficial. Food supplementation with selenium and zinc has already been introduced in different hospitals; this is also true for antioxidant vitamins. However, applying a single antioxidant or a combination of antioxidants in high doses to severely-malnourished patients should be avoided. Many antioxidants can become pro-oxidants—depending on their concentrations and the surrounding metabolic milieu—and no systematic studies have been carried out on such a substitution therapy. The authors' recommendation is therefore to apply a combination of the major antioxidant vitamins and trace elements—as recommended for children of the corresponding age—together with a slowly-increasing protein-containing diet (see Table 17.2). Polyunsaturated fats in excess should be avoided, and infections should be actively treated. In parallel, systematic studies on the pathophysiology, therapy and prevention of PEM must be pushed forward. As described by Golden & Ramdath (1987) iron chelators and allopurinol (as an inhibitor of the ROS-producing enzyme xanthine oxidase) might improve the clinical situation of PEM patients. However, xanthine oxidase also synthesizes uric acid, and it should be taken into account that uric acid, like bilirubin, represents an important physiological antioxidant in blood plasma. Present data also suggest the application of glutathione, which has recently been shown to support the recovery from kwashiokor (Becker et al, unpublished). However, clinical experience with administration, bioavailability and toxicity of glutathione is still limited. For this reason, metabolic precursors of cysteine like N-acetylcysteine, glutathione esters (Meister 1991, Bray & Taylor 1994), and methionine or dithiols like α-lipoic acid should also be considered as possible therapeutic approaches (Goss et al 1994, Packer et al 1995, Roediger 1995). The role of nutritional ergothioneine, a major thiol compound of erythrocytes and liver cells, remains to be studied (Asmus et al 1996).

REFERENCES

Ashour, M.N., Salem, S.I., El-Gadbon, H.M., Elwan, N.M., Basu, T.K. (1999) Antioxidant status in children with protein-energy malnutrition (PEM) living in Cairo, Egypt. *Eur J Clin Nutr*, 53, 669–673.

Aruoma, O.I. (1994) Nutrition and health aspects of free radicals and antioxidants. *Fd Chem Toxic*, 32, 671–683.

Asmus, K.D., Bensasson, R.V., Bernier, J.L., Houssin, R., Land, E.J. (1996) One-electron oxidation of ergothioneine and analogues investigated by pulse radiolysis: Redox reactions involving ergothioneine and vitamin C. *Biochem J*, 315, 625–629.

Avery, M.E., Lewis, R. (1994) *Pediatric Medicine*, 2nd edn. Baltimore: Williams & Wilkins.

Baker, D.H. (1987) Construction of assay diets for sulfur-containing amino acids. *Methods Enzymol*, 143, 297–307.

Bates, C. (1992) Riboflavin. *Internat J Vit Nutr Res*, 63, 274–277.

Beau, J.P., Sy, A. (1996) Vitamin E supplementation in Senegalese children with kwashiorkor. *Sante*, 6, 209–212.

Becker, K., Bötticher, D., Leichsenring, M. (1994a) Antioxidant vitamins in malnourished Nigerian children. *Internat J Vitam Nutr Res*, 64, 306–310.

Becker, K., Bötticher, D., Leichsenring, M. (1995a) Ubiquinone-10 plasma concentrations in healthy European children. *Redox Report*, 1, 97–98.

Becker, K., Gromer, S., Schirmer, R.H., Müller, S. (2000) Thioredoxin reductase as a patho-physiological factor and drug target *Eur J Biochem*, 267, 6118–6125.

Becker, K, Krebs, B., Schirmer, R.H. (1991) Protein-chemical standardization of the erythrocyte glutathione reductase activation test (EGRAC test). Application to riboflavin deficiency and hypothyroidism. *Internat J Vitam Nutr Res*, 61, 180–187.

Becker, K., Leichsenring, M., Gana, L., Bremer, H.J., Schirmer, R.H. (1995b) Glutathione and associated antioxidant systems in protein energy malnutrition: Results of a study in Nigeria. *Free Rad Biol Med*, 18, 257–263.

Becker, K., Wilkinson, A. (1993) Flavin adenine dinucleotide levels in erythrocytes of very low birth weight infants under vitamin supplementation. *Biol Neonate*, 63, 80–86.

Beutler, E., Dale, G.L. (1988) Erythrocyte glutathione: Function and Metabolism. In: Dolphin, D., Avramovic, O., Poulson, R. (eds.) *Coenzymes and Cofactors* vol. III Part B, Chapter 8, pp. 291–317. New York: Wiley and Sons.

Beyer, R.E. (1990) The participation of coenzyme Q in free radical production and antioxidation. *Free Rad Biol Med*, 8, 545–565.

Bowry, V.W., Stocker, R. (1993) Tocopherol-mediated peroxidation. The prooxidant effect of vitamin E on the radical-initiated oxidation of human low-density lipoprotein. *J Am Chem Soc*, 115, 6029–6044.

Bray, T.M., Taylor, C.G. (1993) Tissue glutathione, nutrition, and oxidative stress. *Can J Physiol Pharmacol*, 71, 746–751.

Bray, T.M., Taylor, C.G. (1994) Enhancement of tissue glutathione for antioxidant and immune functions in malnutrition. *Biochem Pharmacol*, 47, 2113–2123.

Dempster, W.S., Sive, A.A., Rosseau, S., Malan, H., Heese, H.V. (1995) Misplaced iron in kwashiorkor. *Eur J Clin Nutr*, 49, 208–210.

Dringen, R., Gutterer, J.M., Hirrlinger, J. (2000) Glutathione metabolism in brain. Metabolic interactions between astrocytes and neurons in the defense against reactive oxygen species. *Eur J Biochem*, 267, 4912–4916.

El Ghazali, S., Mikhail, M., Awadallah, M., Shatla, H. (1990) Significant increase of chromosomal damage in protein energy malnutrition. *J Trop Med Hygiene*, 93, 372–376.

Erinoso, H.O., Akinbami, F.O., Akinyinka, O.O. (1993) Prognostic factors in severely malnourished hospitalized Nigerian children. Anthropometric and biochemical factors. *Trop Geogr Med*, 45, 290–293.

Fechner, A., Böhme, C.C., Gromer, S., Funk, M., Schirmer, R.H., Becker, K. (2001) Antioxidant status and nitric oxide in the malnutrition syndrome kwashiorkor. *Pediatr Res*, 49, in press.

Folkers, K., Brown, R., Judy, W.V., Morita, M. (1993) Survival of cancer patients on therapy with coenzyme Q10. *Biochem Biophys Res Commun*, 192, 241–245.

Fondu, P., Hariga-Muller, C., Mozes, N., Nene, J., Van Steirteghem, A., Mandelbaum, I.M. (1978) Protein-energy malnutrition and anemia. *Am J Clin Nutr*, 31, 46–56.

Geigy Scientific Tables. (1985) Lentner C, editor. 8th edn. Basle: Ciba-Geigy Limited.

Golden, M.H.N. (1994) Issues in kwashiorkor. *Lancet*, 343, 292.

Golden, M.H.N., Golden, B.E., Jackson, A.A. (1980) Albumin and nutritional oedema. *Lancet*, I, 114–116.

Golden, M.H.N., Ramdath, D. (1987) Free radicals in the pathogenesis of kwashiorkor. *Proc Nutr Soc*, 46, 53–68.

Goss, P.M., Bray, T.M., Nagy, L.E. (1994) Regulation of hepatocyte glutathione by amino acid precursors and cAMP in protein-energy malnourished rats. *J Nutr*, 124, 323–330.

Halliwell, B. (1988) Albumin—an important extracellular antioxidant? *Biochem Pharmacol*, 37, 569–571.

Halliwell, B. (1996) Vitamin C: Antioxidant or prooxidant in vivo? *Free Rad Res*, 25, 439–454.

Halliwell, B., Gutteridge, J.M., Cross, C.E. (1992) Free radicals, antioxidants, and human disease: Where are we now? *J Lab Clin Med*, 119, 598–620.

Hemalatha, P., Bhaskaram, P., Khan, M.M. (1993) Role of zinc supplementation in the rehabilitation of severely malnourished children. *Eur J Clin Nutr*, 47, 395–399.

Hendrickse, R.G. (1988) Kwashiorkor and aflatoxins. *J Ped Gastroenterol Nutr*, 7, 633–636.

Househam, K.C., Hundt, H.K. (1991) Aflatoxin exposure and its relationship to kwashiorkor in African children. *J Trop Pediatr*, 37, 300–302.

Huang, C.J., Fwu, M.L. (1992) Protein insufficiency aggravates the enhanced lipid peroxidation and reduced activities of antioxidant enzymes in rats fed diets high in polyunsaturated fat. *J Nutr*, 122, 1182–1189.

Kaplay, S.S. (1978) Erythrocyte membrane Na^+ and K^+ activated adenosine triphosphatase in protein-calorie malnutrition. *Am J Clin Nutr*, 31, 579–584.

Leichsenring, M., Sütterlin, N., Less, S., Bäumann, K., Anninos, A., Becker, K. (1995) Polyunsaturated fatty acids in erythrocyte and plasma lipids of children with severe protein-energy malnutrition. *Acta Paediatr*, 84, 516–520.

Lenhartz, H., Ndasi, R., Anninos, A., Boetticher, D., Mayatepek, E., Tetanye, E., Leichsenring, M. (1998) The clinical manifestation of the kwashiorkor syndrome is related to increased lipid peroxidation. *J Pediatr*, 132, 879–881.

Levander, O.A., Beck, M.A. (1999) Selenium and viral virulence. *Br Med Bull*, 55, 528–533.

Macdougall, L.G., Moodley, G., Eyberg, C., Quirk, M. (1982) Mechanisms of anemia in protein-energy malnutrition in Johannesburg. *Am J Clin Nutr*, 35, 229–235.

Mayatepek, E., Becker, K., Gana, L., Hoffmann, G.F., Leichsenring, M. (1993) Leukotrienes in the pathophysiology of kwashiorkor. *Lancet*, 342, 958–960.

Mayatepek, E., Leichsenring, M., Ahmed, H.M., Lareya, M.D., El-Karib, A.O., Bremer, H.J. (1991) Vitamin A supplementation in malnourished Sudanese children. *Internat J Vit Nutr Res*, 61, 268–269.

Meister, A. (1991) Glutathione deficiency produced by inhibition of its synthesis, and its reversal; applications in research and therapy. *Pharmac Ther*, 51, 155–194.

Navarro, F., Navas, P., Burgess, J.R., Bello, R.I., De Cabo, R., Arroyo, A., Villalba, J.M. (1998) Vitamin E and selenium deficiency induces expression of the ubiquinone-dependent antioxidant system at the plasma membrane. *FASEB J*, 12, 1665–1673.

Packer, L., Witt, E.H., Tritschler, H.J. (1995) Alpha-lipoic acid as a biological antioxidant. *Free Rad Biol Med*, 19, 227–250.

Patrick, J., Golden, M. (1977) Leukocyte electrolytes and sodium transport in protein energy malnutrition. *Am J Clin Nutr*, 30, 1478–1481.

Persson-Moschos, M., Huang, W., Srikumar, T.S., Akesson, B., Lindeberg, S. (1995) Selenoprotein P in serum as a biochemical marker of selenium status. *Analyst*, 120, 833–836.

Phadke, M.A., Khedkar, V.A., Pashankar, D., Kate, S.L., Mokashi, G.D., Gambhir, P.S., Bhate, S.M. (1995) Serum amino acids and genesis of protein energy malnutrition. *Indian Pediatr*, 32, 301–306.

Ramdath, D.D., Golden, M.H.N. (1993) Elevated glutathione S-transferase activity in erythrocytes from malnourished children. *Eur J Clin Nutr*, 47, 658-665.

Roediger, W.E. (1995) New views on the pathogenesis of kwashiorkor: Methionine and other amino acids. *J Pediatr Gastroenterol Nutr*, 21, 130–136.

Salih, M.A., Mohamed, E.F., Galgan, V., Jones, B., Hellsing, K., Bani, I.A., Alasha, E. (1994) Selenium in malnourished Sudanese children: Status and interaction with clinical features. *Ann Nutr Metab*, 38, 68–74.

Sies, H. (1991) *Oxidants and Antioxidants*. London: Academic Press Limited.

Sive, A.A., Subotzky, E.F., Malan, H., Dempster, W.S., Heese, H.D. (1993) Red blood cell antioxidant enzyme concentrations in kwashiorkor and marasmus. *Ann Trop Paediatr*, 13, 33–38.

Smith, F.R., Goodman, D.S., Zaklama, M.S., Gabr, M.K., Maraghy, S.E., Patwardhan, V.N. (1973) Serum vitamin A, retinol-binding protein, and prealbumin concentrations in protein-calorie malnutrition. I. A functional defect in hepatic retinol release. *Am J Clin Nutr*, 26, 973–981.

Stocker, R., Bowry, V.W., Frey, B. (1991) Ubiquinol-10 protects low density lipoprotein more efficiently against lipid peroxidation than does α-tocopherol. *Proc Natl Acad Sci*, 88, 1646–1650.

Suskind, D., Murthy, K.K., Suskind, R.M. (1990) *The Malnourished Child*. New York: Raven Press.

Thomas, A.G., Miller, V., Shenkin, A., Fell, G.S., Taylor, F. (1994) Selenium and glutathione peroxidase status in paediatric health and gastrointestinal disease. *J Pediatr Gastroenterol Nutr*, 19, 213–219.

Wellcome Trust Working Party. (1970) Classification of infantile malnutrition. *Lancet*, II, 302–303.

Williams, C.D. (1935) Kwashiorkor: A nutritional disease of children associated with a maize diet. *Lancet*, II, 1151–1152.

Winkler, B.S., Orselli, S.M., Rex, T.S. (1994) The redox couple between glutathione and ascorbic acid: A chemical and physiological perspective. *Free Rad Biol Med*, 17, 333–349.

Wolff, J.A., Margolis, S., Bujdoso-Wolff, K., Matusick, E., MacLean, W.C. Jr. (1984) Plasma and red blood cell fatty acid composition in children with protein energy malnutrition. *Pediatr Res*, 18, 162–167.

van Dusseldorp, M., Poortvliet, E.J., de-Waart, F.G., Kok, F.J., Alexandrov, A.A., Mazaev, V., Katan, M.B. (1996) Antioxidant vitamin status of Russian children and elderly. *Eur J Clin Nutr*, 50, 195–196.

Zhang, H., Olejnicka, B., Öllinger, K., Brunk, U.T. (1996) Starvation-induced autophagocytosis enhances the susceptibility of insulinoma cells to oxidative stress. *Redox Report*, 2, 235–247.

18

Vitamin supplementation in developing countries

Christine A. Northrop-Clewes

Abbreviations

VAD	Vitamin A deficiency
IU	International Units
XN	night-blindness
X1B	Bitot's spots
RR	Relative risk
HIV	Human immunodeficiency virus
AIDS	Autoimmune deficiency syndrome
TE	Tocopherol equivalents
PUFA	Polyunsaturated fatty acids
i.m.	Intramuscularly
i.v.	Intravenously
RNI	Reference nutrient intake
NE	Niacin equivalents
RE	Retinol equivalents
APP	Acute phase protein
NNIPS	Nepal Nutrition Intervention Project Sarlhi
FAO/	Food and Agriculture Organization/World
WHO	Health Organization

Introduction

Vitamins have been defined classically as a group of organic compounds required in very small amounts for the normal development and functioning of the body. They are not synthesized by the body, or are done so only in insufficient amounts, and are mainly obtained through food (Hoffmann-La Roche 1994).

There are 13 vitamins: four are fat-soluble, namely vitamins A, D, E and K, and nine are water-soluble, vitamin C and the B-complex made up of vitamins B1, B2, B6, B12, folic acid, biotin, niacin and pantothenic acid. No single food contains all of the vitamins and therefore a balanced and varied diet is necessary for an adequate intake.

Some vitamin deficiencies have had a major clinical impact on the health of many developing countries. However, they occurred before pure vitamins were readily available. Hence there have been relatively few vitamin supplementation studies in developing countries apart from the work on vitamin A.

Vitamin A deficiency (VAD) still affects over 200 million pre-school children in 90 countries in the developing world, and is the leading cause of paediatric blindness with 5–10 million children developing xerophthalmia each year. In 43 affected countries, the deficiency was severe enough to cause clinical eye damage in 3 million children and blindness in up to 500,000 of them. Hence a major emphasis in this chapter is placed on vitamin A.

Historical understanding of the role of vitamins

The ability of foods to cure disease has been known for a considerable time. Night-blindness (XN) and its successful treatment with animal liver was known to the ancient Egyptians at least 3500 years ago (Ebers Papyrus 1600). Scurvy was treated with pine needle extracts (American Indians 16th Century) and citrus fruits (Europeans 17th Century). However, the concept of dietary deficiency diseases only began about a century ago in Asia with an observation with respect to the paralytic disease beriberi. Polished rice (with the husks removed) was a staple diet in the region and it was found that the husks or bran from rice contained a substance that relieved the paralysis (Sinclair 1982). Funk (1911) reasoned that beriberi and three other nutritional diseases, pellagra, rickets and scurvy, all resulted from the lack of a dietary trace substance, which he called *vitamine* (literally, amine of life) (Sinclair 1982). This led to the adoption of the generic term, vitamin. Thiamin was the component of rice bran that was deficient in beriberi, and subsequently the vitamin deficiencies associated with pellagra, rickets and scurvy were related to vitamins B6, D and C respectively.

Practice and procedures

Vitamin A

Vitamin A was discovered in 1913 by McCollum. It is a lipid-soluble essential nutrient found in animal and dairy products (e.g., milk, cheese, egg yolks, meat, fish). Vitamin A is stored in the liver as retinyl palmitate, hence liver and cod liver oil are rich sources of the vitamin. Orange and yellow fruits and vegetables, dark green leafy vegetables and red palm oil contain α and β-carotene and β-cryptoxanthin, which can be metabolized by enzymes in the gut to form retinol. The efficiency of conversion is very variable and dependent on many different factors such as dietary fat content and accessibility of dietary carotenoids (Bates 1995). Vitamin A levels in the diet are expressed as retinol equivalents (RE) i.e., 6 μg β-carotene or 1 μg retinol or 3.33 international units (IU) retinyl palmitate equals 1 RE. The reported range for levels of pre-formed vitamin A in breast milk is extremely wide, 0.15–2.26 mg/L (0.53–7.9 μmol/L), which could reflect maternal intake (Moran et al 1983, Scharz

Table 18.1 — Estimated requirements for vitamin A (µg RE/day)

Group	Age (years)	Basal requirement★		Safe intake level★	
		µg/day	µg/ kg	µg/day	µg/kg
Both sexes	0–1	180	40–20	350	78–39
	1–6	200	13	400	26
	6–10	250	10	400	16
	10–12	300	8.3	500	14
	12–15	350	7.8	600	12
Women	18+	270	4.8	500	9.3
Pregnancy		370		600	
Lactation		450		850	

★These values are due to be reviewed by a joint FAO/WHO expert consultation in 1998 (in press 2001). From Report of a joint FAO/WHO Expert Consultation (1988).

1989). The influence of maternal intakes of vitamin A on levels in breast milk is uncertain, because the majority of maternal supplementation studies have been carried out in communities where maternal intakes are low but in which other factors such as infection may have influenced the association (Kim et al 1990). Required intake of vitamin A during pregnancy and lactation and the basal requirements and safe level of intake for vitamin A by age group are given in Table 18.1.

Vitamin A deficiency (VAD)

Risk factors for VAD include:

- Early cessation and low frequency of breastfeeding;
- Provision of complementary foods of low vitamin A content to weaning infants;
- High levels of infection that exacerbate nutritional demands.

VAD occurs when body stores are depleted to the extent that physiological functions are impaired. Even before eye signs are evident, the integrity of epithelial barriers and the immune system are compromised and there is increased severity of some infections as well as an increased risk of death, especially amongst children (Ross & Hammerling 1994). Thus, it is now recognized that the health of pre-school and perhaps older children as well as that of pregnant and lactating women is compromised by VAD, even at moderate and possible mild sub-clinical levels (Beaton et al 1993). VAD can easily be prevented by direct periodic supplementation, food fortification and/or dietary change.

Supplementation trials

Studies by Sommer et al (1983) in Indonesia reported

that children with mild *xerophthalmia*, classified as night-blindness (XN) and/or Bitot's spots (X1B), died at much higher rates than those without xerophthalmia. Children with XN died at roughly three times the rate of non-xerophthalmic children; children with X1B died at six times the rate; and children with both died at nine times the rate (Sommer et al 1983). Hence, the more severe the xerophthalmia the greater the risk of dying. Because proof that this is a causal relationship is required, many controlled trials have been carried out since. Vitamin A supplements have been shown to be particularly effective against diarrhoea (Beaton et al 1993) and more recently malaria (Shankar et al 1997).

Supplementation trials with mortality as their end-point

The Aceh Study Group in Indonesia carried out the first of several controlled double-blind supplementation trials (Sommer et al 1986). Pre-school children were selected randomly by village to receive 200,000 IU of vitamin A once every 6 months. The control group received nothing. The outcome was a significant 27% relative reduction in mortality from all causes in the vitamin-A-supplemented villages. Within 6 years, eight major vitamin-A-supplementation trials in children were completed. Table 18.2 summarizes the main features and outcomes of the studies.

A meta-analysis, which combined the results of all eight studies (Beaton et al 1993), concluded that improving vitamin A status of deficient children significantly reduced their overall mortality by 23% (P < 0.0001). In addition, there was significantly reduced mortality from diarrhoeal disease (relative risk (RR) compared with controls 0.71; P < 0.002), but no effect

Table 18.2 — Effect of vitamin A supplements on mortality of young children in developing countries

Country	Number enrolled in study	Vitamin A dose IU[*]	Interval between doses (months)	Outcome #Relative Risk (mortality)	P	Reference
Indonesia – Aceh	25,200	200,000	6	0.73	0.024	Sommer et al 1986
Nepal – NNIPS 1	28,630	≤ 200,000 (age-graded)	4	0.71	0.003	West et al 1991
Nepal – (highland)	7197	≤ 200,000 (age-graded)	Once	0.74	0.058	Daulaire et al 1992
India – Tamil Nadu	15,419	8333	0.25	0.46	0.01	Rahmathullah et al 1990
India – Andhra Pradesh	15,775	200,000	6	0.94	0.82	Vijayaraghavan et al 1990
Ghana Vast Study	21,906	≤ 200,000 (age-graded)	4	0.81	0.03	Ghana VAST study team 1993
Sudan[1]	28,492	200,000	6	1.06	0.76	Herrera et al 1992
Indonesia	11,200	Fortified MSG	Diet	0.70	0.05	Muhilal et al 1988

[*]1 IU vitamin A = 0.3 µg retinol = 1.05 nmol retinol. # Relative risk, ratio of treated: control mortality rates; P, probability that treated and control group mortalities were equal, value < 1 indicates a positive effect of supplements; [1] This study found a highly-significant inverse correlation between dietary vitamin A intake and risk of mortality in children in the same community. MSG = monosodium glutamate. Modified from Bates (1995).

Table 18.3 — Universal vitamin A distribution schedule for pre-school children and lactating mothers

Group	Vitamin A supplementation dose
Infants < 6 months (not breastfed)	50,000 IU of vitamin as a single dose or as divided doses of 25,000 IU before the infant reaches 6 months.
Infants 6–11 months (breastfed)	100,000 IU of vitamin A orally every 3–6 months. Immunization against measles (at about 9 months) provides a good opportunity to give one of these doses.
Children 1–6 years	200,000 IU of vitamin A contained in a gelatinous capsule or as an oily solution, orally every 3–6 months.
Lactating mothers	200,000 IU of vitamin A orally once: at delivery or during the first 8 weeks post-partum if breastfeeding or during the first 6 weeks if not breastfeeding to protect the mother and raise breast milk vitamin A levels to protect the breastfed infant.

Modified from Sommer & West (1996).

on mortality from respiratory infection (RR 0.94; P < 0.94). However the supplementation of young infants is still somewhat controversial. Data from the NNIPS-1 study suggested that a very large dose (100,000 IU vitamin A in a single bolus) might be detrimental during the first few months of life, becoming protective only at the fourth or fifth month (West et al 1991). The safety and value of directly dosing newborns was supported by data from a clinical trial in Indonesia, where newborn infants received either 50,000 IU

vitamin A or a placebo within 1–3 days of birth (Humphrey et al 1994). The benefit of the supplement was most apparent during months 2–4 of life. Table 18.3 summarizes the current universal recommendations for supplementation of lactating mothers and pre-school children (Sommer & West 1996).

Measles

Measles not only accounts for a large proportion of

preventable childhood blindness, particularly in Africa, but acute and delayed mortality as well. Three controlled treatment trials, in London (Ellison 1932), Tanzania (Barclay et al 1987) and South Africa (Hussey & Klein 1990) demonstrated that vitamin A treatment after the onset of measles reduced associated mortality. A fourth study by Coutsoudis et al (1991) carefully assessed the impact of treatment on morbidity and found vitamin A to exert a powerful influence in reducing the severity and complications of measles. The full xerophthalmic treatment of children with complicated measles from VAD communities is recommended (Table 18.4):

Table 18.4 — Treatment of children with complicated measles from VAD

Time	< 1 year of age (IU)	> 1 year of age (IU)
Immediately	100,000	200,000
Next day	100,000	200,000
2–4 weeks later	100,000	200,000

Modified from Sammer & West (1996).

HIV

In contrast to measles where vitamin A treatment appears to be unquestionably beneficial, the role of vitamin A in HIV is controversial. The work of Semba et al (1994), who reported an apparent beneficial effect of vitamin A in preventing vertical transmission of HIV from mother-to-child in Africa, has been followed up by a number of studies in both the developed and developing world; these show no conclusive evidence of any association between vitamin A status and progression to AIDS (Blaner et al 1997, Burri et al 1997, Filteau et al 1997, Stallings et al 1997). However, further work by Semba et al (1997) reported a 30% reduction in low-birth-weight infants and, at 6-weeks' postpartum, breast-milk vitamin A levels were 41% higher following treatment of Malawian pregnant HIV+ women with 10,000 IU/day vitamin A together with iron and folate. In addition, work by Coutsoudis et al (1995) showed that infants in South Africa who were born to HIV-infected mothers who received 50,000 IU of vitamin A showed a 49% reduction in diarrhoeal episodes, a 56% reduction in severe diarrhoea and increased counts of lymphocytes CD4, CD56 and CD29 compared to those on placebo.

Vitamin A and epithelial integrity

Vitamin A is known to have a role in maintaining the integrity of epithelial tissues and in reducing the body's response to inflammatory stress. Infants from developing countries show pronounced growth faltering that is closely correlated to gut mucosal damage (Lunn et al 1991). Data from the Gambia has shown an improvement in gut integrity and in acute phase proteins (APP) associated with an increased intake of pro-vitamin A from mangoes (Northrop-Clewes et al 1997). Studies in rural Indian infants during the rainy season showed 16,000 IU retinyl palmitate given weekly produced a significant improvement in gut mucosal integrity at 4 and 8 weeks, in addition haemoglobin levels were maintained, whereas those in the placebo group fell (Northrop-Clewes et al 1997). The results suggest that vitamin A helps to restore gut integrity and increases resistance to infection, resulting in a down-regulation of the APP and stimulating the release of iron for haemoglobin synthesis.

Vitamin A and respiratory disease

Observational studies all show an association between VAD and increased respiratory infection. However, the meta-analysis (see p 174) showed a lack of impact of vitamin A supplementation on respiratory infections, although there were some indications of reduced severity and possibly reduced duration of respiratory symptoms. Furthermore, some have suggested that the increased strength of cough following supplementation may be indicative of greater mucous production and removal of infective material (Herrera et al 1996). A promising method of treating respiratory infection using organ-specific targeting was suggested by Biesalski (1996). Direct inhalation of 3000 IU retinyl esters produced an increase in plasma retinyl esters from 45 µg/L (0.16 µmol/L) to 190 µg/L (0.66 µmol/L) with no side effects.

The delivery of supplements

Community trials have shown mortality in mal-nourished, pre-school children can be reduced by 25–30% when children > 5 months of age are supplemented with vitamin A, thus saving 2.5 million child deaths due to underlying VAD. Administration of supplements is an effective way to correct existing deficiencies rapidly or to avoid their development in high-risk populations. However, it is important that supplementation be replaced by a sustainable strategy such as dietary diversification and food fortification (Blum 1997). Table 18.5 summarizes important

Table 18.5 — Points to target when planning a supplementation programme

- Educate community leaders to win them as allies;
- Rank target groups and try to reach highest priority groups first;
- Induce families to come to clinics by marketing 'the supplement' as health-promoting rather than as prevention for blindness;
- Extend the programme beyond clinics, the Expanded Programme on Immunization can be useful (e.g., giving vitamin A supplements at the time of measles) immunization;
- Deliver supplies on time and in the right amounts;
- Make sure health care providers know exactly what to do and why;
- Train and supervise for improved understanding and motivation;
- Schedule regular weeks or months for supplements to ease management problems;
- Keep supplementation records and check supplementation status whenever a target-group member appears at a clinic;
- Educate families about giving vitamin A-rich foods to young children and pregnant and lactating women and include breastfeeding promotion in this;
- Integrate supplements with the development of longer-term more sustainable solutions.

points to target when planning a supplementation programme.

Other fat soluble vitamins

Vitamin E

There are eight tocopherols and tocotrienols with vitamin E activity, of which α-tocopherol is the most active. Dietary sources of vitamin E are vegetable oils, and the recommended daily dietary intake is about 5 mg α-tocopherol. Breast milk α-tocopherol concentrations in healthy mothers is in the range of 1.1–8 mg D α-tocopherol equivalents (TE)/L, the value being dependent on the time during lactation, early milk has higher concentrations than late milk. β and γ forms of tocopherol are higher in mature milk compared with colostrum or transitional milk (Powers 1997). Protein energy malnutrition is associated with low vitamin E status, and secondary deficiency may occur in coeliac disease, cystic fibrosis, bilary atresia and abetalipoproteinaemia. Vitamin E is well absorbed from the gastrointestinal tract, even in low-birth-weight infants, but has little biological activity when given parenterally. Vitamin E requirements are highly influenced by the polyunsaturated fatty acid (PUFA) content of the tissues, which is itself influenced by dietary intake. It is not clear which factor should be used to express tocopherol requirements relative to dietary PUFA. The UK Department of Health (1991) recommends 0.4 mg α-TE/g PUFA for formula milk. There is no information on supplementation in developing countries.

Vitamin K (phylloquinone)

Vitamin K is quite widely distributed in a large variety of common foods, for example green leafy vegetables, fruits, cereals, meat and dairy products. There is little information about the concentration of vitamin K in mature breast milk. Reports suggest values between 1 and 10 µg/L (Powers 1997). Deficiency of vitamin K is usually secondary to disease or drug therapy. Haemorrhagic disease of the newborn has been attributed to vitamin K deficiency in breastfed infants 2–5 days following birth, and is sometimes observed in breastfed infants at 4–6 weeks of age (Powers 1997). Pietschnig et al (1993) were unable to show a beneficial effect of long-term supplements of the maternal diet (88 µg) on breast milk, while other workers have shown single doses of 0.5–3.0 mg can produce an increase in breast milk vitamin K (Powers 1997). There is no evidence of vitamin K supplements being given in developing countries.

Vitamin D

The greatest period of demand for vitamin D in childhood is between 6 months and 3 years of age when the rate at which calcium is laid down in the bone is highest (Belton 1986). The two main forms of vitamin D are ergocalciferol (D_2), mainly from plants, and cholecalciferol (D_3), synthesized by the action of ultraviolet light on 7-dehydrocholesterol in the skin. Vitamin D is present in human milk as ergocalciferol (0.3 µg/L), cholecalciferol (0.04 µg/L) and 25-hydroxyvitamin D (0.16 µg/L) (Reeve et al 1982). There is a seasonal variation in the levels of vitamin D and metabolites in breast milk, most especially in the northern latitudes (Markestad 1984). The feeding of infants post-natally is a factor in the pathogenesis of rickets. Hypocalcaemia and rickets secondary to vitamin D deficiency have been found in exclusively breastfed non-white infants who receive inadequate exposure to sunlight due to swaddling or to the purdah system where infants are kept indoors with their mothers (Chang et al 1992). Countries where this is most likely to happen include most of the Middle East, North and South Africa, Pakistan and China where the incidence has been shown to be 25% or higher (Chen et al 1988). At risk communities benefit from supplementation with vitamin D (400 IU or 10 µg/day), beginning during pregnancy. Supplementation may be weekly using a single capsule (75 µg) or less frequently such as the parenteral 'depot' doses in Saudi Arabia where up to 300,000 IU (7500 µg) are given to pregnant mothers (Belton & Hambridge 1991). Alternative approaches have been to fortify milk or other foods such as chapatti flour.

Water-soluble vitamins

Water-soluble vitamins have no storage depot and therefore vitamin depletion can occur rapidly during a period of low dietary intake. Materno-foetal transport favours active accumulation of these vitamins through gestation, and at birth, circulating levels are often higher in the infant than in the mother. Levels in the circulation fall fairly rapidly during the neonatal period if intake is not maintained (Greene 1982).

Reasons for vitamin B deficiency

Dietary sources of the B vitamins include meat (B1, B6, B12, niacin), milk (B2, B12, niacin), whole grain cereals (B1, B2, B6, niacin), green leafy vegetables (folate, pantothenate), and with a few exceptions, fruits and vegetables have a low content of thiamin, riboflavin and vitamin B6.

Important losses of B vitamins occur during food storage, processing and preparation. Eighty percent of thiamin, riboflavin and vitamin B6 in whole grain is lost during milling. Significant losses of folate and thiamin occur during steaming, blanching or boiling of vegetables. The global prevalence of B vitamin deficiency has not yet been established, and although frank deficiencies are no longer common, marginal deficiencies may still be widespread. Pellagra and beriberi occur sporadically in refugee camps and other severely-deprived communities, and sub-clinical deficiencies are found in populations that do not regularly consume milk, meat and dairy products (Blum 1997).

Vitamin B1 (thiamin)

Women from developing and developed countries have similar thiamin breast milk levels (0.15 mg/L, 0.45 µmol/L), even though there is evidence of lower thiamin intakes amongst women from some developing countries (e.g., The Gambia, India and Kenya) (Macy 1949, Department of Health and Social Security 1977). The concentration of total thiamin is generally one order of magnitude lower in colostrum and transitional milk than in mature milk, but levels progressively increase during lactation. Evidence suggests that breast-milk thiamin is insensitive to maternal dietary intake, although it has been shown that maternal supplements early in lactation can increase breast milk levels (Nail et al 1980, Thomas et al 1980). Infantile beriberi is seen in breastfed infants of thiamin-deficient mothers usually between the first and fourth months of life. The disease may occur even if the nursing mother appears to be healthy. Infantile beriberi occurs rapidly and is characterised by hypotonia, vomiting, abdominal pain, aphonia (soundless cry) and tachycardia, which may progress to cardiac failure. There is a dramatic improvement within a few hours of giving 50–100 mg thiamin hydrochloride intramuscularly (i.m.) or intravenously (i.v.) followed by 5–10 mg/day orally for several days. The thiamin status of the mother should also be checked and treated. Other than levels in human milk, very few data exist on which to base requirements for thiamin in infancy. The most recent recommended reference nutrient intake (RNI) of thiamin in infants up to 12 months old is 0.3 mg/1000 kcal (0.3 mg/4.2 Mjoule) (Table 18.6) (Department of Health 1991).

Vitamin B2 (riboflavin)

Riboflavin plays a key role in respiratory enzymes, in systems responsible for activation and metabolism of iron, pyridoxine, and folate, and in systems protecting against peroxidation. Riboflavin deficiency is a widespread endemic condition in most developing countries, particularly where the diet is based on rice. However, the overall physiological importance of riboflavin deficiency is still largely unknown. Riboflavin deficiency can result in impaired growth with clinical signs such as angular dermatitis and corneal vascularization. Average levels in mature breast milk of mothers in industrialized countries are between 0.2–0.8 mg/L (0.53–2.12 µmol/L) (Ford et al 1983). However where riboflavin intakes are low, babies are born with biochemical evidence of riboflavin deficiency and the breast milk content is often insufficient to correct the riboflavin deficiency (Bates

Table 18.6 — UK Reference nutrient intakes for vitamins

Age	0–3 months	4–6 months	7–9 months	10–12 months	1–2 years	Lactation
Thiamin mg/day	0.2	0.2	0.2	0.3	0.5	1.0
Riboflavin mg/day	0.4	0.4	0.4	0.4	0.6	1.6
Vitamin B6 mg/day[1]	0.2	0.2	0.3	0.4	0.7	1.2
Vitamin B12 µg/day	0.3	0.3	0.4	0.4	0.5	2.0
Folate µg/day	50	50	50	50	70	260
Niacin mg NE/1000 kcal	6.6	6.6	6.6	6.6	6.6	8.9
Pantothenic Acid mg/day[2]	1.7	1.7	1.7	1.7	1.7	3.4–5.3
Biotin	N/A	N/A	N/A	N/A	N/A	N/A
Vitamin C mg/day	25	25	25	25	30	70
Vitamin E mg α-TE/100 ml milk	0.32	0.32	0.32	0.32	0.32	3.0 mg α-TE/d
Vitamin A µg/day	350	350	350	350	400	950
Vitamin D µg/day	8.5	8.5	7	7	7	10
Vitamin K µg/day	10	10	10	10	10	1 µg/kg/day

[1]Based on protein providing 14.7% of estimated average requirement for energy; [2]No biochemical method has yet been established for pantothenic acid. There are no signs of deficiency in the UK population therefore requirements are based on UK intakes; N/A, data not available. Modified from Department of Health (1991).

et al 1982a). In The Gambia, riboflavin deficiency is both common and severe and babies are born deficient. A weaning food supplement containing 0.15–0.2 mg riboflavin was given to infants 3–12 months of age, in addition to breast milk and locally-available weaning foods, which provided 0.13–0.21 mg/day. Riboflavin status fell within normal limits while the supplement was continued, but once stopped it again deteriorated. The results confirm that daily requirements for infants up to 12 months are probably about 0.4 mg/day. Clinical signs in lactating mothers were corrected by a 2 mg daily riboflavin supplement added to the approximate 0.5 mg daily intake from local home foods. Breast milk riboflavin was moderately increased by these supplements and Bates et al (1982b) concluded that a total riboflavin intake of about 2.5 mg/day during lactation is sufficient to maintain normal biochemical status. UK RNI values are quoted in Table 18.6.

Vitamin B6 (pyridoxine)

Gross clinical deficiency of vitamin B6 is rare. There has never been a major deficiency disease associated with pyridoxine deficiency, although it is reported in India in association with riboflavin deficiency. Maternal intake of B6 influences breast milk levels, and values in mature breast milk range from 34–145 nmol/g protein in women from low socio-economic status in developed countries. This does not appear to be associated with clinical deficiency of mother or infant. B6 is of special interest as it is required for the metabolism of protein, carbohydrate and lipids. Metabolism of all three are accelerated during pregnancy. B6 is also important for normal brain development both before and after birth. However, the amounts to be recommended for daily intake remain controversial. The optimal amounts for pregnancy and lactation remain unknown, but human studies suggest that insufficient B6 may be associated with subtle neurological damage of the infant. The current UK RNI for infants is shown in Table 18.6.

Vitamin B12 (cobalamin)

B12 is actively transported across the placenta and stored in the foetal liver. The stores of B12 in the term infant are estimated to be approximately 25 µg, which deplete gradually during the first 6 months of life and are re-plenished when solid food is introduced (Luhby 1961). In human milk, colostrum contains around 2.4 µg/L (1.77 nmol/L) of B12, with mean concentrations of 0.2–1.3 µg/L (0.15–0.96 nmol/L) in the mature milk of well-nourished mothers. Deficiencies due to inborn errors of B12 metabolism cause lack of intrinsic factor, haptocorrin or transcobalamin II, resulting in hypotonia, lethargy or irritability, loss of developmental milestones and anaemia. The latter usually appear during the first year of life. However, cases have been reported of exclusively breastfed infants of vegan mothers or mothers with pernicious anaemia presenting with serious neurological abnormalities due to dietary deficiency, the milk content of B12 being as low as 0.06 µg/L (0.04 nmol/L) (Higginbottom et al 1978, Gambon et al 1986). Immediate treatment is usually about 100 µg B12 i.m., although daily intakes of 0.1µg have been reported to be adequate (Jadhav et al 1962). The current lower RNI has been set at 0.1µg/day based on the dose used to correct megoblastic anaemia in infants receiving inadequate amounts of B12 in breast milk (Jadhav et al 1962). The UK RNI is shown in Table 18.6.

Folate

Folate has an important role as a co-enzyme donating single carbon units to a variety of molecules for cell replication and protein synthesis, thus there is an increased requirement for folate during pregnancy, lactation and infant growth. The foetus begins to store folate in the liver late in pregnancy. These reserves can be depleted, however, in 4–12 weeks with inadequate folate intake (Gallagher & Ehrenkranz 1995). Folic acid deficiency due to malnutrition is the commonest cause of megoblastic anaemia in the world. Other causes include congenital folate malabsorption, inborn errors of metabolism or defective cellular uptake. During lactation, folate is probably preferentially partitioned to mammary tissue, suggesting that folate in breast milk remains adequate even though the mother's status may be compromised (Metz 1970). Only in severe deficiency is breast-milk folate adversely affected by maternal status. However, the amount of folate required to maintain maternal folate status during lactation is unknown (Picciano 1995). Recent studies suggest 200 µg/day supplemental folate or a total intake of 500 µg/day folate is necessary to maintain status in healthy lactating women (Picciano 1995).

A number of studies involving small numbers of malnourished infants supplemented with folic acid in formula feed or by injection provided the basis of early estimates of infant requirements (Waslien 1977, Rodriguez 1980). Current recommendations for infants are shown in Table 18.6 and are based on the amount of dietary folate ingested by healthy infants from the breast milk of healthy mothers (Department of Health 1991). The calculation is made from assumptions concerning the quantity of milk ingested, approximately 600 ml/day, which contains 100 µg folate/L. The contribution from other foods is often neglected. Dietary assessments of infants in the first year of life show that, following the introduction of supplemental foods, the contribution of milk to total

kilocalories declines and that for infants fed mixed diets at 9 and 12 months, the majority of dietary folate was provided by foods other than milk (Smith 1985). However, during prolonged lactation, folate levels increase significantly (Ford et al 1983). Deficient intake of folate is often associated with poverty, artificial feeding or excessive loss of folate due to overheating of food, and may lead to growth retardation, deranged function of the bone marrow, delayed maturation of the central nervous system, functional changes in the gastrointestinal tract and an increased susceptibility to infections. Treatment with folate to recommended levels resolves symptoms in 1–2 months.

Vitamin B5 (niacin)

Pellagra, the disease of niacin deficiency, is widespread in the poorer classes where the diet is low in animal and high in vegetable protein. However, it is particularly associated with eating maize or sorghum in India. Historically, pellagra was found in Europe and America but today it remains a problem in India, parts of Africa, the Middle East and China. A deficiency of niacin is characterized by a photosensitive dermatitis, inflammation of mucous membranes, diarrhoea and vomiting. Severe deficiency can be fatal. High intakes (1 g/day) result in hepatotoxicity (Powers 1997).

Biosynthesis of niacin from the amino acid tryptophan occurs in man, but the conversion is poor (1 mg niacin from 60 mg tryptophan) and usually insufficient to meet requirements. However, it has been estimated that tryptophan in human milk could contribute 70% of niacin equivalents (NE) and could supply as much as 3.67 mg niacin/L. The conversion factor in infants is not known nor is the proportion of milk tryptophan that undergoes this conversion. The average pre-formed niacin content of mature breast milk of healthy mothers is about 1.8–2.3 mg/L (14.8–18.7 nmol/L) providing 1.4–1.8 mg/day niacin (Ford et al 1983). Maternal supplements can raise low breast milk levels in malnourished mothers (Prentice et al 1983). Requirements for niacin are linked to energy expenditure, and intakes in infants are expressed as NE/1000 kcal (see Table 18.6).

Pantothenic acid

There is currently no satisfactory biochemical method for determining pantothenic acid status in humans, and no experimental data from human studies on which to base recommendations for infants. Deodhar et al (1964) supplemented Indian mothers with 50 mg/day and increased breast milk levels from 1 to 3 mg/L, but Song et al (1984) have shown that the analytical methods used influenced the results obtained.

Biotin

During the first days of lactation, biotin is almost completely absent, even from the milk of well-nourished mothers (Dostalova 1982). From the second week post-partum, the biotin content of breast milk, as assessed in a small number of studies, is in the range of 5.2–11 µg/L (0.02–0.05 µmol/L)(Prentice et al 1983, Hirano et al 1992, Mock et al 1992). However, if the mother has a poor nutritional status, the biotin content of the milk is reduced (Deodhar et al 1964). Maternal supplements of 7.4 µg/day to Gambian women showed no change in the average breast milk concentration of 9 µg/L, but supplements of 0.25 mg/day to Indian mothers increased milk levels from 1.6 µg/L to 5.0 µg/L (Deodhar et al 1964).

Vitamin C (ascorbate)

There is little information about the body pool and turnover rates for vitamin C in infants. However, daily intakes of 7–12 mg have been shown to be enough to protect infants from scurvy (Rajalakshmi et al 1965). Plasma vitamin C levels of term and premature babies fall immediately after birth but as breastfeeding becomes established, levels rise to values seen in adults. It is probable that vitamin C is transported exclusively from the plasma to the mammary gland and is present as ascorbic acid in a concentration in the range of 33–110 mg/L (0.18–0.63 mmol/L), which would supply 25–75 mg/day to the infant (Bates et al 1994). Supplementation of malnourished mothers has been shown to increase vitamin C levels in milk (Bates et al 1983), but supplements of up to 1000 mg/day for 2 days to well-nourished mothers have been reported to have no effect (Byerley & Kirksey 1985). It appears that the secretion of ascorbate into breast milk is actively regulated and that there may be disadvantages of very high intakes during infancy. Clinical deficiency of vitamin C has not been reported in breastfed infants.

Acknowledgements

I would like to thank Dr. Petroni, Dr. Cori and Dr. Nilson of Hoffmann La-Roche for the useful literature that they supplied.

References

Barclay, A.J.G., Foster, A., Sommer, A. (1987) Vitamin A supplements and mortality related to measles: A randomised clinical trial. *BMJ*, 294, 294–296.

Bates, C.J. (1995) Vitamin A. *Lancet*, 345, 31–35.

Bates, C.J., Prentice, A., Paul, A.A. (1994) Seasonal variation in vitamins A, C, riboflavin and folate intakes and status of pregnant and lactating women in a rural Gambian community: Some possible implications. *Eur J Clin Nutr*, 48, 660–668.

Bates, C.J., Prentice, A.M., Paul, A.A., Prentice, A., Sutcliffe, B.A., Whitehead, R.G. (1982a) Riboflavin status in infants born in rural Gambia, and the effects of a weanling food supplement. *Trans R Soc Trop Med & Hyg*, 76, 253–258.

Bates, C.J., Prentice, A.M., Prentice, A., Lamb, W.H., Whitehead, R.G. (1983) The effect of vitamin C supplementation on lactating women in Keneba, a West African rural community. *Int J Vit Nutr Res*, 53, 68–76.

Bates, C.J., Prentice, A.M., Watkinson, M., Morrell, P., Sutcliffe, B.A., Foord, F.A. (1982b) Riboflavin requirements of lactating Gambian women: A controlled supplementation trial. *AJCN*, 34, 701–709.

Beaton, G.H., Martorell, R., Aronson, K.J., Edmonston, B., McCabe, G., Ross, A.C., Harvey, B. (1993) *Effectiveness of Vitamin A Supplementation in The Control of Young Child Morbidity and Mortality in Developing Countries. State of The Art Series Nutrition Policy Discussion Paper No 13.* Geneva, Switzerland: ACC/SCN.

Belton, N.R. (1986) Rickets — Not only the 'English disease'. *Acta Paediatr Scand*, 323(suppl), 68–75.

Belton, N.R., Hambridge, K.M. (1991) Essential Element Deficiency and Toxicity. In: McLaren, D.S., Burman, D., Belton, N.R., Williams, A.F. (eds.) *Textbook of Paediatric Nutrition*, 18, pp. 429–444, 3rd edn. Edinburgh: Churchill Livingstone.

Biesalski, H.K. (1996) *Efficient Vitamin A Supply through Inhalation. Report of the XVII IVACG Meeting, Guatemala City, Guatemala.* Washington DC: IVACG Secretariat.

Blaner, W.S., Gamble, M.V., Burger, H., Kovacs, A., Weiser, B., Grimson, R., Nachman, S., Trooper, P., van Bennekum, A., Elie, M. (1997) *Maternal Serum Vitamin A Are Not Associated with Mother-To-Child Transmission of HIV-1 in The United States. Report of the XVIII IVACG Meeting, Cairo, Egypt.* Washington, DC: IVACG Secretariat.

Blum, M. (1997) Food fortification: A key strategy to end micronutrient malnutrition. *Nutriview*, 1–22.

Burri, B.J., Nimmagadda, A.P., Neidlinger, W.A., O'Brian, M.B., Goetz, M.B. (1997) *HIV Progression Was Not Influenced by Vitamin A Status Or Beta-Carotene Supplementation in Well-Nourished American Men. Report of The XVIII IVACG Meeting, Cairo, Egypt.* Washington, DC: IVACG Secretariat.

Byerley, L.O., Kirksey, A. (1985) Effects of different levels of vitamin C intake on vitamin C concentration in human milk and the vitamin C intakes of breast fed infants. *AJCN*, 41, 665–671.

Chang, Y.T., Germain-Lee, E.L., Doran, T.F., Migeon, C.J., Levine, M.A., Berkovitz, G.D. (1992) Hypocalcemia in non-white breast fed infants: Vitamin deficiency revisited. *Clin Pediatr*, 31, 695–698.

Chen, X., Li, R.W., Yen, H.C., Xu, Q.M., Liu, D.S. (1988) Studies of Rickets and Its Prevention in Beijing, China. In: Norman, A.W., Schaefer, K., Grigoleit, H., Herrath, D. (eds.) *Vitamin D. Molecular, Cellular and Clinical Endocrinology*, pp. 664–665. Berlin: De Gruyter.

Coutsoudis, A., Bobat, R.A., Coovadia, H.M., Kuhn, L., Tsai, W., Stein, Z.A. (1995) The effects of vitamin A supplementation on the morbidity of children born to HIV-infected women. *Am J Public Health*, 85, 1076–1081.

Coutsoudis, A., Kiepiela, P., Coovadia, H.M., Broughton, M. (1991) Vitamin A supplementation reduces measles morbidity in young African children: A randomised placebo controlled double blind trial. *AJCN*, 54, 890–895.

Deodhar, A.D., Rajalakshmi, R., Ramakrishnan, C.V. (1964) Studies on human lactation. 3. Effect of dietary vitamin supplementation on vitamin content of breast milk. *Acta Paediatr Scand*, 53, 42–48.

Department of Health. (1991) *Dietary Reference Values for Food Energy And Nutrients for The United Kingdom. Report of The Panel on Dietary Reference Values of The Committee on Medical Aspects of Food Policy. Reports on Health and Social Subjects No. 41*. London: HMSO.

Department of Health and Social Security. (1977) *The Composition of Mature Human Milk. Reports on Health and Social Subjects No. 12*. London: HMSO.

Dostalova, L. (1982) Correlations of the vitamin status between mother and newborn during delivery. *Dev Pharmacol Ther*, 4(suppl), 45–57.

Egypt. (1600) *The Ebers Papyrus*.

Ellison, J.B. (1932) Intensive vitamin therapy in measles. *BMJ*, 2, 708–711.

Food and Agriculture Organization (1988) Requirements of vitamin A, folate and vitamin B12. Report of a joint FAO/WHO Expert Consultation, FAO Food and Nutrition Series No 23 Rome, Italy. FAO press, 107.

Filteau, S.M., Maude, G.H., Raynes, J.G., Whitworth, J., Quigley, M. (1997) *The Association between Serum Retinol Concentrations And HIV in Adult Ugandans: A Preliminary Study. Report of the XVIII IVACG Meeting, Cairo, Egypt*. Washington, DC: IVACG Secretariat.

Ford, J.E., Zechalko, A., Murphy, J., Brooke, O.J. (1983) Comparison of the B vitamin composition of milk from mothers of preterm and term babies. *Arch Dis Childhd*, 58, 367–372.

Gallagher, P.G., Ehrenkranz, R.A. (1995) Nutritional anemias in infancy. *Clinics Perinatol*, 22, 671–692.

Gambon, R.C., Lentze, M.J., Rossi, E. (1986) Megoblastic

anaemia in one of monozygous twins breast fed by their vegetarian mother. *Eur J Pediatr*, 45, 570–571.

Greene, H.L. (1981) Gastrointestinal Development and Perinatal Nutrition. In: Lebenthal, E. (ed.) Textbook of Gastroenterology and Nutrition in Infancy, 50, pp. 585–593, water-soluble vitamins 1st edn. New York: Raven Press.

Herrera, M.G., Fawzi, W.W., Nestel, P., El Amin, A., Mohamed, K.A. (1996) *Effect of Vitamin A on The Incidence of Cough, Diarrhoea And Fever. Report of The XVII IVACG Meeting, Guatemala City, Guatemala*. Washington DC: IVACG Secretariat.

Higginbottom, M.C., Sweetman, L., Nyhan, W.L. (1978) A syndrome of methylmalonic aciduria, homocsyteinuria, megoblastic anemia and neurological abnormalities in a vitamin B deficient breast fed infant of a strict vegetarian. *N Engl J Med*, 299, 317–323.

Hirano, M., Honma, K., Daimatsu, T., Hayakawa, K., Oizumi, J., Zaima, K., Kanke, Y. (1992) Longitudinal variations of biotin content in human milk — Research note. *Int J Vit Nutr Res*, 62, 281–282.

Hoffmann-La Roche. (1994) *Vitamins*, 1st edn. Basel, Switzerland: F. Hoffmann-La Roche.

Humphrey, J.H., Agoestina, T., Taylor, G., Usman, A., West, K.P.J., Sommer, A. (1994) *Acute and Long Term Risks And Benefits to Neonates of 50,000 IU Oral Vitamin A. Report of The XVI IVACG Meeting Chiang Rai, Thailand*. Washington DC: The Nutrition Foundation.

Hussey, G.D., Klein, M. (1990) A randomised controlled trial of vitamin A in children with severe measles. *N Eng J Med*, 323, 160–164.

Jadhav, M., Webb, J.K.G., Vaishnava, S., Baker, S.J. (1962) Vitamin-BA deficiency in Indian infants. A clinical syndrome. *Lancet*, ii, 903–907.

Kim, Y., English, C., Reich, P., Gerber, L.E., Simpson, K.L. (1990) Vitamin A and carotenoids in human milk. *J Agric Food Chem*, 38, 1930–1933.

Luhby, A.L., Cooperman, J.M., Stone, M.L., Slobody, L.B. (1961) Physiology of vitamin B in pregnancy the placenta and the newborn. *Am J Dis Child*, 102, 753–754.

Lunn, P.G., Northrop-Clewes, C.A., Downes, R.M. (1991) Intestinal permeability, mucosal injury and growth faltering in Gambian infants. *Lancet*, 338, 907–910.

McCollum, E.V., Davis, M. (1913) The necessity of certain lipins in the diet during growth. *J Biol Chem*, 15, 167–175.

Macy, I.G. (1949) Composition of human colostrum and milk. *Am J Dis Child*, 78, 589–603.

Markestad, T., Kolmannskog, S., Arntzen, E., Toftegaard, L., Haneberg, B., Aksnes, L. (1984) Serum concentrations of vitamin D metabolites in exclusively breast fed infants at 70 north. *Acta Paediatr Scand*, 73, 29–32.

Metz, J. (1970) Folate deficiency conditioned by lactation. *AJCN*, 23, 843–847.

Mock, D.M., Mock, N.I., Dankle, J.A. (1992) Secretory patterns of biotin in human milk. *J Nutr*, 122, 546–552.

Moran, J.R., Vaughan, R., Stroops, S., Coy, S., Johnston, H., Greene, H.L. (1983) Concentrations and total daily output of micronutrients in breast milk of mothers delivering preterm: A longitudinal study. *J Pediatr Gastroenterol Nutr*, 2, 629–634.

Nail, P.A., Thomas, M.R., Eakin, R. (1980) The effect of thiamin and riboflavin supplementation on the level of those vitamins in human breast milk and urine. *AJCN*, 33, 198–204.

Northrop-Clewes, C.A., McCullough, F.S.W., Das, B.S., Lunn, P.G., Downes, R.M., Thurnham, D.I. (1997) *Improvements in Vitamin A Intake Influence Gut Integrity in Infants. Report of The XVIII IVACG Meeting, Cairo, Egypt.* Washington, DC: IVACG Secretariat.

Picciano, M.F. (1995) Folate Nutrition in Lactation. In: Bailey, B.B. (ed.) *Folate in Health and Disease*, pp. 153–169, 1st edn. New York: Mecel Dekker.

Pietschnig, B., Haschke, F., Vanura, H., Shearer, M., Veitl, V., Kellner, S., Schuster, E. (1993) Vitamin K in breast milk: No influence of maternal dietary intake. *Eur J Clin Nutr*, 47, 209–215.

Powers, H.J. (1997) Vitamin requirements for term infants: Considerations for infant formulae. *Nutr Res Rev*, 10, 1–33.

Prentice, A.M., Roberts, S.B., Prentice, A., Paul, A.A., Watkinson, M., Watkinson, A.A., Whitehead, R.G. (1983) Dietary supplementation of lactating Gambian women. I. Effect on breast milk volume and quality. *Human Nutr Clin Nutr*, 37C, 53–64.

Rajalakshmi, R., Deodhar, A.D., Ramakrishnan, C.V. (1965) Vitamin C secretion during lactation. *Acta Paediatr Scand*, 54, 375–382.

Reeve, L.E., Chesney, R.W., DeLuca, H.F. (1982) Vitamin D of human milk: Identification of biologically active forms. *AJCN*, 36, 122–126.

Rodriguez, M.S. (1980) A Conspectus of Research on Folacin Requirements of Man. In: Irwin, M.I., Hegsted, D.M. (ed.) *Nutritional Requirements of Man: A Conspectus of Research*, pp. 397–489. New York: The Nutrition Foundation Inc.

Ross, A.C., Hammerling, U.G. (1994) Retinoids and The Immune System. In: Sporn, M.B., Roberts, A.B. and Goodman, D.S. (eds.) *The Retinoids: Biology, Chemistry and Medicine*, pp. 521–543, 2nd edn. New York: Raven Press.

Scharz, K.B. (1989) Requirements And Absorption of Fat-Soluble Vitamins during Infancy. In: Lebenthal, E. (ed.) *Textbook of Gastroenterology and Nutrition in Infancy*, 28, pp. 347–366, 2nd edn. New York: Raven Press.

Semba, R.D., Miotti, P.G., Chiphangwi, J.D., Saah, A.J., Canner, J.K., Dallabetta, G.A., Hoover, D.R. (1994) Maternal vitamin-A-deficiency band mother-to-child transmission of HIV-1. *Lancet*, 343, 1593–1597.

Semba, R.D., Miotti, T.E., Taha, N., Kumwenda, L., Mtimavalye, R., Broadhead, A. et al (1997) *Maternal Vitamin A Supplementation And Mother-To-Child Transmission of HIV. Report of The XVIII IVACG Meeting, Cairo, Egypt.* Washington, DC: IVACG Secretariat.

Shankar A. H., Genton, B., Semba, R.D. Tielsch J., West K.P., Jr. (1997) *Vitamin A Supplementation as A Nutrient Based Intervention To Reduce Malaria-Related Morbidity. Report of The XVIII IVACG Meeting, Cairo, Egypt.* Washington, DC: IVACG Secretariat.

Sinclair, H.M. (1982) Thiamin. In: Barker, B.M. and Bender, D.A. (eds) vitamins in medicine volume 2, chapter 4, pp 114–167 4th edn. London: W Heinemann Medical Books Ltd.

Smith, A.M., Picciano, M.F., Deering, R.H. (1985) Folate intake and blood concentrations in term infants. *AJCN*, 41, 590–598.

Sommer, A. (1983) Mortality associated with mild untreated xerophthalmia (thesis). *Trans Am Ophthamol Soc*, 81, 825–853.

Sommer, A., Hussaini, G., Tarwotjo, I., Susanto, D. (1983) Increased mortality in children with mild vitamin A deficiency. *Lancet*, ii, 585–588.

Sommer, A., Tarwotjo, I., Djunaedi, E. (1986) Impact of vitamin A supplementation on childhood mortality: A randomised controlled community trial. *Lancet*, i, 1169–1173.

Sommer, A., West, K.P.J. (1996) V. Assessment and Prevention. In: Anonymous (ed.) *Vitamin A deficiency: Health, Survival and Vision*, pp. 388–409, 1st edn. New York: Oxford University Press.

Song, W.O., Chan, G.M., Wyse, B.W., Hansen, R.G. (1984) Effect of pantothenic acid status on the content of the vitamin in human milk. *AJCN*, 40, 317–324.

Stallings, R.Y., Stoltzfus, R.J., Schulze, K., Miotti, P. (1997) *Negative Association of An Acute Phase Protein with Maternal Serum Retinol in HIV Infection. Report of The XVIII IVACG Meeting, Cairo, Egypt.* Washington, DC: IVACG Secretariat.

Thomas, M.R., Sneed, S.M., Wei, C., Nail, P.A., Wilson, M., Sprinkle, E.E. (1980) The effects of vitamin C, vitamin B6, vitamin B12, folic acid, riboflavin and thiamin on the breast milk and maternal status of well-nourished women at 6 months post partum. *AJCN*, 33, 2151–2156.

Waslien, C.I. (1977) Folate requirements of infants. In: *Folic Acid: Biochemistry and Physiology in Relation to The Human Nutrition Requirement*, 21, pp. 232–246. Washington, DC: Food and Nutrition Board, National Research Council, National Academy of Sciences.

West, K.P., Pokhrel, R.P., Katz, J. (1991) Efficacy of vitamin A in reducing preschool child mortality in Nepal. *Lancet*, 338, 67–71.

19

Mass nutritional supplementation

Christine A. Northrop-Clewes

Abbreviations

ACC/SCN	Administrative Co-ordination Committee/Subcommittee on Nutrition
INCAP	Institute of Nutrition of Central America and Panama
WHO	World Health Organisation
UNICEF	United Nations Children's Fund
IDD	iodine deficiency disorder
FAO/WHO	Food and Agricultural Organisation/World Health Organisation
QC	quality control
ppm	parts per million
KIO_3	potassium iodate
KI	potassium iodide
IDA	iron deficiency anaemia
MSG	monosodium glutamate
RE	retinol equivalents
SMHP	sodium hexameta-phosphate
NIN	Nutrition Institute of Nutrition
RDA	recommended dietary allowance
USAID	Unites States Agency for International Development
VAD	vitamin A deficiency

Introduction

The problem of micro-nutrient malnutrition

A significant proportion of the world's population suffers from or is at risk of deficiencies of vitamins and minerals. Adequate intake and availability of these essential vitamins and minerals are closely related to survival, physical and mental development, general good health and the overall well being of all individuals and populations (Lofti et al 1996).

Historical background

History of fortification

The scientific rationale, including technology, stability, interactions and effectiveness, for fortifying staple foods was developed early in the twentieth century (Nilson & Piza 1997). In 1923, Switzerland was the first country to fortify salt with iodine to prevent goitre and cretinism because iodine deficiency was widespread throughout the alpine region. The United States followed the Swiss initiative in 1930 (Blum 1997). Also in 1923, the United Kingdom and United States began fortifying milk with vitamin D to prevent rickets, which were common at that time in the northern hemisphere due to poor socio-economic conditions and the lack of sunshine in the winter months (Blum 1997). In 1944, the government of Canada started the fortification of white wheat flour with iron, thiamin (B1), riboflavin (B2) and niacin and of margarine with vitamin A. Results were remarkable, and symptoms of vitamins A and B deficiencies were substantially reduced or eliminated. Beriberi was eliminated completely and infant mortality in Canada during the first year of life fell from 102/1000 live births in 1944 to 61/1000 in 1947 (Nilson & Piza 1997).

The introduction of polished rice into the Philippines at the turn of the twentieth century was associated with widespread beriberi. However, in October 1948 thiamin-fortified rice was distributed, which led, for example in Bataan province, to a spectacular reduction in death from beriberi from 194 in 1948 to 20/100,000 in 1950 (Williams 1961).

Fortification of sugar with vitamin A in Guatemala in 1974 reduced the prevalence of low plasma retinol levels (< 0.35 μmol/L) from 3.3% to 0.2% within 2 years. The Institute of Nutrition of Central America and Panama (INCAP) used sugar because there was no other staple food reaching all the target groups in the country (Arroyave 1971).

In 1993, Venezuela began fortifying pre-cooked yellow and white corn flour with vitamins A, B1, B2, niacin and iron, and wheat flour was fortified with B1, B2, niacin and iron. The two cereals represented 45% of the calorie intake of the population. Evidence of a reduction in the prevalence of iron deficiency from 37 to 19% and anaemia from 15 to 10% was shown in a study of 397 children (Layrisse et al 1996). In 1994, the government of Guatemala reviewed the fortification of wheat flour and included folic acid, because a high prevalence of deficiency of this vitamin existed and its potential importance in preventing anaemia was recognized. Columbia, Bolivia and Ecuador followed the example of Guatemala in 1996 and fortified their flour with folate. In 1998, the United States also added folic acid to their wheat flour (1.54 mg/kg flour), however this was to prevent the high prevalence of pregnancies affected by spina bifida and other neural tube defects. The US Public Health Service recommend that women of child-bearing age should eat at least 400 μg of folic acid daily to prevent neural tube defects (US Federal Register 1996).

Developing countries

Clinical deficiencies in developing countries have been treated using supplementation programmes. The most challenging problems have been xerophthalmia, anaemia and goitre because:

1. Vitamin A, iron and iodine deficiencies are highly prevalent in the world;

2. There are serious adverse consequences of these deficiencies for physical and mental health, education, work capacity and economic efficiency;

3. The extent of these deficiencies at population and individual levels can be measured relatively accurately;

4. Solutions for eliminating these deficiencies are known and fairly easy to implement.

Other micro-nutrients have received little attention. The prevalence rates of iron, iodine and vitamin A deficiencies are much higher in developing relative to developed countries (Table 19.1). The latest estimations show that 254 million children suffer from clinical and marginal vitamin A deficiency, resulting in 1 million childhood deaths annually (WHO 1995). 1.5 billion people suffer from iodine deficiency; it is the leading cause of mental and physical retardation in infants and of increased risk of neonatal mortality (ACC/SCN 1993). 2.2 billion, mainly children and pregnant women, suffer from iron deficiency (The World Bank 1994). Iron deficiency is so prevalent that even in developed nations the rates amongst some pregnant

women may reach levels of public health significance (The World Bank 1994).

Global commitment

Global attention to understand, control and eliminate micro-nutrient deficiencies reached a peak in 1990 when specific goals for the elimination and control of micro-nutrient malnutrition (particularly vitamins A, B-complex, and C, and iron, iodine, zinc, and calcium) by the year 2000 were adopted at the World Summit for Children in New York (123 countries). Subsequent to the commitments made by 159 governments (First International Conference on Nutrition 1993), much groundwork has been done in many countries to accelerate the reduction of micro-nutrient malnutrition by:

1. Direct supplementation of vulnerable populations or groups with micro-nutrient supplements;

2. Dietary improvement;

3. Fortification of common foods with micro-nutrients.

Supplementation

Periodic administration of pharmacological preparations by injections or in the form of capsules or tablets is an effective strategy whereby almost immediate benefits can be brought to the most at-risk groups. However, hard-to-reach at-risk groups and other household and community members who are not targeted to receive

Table 19.1 — Population at risk[1] of and affected by micro-nutrient malnutrition (in millions)

Region[2]	Iodine deficiency disorder (IDD)[3]		Vitamin A deficiency (VAD)[4]		Iron deficient or anaemic[5] population
	At risk IDD	Affected by goitre	Population affected[6]	Prevalence (%)	Population affected
Africa	181	86	53	49	206
Americas	168	63	16.1	20	94
Southeast Asia	486	176	126.5	69	616
East Mediterranean	173	93	16.1	22	149
West Pacific[7]	423	141	42.1	27	1058
Total	1572	655	254		2150

[1]Number of persons living in areas at risk of IDD and the number of pre-school children living in VAD areas; [2]WHO regions; [3]Source WHO 1994; [4]Reflects estimates from data available to WHO 1994 (WHO 1995); [5]Pre-school children only (WHO 1992); [6]Population affected by sub-clinical, severe and moderate deficiencies; [7]Including China.

the supplement may not benefit. Supplementation often requires a large foreign currency input and an elaborate and costly distribution system. In addition, patient compliance is a prerequisite for success

Dietary improvement

The aim here is to increase dietary availability, regular access and consumption of vitamin- and mineral-rich foods in at-risk and micro-nutrient-deficient groups of populations in developing countries. Such efforts require changes in dietary behaviour, which may necessitate changes in food supply and availability. Hence, a long time period to achieve success may be needed.

Fortification of foods

Fortification of foods with micro-nutrients that have been shown to be insufficient in the daily diet has largely been responsible for the elimination of vitamin and mineral deficiencies in the Western World. Margarine containing no 'fat-soluble A' was the first 'imitation' food produced on a large industrial scale. The introduction of margarine as a substitute for butter into the Danish food supply in 1910 led to an epidemic of xerophthalmia in children. The margarine was fortified with vitamin A, eliminating the xerophthalmia (Bloch 1931), and now throughout the world margarine is amongst those items of food that are most frequently fortified with vitamin A (Bauernfeind 1983). In addition, fortification of margarine with vitamin D is thought to have rid Canada and Northern Europe of rickets in the early part of the twentieth century (Bloch 1931). Fortification of refined flour with iron in Sweden and the United States is said to have dramatically reduced iron deficiency anaemia (IDA), and in countries where iodization of salt has been introduced, sustained reductions in the prevalence of iodine deficiency disorder (IDD) have been seen (UNICEF 1995). Enrichment of a staple food improves dietary quality long-term without a change of diet. It should therefore be considered as an alternative to dietary diversity (Flores 1996).

Practice and procedures

Developing a food fortification programme

Definition of food fortification

Food fortification involves the addition of nutrients to food in order to maintain or improve the quality of the diet of a targeted group or population (FAO/ WHO ad hoc Expert Committee 1971, Crowley 1974). Food fortification can be used to correct a demonstrated dietary deficiency, to restore nutrients lost during food processing, to increase the nutritional quality of manufactured food products used as a sole source of nourishment (e.g., infant formula), or to ensure that when manufactured foods substitute for other foods the nutritional content remains constant. The important steps in the development of and the conditions for a successful food fortification programme are summarized in Table 19.2.

Selection of a food vehicle

Selection of the right food ingredient or food to act as a carrier (food vehicle) of the specific micro-nutrient (fortificant) is important for compliance. There are a number of criteria that must be met for the food to be a vehicle (Lofti et al 1996, Nilson & Piza 1997):

- A high proportion of the target population must consume the food;
- The food should be eaten regularly, in relatively constant amounts and the upper and lower levels of intake should be known;
- There should be little variation in consumption patterns between individuals and between regions;
- The normal serving size should meet a significant part of the daily dietary requirement;
- All the population should be able to afford to buy the food, i.e. the additional cost of fortification should be reasonable for the consumer;
- The probability of excessive intake is minimal (i.e., risk of toxicity is low);
- There should be no change in acceptability of the product or change in the quality of the product as a result of fortification.

Processing/storage

Ideally, a central processing plant should carry out the fortification process. It should be a simple process using low-cost technology suitable for a developing-world situation. The food may need to have a dark colour and/or strong odour to mask slight changes to the colour or odour of the food by the fortificant. The vehicle and fortificant should be stable, with no micro-nutrient interaction, and remain mixed even after storing.

Stability and marketing

Nilson & Piza (1997) recommend that the nutrient(s) added should be sufficiently stable in the food using

Table 19.2 — Development of a food fortification programme

Steps in the development of a food fortification programme	Conditions necessary for the success of food fortification programmes
Determine the prevalence of the micro-nutrient deficiency	Political support
Determine the micro-nutrient intake from a dietary survey	Industry support
Obtain consumption data for potential vehicles	Adequate application of legislation including external quality control
Determine the micro-nutrient availability from the typical diet	Good bioavailability of the compound
Seek government support	Human resource training at industry and marketing level
Seek food industry support	No inhibitory effect of the common diet
Assess status of potential vehicles and the processing industry chain (suppliers)	Adequate laboratory assessment of micro-nutrient status
Determine the type and amount of micro-nutrient fortificant	No cultural or other objection against fortified foods
Develop fortification technology	Consumer acceptability
Study interactions, potency, stability, organoleptic quality of fortified food	Adequate study design or statistical evaluation
Determine bioavailability of fortified foods	Absence of parasitism or other non-dietary causes of iron deficiency anaemia
Develop standards for the fortified foods	No constraint on obtaining micro-nutrients
Define final product, packaging and labelling requirements	
Develop legislation and regulation for mandatory compliance	
Promote campaigns to improve consumer acceptance.	

Modified from Lofti et al (1996).

customary conditions of packing, storage, distribution and use. As well, they state that: 1) the product should be labelled according to the standards of the country; 2) there should be an adequate turnover of the product; 3) Oxygen, humidity, heat, acids, redox agents and light can affect vitamins, and other components can interfere with the stability, like heavy metals; 4) technology exists to prevent losses, but losses cannot be totally avoided; and 5) in order to ensure that when the food is ingested the vitamin content is as described on the label, the food industry should compensate for losses during processing and during storage of the finished product.

Selection of fortificants

- The fortificant must have good bioavailability during the normal shelf life of the fortified food;
- It should not interact with the flavour, taste, texture, colour or cooking properties of the vehicle and should not shorten the shelf life of the vehicle;
- The fortified product should be offered at a price that is affordable;
- The fortificant should be a suitable colour and have the right solubility and particle size for mixing with the vehicle;
- There should be a commercial source of the food-grade fortificant;
- It should be commercially possible to add the fortificant to the vehicle (Lofti et al 1996, Nilson & Piza 1997).

The following fortification technologies are already in use and widely applied:

1. Iodization of salt to combat IDD;
2. Fortification of oil, fat, sugar, milk, dairy products and cereals with vitamin A;

Table 19.3 — Opportunities for food fortification

Food		β-carotene	A	D	E	B1	B2	B6	C	Folate + B12	Fe	Ca	I
						Vitamins						Minerals	
Milk:	Liquid	+	+	+	+	+	+	+	+	+	T	+	+
	Powder	+	+	+	+	+	+	+	+	+	+	+	+
	With cereal	+	+	+	+	+	+	+	+	+	+	+	+
Flour:	Wheat	T	+	+	+	+	+	+	X	+	+	+	+
	Corn	T	+	+	+	+	+	+	T	+	+	+	+
	Rice	T	+	+	+	+	+	+	+	+	+	+	+
Rice		T	+	+	+	+	+	+	+	+	+	+	T
Snacks		T	+	+	+	+	+	+	+	+	+	+	T
Corn flakes		T	+	+	+	+	+	+	+	+	+	+	T
Oil		+	+	+	+	X	X	X	T	T	T	T	X
Margarine		+	+	+	+	T	T	T	T	T	X	T	X
Sugar		X	+	T	T	X	X	X	X	T	+	T	+
Salt		X	T	X	X	X	X	X	X	X	+	+	+

+, Possible; X, not possible; T, trials needed; Fe, iron; Ca, calcium; I, iodine. Modified from Lofti et al (1996).

3. Fortification of flour, cereals, weaning foods and biscuits with iron.

Other possibilities for fortification are listed in Table 19.3.

Fortification technology

For most foods, technology is quite simple. For example, vitamins that are soluble in water can be dissolved in water and added to liquid foods like dairy products, fruit juices and beverages. In powder form, they can be mixed directly with foods like wheat flour, corn flour, corn starch and dry milk. The fat-soluble vitamins can be added directly to the oily phase of foods like margarine, mayonnaise and re-combined milk. The industry can micro-encapsulate fat-soluble vitamins in order to mix them with powders, water-soluble products or to protect them from oxygen and other harmful components (Nilson & Piza 1997).

Fortification of rice and sugar requires more complex technologies. Vitamin A in powder form is adhered with vegetable oil to the sugar crystals by embedding a beadlet of retinyl palmitate, plus antioxidant, in a gelatin matrix that transforms the liposoluble and liquid vitamin into a dry water-dispersible powder. Rice is fortified by spraying the vitamins onto rice kernels and then coating with food grade resins to avoid leaching when washing the rice before cooking (Sommer & West 1996).

Fortification costs

Compared to the social and health costs of micro-nutrient deficiencies, the direct cost of delivering nutrients in foods is remarkably low (Nilson & Piza 1997). The cost of fortification includes the cost of the fortificant, labour costs for processing, transport and quality control (QC). In addition, depending on the type of food to be fortified, the level of fortification, and the technology needed, the final cost of fortification can vary widely. In most cases, it costs less than $1.00 US per year to protect a child against deficiency of vitamin A, iron and iodine with food fortification (The World Bank 1994). The cost of fortification to protect an individual for 1 year against vitamin A deficiency is < $0.30 US and for iron < $0.10 US (Table 19.4). These are approximate costs and indicate the price for the actual processing and chemical costs at source. They exclude costs related to programme management, product promotion, marketing and monitoring. The ultimate cost to the consumer is progressively inflated as the fortified food passes from producer to retailer (Lofti et al 1996). These inflated costs to the consumer are an economic question, which should be looked at on a country-to-

Table 19.4 — Examples of the concentration of fortificant used and approximate cost of fortification in a number of countries

Vehicle	Fortificant	Concentration	Cost (range)/person/ year (US cents)	Country
Salt	K–iodate	50–80 ppm I_2	2–6 (1992)	Several
	Fe(II) sulphate +	1000 ppm Fe+	12–18 (1991)	India
	Na-acid pyrophosphate	2500 ppm +		
	+ Na-acid sulphate	5000 ppm		
	K–iodide +	50 ppm I_2 +	12–20 (1990)	India
	Fe (II) fumarate	1000 ppm Fe		
	K–iodate +	20 ppm I_2	12–20 (1992)	India
	Fe(II) sulphate +	1000 ppm Fe +		
	Na-polyphosphate	10 ppm Na-polyphosphate		
Sugar	Vitamin A 250 cold water storage (CWS)	15,000 IU/kg	29 (1994)	Guatemala
	NaFeEDTA	3 ppm Fe	10 (1981)	Guatemala
Wheat flour	Elemental iron	25–35 ppm	1.5 (1980)	Several
Cooking fat	Vitamin A	50,000 IU/kg	30–40 (1988)	Several
Biscuits	Haem-iron concentrate	1.8 gHb/30g	108 (1981)	Chile
Edible oil	Vitamin A	20 IU/g	n/a	Pakistan
Margarine	Vitamin A	375 RE/15g	20 (1994)	Philippines
Fish sauce	NaFeEDTA	1 mg Fe/ml	5–15 (1970)	Thailand
MSG[1]	Vitamin A palmitate 250 CWS	175,000 IU/kg	6 (1988)	Indonesia
Corn flour/ wheat flour	Iron	20–50 mg/kg	7–8 (1994)	Venezuela
	Vitamin A (+ niacin, thiamin, riboflavin)	39,000 IU/kg		

n/a, not available; [1]monosodium glutamate.

country basis. If fortification is introduced, then the cost increase related to fortification perhaps should be subsidized initially by the government and gradually passed onto the consumer.

Bioavailability of the micro-nutrients

The term *bioavailability* generally refers to the extent to which a nutrient is capable of being absorbed (i.e., enters the blood stream) to be used by the body. Bioavailability of a nutrient in the diet is a function of (Lofti et al 1996):

- The form in which the nutrient is ingested (i.e., the nutrient must be in a form that can either be transported directly through the intestinal mucosa or can easily be converted to a form that can be transported through the mucosa);
- The extent of conversion of the nutrient into absorbable forms and the absorbed form of the nutrient must be able to be metabolized;

- The composition of the diet (i.e., other constituents in the diet can inhibit or enhance the transport of the micro-nutrient through the mucosa, for example, phytate [found in major cereals and legumes] and polyphenols [found in sorghum] diminish iron absorption, whereas vitamin C enhances it) (Hurrell 1997);
- The physiological status and integrity of the gut can affect how much of the nutrient is absorbed and how efficiently it is absorbed. For example, the presence of infection depresses the concentration of existing iron and vitamin A in the circulation (Thurnham & Singkamani 1991), gastrointestinal motility affects transit time (Elia et al 1987), and the immaturity of intestinal function in infants may reduce absorption (Thompson et al 1998);
- The proportion of the nutrient that is absorbed may be affected by the concentration of the nutrient (i.e., whether it is in physiological or

pharmacological doses or by taking certain drugs concurrently).

Therefore, when considering a food fortification programme, the bioavailability of the fortificant in relation to the type of diet consumed by the target population and the overall health of the population should be considered.

Legislation and regulations for food fortification

The food industry has in some cases voluntarily fortified products. However, the development of voluntarily fortified foods has been impaired in some countries because of consumer and government lack of awareness of the prevalence of micro-nutrient deficiencies and their impact on health (Nilson & Piza 1997). To be effective, and to raise awareness of consumers and health policy makers, fortification programmes need to be supported by suitable legislation and/or regulations. It is essential to have in place the mechanisms through which the entire fortification programme can be controlled. Once policy makers are aware of the health problems of their population, and are motivated to instigate regulations and/or legislation for a fortification programme, then they are in a position to accelerate the fortification process and to protect the consumer from harmful practices, such as technical inadequacies in the fortification process (Lofti et al 1996).

Current practices in micro-nutrient fortification

Iodine

Salt

The single fortification of salt with iodine occurs in both developed and developing countries. Salt fulfils nearly all the characteristics of a suitable food vehicle and is one of the few commodities consumed by all members of a community regardless of social class. The two principal fortificants are potassium iodide (KI) and potassium iodate (KIO_3), neither of which transmit any colour or odour to the salt. Therefore, iodized salt is not distinguishable from non-iodized salt and is fully acceptable to the consumers. The current level of iodization varies from country to country, and ranges from 20–165 parts per million KIO_3 (ppm) supplying 12–100 ppm iodine (Lofti et al 1996) (see Table 19.4). The level of fortification may be changed over time and is calculated using the following equation (Mannar & Dunn 1995):

Assuming a requirement of iodine of 200 µg/day and salt consumption is 10 g/day

Level of iodine required is 200/10 = 20 µg/g salt or	20 ppm
Compensation for transit and storage losses	20 ppm
Fixed level of iodization required	40 ppm iodine $\equiv 40 \star 1.685^a =$ 67 ppm KIO_3

[a]ratio of molecular weight of KIO_3/I_3, i.e., 214/127 = 1.685

Water

The potential of using community drinking water as a carrier of iodine has been of interest for several decades, and experimental systems for iodizing town and school water supply systems have been tried in the Central African Republic, Italy, Mali, Malaysia and Thailand (Lofti et al 1996). Iodization of public water systems is achieved by diverting a small amount of water through a canister containing crystals of iodine and then re-introducing the iodized water into the main supply at a concentration of 50–200 µg/L of water.

In Thailand, an iodine solution is prepared in small dropper bottles and distributed to schools and households for direct addition to drinking water (Lofti et al 1996). The experience in Thailand of using institutional settings like schools where a water distribution system exists perhaps should be considered in other populations. A French company, Rhone-Poulenc, developed a method that involved placing an iodine-silicone polymer in a basket at the bottom of a tube-well, which released iodine slowly into the water over 12 months (diffuser). Mannar & Stone (1993) looked at some practical difficulties in using diffusers and concluded the following:

1. Rural populations might use water from other sources (e.g., streams, rainwater or open wells rather than tubewells);

2. The amount of polymer required had to be calculated in terms of the average number of persons using the well and the water consumption /person. Therefore, the appropriate dose/well required preliminary studies;

3. Routine monitoring of iodine levels could be costly;

4. The silicone-iodine polymer has to be replaced annually, and this could be more expensive than capsule distribution;

5. The population would probably not be able to afford to cover the costs.

Bread

In 1966, wheat flour used for bread in Tasmania was fortified with KIO_3 at a concentration of 2 ppm. Based on estimates of bread consumption according to age, average iodine daily consumption was very variable (Clements 1979):

Age 1–3 years	81 µg
Age 7–11 years	187 µg
Age 15–18 years	270 µg

Brick tea

This is fortified with iodine in Tibet and West China (Lofti et al 1996).

Sweets

Trials to fortify sweets have been carried out in the Middle East (Lofti et al 1996).

Sugar

Iodization was tested in the Sudan but abandoned. Because sugar is rationed and controlled, it was found that a huge black market developed, which led to a sugar shortage in western Sudan where IDD is endemic and an over-spill into Khartoum where IDD is not a problem.

Milk

The iodine content of milk is influenced by the husbandry of dairy cattle. Cattle are exposed to iodine in water, forage, feed supplements, salt blocks and veterinary medications. The milk is exposed to iodine contamination from iodophor sanitizing solutions used as disinfectants on the cattle, milking equipment, vats and other milk containers. Variation in husbandry practices and in seasonal and regional factors result in variations in iodine concentrations in milk. In the United States, the average iodine content of milk is 23 ($\pm$ 9) µg/100 g milk, which is calculated to be equivalent to 37% of the RDA for adults from one cup of milk (Lofti et al 1996).

Iron

Bioavailability of a single iron source is difficult to predict because it can vary considerably due to the enhancing or inhibitory effects of other food components on absorption (Hurrell 1984). With this in mind, iron fortification is considered to be a long-term approach to combating iron deficiency anaemia.

Infant food and formulas

Breastfeeding is recommended as the best food for infants up to 6 months of age. Cow's milk should not be given to a child < 1 year of age as it contains little vitamin D and iron and can cause occult blood loss due to damage to the gut caused by dietary protein sensitization or lactose intolerance (Sullivan 1993). After 6 months, breast milk should be supplemented with additional food because infants reach a critical stage when there is an increased demand for higher energy and iron for growth.

In developed countries, and where it can be afforded in developing nations, manufactured infant cereals, which meet the solid food requirement, can be used as a supplement. Infant cereals were mainly designed for weaning infants, however other risk groups such as pregnant and lactating women and children in developing countries may benefit from eating infant cereals.

Characteristics of iron compounds used in fortification of foods

The iron compounds used for food fortification have to meet certain requisites related to their bioavailability, absorption mechanism and toxicity (Boccio et al 1998). The choice of iron compound depends on its solubility in gastric juice and on the presence of activators or inhibitors (Boccio et al 1997). The most common iron fortification compounds can be classified into 4 groups:

1. **Freely water–soluble iron** (ferrous sulphate, ferrous gluconate and ferrous lactate). Very bioavailable, however they tend to interact with the fortified food altering its sensory properties (e.g., provoking fat rancidity);

2. **Poorly water–soluble or soluble in dilute acids** (ferrous fumarate, ferrous succinate). Good bioavailability but tend only to be used in solid dehydrated foods;

3. **Water-insoluble or poorly-soluble forms of iron in dilute acids** (ferric orthophosphate, ferric pyrophosphate, elemental iron). Do not change the sensory properties or nutritional value of the food but have low bioavailability;

4. Recently, a product containing **ferrous sulphate micro-encapsulated with lecithin** has been produced. This product has the same bioavailability as ferrous sulphate but the coat of phospholipids keeps the iron from coming in contact with the food vehicle thereby preventing undesirable inter-actions seen with conventional ferrous sulphate.

Fortificants in infant formula

Infant formulas are usually milk based with added vegetable oils, minerals and vitamins. Iron is nearly always added as ferrous sulphate (5–12 mg/L), and its absorption can be improved considerably with the addition of 100–200 mg vitamin C/L (Hurrell 1997). The absorption of iron from fortified formulas has been found to be between 3–10% of the dose, which is very low in comparison to breast milk where absorption is 49–70% (Hurrell 1984). The reason for this discrepancy is not known, but it does not appear to be due to lactoferrin (Kushner 1982). However it could possibly be due to chelating agents in breast milk, which keep iron soluble during digestion (Hurrell 1984), or to the presence of calcium and the milk protein, casein, in formula, which act as inhibitory factors (Hurrell 1997).

Fortificants in infant cereals

The manufacturers of infant cereals have a problem because the iron compounds, which have the best availability, reduce the product quality and shelf life. The use of less effective iron sources may satisfy label claims and regulations, but there is a question about their bioavailability. The most commonly-used fortificants are elemental iron, ferric pyrophosphate, ferric orthophosphate, ferrous succinate and ferrous fumarate. All have lower bioavailability than ferrous sulphate. The best researched of the fortificants is elemental iron, which is used for infant cereal fortification in the United States. Ferrous fumarate is often used in corn soy milk and wheat-soy blend as the reddish-brown colour of fumarate is compatible with the yellowish-brown colour of the vehicles. Ferrous succinate appears to be just as suitable as fumarate without causing fat oxidation and discolouration (Hurrell et al 1989). Hence, the main technological problems with iron fortification of infant cereal concerns colour, bioavailability and off-flavour due to fat oxidation. To reduce the technological problems, research into the encapsulation of ferrous sulphate has been underway for some time (see above).

Iron fortification levels of infant foods

The Codex Alimentarius (1981) sets the minimal fortification level of iron in infant foods at 1 mg iron/100 kcal, equivalent to 7 mg iron/L formula. Fortification levels vary from country to country: in the United States the upper limit is 3 mg iron/100 kcal ($\equiv$ 20 mg/L), the maximum level in the United Kingdom is 1 mg iron/100 kcal, and in France it is 1.5–2 mg iron/100 kcal (Lofti et al 1996). In most studies, fortification levels are about 12 mg iron/L formula (range 10–17 mg/L) and 0.15–0.5 mg iron/g cereal. However, in Europe, lower levels are common with more efficient use of iron from foods with lower

fortification levels. Recently, Haschke et al (1993) found 3 mg ferrous sulphate/L whey-predominant formula was sufficient to protect infants aged 3–6 months from deficiency.

Possibly a more important reason to minimize iron fortification is the effect of iron on the absorption of copper and zinc. Iron competes with copper and zinc for absorption. However, the Committee on Nutrition (1989) claimed that iron fortification of infant formulas does not impair the absorption of zinc or copper enough to affect nutritional status. This has been confirmed by other studies, which have also shown no effect of iron fortification of infant cereals on zinc absorption (Davidsson et al 1995, Fairweather-Tate et al 1995, Polberger et al 1996).

Other vehicles used in iron fortification

A number of other vehicles have been used, including wheat flour biscuits in Chile (Asenjo et al 1985), rice flour in Argentina and Chile (Lofti et al 1996), salt in India and Thailand (see *Double fortification* below), fish sauce (nampla) in Thailand (INACG 1993), and curry powder in South Africa (INACG 1993).

Double fortification

Iodine and iron

Double fortification of salt with iron and iodine has been considered in Thailand, India and Canada. The product was viewed as potentially useful for large populations or perhaps to be targeted at pregnant women and young children through special delivery channels (Lofti et al 1996).

Mannar et al (1991) reported that a combination of ferrous fumarate 3200 ppm (iron content 1000 ppm) and KI 65 ppm (iodine content 50 ppm) were a workable combination of compounds that would not need added stabilisers. The salt does become light brown in colour but does not deteriorate if sealed in waterproof packaging. Rao (1994) proposed a combination of ferrous sulphate 3200 ppm (iron content 1000 ppm), KI 40 ppm (iodine content 20 ppm) and a stabiliser 1% sodium hexameta-phosphate (SMHP), which acts as a chelator. The bioavailability and stability of the double-fortified salt were found to be acceptable. The National Institute of Nutrition (NIN) (The micro-nutrient initiative 1996) in India has reported a dry mixing technique to mix ferrous sulphate and SHMP with salt to be successful. However, Diosady (1996) in Canada found that there were heavy losses of iodine due to the presence of magnesium chloride, an impurity of salt. The Canadian group developed a new technique of dextrin micro-encapsulation to create a barrier between the iron and iodine compounds, which helps to retain them in a stable form. A pilot fortification programme in the north-east of Thailand was proposed in 1979, but its implementation was never reported. The NIN have proposed to use multi-centre trials in India to test the impact of the double-fortified salt and its acceptability and bioavailability (Lofti et al 1996).

Vitamin A

Experiences in developing countries with vitamin A fortification highlight the nutritional benefits that can be gained, but also some of the problems faced by fortification. Developing countries reporting commercial production of foods fortified with vitamin A or high-retinol foods are shown in Table 19.5. Vitamin A fortified mono sodium glutamate (MSG) (Indonesia, The Philippines) and sugar (Central America) stand out as products that have undergone extensive testing, have been widely distributed in-country and have been evaluated for their public health impact (Sommer & West 1996). In a large number of developed (24) and only a few developing countries (5), vitamin A (average amount 30,000 IU/kg) has been added to margarine for many years. However, the same technology has now been used on other processed oils and fats, which are increasingly becoming affordable to lower socio-economic markets and may therefore be suitable carriers of vitamin A. An outstanding example is a popular margarine in the Philippines that has been highly hydrogenated (so that it does not need refrigeration) and that is consumed weekly by ~ 40% of children under 6 years. Two tablespoons of a fortified version of the margarine provided 430 µg retinol equivalents (RE) vitamin A/day, and increased mean serum retinol levels in pre-school children by 3 µg/dl (0.1 µmol/L) (Sommer & West 1996). Fats and oils are used directly or as food ingredients and are suitable vehicles for vitamin A because:

- Vitamin A and pro-vitamin A compounds are highly fat-soluble and when added to fats or oils, distribute evenly;
- Vitamin A and pro-vitamin A compounds are stable in fats and oils as they are protected from the air and hence oxidation is delayed;
- The absorption of vitamin A is enhanced in the presence of dietary fats;
- High coverage of populations can be achieved as fats and oils are used directly or indirectly in most diets.

Sugar

In the early 1970s white refined sugar was identified as a potentially-fortifiable food carrier for vitamin A in Central and South America. Tests in Chile (Toro et al 1975) and Guatemala (Arroyave 1971, Pineda 1993) found vitamin A fortified sugar to be bioavailable, organoleptically acceptable, and stable under ambient humid conditions (90% retention after 6–8 months) and after cooking (85–99% retention in a wide range of products). Continued testing during the 1990s showed 50–85% vitamin A potency after 9 months (Dary 1994).

GUATEMALA. Sugar fortification was mandated in Guatemala in 1974, and the twice-yearly nutritional surveillance during the first 2 years provided strong evidence that the programme was achieving an impact on vitamin A status. Increases in serum retinol were observed in wasted and non-wasted children, indicating the sugar was reaching the most disadvantaged (Arroyave et al 1979). In addition, breast-milk retinol levels rose from a mean of 0.75 µmol/L to 1.2 µmol/L, which was estimated to provide a dietary increment to the breastfed infant of 2.7 RE/day (~ 60% increase to infants consuming 600 ml breast milk/day).

Unfortunately, sugar fortification in Guatemala was suspended for almost 8 years due to civil conflict, lack of enforcement of the fortification law, a glut in the international sugar market (reduced profits) and a rise in the Swiss franc, which raised the price of the vitamin A (Sommer & West 1996). Sugar manufacturers were required by law to absorb the cost of fortification, thus when the fortificant was too expensive, the programme stopped. This example illustrates that to sustain a fortification programme the consumers must ultimately bear the real cost of the fortification. Fortification also ceased in El Salvador, Panama and, to some extent, in Honduras for the same reasons as Guatemala. It ceased in Costa Rica because dietary surveys suggested that sugar fortification was unnecessary.

The sugar fortification programme was re-started in Guatemala in 1987–1988 as a universal programme, that is to fortify all sugar regardless of final destination either for domestic or industrial use (Dary 1998). The strategy was selected to ensure there would be no 'cracks' in the system, but it generated opposition from industry because of a 2% price increase caused by the fortification with no clear benefit to the marketing of their products. To overcome the opposition, the sugar fortification law was revised to exempt sugar intended for industrial use. However, producers still have to shoulder the costs of fortifying the sugar at a cost of $0.37 US/per person/year.

Table 19.5 — Countries reporting programmes for commercial production of fortified and high retinol foods

Region	Countries with programmes	Commodity fortified	Programme status
Africa	Botswana	Weaning food (Tsabana)	Implemented
	Ethiopia	Weaning food	Implemented
	Kenya	Sugar and oil	In preparation
	Malawi	Maize meal	Investigating feasibility
	Mozambique	Sugar	In preparation
	South Africa	Maize meal	In preparation
		Sugar	Investigating feasibility
	Tanzania	Palm oil (unfortified)	Implemented
		Fortified orange drink	Experimental
	Zambia	Palm oil (unfortified)	In preparation
	Namibia	Wheat flour	In preparation
	Senegal	Dried mango (unfortified)	Implemented
	Nigeria	Food flavouring cubes	Investigating feasibility
South Asia	Bangladesh	Sugar	Investigating feasibility
	India	Dairy & vegetable fat	Implemented
		Sugar	Investigating feasibility
	Pakistan	Vegetable fat	Implemented
	Sri Lanka	Margarine	In preparation
East Asia and Pacific	Indonesia	MSG	In preparation
	Philippines	Wheat	In preparation
		Margarine	Implemented
		Sugar	Investigating feasibility
	Thailand	Condensed milk	Implemented
		Instant noodles	Experimental
	China	Dairy & vegetable oils	Implemented
	Papua New Guinea	Sugar	Investigating feasibility
Latin and Caribbean	Cuba	Milk & other basic foods	Proposed
	Dominican Republic	Sugar	Proposed
	El Salvador	Sugar	Implemented (mandatory)
	Guatemala	Sugar	Implemented (mandatory)
	Haiti	Dried mango (unfortified)	Implemented
	Honduras	Sugar	Implemented (mandatory)
	Bolivia	Sugar	Pilot
	Venezuela	Enriched formula whole milk powder maize flour	Implemented
	Brazil	Sugar	Pilot
	Mexico	Chocolate drink mix	Implemented
	Nicaragua	Sugar	Implemented
	Ecuador	Sugar	Implemented
	Colombia	Sugar	In preparation

Modified from UNICEF 18 Nations fortify food (1997) Field Office and UNICEF Nutrition Section Report 1996.

Unfortunately, it is essential that fortification programmes are effectively monitored, and QC in the sugar mills is necessary to ensure that levels of the fortificant are reached and maintained. Not all of the Guatemalan sugar mills had QC procedures installed, but household surveys reported 96% of households used fortified sugar and 75% of the sugar had a vitamin A content greater than 5 mg/kg sugar

(Dary 1998). However, when plasma retinol levels were measured as an indicator of vitamin A status, children aged 12–24 months were still showing biochemical VAD. The low sugar intake by infants aged 6–24 months meant the nutritional goal of 50% of the RDA could not be achieved (Dary 1997). Complementary measures such as promotion of breastfeeding, development of weaning foods rich in vitamin A, and periodic (at least every 6 months) supplementation with pharmaceutical preparations were implemented for these infants. A survey by the International Eye Foundation in 1996 reported that the distribution of vitamin A capsules to infants brought the number of children reaching the RDA to almost 100% (Clement et al 1998).

HONDURAS. In Honduras, a targeted fortification programme was adopted in which only sugar destined for direct domestic use (i.e., 40% of total sugar) is fortified (Dary 1998). A special type of labelling was introduced to identify fortified sugar, and a QC programme monitored the fortification. The outcome was that 90% of sugar samples had a vitamin A content higher than 10 mg/kg and 82% of sugar at household level was fortified. The cost was no more than $0.40 US/person/year. However, following the initial success of the Honduran programme, the system was tested again in 1997, when the QC programme had been discontinued. Only 70% of sugar in the household was fortified, and the amount of sugar with retinol values > 5 mg/kg decreased from 64 to 27%, equivalent to a change from 6.6 to 3.7 mg retinol/kg/household. In addition, part of the fortified sugar was being illegally exported, which caused a sugar shortage leading to price rises and the purchase of cheaper, imported non-fortified sugar. Hence, the marketing of staple foods is not driven by quality but by economic gain and consumer affordability.

The universal fortification of carrier is not a requirement to achieve a nutritional goal. However, if targeted fortification is to be used, there must be good QC, a good labelling system, a reliable distribution system and a policy of food-price control to avoid commercial competition with the non-fortified product (Dary 1998).

Monosodium glutamate (MSG)

The use of MSG for vitamin A fortification was pioneered in The Philippines where 47% of children (aged 1–16 years) had low or deficient retinol levels (Solan et al 1985).

In Indonesia, a national xerophthalmia survey in 1978 found that the majority of children had low vitamin A status. As a result, the government decided that fortification of a commonly-consumed dietary item with vitamin A might prove an effective way of controlling VAD (Muhilal et al 1988). Pre-school children were found to consume 0.2–0.3 g/day of MSG, and the fortification levels would provide half an RDA (810 µg RE/g). A controlled trial using MSG fortified with 810 µg RE vitamin A/g or non-fortified MSG was carried out in 10 villages (Muhilal et al 1988). The fortified MSG retained 84% of its potency after 4 months and 57% after 11 months in the market place. Serum retinol levels in pre-school children in the programme area, increased significantly (p < 0.001) as did breast milk levels (p < 0.05). There were no changes in the control villages. Unfortunately, the yellow colour of the fortificant caused some dis-colouration of the MSG. The MSG manufacturers and government officials decided that the colour of the fortified MSG must not deviate from the unfortified MSG because it is marketed in clear, multi-laminate packages showing its whiteness and purity. Between 1988–1993 a number of different techniques were used to try to mask the colour. In April 1993, a vitamin A palmitate coated beadlet of unknown matrix was produced. The appearance stability was greater than 25 weeks and the vitamin A chemical stability was good. Unfortunately, the technical difficulties associated with the purity of the colour increased the resistance of the major MSG manufacturers to collaborate (Sommer & West 1996). In addition, funding was withdrawn by USAID because the production of the fortificant had taken too long (Murphy 1996). A national pilot field trial has never taken place.

Other vehicles for vitamin A fortification

Table 19.5 lists some of the countries where foods fortified with retinol are being produced commercially or experimentally. In addition to this list, other vehicles may offer opportunities for fortification. These include rice, tea, salt and biscuits.

RICE. Rice is consumed by half the world's population as a staple grain. The main limitation to its use is that the rural poor often produce their own rice or buy from local millers, precluding it from careful fortification. Fortification of rice may be effective and practical when centrally processed or when distributed to the poor as part of government food-for-work programmes, subsidized ration outlets or refugee feeding. Otherwise, feasibility, cost, and QC pose major challenges (Sommer & West 1996).

WHEAT FLOUR. Wheat consumption is increasing in

many developing countries in response to such factors as constraints in the supply of rice and the development of affordable wheat products (Sommer & West 1996). Fortified wheat may provide a growing opportunity to improve vitamin A intake in the poor. Many tropical countries import wheat either commercially or via food aid, the latter being targeted at the needy. Imported wheat is often milled at government or a limited number of private mills, making the central fortification process possible. Locally-grown and milled wheat suffers the same practical problems as rice. Vaghefi & Delgosha (1975) proposed that vitamin A should be added to baker's yeast tablets. The tablets were produced in Iran's only yeast plant, thus serving the centralized and QC needs of fortification. Although yeast may be a poor matrix to standardize for this purpose, tests did show ~70% vitamin A retention in bread baked by this method. This idea has not been pursued.

TEA. The idea of fortifying tea was patented in 1943 (Buxton & Harrison 1943 US patent). In India (Brooke & Cort 1972) and Pakistan (Fuller et al 1974), tea was successfully fortified with vitamin A (~125–250 IU/g or 375–750 IU/brewed 150 ml cup). Stability was excellent even after boiling for 1 hour. The option was not pursued because the youngest children did not consume enough tea to make the fortification effective. However it is possible that this method may have a beneficial effect by raising the retinol levels amongst women of child-bearing age (Sommer & West 1996). In Tanzania, a tea-fortification project is being formulated. One note of caution is that drinking tannin-containing beverages with meals may contribute to iron deficiency, particularly if the diet consists largely of vegetables (Disler et al 1975).

BISCUITS. In 1995, a randomized control trial among lactating women in Indonesia demonstrated the value of feeding wafers fortified with β-carotene (DePee et al 1995). Daily consumption of these wafers, containing 3.5 mg or 585 μg RE/day, resulted in a significant rise in serum β-carotene, and both serum and breast-milk retinol compared with controls.

Discussion

The global control of micronutrient deficiencies is a realizable goal. However, it is an enormous task and there remain many challenges and constraints to be resolved to reach the target population (Lofti et al 1996). Food fortification clearly can be effective and should be pursued as a potential intervention strategy. Implementing a national fortification programme is a major undertaking that requires sound scientific rationale, industrial capacity, training, advocacy, adequate legislation, economic viability, community acceptance and long-term sustainability, monitoring and control (Sommer & West 1996).

References

ACC/SCN Consultative Group. (1993) Focus on micronutrients. *SCN News*, 9, 11–16.

Arroyave, G. (1971) Distribution of vitamin A to population groups. *Proc West Hemsph Nutr Congr*, 3, 68–79.

Arroyave, G. (1979) Evaluation of sugar fortification with vitamin A at the national level. Pan American Health Organisation, Scientific Publication, 384.

Asenjo, J.A., Amar, M., Cartagena, N., King, J., Hiche, E., Stekel, A. (1985) Use of a bovine haem iron concentrate in the fortification of biscuits. *J Food Science*, 50, 795–799.

Bauernfeind, J.C. (1983) Vitamin A: Technology and applications. *World Rev Nutr Diet*, 41, 110–199.

Bloch, C.E. (1931) Effects of deficiency in vitamins in infancy. *Am J Dis Child*, 42, 271–275.

Blum, M. (1997) *Status Paper: Food Fortification, A Key Strategy to End Micronutrient Malnutrition. NUTRIVIEW 97/Special Issue*. Basel, Switzerland: Hoffmann-La Roche Ltd.

Boccio, J.R., Zubillaga, M.B., Caro, R.A., Gotelli, C.A., Gotelli, M.J., Weill, R. (1997) A new procedure to fortify fluid milk and dairy products with high bioavailable ferrous sulfate. *Nutr Rev*, 65, 240–246.

Boccio, J.R., Zubillaga, M.B., Caro, R.A., Lysionek, A., Gotelli, C.A., Gotelli, M.J., Weill, R. (1998) Bioavailability, absorption mechanism and toxicity of microencapsulated iron (I) sulfate. *Biological Trace Element Research*, 62, 65–73.

Brooke, C.L., Cort, W.M. (1972) Vitamin A fortification of tea. *Food Technology*, 26, 50–52.

Clement, L.R., Piedrasanta, M.B., Matute, J. (1998) *The Contribution of Vitamin A Capsules and Sugar Fortification to The Daily Vitamin A Intake of Guatemalan Children*, 4/98 edn. Basel, Switzerland: Hoffmann-la Roche.

Clements, F.W. (1979) Should Australian white flour be enriched? *Food Technology in Australia*, 506–508.

Committee on Nutrition. (1989) Iron fortified infant formulas. *Pediatr*, 84, 1114–1115.

Crowley, P.R. (1974) *Current Approaches for The Prevention of Vitamin A Deficiencies—Food Fortification*. Jakarta, Indonesia: World Health Organisation.

Dary, O. (1994) Avances en el proceso de fortificacion de azucar con vitamina A en Centro america. *Boletin de la Oficiana Sanitaria Pan Americana*, 117, 529–536.

Dary, O. (1997) Sugar fortification with vitamin A (A key factor toward the elimination of vitamin A deficiency in Central America). Personal communication.

Dary, O. (1998) *Universal vs. Targeted Coverage Vitamin A-Fortified Sugar.* Arkansas, USA: International workshop of Micronutrient Enhancement of Rice in developing Countries.

Davidsson, L., Almgren, A., Sandstrom, B., Hurrell, R.F. (1995) Zinc-absorption in adult humans—the effect of iron fortification. *Br J Nutr*, 74, 417–425.

DePee, S., West, C.E., Muhilal, Karyadi, D., Hautvast, J.G.A.J. (1995) Increased consumption of dark leafy vegetables does not improve vitamin A status of anaemic breast-feeding women in Indonesia. *Lancet*, 346, 75–78.

Diosady, L.L. (1996) Personal communication to The Micronutrient Initiative.

Disler, P.B., Lynch, S.R., Charlton, R.W., Bothwell, T.H., Mayet, F. (1975) The effect of tea on iron absorption. *Gut*, 16, 193–200.

Elia, M., Behrens, R., Northrop, C.A., Wraight, P., Neale, G. (1987) Evaluation of mannitol, lactulose and 51Cr-labelled Ethylenediaminetetra-acetate in man. *Clin Sci*, 73, 197–204.

Fairweather-Tate, S.J., Wharf, S.G., Fox, T.E. (1995) Zinc absorption in infants fed iron-fortified weaning food. *Am J Clin Nutr*, 62, 785–789.

FAO/WHO ad hoc expert committee. (1971) Rome: Food and Agricultural Organisation/World Health Organisation.

FAO/WHO International Conference on Nutrition Rome 1992.

FAO/WHO Food Standards/Cadex Alimentarius commision (1981) Cadex standards for foods for infants and children. Rome: FAO.

Flores, H. (1996) *Fortification of Rice with Vitamin A. NUTRIVIEW 3/96.* Basel, Switzerland: Hoffmann-La Roche.

Fuller, C.E., Nelson, J.H., Smith, D.E., Crowley, P.R. (1974) A technology for the fortification of tea with vitamin A. *Proceedings of the IV International Congress of Food Science Technology*, 5, 180–189.

Haschke, F., Vanura, H., Male, C., Owen, G., Pietschnig, B., Schuster, E., Krobath, E., Huemer, C. (1993) Iron nutrition and growth of breast- and formula-fed infants during the first 9 months of life. *J Pediatr Gastroenterol Nutr*, 16, 151–156.

Hurrell, R.F. (1984) Bioavailability of Different Iron Compounds Used to Fortify Formulas And Cereals: Technological Problems. In: Stekel, A. (ed.) *Iron Nutrition in Infancy And Childhood* pp. 147–178. New York: Raven Press.

Hurrell, R.F. (1997) Preventing iron deficiency through food fortification. *Nutr rev*, 55, 210–222.

Hurrell, R.F., Lynch, S.R., Trinidad, T.P. (1989) Iron absorption in humans as influenced by bovine milk proteins. *Am J Clin Nutr*, 49, 546–552.

International Anaemia Consultative Group (INACG). (1993) *Iron EDTA for Food Fortification: A Report of The INACG.* Washington, DC: INACG.

Kushner, I. (1982) The phenomenon of the acute phase response. *Ann New York Acad Sci*, 389, 39–48.

Layrisse, M., Chaves, J.F., Mendez-Castellano, H., Bosch, V., Tropper, E., Bastardo, B., Gonzalez, E. (1996) Early response to the effect of iron fortification in the Venezuelan population. *Am J Clin Nutr*, 64, 903–907.

Lofti, M., Mannar, M.G.V., Merx, R.J.H.M., Naber-van Heuvel, P. (1996) *Micronutrient Fortification of Foods. Current Practices, Research And Opportunities.* Ottawa, Canada: The Micronutrient Initiative and Wageningen, The Netherlands: International Agricultural Centre.

Mannar, M.G.V. (1991) Double fortification of salt with iron and iodine. Status review and blueprint for action. United Nations Childrens Fund (UNICEF) New York, NY, USA.

Mannar, M.G.V., Dunn, J.T. (1995) Salt iodization for the elimination of iodine deficiency. MI/ICCIDD/WHO/UNICEF. Ottawa, Canada: Micronutrient Initiative.

Mannar, M.G.V., Stone, T. (1993) Status of national programs for IDD in Africa and Asia. Hull, Canada: Canadian International Development Agency.

Muhilal, Permeisih, D., Idjradinata, Y.R., Muherdiyantingsih, Karyadi, D. (1988) Vitamin A-fortified monosodium glutamate and health, growth and survival of children: A controlled field trial. *Am J Clin Nutr*, 48, 1271–1776.

Murphy, P.A. (1996) Technology of vitamin A fortification of foods in developing countries. *Food Technology*, 50(9), 69–74.

Nilson, A., Piza, J. (1997) *Food Fortification: A Tool for Fighting Hidden Hunger.* Latin America Congress of Nutrition, Guatemala.

Pineda, O. (1993) Fortification of sugar with vitamin A. Basel, Switzerland: Human Nutrition Communications, Hoffmann-La Roche. *Nutriview*, 2, 6–7.

Polberger, S., Fletcher, M.P., Graham, T.W., Vruwink, K., Gershwin, M.E., Lonnerdal, B. (1996) Effect of infant formula zinc and iron level on zinc absorption, zinc status and immune function in infant rhesus monkeys. *J Pediatr Gastroenterol Nutr*, 22, 134–143.

Rao, B.S.N. (1994) Fortification of salt with iron and iodine to control anemia and goitre: Development of a new formula with good stability and bioavailability of iron and iodine. *Food Nutrition Bulletin*, 15, 32–39.

Solan, F.S., Latham, M.C., Guirriec, R., Florentino, R., Williamson, D.F., Aguilar, J.R. (1985) Fortification of MSG with vitamin A: The Philippines experience. *Food Technology*, 39, 71–79.

Sommer, A., West, K.P.J. (1996) Fortification of Dietary Items with Vitamin A. In: Sommer, A., West, K.P.J. (eds.) *Vitamin A Deficiency: Health, Survival and Vision*, 15, pp. 410–431, 1st edn. New York: Oxford University Press.

Sullivan, P. (1993) Cow's milk induced intestinal bleeding in infancy. *Arch Dis Child*, 68, 240–245.

Thompson, F.M., Catto-Smith, A.G., Moore, D., Davidson, G., Cummins, A.G. (1998) Epithelial growth of the small intestine in human infants. *J Pediatr Gastroenterol Nutr*, 26, 506–512.

Thurnham, D.I., Singkamani, R. (1991) The acute phase response and vitamin A status in malaria. *Trans R Soc Trop Med & Hyg*, 85, 194–199.

Toro, O., de Pablo, S., Aguayo, M., Gattan, M., Contreras, V., Monckeberg, F. (1975) Prevention of vitamin A deficiency by fortificaton of sugar. A field study. *Archives Latinoamericos Nutricion*, 169–179.

United Nations Children's Fund (UNICEF) (1995) *The State of The World's Children 1995*. New York: Oxford University Press.

US Federal Register. (1996) 61, 173.

Vaghefi, S.B., Delgosha, M. (1975) Fortification of Persian-type bread with vitamin A. *Cereal Chem*, 52, 753–756.

Williams, R.R. (1961) The Bataan Experiment And Present Status of Beriberi in The Philippines. In: Williams, R.R. (ed) *Towards The Conquest of Beriberi*, XI, pp. 190–219. Cambridge: Harvard University Press.

The micronutrient initiative (1996) Opportunities for multiple fortification In: Lofti, M., Mannar, M.G.V., Merx, J.H.M. and Naber-van den Heuval, P. (eds) Micronutrient fortification of foods: Current Practice, Reserach and Opportunities, 8, 81–96. Ontario: The micronutrient initiative.

The World Bank. (1994) *Development in Practice Enriching Lives: Overcoming Vitamin And Mineral Malnutrition in Developing Countries*, pp. 1–73. Washington DC: USA.

World Health Organisation (WHO). (1995) *Prevalence of Vitamin A Deficiency. Micronutrient Deficiency Information System (MDIS) Working Paper Number 2*. Geneva: WHO.

20

Dietary fibre in childhood

Beth H. Olson and Barbara O. Schneeman

Introduction

Dietary fibre is composed of materials in food that are not digested in the human small intestine. These materials are primarily non-starch polysaccharides of plant cells. Therefore, breast milk and infant formula are not sources of dietary fibre. However, dietary fibre is apparently unnecessary, as normal bowel patterns range from two to three movements per day for breastfed infants, and one per day for formula-fed infants (Ekvall 1992). As older infants and toddlers are introduced to the full range of foods available in the diet, dietary fibre intakes increase. Few studies have been conducted to determine the health benefits of dietary fibre in children, although data indicate dietary fibre may be beneficial for laxation and for lowering cholesterol in children who are high risk. In addition, dietary patterns that are established in childhood may continue into adulthood, and thus a diet that contains a variety of fibre-containing foods such as cereals, whole grain breads, legumes, fruits and vegetables reduces the risk of chronic disease if established early and maintained.

This chapter discusses current and recommended intakes of fibre for children, definition and analysis of dietary fibre, and physiological responses to dietary fibre intakes. Much of the data on physiological responses is the result of research done on adults, although a few studies in children are presented. Finally, implications for the diets of children are addressed.

Historical background

Dietary fibre intakes and recommendations

Data from the first phase of the US National Health and Nutrition Examination Survey III, 1989–1991, indicate that both adults and children have low fibre intakes. Men aged 20 years and older have mean intakes of 16.6–20 g of dietary fibre/day and women have between 12.5–14.7 g/day (Alaimo et al 1994), both of which are well below the National Cancer Institute's recommendation of 20–30 g/day (Butrum et al 1988). Children have mean intakes of 4.4, 8.5, 10.7, 12.5, 13.3 and 15.0 g/day at ages 2–11 months, 1–2, 3–5, 6–11, 12–15 and 16–19 years, respectively.

The American Academy of Pediatrics Committee on Nutrition recommends that children consume 0.5 g fibre/kg body weight (American Academy of

Pediatrics 1993). This formula is not applied easily, however, and levels of recommended intake for older, heavier adolescents could be unreasonably high. Adult recommendations applied on a kcal basis to children could result in recommended intakes too high for pre-school-aged children. The American Health Foundation (AHF) has developed a recommendation for children that is easy to use and that allows children 3–20 years to increase fibre intakes gradually throughout childhood to the levels recommended for adults (Williams et al 1995). The AHF's 'Age + 5' recommendation is for a minimum fibre intake of the child's age + 5 g; thus an 8-year-old child would have a minimum recommended intake of 13 g and by 20 years the recommended intake would be 25 g.

Using the 'Age + 5' formula, Mueller et al (1997) analysed intakes of children versus this recommended level using the US Department of Agriculture's Continuing Survey of Food Intakes by Individuals for 1989–1991. Although many children are achieving recommended levels of intakes from ages 3–6 years, by 7 years intakes are falling below recommended levels (Fig. 20.1). Intakes of fibre do not increase substantially through adolescence, such that by age 20, only 15% of males and 2% of females are achieving recommended intakes. An analysis of the types of foods consumed by children found that intakes of fibre fall further from recommendations in older children due to lower intakes of cereals, fruits, and vegetables and greater intakes of foods such as sandwiches, pizza, potatoes, and pastries (Mueller et al 1997).

For children under 2 years of age, high-fibre low-fat, and low-calorie diets are not recommended. Adequate fat and calories are needed for growth and development at this age (American Academy of Pediatrics 1993; American Dietetic Association 1993). Rather, as a child's developmental and nutritional needs outgrow exclusive breast or formula feedings, supplemental

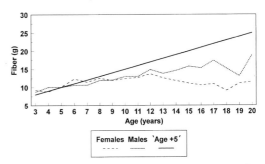

Figure 20.1 — Dietary fibre intakes versus 'age + 5' recommendation.

feeding with low-to-moderate fibre intake can be introduced, such as infant rice cereal and pureed fruits and vegetables. During this transition from formula or breast milk in infancy to the inclusions of fruits, vegetables and grains, carbohydrates increase from 42% to 52% of calories (Baker 1994).

Definition

Whereas the term *fibre* has been used since the 1800s, the term *dietary fibre* was coined in 1953 to refer to the non-digestible residue in foods (Hipsley 1953). Southgate (1978) subsequently proposed that Trowell's definition of dietary fibre as plant polysaccharides and lignin that are not digested by enzymes of the human gastrointestinal tract was a more physiological one. It includes not only structural materials of the cell wall, such as cellulose, hemicellulose and pectins but also non-structural components such as gums and mucilages. Other components are food additives—certain gums, algal polysaccharides and modified celluloses (Southgate 1978). Starch may also escape digestion in the small intestine (Stephen et al 1983, Englyst & Cummings 1985), and this has been called *resistant starch*. By escaping digestion in the small intestine, resistant starch may behave physiologically like dietary fibre. Differentiation between resistant starch and non-starch polysaccharides in relation to the physiological events traditionally attributed to dietary fibre helps to determine health benefits associated with resistant starch. This topic has been reviewed recently (Muir et al 1993).

Analysis

Dietary fibre is a heterogeneous mix of compounds that are different chemically and physiologically. In addition, foods contain a mixture of various types of dietary fibre. Consequently, chemical analytic methods may provide information on fibre content but not on the physiological properties important for health benefits of fibre. In the United States and several other countries, the most commonly-accepted method of analysis is an AOAC-accepted enzymatic-gravimetric assay for total dietary fibre (Prosky et al 1984, Prosky et al 1985). This method has also been accepted in the United States for the purposes of food labelling (Schweizer 1990). The method has been criticized for including lignin and maillard products as well as some starch in the measurement. The issue of compounds that are or should be included in dietary fibre analysis is still debated (Englyst et al 1987, Asp et al 1988).

The terms *soluble* and *insoluble fibre* were introduced based on the properties of fibre in water, although soluble fibres do not dissolve in water but rather form a dispersion. More recently, modifications of the Prosky AOAC method for total dietary fibre have been developed and tested in inter-laboratory studies to analyse soluble and insoluble fibre. Good correlations have been found between the sum of the soluble and insoluble fibres analysed and the total dietary fibre analysed by these methods (Prosky et al 1988, Prosky 1990, Lee et al 1992). Marlett et al (1992) have demonstrated that soluble fibre measured in various foods is a reflection of the method used. Therefore, care must be taken in evaluating studies to interpret data in view of the method used to determine soluble fibre.

The terms soluble and insoluble fibre are used, sometimes inappropriately, to simplify the categorization of dietary fibre, especially in an attempt to correlate solubility with physiological effects. However, fibre sources are a mix of soluble and insoluble. In addition, this simple characterization does not always predict accurately the behaviour of the sources of fibre in the human body. Many other properties of fibre may be needed in order to understand its physiological actions. These properties include chemical composition, structure, particle size, binding of organic compounds, ion exchange, viscosity, water-holding capacity and fermentability. Relationships of these properties to physiological effects contribute more to the understanding of the health benefits of fibre than do chemical measures of fibre content alone. These properties are related to gastrointestinal function and perhaps to subsequent effects on glucose and lipid metabolism as well as chronic diseases such as obesity, heart disease and colon cancer.

Physiological responses

Gastrointestinal effects

Dietary fibre affects gastric emptying, intestinal transit and faecal bulking and fermentation in the large intestine. Soluble, or viscous fibre sources, have been reported to delay gastric emptying and slow transit time in the small intestine, whereas insoluble, or less viscous fibre sources, increase transit time in the large intestine. Because the large intestinal phase is by far the longest part of intestinal transit, soluble fibre sources may have no or a small effect in increasing overall intestinal transit time, whereas insoluble fibre sources may significantly decrease intestinal transit time. Soluble fibre sources are more fermented in the large intestine and insoluble sources contribute more to faecal bulking.

Harju (1985) used a polyethylene glycol (PEG) marker in a test meal (yoghurt, orange juice, wheat bread and butter) to test whether 5 g of guar gum or 5 g placebo raised the viscosity of stomach contents and lowered gastric emptying rates in human subjects. Compared to placebo, guar gum in a test meal lowered the rate of gastric emptying. The results of Holt et al (1979) suggested that guar gum and pectin slowed the gastric emptying of glucose. In contrast, both Chang & Li (1984) and Ebihara & Kiriyama (1982) did not find that cellulose, an insoluble fibre source, affected stomach emptying.

Jenkins et al (1978) fed subjects a test drink (glucose, xylose, lactulose, lemon juice and water) supplemented with various fibre sources (wheat bran, methylcellulose, pectin, guar gum, gum tragacanth or cholestyramine) and measured breath hydrogen. Hydrogen gas, a microbial fermentation product, can be absorbed from the lower intestine and into the lungs where it is expired as breath. An earlier measurement of breath hydrogen when fibre was fed versus a fibre-free meal was taken to indicate decreased intestinal transit time due to fibre. Insoluble fibre sources decreased mouth-to-caecum transit time, whereas sources of soluble fibre increased it. The transit time correlated with fibre viscosity. Similar results were found by Hanson & Winterfeldt (1985) where test meals of pancakes with varying sources of soluble fibre such as oat bran and insoluble fibre such as wheat bran were used to look at breath hydrogen and intestinal transit time. Wheat bran decreased mouth-to-caecum transit time. In addition, the researchers found increased hydrogen concentrations for oat bran versus wheat bran, and concluded that oat bran was more fermented than wheat bran. Decreased mouth-to-caecum time with wheat bran versus guar gum has been shown in rats (Tinker & Schneeman 1989).

Dietary fibre (as well as resistant starch) that passes into the large intestine is subject to the metabolism of colonic micro-flora, and is a major source of energy for that micro-flora. The more viscous fibres are more extensively fermented and lose their structure and water-holding capacity (McBurney et al 1985). Although this loss of water-holding capacity may decrease the ability of viscous fibres to contribute to faecal bulk, this may be offset in part by the increased bacterial mass resulting from the fermentation. The less viscous fibres, such as wheat bran, may retain their structure and contribute significantly to faecal bulk. In studies on rats, Nyman & Asp (1982) found lower faecal bulking in rats fed pectin, a viscous fibre source, than those fed wheat bran. Jenkins et al (1987) quantified the effect of wheat bran in men and women using various wheat-bran-containing ready-to-eat cereals and found that 1 g of total dietary fibre from wheat bran caused an increase in faecal weight of 2.7 g. Cummings (1993) summarized the literature on the effects of various sources of dietary fibre on faecal bulk and composition. The average increase in faecal output per g fibre fed ranged from 5.4–1.2 g/g. The order of fibre effect from greatest to least faecal bulking was: wheat bran, fruits and vegetables, gums and mucilages (especially psyllium), cellulose, oats, corn, legumes and pectin. Wheat bran, which is by and large insoluble, not viscous, and not greatly fermented, results in the greatest increase in faecal bulk. Pectin, which is more viscous and greatly fermented, contributed much less to faecal bulk. Other sources of fibre are a mixture of fibre types but all contribute to faecal bulking. The intake of non-starch polysaccharides are the only dietary components that increase faecal weight, and thus they are a necessary component of the diet for normal laxation (Cummings et al 1992).

Fermentation of dietary fibre in the large intestine by colonic micro-flora leads to the production of short-chain fatty acids (SCFA), primarily acetate, propionate and butyrate in the approximate molar ratios 60:25:15 (Cummings et al 1987). Gases are also produced, including hydrogen, methane and carbon dioxide. A significant portion of the butyrate is used by the colonic cells for fuel (Bergman 1975). The absorbed butyrate as well as propionate are cleared by the liver, with little appearing in peripheral blood. SCFA have been measured in the terminal ileum and colon and in portal, hepatic and peripheral venous blood in sudden death victims. The authors of the study determined greater uptake of butyrate by the colonic epithelium and propionate by the liver (Cummings et al 1987). Acetate passes in the circulation to peripheral tissues, where it is utilized by muscle cells (Pomare et al 1985, Venter and Vorster 1989). It has been suggested that the propionate cleared by the liver affects hepatic cholesterol metabolism.

SCFA production yields energy for metabolism, although the exact amount is uncertain and varies with the type of fibre and extent of fermentation. The average apparent digestibility of non-starch polysaccharides and resistant starch in humans consuming mixed diets has been estimated at 6 KJ/g (1.5 kcal/g). The energy value for each individual type of dietary fibre would, of course, differ (Livesey 1995).

Diets high in grains, fruits and vegetables are associated epidemiologically with a lower risk of colon cancer (MacLennan et al 1995, Shannon et al 1996). Studies using animal models with chemically-induced tumours or aberrant crypts have demonstrated a decreased incidence with consumption of fibre sources such as wheat bran or psyllium as compared to low-fibre diets (Calvert et al 1987, Alabaster et al 1993). As well, studies in humans have shown fibre from wheat bran can reduce the number or size of colorectal adenomas, which are precursors to colorectal cancer (DeCosse et al 1989, MacLennan et al 1995). The production of butyrate may be protective against the development of cancer, but other protective mechanisms have also been suggested, such as the dilution of bile acids, the conversion of primary to secondary bile acids, or the presence of other phytochemicals.

Nutrient digestion and absorption

Dietary fibre delays or decreases the absorption of nutrients from the small intestine, including dietary lipids. They may bind or entrap bile acids, which may interfere with the formation of micelles and thus the digestion and absorption of triglycerides and cholesterol. Viscosity is another property of some dietary fibres which may play an important role in their hypocholesterolemic effects. Gallaher et al (1993) have demonstrated that fibres with high, versus low, viscosity in the small intestinal contents are better at reducing plasma and liver cholesterol in hamsters. Wang et al (1992) reported similar results when comparing the cholesterol reducing ability of barley versus corn-soybean diets. Chicks were fed diets of either barley, barley treated with β-glucanase, or corn-soybean. Plasma cholesterol was lowest in the barley group, intermediate in the enzyme-treated group and highest in the corn-soybean group. Small intestinal digesta viscosity was negatively correlated with plasma and LDL cholesterol. Tietyen et al (1991) reported similar results when oat bran or oat bran treated with β-glucanase was fed to rats. Rats fed oat bran had the lowest total cholesterol pool (plasma plus liver cholesterol), the enzyme treated group was intermediate and the cellulose control group had the highest total pool of cholesterol. In humans, a fibre mixture with higher viscosity (psyllium, pectin, guar gum and locust bean gum) was found to lower plasma cholesterol, whereas a fibre with lower viscosity (acacia gum) did not (Jensen et al 1993).

The viscosity of the fibres, particularly soluble fibres, may slow small intestinal transit time and interfere with digestive enzyme activity. There may also be a slowed diffusion of nutrients to the absorbing surface. Between the intestinal lumen and the brush border exists an intestinal diffusion barrier that is referred to as the *unstirred layer*. Viscous fibres enlarge the apparent thickness of the layer, increasing resistance to diffusion and absorption, which may reduce the absorption of fatty acid and glucose in rats and humans (Fuse et al 1989). This may result in more lipid being carried to the lower half of the small intestine, a slower appearance of lipids in the blood following a meal, and perhaps differences in the properties of those lipids with subsequent alterations in their metabolism. However, an animal study laboratory has indicated that although chronic fibre feeding may alter some aspects of lipid metabolism, alterations in post-prandial lipaemia require the presence of fibre in the meal (Redard et al 1992). In addition, merely the presence of nutrients in the lower half of the small intestine of rats was insufficient to cause alterations in fasting plasma lipids (Middleton & Schneeman 1995).

Dietary fibres may interfere with and delay lipid digestion, but do not decrease lipid absorption overall. In humans, ileostomy patients have been used as a model to determine the effect of fibre on lipid digestion. In ileostomy patients, guar and pectin have been shown to increase lipid in ileostomy fluid whereas wheat bran has not (Sandberg et al 1981, Higham & Read 1992). More fat was also excreted in the ileostomy fluid of subjects consuming a brewer's spent grain (primarily barley fibre) compared to consumption of a low-fibre diet (Zhang et al 1991). Ebihara & Schneeman (1989) reported triolein higher in intestinal contents versus tissue of rats 2.5 h after a test meal containing guar gum or glucomannan versus cellulose. Gallaher & Schneeman (1985) found that cellulose did not decrease the total amount of lipid that disappeared from the small intestine of rats, but shifted triglyceride absorption so that it occurred in the ileum as well as the jejunum. Vahouny et al (1988) fed rats various fibre supplements or cholestyramine for 2 weeks and then fitted them with lymphatic catheters. After duodenal administration of a lipid emulsion, absorption rates of cholesterol and oleic acid were determined. Although several soluble fibres decreased oleic acid recovery relative to rats pre-fed a fibre-free diet, there was no decrease at 24 h except in the psyllium group. A review by Vahouny & Cassidy (1986) reported that apparent fat digestibility was lowered by less than 4% by a high-fibre diet.

If fibre can delay lipid digestion and absorption, one would expect the appearance of nutrients in the plasma following a fibre-containing meal to be delayed and prolonged relative to a meal without fibre. Several fibres have been shown to delay the appearance of glucose in the blood when incorporated into a test meal. Tinker & Schneeman (1989) measured the disappearance of radio-labelled starch from the small intestines of rats fed a meal containing guar gum or wheat bran, compared to a fibre-free control. Starch disappearance was delayed in the rats fed the guar-gum containing meal, but not in those fed wheat bran. Leclere et al (1994) found that high-viscosity guar gum resulted in lower glucose and insulin responses compared to low-viscosity guar gum when consumed with a cornstarch containing meal. Guar incorporated into a wheat-flake cereal also reduced glucose and insulin responses following a meal compared to the meal without guar in normal healthy-weight adults (Fairchild et al 1996). β-glucan was incorporated into breakfast cereals at three dose levels and consumed by non-insulin diabetic subjects. A linear inverse relationship was seen between the β-glucan level and both the plasma glucose peak and the area under the glucose curve (Tappy et al 1996). Psyllium incorporated into or sprinkled on top of a wheat-bran-flake cereal reduced the glycaemic response compared to the bran-flake cereal alone (Wolever et al 1991). Beans have also been shown to result in a lower glycaemic response when compared to other foods, including potatoes (Jenkins et al 1980, Tappy et al 1986, Wursch et al 1988). It has been suggested that incorporation of such low-glycaemic index foods into the diets of diabetics may be effective in helping to control blood glucose (Wolever et al 1992). In addition, a recent epidemiological study found a correlation between low-glycaemic index diets and high-cereal-fibre diets and a delayed risk of onset of type II diabetes (Salmeron et al 1997).

Several studies have been conducted in humans to determine if fibre attenuates the appearance of triglycerides in the plasma following a meal. No difference in lipaemia was reported in a study where bran or psyllium was added to a bolus of cream. However, the number of subjects was small and the bolus of cream not representative of a typical fibre-containing meal (Miettinen 1987). Irie et al (1982) found 8 g guar gum added to a high-fat test meal resulted in lower plasma triglyceride at 2 and 4 h post-meal compared to the meal without guar gum. Again, the high-fat meal, containing 91% energy from fat, is not a typical fibre-containing mixed meal. Using

six normal male subjects, Cara et al (1992) found that oat bran, wheat fibre or wheat germ added to a test meal blunts the increase in post-prandial triglyceride compared to a low-fibre test meal. Gatti et al (1984) compared a regular pasta to one enriched with guar in ten normal subjects, eight men and two women. The guar pasta prevented the post-prandial triglyceride increase, even though 50% of the energy was from fat. The processing of guar into pasta may have altered the properties of guar. Other investigators have reported that certain dietary fibres actually enhanced post-prandial lipaemia. Jenkins et al (1978) gave subjects Lundh test meals with and without 12 g dietary fibre from wheat bran, pectin or guar gum. With both pectin and guar gum, the rises in serum triglyceride were significantly above the control during the first 3 h. This led the authors to suggest that there may have been a decreased clearance of chylomicrons secondary to a flatter glucose and insulin response. In a subset of subjects fed a high-soluble fibre diet or high-insoluble fibre diet in a crossover design, Jenkins et al (1993) quantified the area under the chylomicron triglyceride response curve following a fat tolerance test. Although dietary fibre was not included in the test, the subjects had a smaller chylomicron triglyceride response following the soluble fibre diet than the insoluble fibre diet. In a previous study from this laboratory, Redard et al (1990) also found that guar gum and oat bran added to a high-fat test meal resulted in an enhanced lipaemia in women relative to a low-fibre meal. There was a trend to enhanced lipaemia in men, but this did not reach significance, leading the authors to suggest that the effect of fibre on post-prandial lipaemia may be influenced by gender.

The differences in the effect of fibre on post-prandial lipaemia in the above studies might be explained by different actions of soluble, or viscous, fibres versus the less viscous fibres. The studies of Jenkins et al (1978, 1993) and Redard et al (1990) suggest that the viscous fibres enhance post-prandial lipaemia, perhaps through alterations in clearance of post-prandial lipoproteins. Conditions associated with increased insulin levels, such as obesity or a post-prandial state, correlate with increased lipoprotein lipase (LPL) activity in adipose tissue. Conversely, untreated diabetics exhibit low levels of LPL (Pykalisto et al 1975, Enerback & Gimble 1993). In isolated adipocytes, it has been demonstrated that glucose is required for insulin to increase the synthesis and secretion of LPL (Olivecrona et al 1987). A delay in the digestion and absorption of carbohydrate due to the presence of viscous fibre in a meal leads to delayed presence of glucose in the plasma. A subsequent delay in insulin secretion may then result in lower LPL activity and triglyceride clearance, and therefore an enhanced lipaemia. The study of Cara et al (1992) suggests that a blunting of lipaemia occurs when less viscous fibres are fed, perhaps due to lipase inhibitors that may slow the digestion and absorption of triglyceride.

Lipid metabolism

In rats, oat bran feeding resulted in higher portal vein concentrations of SCFA than cellulose feeding in two studies (Illman & Topping 1985, Chen & Anderson 1986), but not in a third (Illman & Topping 1985). Several fibres resulted in an increased caecal SCFA pool in rats, but the more-soluble fibres (soluble or internal portion of pea fibre and sugar beet fibre) increased the SCFA pool more than the less-soluble fibres (oat hull and insoluble or external pea fibre) (Remesy et al 1992). Propionate has also been fed to rats directly, leading to significant reductions in cholesterol (Chen et al 1984, Illman et al 1988). Pharmacological doses of propionate have been used to obtain inhibition of hepatic lipid regulatory enzymes *in vivo* and *in vitro*. Nishina & Freedland (1990b) measured sterol synthesis in isolated rat hepatocytes by tritium incorporation and found overall sterol synthesis, as measured by tritium incorporation, unaffected by physiological levels of propionate. These authors suggested that the inhibition of sterol synthesis from $1\text{-}^{14}\text{C}$-acetate that was demonstrated by themselves and Anderson & Bridges (1984) was peculiar to $1\text{-}^{14}\text{C}$-acetate. It is possible that although propionate decreases acetate incorporation into cholesterol, overall acetate availability is not limiting for cholesterol synthesis. Nishina & Freedland (1990b) demonstrated that fatty acid synthesis from tritiated water was inhibited in the presence of propionate. This effect on fatty acid synthesis may be a more important factor than the inhibition of cholesterol synthesis in the cholesterol-lowering effects of soluble fibre. Although dietary fibre intake does appear to increase SCFA production in the gut and SCFA concentrations in the blood, there is very limited evidence that SCFA inhibits cholesterol synthesis in the liver.

It has been hypothesized that dietary fibre may bind or sequester bile acids and increase their excretion in the faeces. The increased demand by the bile acid synthetic pathways in the liver is met by removal of cholesterol from the blood, reducing plasma cholesterol. Early work by Eastwood & Hamilton (1968) indicated that vegetable fibres bind bile acids. More recently, Vahouny et al (1980) prepared mixed micelles with either taurocholate or taurochenodeoxycholate and incubated them with various resins and dietary fibres.

Two viscosity grades of guar gum bound 20–38% of each micellar components, but cellulose bound only 0.5–7.5% and wheat bran bound 0–12.1%. Bile acid binding or sequestering by dietary fibres has also been demonstrated in animal models. Ebihara & Schneeman (1989) found that guar gum, konjac mannan and chitosan bound or sequestered bile acids in rats fed these fibres at 5% in a test meal, compared to rats fed cellulose, which has been shown not to bind bile acids. These three fibres have also been shown to lower plasma cholesterol. De Schrijver et al (1992) found 30% oat bran, baked or non-baked, lowered plasma cholesterol in rats and increased faecal bile acid excretion relative to fibre-free controls. They also found a linear relationship between plasma cholesterol and faecal bile acid excretion. Amigo et al (1992) fed whole bean, bean starch and bean fibre diets to rats and found that the whole bean and bean starch resulted in higher bile acid and cholesterol excretion compared to controls that were fed casein, whereas bean fibre did not. However, the authors acknowledged the bean starch may have contained soluble fibre, whereas the bean fibre was largely insoluble. Generally, the more insoluble fibres have not been shown to bind bile acids nor to lower blood cholesterol. Kingman et al (1992) fed hypercholesterolaemic pigs four types of legumes. Relative to a hypercholesterolaemic cellulose-fed control, all four groups consuming legumes had lower total plasma cholesterol but not significantly different faecal excretion of bile acids. McCall et al (1992) found that monkeys fed psyllium for 3.5 years did not have an increase in neutral steroid excretion.

Everson et al (1992) followed 20 males with moderate hypercholesterolaemia consuming either 15 g/day of psyllium or a cellulose placebo in a crossover design. Psyllium resulted in an increased fractional turnover of chenodeoxycholic and cholic acid relative to both baseline and the placebo. In addition, the decrease in LDL-C during the use of psyllium was directly correlated with an increase in total bile acid synthesis. However, the increase in the bile acid turnover alone was not sufficient to result in the amount of LDL-C lowering. Jenkins et al (1993) studied 43 hypercholesterolaemic men and women consuming high-soluble and high-insoluble fibre diets in a crossover study. Total, LDL and HDL cholesterol was lower when the soluble fibre period was compared to the insoluble fibre period. In addition, the loss of faecal bile acids was 83% greater during the soluble versus insoluble fibre period. Although this increase in bile acid loss may be sufficient to account for the cholesterol-lowering of the soluble fibre diet, the amount of total fibre intake was higher than is generally recommended or consumed—49.8 g (24.7 g/1000 kcal) with 16.1 g of soluble fibre. Abraham & Mehta (1988) were not able to detect any differences in faecal steroid excretion with psyllium supplementation compared to a usual diet in men, although plasma cholesterol was reduced. There is not consistency between the ability of the dietary fibres to bind bile acids and their cholesterol-lowering effects. Fibre sources that increase viscosity, such as oat bran, pectin and psyllium, generally lower plasma cholesterol and increase faecal bile acid excretion. Nishina & Freedland (1990a) found that rats fed pectin had an increased rate of sterol synthesis compared to those fed a fibre-free diet. This higher synthesis rate corresponded to an increase in 3-hydroxy-3-methylglutaryl co-enzyme A reductase activity (HMGCoA reductase). This suggests that pectin may have increased bile acid excretion, resulting in an increased need for cholesterol synthesis and therefore an increased activity of HMGCoA reductase. Arjmandi et al (1992) also found that rats fed various soluble fibres (psyllium, oat bran or pectin) had higher rates of hepatic cholesterol synthesis, as measured by incorporation of tritiated water, compared to rats fed cellulose. Beans also lower plasma cholesterol but with much smaller effects on faecal bile acid excretion. In general, the amount of bile acid excretion resulting from soluble fibre intake may contribute to the cholesterol-lowering properties of some soluble fibres, but is insufficient to account for all of the lowering (Vahouny & Cassidy 1986). In addition, dietary fibre may affect the ratio of primary:secondary bile acids (Story et al 1985) or the amounts of the different bile acids or their conjugates (Turley et al 1991, Trautwein et al 1993), which may affect bile acid metabolism and plasma cholesterol levels.

Several studies have shown that increased fibre intake leads to increased faecal excretion of SCFA (Cummings et al 1976, Spiller et al 1980, Ehle et al 1982, Fleming & Rodriguez 1983). In addition, researchers from the Dunn Clinical Nutrition Centre in Cambridge have shown that pectin intake results in elevated blood acetate levels from 6 h through 18 h (Pomare et al 1985).

Practice and procedures

Health conditions

Obesity

Viscous fibres have been suggested to increase feelings of fullness, or satiety, following meals in which they are consumed. Insulin rises to a lesser degree with foods that elicit a lower, versus higher, blood glucose response. Holt & Brand Miller (1995) found a significant negative association between insulin and satiety responses when comparing ordinary and quick-cooking rice and high- and low-amylose puffed rice. This same research group reported some, but not all foods, high in viscous fibres were associated with increased satiety. This high satiety value may make foods high in viscous fibre useful in diets used to treat obesity. In addition, higher-fibre diets tend to be lower in total fat and dietary fat correlates with incidence of obesity. Children with dietary intakes from the Bogalusa Heart Study were stratified into quartiles of fibre intake per 1000 kcal; the percent energy of total and saturated fat was lower in children with higher intakes of fibre (Nicklas et al 1995).

Cholesterol lowering and heart disease

The cholesterol-lowering effect of these dietary fibres has been thoroughly reviewed by Anderson et al (1990) and more recently by Glore et al (1994). Glore reviewed 77 human studies published through 1992 on legumes, oats, pectin, gums, psyllium and other fibres. A statistically-significant reduction in total cholesterol was found in 68 of the 77 studies (88%). Of those reporting LDL-C, 41 of 49 (84%) reported significant lowering. The average total cholesterol lowering for subjects with hypercholesterolaemia and normocholesterolaemia were 10.9% and 10.6%, respectively. For LDL-C, the average reduction for subjects with hypercholesterolaemia was 13.6%, and for those with normal cholesterol levels it was 9.9%. The majority of these studies showed the potential of soluble fibres to lower total and LDL cholesterol levels. Fewer studies have been done with children as subjects. The National Cholesterol Education Program recommends that all children consume a diet moderately-reduced in fat and cholesterol with an increased intake of complex carbohydrates (National Cholesterol Education Program 1992). Children at high risk due to a family history should be screened and treated with diet. A possible adjunct to this dietary management is the addition of water-soluble or viscous fibre sources. In a summary of seven studies of children fed varying amounts of fibre sources, including oat bran, psyllium and locust bean gum, LDL cholesterol was lowered by 0–23% (Kwiterovich 1995) (Table 20.1). Total and LDL-C was lowered more effectively when diets were higher in dietary fat, similar to studies in adults. Increasing

Table 20.1 — Studies on the effect of a low-fat, high-fibre diet in Hypercholesterolaemic children

Study	n	Age (y)	Fiber Source	% LDL Change
Gold et al	49	10	oat bran (28g/day)	−6
Williams et al	48	2–11	psyllium (6.4 g/day)	−16
Dennison & Levine	20	5–18	psyllium (6 g/day), wheat (5 g/day)	nc
Glassman et al	36	3–17	psyllium (5–10 g/day)	−23
Blumenschein et al	20	5–12	oat bran (1g/kg/day)	−7
Taneja et al	11	16–18	psyllium (25 g/day)	−7
Zavoral et al	11	10–18	locus bean gum (10–20 g/day)	−19

Adapted from Kwiterovich (1995).

dietary fibre intakes of children to recommended levels using foods such as cereals, fruits and vegetables increases soluble fibre intakes as well, and may be a helpful addition in managing blood cholesterol levels.

Laxation

Constipation is a common problem in childhood associated with the retention and passage of very large stools. Incomplete rectal emptying leads to chronic over-distension and then to an insensitivity to the need to empty the rectum (Leoning-Baucke 1984). Treatment is aimed at re-establishing normal colonic muscular tone and establishing a diet that promotes the passage of more frequent, softer stools. Dietary recommendations include an increased intake of dietary fibre and fluids. For the reasons discussed above, increased intake of foods higher in dietary fibre increases the intake of both soluble and insoluble fibre—both of which may help in promoting laxation in children.

Safety of fibre intakes for children

There is concern that diets high in fibre may not be safe for children. It has been suggested that a diet high in fibre may be of low-energy density, compromising growth and development. In addition, dietary fibre or components of fibre may bind minerals, which may be low in the diets of some children, particularly adolescents.

Diets high in dietary fibre may increase the amount of faecal energy. In adults, this amount of energy has been found to be relatively small, about 1% of energy for each 6 g of fibre added to the diet in a study of young women (Southgate & Durnin 1970), and an increase from 96 to 159 kcal/day in another study of women 22–38 years of age (Stevens et al 1987). Children have been studied less, with a more recent study conducted in Peruvian children 10–38 months of age. Although faecal energy loss doubled (52–118 g/day), fibre doses were fairly high, up to 22 g/day, and overall weights and heights were low, indicating malnourishment (Hamaker et al 1991).

Foods high in dietary fibre may contain phytate or oxalate, both of which have been shown to bind minerals such as calcium, iron and zinc, making them unavailable for absorption. The body is capable of adapting to high amounts of fibre with compensatory physiological mechanisms to make the absorption of such minerals more efficient (Walker et al 1948, Cullumbine et al 1950). Recent studies have also shown that with fermentation, minerals are released from foods containing dietary fibre and absorbed (Trinidad et al 1996a, 1996b). Therefore, although high-fibre low-fat diets are not recommended for children under the age of 2, for older children this may primarily be a concern where mineral intakes are inadequate from the start. Many fibre-rich foods such as fortified cereal products and other grains, fruits, vegetables, legumes and beans are good sources of such minerals. In addition, other foods appropriate for children provide highly-bioavailable sources of minerals (e.g., lean meats, dairy products), and should provide a complement to other, higher-fibre foods (Drews et al 1979).

Discussion

Dietary fibre has an important role in the health of children. It helps to promote normal laxation and may help to lower cholesterol in children with elevated levels. Due to their bulk, fibre-containing foods may help promote satiety and prevent the development of obesity with its associated increased risk of diabetes and cancer. Although young children < 7 years of age may consume adequate amounts of dietary fibre, intakes do not increase sufficiently as children age. Intakes of dietary fibre should be increased to the 'Age + 5' guideline by encouraging the consumption of grains and cereals, especially cereals, whole grain breads, legumes, fruits and vegetables. If close attention is paid to the overall diet, there is little risk of adverse effects of fibre to the levels recommended by Age + 5, and the health benefits and establishment of good eating patterns benefit the child through to adulthood.

References

Abraham, Z.D., Mehta, T. (1988) Three-week psyllium-husk supplementation: Effect on plasma cholesterol concentrations, fecal steroid excretion, and carbohydrate absorption in men. *Am J Clin Nutr*, 47, 67–74.

Alabaster, O., Tang, Z.C., Frost, A., Shivapurkar, N. (1993) Potential synergism between wheat bran and psyllium: Enhanced inhibition of colon cancer. *Cancer Letters*, 75, 53–58.

Alaimo, K., McDowell, M.A., Briefel, R.R., Bischof, A.M., Caughman, C.R., Loria, C.M., Johnson, C.L. (1994) Dietary intake of vitamins, minerals, and fiber of persons ages 2 months and over in the United States: Third National Health and Nutrition Examination Survey, Phase 1, 1988–1991. *Advance data from vital and health statistics*, 258, 1–27.

American Academy of Pediatrics (1993) Carbohydrate And Dietary Fiber. In: Barness, L. (ed.) *Pediatric Nutrition Handbook*, pp. 100–106, 3rd edn. Elk Grove Village: American Academy of Pediatrics.

American Dietetic Association. (1993) Health implications of dietary fiber. *J Am Diet Assoc*, 93, 1446–1447.

Amigo, L., Marzolo, M.P., Aguilera, J.M., Hohlberg, A., Cortes, M., Nervi, F. (1992) Influence of different dietary constituents of beans (Phaseolus vulgaris) on serum and biliary lipids in the rat. *J Nutr Biochem*, 3, 486–490.

Anderson, J.W., Bridges, S.R. (1984) Short-chain fatty acid fermentation products of plant fiber affect glucose metabolism of isolated rat hepatocytes. *Proc Soc Exp Biol Med*, 177, 372–376.

Anderson, J.W., Deakins, D.A., Floore, T.L., Smith, B.M., Whitis, S.E. (1990) Dietary fiber and coronary heart disease. *Crit Rev Food Sci Nutr*, 29, 95–147.

Arjmandi, B.H., Craig, J., Nathani, S., Reeves, R.D. (1992) Soluble dietary fiber and cholesterol influence in vivo hepatic and intestinal cholesterol biosynthesis in rats. *J Nutr*, 122, 1559–1565.

Asp, N-G., Furda, I., DeVries, J., Schweizer, T.F., Prosky, L. (1988) Dietary fiber definition and analysis (letter). *Am J Clin Nutr*, 47, 688–690.

Baker, S.S. (1994) Introduce Fruits, Vegetables And Grains, But Don't Overdo High-Fiber Foods. In: *Dietary Guidelines for Infants. Pediatric Basics No. 69.* Fremont, MI: Gerber Products Company.

Bergman, E.N. (1975) Production And Utilization of Metabolites by The Alimentary Tract As Measured in Protal And Hepatic Blood. In: McDonald, I.W., Warner, A.C.I. (eds.) *Digestion And Metabolism in The Ruminant*, pp. 292–305. Sydney, Australia: University of New England Publishing Unit.

Butrum, R.R., Clifford, C.K., Lanza, E. (1988) NCI dietary guidelines: Rationale. *Am J Clin Nutr*, 48, 888–895.

Calvert, R.J., Klurfeld, D.M., Subramaniam, S., Vahouny, G.V., Kritchevsky, D. (1987) Reduction of colonic carcinogenesis by wheat bran independent of fecal bile acid concentration. *J Natl Cancer Inst*, 79, 875–880.

Cara, L., Dubois, C., Borel, P., Armand, M., Senft, M., Portugal, H., Paulie, A-M., Bernard, P-M., Lairon, D. (1992) Effects of oat bran, rice bran, wheat fiber, and wheat germ on postprandial lipemia in healthy adults. *Am J Clin Nutr*, 55, 81–88.

Chang, M.L.W., Li, B.W. (1984) Effect of gel-forming undigestible polysaccharides versus cellulose on intestinal sugar concentrations and serum glucose level in rats. *Nutr Rep Intl*, 30, 789–796.

Chen, W-J.L., Anderson, J.W. (1986) Hypocholesterolemic Effects of Soluble Fibers. In: Vahouny, G.V., Kritchevsky, D. (eds.) *Dietary Fiber: Basic And Clinical Aspects*, pp. 275–286. New York: Plenum Press.

Chen, W-J.L., Anderson, J.W., Jennings, D. (1984) Propionate may mediate the hypocholesterolemic effects of certain soluble plant fibers in cholesterol-fed rats. *Proc Soc Exp Biol Med*, 175, 215–218.

Cullumbine, H., Basnayake, V., Lemottee, J. (1950) Mineral metabolism of rice diets. *Br J Nutr*, 4, 101–111.

Cummings, J.H. (1993) The Effect of Dietary Fiber on Fecal Weight And Composition. In: Spiller, G.A. (ed.) *Dietary Fiber in Human Nutrition*, pp. 263–349. Boca Raton: CRC Press.

Cummings, J.H., Bingham, S.A., Heaton, K.W., Eastwood, M.A. (1992) Fecal weight, colon cancer risk, and dietary intake of nonstarch polysaccharides (dietary fiber). *Gastroenterol*, 103, 1783–1789.

Cummings, J.H., Hill, M.J., Jenkins, D.J.A., Pearson, J.R., Wiggins, H.S. (1976) Changes in fecal composition and colonic function due to cereal fiber. *Am J Clin Nutr*, 29, 1468–1473.

Cummings, J.H., Pomare, E.W., Branch, W.J., Naylor, C.P.E., MacFarlane, G.T. (1987) Short chain fatty acids in human large intestine, portal, hepatic, and venous blood. *Gut*, 28, 1221–1227.

DeCosse, J.J., Miller, H.H., Lesser, M.L. (1989) Effect of wheat fiber and vitamins C and E on rectal polyps in patients with familial adenomatous polyposis. *J Natl Cancer Inst*, 81, 1290–1297.

De Schrijver, R., Fremaut, D., Verheyen, A. (1992) Cholesterol-lowering effects and utilization of protein, lipid, fiber, and energy in rats fed unprocessed and baked oat bran. *J Nutr*, 122, 1318–1324.

Drews, K.M., Kies, C., Fox, H.M. (1979) Effect of dietary fiber on copper, zinc, and magnesium utilization by adolescent boys. *Am J Clin Nutr*, 49, 471–475.

Eastwood, M.A., Hamilton, D. (1968) Studies of the adsorption of bile salts to non-absorbed components of diet. *Biochim Biophys Acta*, 152, 165–173.

Ebihara, K., Kiriyama, S. (1982) Comparative effects of water-soluble and water-insoluble dietary fibers on various parameters relating to glucose tolerance in rats. *Nutr Rep Intl*, 26, 193–201.

Ebihara, K., Schneeman, B.O. (1989) Interaction of bile acids, phospholipids, cholesterol and triglyceride with dietary fibers in the small intestine of rats. *J Nutr*, 119, 1100–1106.

Ehle, F.R., Robertson, J.B., Van Soest, P.J. (1982) Influence of dietary fibers on fermentation in the human large intestine. *J Nutr*, 112, 158–166.

Ekvall, S.W. (1992) Constipation and Fiber. In: Ekvall, S.W. (ed.) *Pediatric Nutrition in Chronic Diseases and Developmental Disorders. Prevention, Assessment, And Treatment*, pp. 301–309. New York: Oxford University Press.

Enerback, S., Gimble, J.M. (1993) Lipoprotein lipase gene expression: Physiological regulators at the transcriptional and post-transcriptional level. *Biochim Biophys Acta*, 1169, 107–125.

Englyst, H.N., Cummings, J.H. (1985) Digestion of the polysaccharides of some cereal foods in the human small intestine. *Am J Clin Nutr*, 42, 778–787.

Everson, G.T., Daggy, B.P., McKinley, C., Story, J.A. (1992) Effects of psyllium hydrophilic mucilloid on LDL-cholesterol and bile acid synthesis in hypercholesterolemic men. *J Lipid Res*, 33, 1183–1192.

Fairchild, R.M., Ellis, P.R., Byrne, A.J., Luzio, S.D., Mir, M.A. (1996) A new breakfast cereal containing guar gum reduces postprandial plasma glucose and insulin concen-trations in normal-weight human subjects. *Br J Nutr*, 76, 63–73.

Fleming, S.E., Rodriguez, M.A. (1983) Influence of dietary fiber on fecal excretion of volatile fatty acids by human adults. *J Nutr*, 113, 1613–1625.

Fuse, K., Bamba, T., Hosada, S. (1989) Effects of pectin on fatty acid and glucose absorption and on thickness of unstirred water layer in rat and human intestine. *Dig Dis Sci*, 34, 1109–1116.

Gallaher, D.D., Hassel, C.A., Lee, K-J., Gallaher, C. (1993) Viscosity and fermentability as attributes of dietary fiber responsible for the hypocholesterolemic effect in hamsters. *J Nutr*, 123, 244–252.

Gallaher, D., Schneeman, B.O. (1985) Effect of dietary cellulose on site of lipid absorption. *Am J Physiol*, 249, G184–G191.

Gatti, E., Catenazzo, G., Camisasca, E., Torri, A., Denegri, E., Sirtori, C.R. (1984) Effects of guar-enriched pasta in the treatment of diabetes and hyperlipidemia. *Ann Nutr Metab*, 28, 1–10.

Glore, S.R., Van Treeck, D., Knehans, A.W., Guild, M. (1994) Soluble fiber and serum lipids: A literature review. *J Am Diet Assoc*, 94, 425–436.

Hamaker, B.R., Rivera, K., Morales, E., Graham, C.G. (1991) Effect of dietary fiber on fecal composition in preschool Peruvian children consuming maize, amaranth, or cassava flours. *J Pediatr Gastroenterol Nutr*, 13, 59–66.

Hanson, C.F., Winterfeldt, E.A. (1985) Dietary fiber effects on passage rate and breath hydrogen. *Am J Clin Nutr*, 42, 44–48.

Harju, E. (1985) Increases in meal viscosity caused by addition of guar gum decrease postprandial acidity and rate of emptying of gastric contents in healthy subjects. *Panminerva Med*, 27, 223–232.

Higham, S.E., Read, N.W. (1992) The effect of ingestion of guar gum on ileostomy effluent. *Br J Nutr*, 67, 115–122.

Hipsley, E.H. (1953) Dietary fibre and pregnancy toxaemia. *Br Med J*, 2, 420–422.

Holt, S.H.A., Brand Miller, J. (1995) Increased insulin responses to ingested foods are associated with lessened satiety. *Appetite*, 24, 43–54.

Holt, S., Heading, R.C., Carter, D.C., Prescott, L.F., Tothill, P. (1979) Effect of gel fibre on gastric emptying and absorption of glucose and paracetamol. *Lancet*, 1, 636–639.

Illman, R.J., Topping, D.J. (1985) Effects of dietary oat bran on faecal steroid excretion, plasma volatile fatty acids and lipid synthesis in rats. *Nutr Res*, 5, 839–846.

Illman, R.J., Topping, D.L., McIntosh, G.H., Trimble, R.P.,

Storer, G.B., Taylor, M.N., Cheng, B-Q. (1988) Hypocholesterolaemic effects of dietary propionate: Studies in whole animals and perfused rat liver. *Ann Nutr Metab*, 32, 97–107.

Irie, N., Hara, T., Goto, Y. (1982) The effects of guar gum on postprandial chylomicronemia. *Nutr Rep Intl*, 26, 207–231.

Jenkins, D.J.A., Peterson, R.D., Thorne, M.J., Ferguson, P.W. (1987) Wheat fiber and laxation: Dose response and equilibration time. *Am J Gastroentrol*, 12, 1259–1263.

Jenkins, D.J.A., Wolever, T.M.S., Leeds, A.R., Gassull, M.A., Haismen, P., Dilawari, J., Goff, D.V., Metz, G.L., Alberti, K.G. (1978) Dietary fibres, fibre analouges, and glucose tolerance: Importance of viscosity. *Br Med J*, 1, 1392–1394.

Jenkins, D.J.A., Wolever, T.M.S., Taylor, R., Barker, H.M., Fielden, H. (1980) Exceptionally low blood glucose response to dried beans: Comparison with other carbohydrate foods. *Br Med J*, 281, 578–580.

Jenkins, D.J.A., Wolever, T.M.S., Venketeshwer, R., Hegele, R.A., Mitchell, S.J., Ransom, T.P.P, Boctor, D.L., Spadafora, P.J., Jenkins, A.L., Mehling, C., Relle, L.K., Connelly, P.W., Story, J.A., Furumoto, E.J., Corey, P., Wursch, P. (1993) Effect on blood lipids of very high intakes of fiber in diets low in saturated fat and cholesterol. *New Eng J Med*, 329, 21–26.

Jensen, C.D., Spiller, G.A., Gates, J.E., Miller, A.F., Whittman, J.H. (1993) The effect of acacia gum and a water-soluble dietary fiber mixture on blood lipids in humans. *J Am Coll Nutr*, 12, 147–154.

Kingman, S.M., Walker, A.F., Low, A.G., Sambrook, I.E. (1993) Comparative effects of four legume species on plasma lipids and faecal steroid excretion in hypercholesterolaemic pigs. *Br J Nutr*, 69, 409–421.

Kwiterovich, P.O., Jr. (1995) The role of fiber in the treatment of hypercholesterolemia in children and adolescents. *Pediatrics*, 96, 1005–1009.

Leclere, C.J., Champ, M., Boillot, J., Guille, G., Lecannu, G., Molis, C., Bornet, F., Krempf, M., Delort-Laval, J., Galmiche, J-P. (1994) Role of viscous guar gums in lowering the glycemic response after a solid meal. *Am J Clin Nutr*, 59, 914–921.

Lee, S.C., Prosky, L., DeVries, J.W. (1992) Determination of total, soluble, and insoluble dietary fiber in foods—enzymatic-gravimetric method, MES-TRIS buffer: Collaborative study. *J AOAC Intl*, 75, 395–416.

Leoning-Baucke, V.A. (1984) Sensitivity of the sigmoid colon and rectum in children treated for chronic constipation. *J Pediatr Gastroenterol*, 3, 454–459.

Livesey, G. (1995) Fiber As Energy in Man. In: Kritchevsky, D., Bonfield, C. (eds.) *Dietary Fiber in Health And Disease*, pp. 46–57. St. Paul: Eagen Press.

McBurney, M.I., Horvath, P.J., Jeraci, J.L., Van Soest, P.J. (1985) Effect of in vitro fermentation using fecal inoculum on the water holding capacity of dietary fiber. *Br J Nutr*, 53, 17–24.

McCall, M.R., Mehta, T., Leathers, C., Forster, D.M. (1992) Psyllium husk I: Effect on plasma lipoproteins, cholesterol metabolism, and atherosclerosis in African green monkeys. *Am J Clin Nutr*, 56, 376–384.

MacLennan, R., Macrae, F., Bain, C., Battistutta, D., Chapuis, P., Gratten, H., Lambert, J., Newland, R.C., Ngu, M., Russell, A., Ward, M., Wahlqvist, M.L. (1995) Randomized trial of intake of fat, fiber, and beta carotene to prevent colorectal adenomas. *J Natl Cancer Inst*, 87, 1760–1766.

Marlett, J.A., Chesters, J.G., Longacre, M.J., Bogdanske, J.J. (1992) Recovery of soluble dietary fiber is dependent on the method of analysis. *Am J Clin Nutr*, 50, 479–485.

Middleton, S.M., Schneeman, B.O. (1995) Nutrient infusion into the illeum of rats does not lower plasma lipids or alter apoliprotein mRNA abundance. *Am J Clin Nutr*, 125, 983–989.

Miettinen, T.A. (1987) Dietary fiber and lipids. *Am J Clin Nutr*, 45, 1237–1242.

Mueller, S., Keast, D.R., Olson, B.H. (1997) Intakes and food sources of dietary fiber in children. *FASEB J*, 11, A187.

Muir, J.G., Young, G.P., O'Dea, K., Cameron-Smith, D., Brown, I.L., Collier, G.R. (1993) Resistant starch — the neglected 'dietary fiber'? Implications for health. *Dietary Fiber Bibliography and Reviews*, 1, 33–47.

National Cholesterol Education Program (1992) Report of the expert panel on blood cholesterol levels in children and adolescents. *Pediatr*, 89(suppl), 525–584.

Nicklas, T.A., Farris, R.P., Myers, L., Berenson, G.S. (1995) Dietary fiber intake of children and young adults: The Bogalusa Heart Study. *J Am Diet Assoc*, 95, 209–214.

Nishina, P.M., Freedland, R.A. (1990a) The effects of dietary fiber feeding on cholesterol metabolism in rats. *J Nutr*, 120, 800–805.

Nishina, P.M., Freedland, R.A. (1990b) Effects of propionate on lipid biosynthesis in isolated rat hepatocytes. *J Nutr*, 120, 668–673.

Nyman, M., Asp, N-G. (1982) Fermentation of dietary fibre components in the rat intestinal tract. *Br J Nutr*, 47, 357–366.

Olivecrona, T., Chernick, S.S., Bengtsson-Olivecrona, G., Garrison, M., Scow, R.O. (1987) Synthesis and secretion of lipoprotein lipase in 3T3-L1 adipocytes: Demonstration of inactive forms of lipase in cells. *J Biol Chem*, 262, 10748–10759.

Pomare, E.W., Branch, W.J., Cummings, J.H. (1985) Carbohydrate fermentation in the human colon and its relation to acetate concentrations in venous blood. *J Clin Invest*, 75, 1448–1454.

Prosky, L. (1990) Collaborative study of a method for soluble and insoluble fiber. *Adv Exper Med Biol*, 270, 193–203.

Prosky, L., Asp, N-G., Furda, I., DeVries, J.W., Schweizer, T.F., Harland, B. (1984) Determination of total dietary fiber in foods, food products and total diets: Interlaboratory study. *J Assoc Off Anal Chem*, 67, 1044–1052.

Prosky, L., Asp, N-G., Furda, I., DeVries, J.W., Schweizer, T.F., Harland, B.F. (1985) Determination of total dietary fiber in foods and food products: Collaborative study. *J Assoc Off Anal Chem*, 68, 677–679.

Prosky, L., Asp, N-G., Schweizer, T.F., DeVries, J.W., Furda, I. (1988) Determination of insoluble, soluble and total dietary fiber in foods and food products: Interlaboratory study. *J Assoc Off Anal Chem*, 71, 1017–1023.

Pykalisto, O.J., Smith, P.H., Brunzell, J.D. (1975) Determinants of human adipose tissue lipoprotein lipase. Effect of diabetes and obesity on basal- and diet-induced activity. *J Clin Invest*, 56, 1108–1117.

Redard, C.L., Davis, P.A., Middleton, S.J., Schneeman, B.O. (1992) Postprandial lipid response following a high fat meal in rats adapted to dietary fiber. *J Nutr*, 122, 219–228.

Redard, C.L., Davis, P.A., Schneeman, B.O. (1990) Dietary fiber and gender: Effect on postprandial lipemia. *Am J Clin Nutr*, 52, 837–845.

Remesy, C., Behr, S.R., Levrat, M-A., Demigne, C. (1992) Fiber fermentability in the rat cecum and its physiological consequences. *Nutr Res*, 12, 1235–1244.

Salmeron, J., Manson, J.E., Stampfer, M.J., Colditz, G.A., Wing, A.L., Willett, W.C. (1997) Dietary fiber, glycemic load, and risk of non-insulin-dependent diabetes mellitus in women. *J Am Med Assoc*, 277, 472–477.

Sandberg, A.S., Andersson, H., Hallgren, B., Hasselblad, K., Isaksson, B., Hulten, L. (1981) Experimental model for in vivo determination of dietary fibre and its effects on the absorption of nutrients in the small intestine. *Br J Nutr*, 45, 283–294.

Schweizer, T.F. (1990) Dietary fiber analysis and nutrition labelling. *Adv Exper Med Biol*, 270, 265–272.

Shannon, J., White, E., Shattuck, A.L., Potter, J.D. (1996) Relationship of food groups and water intake to colon cancer risk. *Cancer Epi Biomarkers Prev*, 5, 495–502.

Southgate, D.A.T. (1978) The definition, analysis and properties of dietary fibre. *J Plant Food*, 3, 9–19.

Southgate, D.A.T., Durnin, J.V.G.A. (1970) Calorie conversion factors. An experimental reassessment of the factors used in the calculation of the energy value of human diets. *Br J Nutr*, 24, 517–535.

Spiller, G.A., Chernoff, M.C., Hill, R.A., Gates, J.E., Nassar, J.J., Shipley, E.A. (1980) Effect of purified cellulose, pectin, and a low-residue diet on fecal volatile fatty acids, transit time, and fecal weight in humans. *Am J Clin Nutr*, 33, 754–759.

Stephen, A.M., Haddad, A.C., Phillips, S.F. (1983) Passage of carbohydrate into the colon. Direct measurement in humans. *Gastroenterol*, 85, 589–595.

Stevens, J., Levitsky, D.A., Van Soest, P.J. (1987) Effect of psyllium hum and wheat bran on spontaneous energy intake. *Am J Clin Nutr*, 46, 812–817.

Story, L., Anderson, J.W., Chen, W-J.L., Karounos, D., Jefferson, B. (1985) Adherence to high-carbohydrate, high-fiber diets: Long-term studies of non-obese diabetic men. *J Am Diet Assoc*, 85, 1105–1110.

Tappy, L., Gugolz, E., Wursch, P. (1996) Effects of breakfast cereals containing various amounts of beta-glucan fibers on plasma glucose and insulin responses in NIDDM subjects. *Diab Care*, 19, 831–834.

Tappy, L., Wursch, P., Randin, J.P., Felber, J.P., Jequier, E. (1986) Metabolic effect of pre-cooked instant preparations of bean and potato in normal and in diabetic subjects. *Am J Clin Nutr*, 43, 30–36.

Tietyen, J. (1991) Hypocholesterolemic potential of oat bran treated with an endobetaglucanase. (Master's thesis, University of California at Davis).

Tinker, L.F., Schneeman, B.O. (1989) The effects of guar gum or wheat bran on the disappearance of 14C-labeled starch from the rat gastrointestinal tract. *J Nutr*, 119, 403–408.

Trautwein, E.A., Siddiqui, A., Hayes, K.C. (1993) Modeling plasma lipoprotein-bile lipid relationships: Differential impact of psyllium and cholestyramine in hamsters fed a lithogenic diet. *Metab*, 42, 1531–1540.

Trinidad, T.P., Wolever, T.M.S., Thompson, L.U. (1996a) Availability of calcium for absorption in the small intestine and colon from diets containing available and unavailable carbohydrates: An in vitro assessment. *Intl J Food Sci Nutr*, 47, 83–88.

Trinidad, T.P., Wolever, T.M.S., Thompson, L.U. (1996b) Effect of acetate and propionate on calcium absorption from the rectum and distal colon of humans. *Am J Clin Nutr*, 63, 574–578.

Turley, S.D., Daggy, B.P., Dietschy, J.M. (1991) Cholesterol-lowering action of psyllium mucilloid in the hamster: Sites and possible mechanisms of action. *Metab*, 40, 1063–1073.

Vahouny, G.V., Cassidy, M.M. (1986) Effect of dietary fiber on intestinal absorption of lipids. In: Spiller, G.A. (ed.) Handbook of Dietary Fiber in Human Nutrition, pp. 121–128. Boca Raton, FL: CRC Press.

Vahouny, G.V., Satchithanandam, S., Chen, I., Tepper, S., Kritchevsky, D., Lightfoot, F.G., Cassidy, M.M. (1988) Dietary fiber and intestinal adaptation: Effects on lipid absorption and lymphatic transport in the rat. *Am J Clin Nutr*, 47, 201–206.

Vahouny, G.V., Tombes, R., Cassidy, M., Kritchevsky, D.,

Gallo, L.L. (1980) Dietary fibers V. Binding of bile salts, phospholipids and cholesterol from mixed micelles by bile acid sequestrants and dietary fibers. *Lipids*, 15, 1012–1018.

Venter, C.S., Vorster, H.H. (1989) Possible metabolic consequences of fermentation in the colon for humans. *Med Hypotheses*, 29, 161–166.

Walker, A.R.P., Fox, F.W., Irving, J.T. (1948) Studies in human mineral metabolism. I. The effect of bread rich in phytate on the metabolism of calcium. *Biochem J*, 42, 452–462.

Wang, L., Newman, R.K., Newman, C.W., Hofer, P.J. (1992) Barley β-glucans alter intestinal viscosity and reduce plasma cholesterol concentrations in chicks. *J Nutr*, 122, 2292–2297.

Williams, C.L., Bollella, M., Wynder, E.L. (1995) A new recommendation for dietary fibre in childhood. *Pediatr*, 96, 985–988.

Wolever, T.M.S., Jenkins, D.J.A., Vuksan, V., Jenkins, A.L., Buckley, G.C., Wong, G.S., Josse, R.G. (1992) Beneficial effect of a low glycaemic index diet in type 2 diabetes. *Diab Med*, 9, 451–458.

Wolever, T.M.S., Vuksan, B., Eshuis, H., Spadafora, P., Peterson, D., Chao, E.S.M., Storey, M.L., Jenkins, D.J.A. (1991) Effect of method of administration of psyllium on glycemic response and carbohydrate digestibility. *J Am Coll Nutr*, 10, 364–371.

Wursch, P., Acheson, K., Boellreutter, B., Jequier, E. (1988) Metabolic effects of instant bean and potato over 6 hours. *Am J Clin Nutr*, 48, 1418–1423.

Zhang, J-X., Lundin, E., Andersson, H., Bosaeus, I., Dahlgren, S., Hallmans, G., Stenling, R., Aman, P. (1991) Brewer's spent grain, serum lipids and fecal sterol excretion in human subjects and ileostomies. *J Nutr*, 121, 778–784.

21

Critical illness: Altered nutritional requirements

A.J. Baker and S.P. Devane

Introduction

Critical illness and trauma have profound effects on metabolism due to hormonal and inflammatory mediators. These effects have been investigated most thoroughly in adult post-operative and infected patients, but some have also been examined in paediatric patients. Infants and older children have different nutrient requirements, metabolic rates, and physiological responses compared with adults. These parameters are even more different in the pre-term infant, making appropriate clinical responses difficult to determine.

Historical background

Metabolism

Since the 1930s, it has been known that trauma and its associated physiological stress lead to a catabolic state, with a breakdown in body proteins, particularly muscle. Releasing amino acids to provide substrates for the production of acute phase proteins has putative short-term advantages for the immune system and for tissue repair (Cuthbertson 1931, Douglas & Shaw 1989). Appetite is lost, probably due to a central effect of cytokines. Basal (minimal energy requirements at rest) energy expenditure is variably increased (Table 21.1). Plasma concentrations of epinephrine, norepinephrine, glucagon and insulin are raised, associated with increased protein breakdown, insulin resistance and hyperlipidaemia. Production of corticosteroids, interleukins, and other metabolites change the pattern of metabolism at a cellular level in favour of whole body catabolism (Schmeling & Coran 1991, Scrimshaw 1991). Changes in production of insulin-like growth factor I (IGF-1), and its two major binding proteins, IGFBP-1 and IGFBP-3, result in a rapid reduction in tissue bioavailability of this anabolic hormone and contribute to growth hormone resistance (Phillips & Unterman 1984, Ross & Buchanan 1990, Ross et al 1991).

Assessing nutritional requirements precisely in adults is difficult, and is even more so in the paediatric patient.

Table 21.1 — Increase in energy expenditure

Sepsis, burns, head injury, organ failure
Up to 50% above basal rate in illness
Increase can be reduced by good care
Persists into convalescence (21 days +)

Early studies led to over-prescribing of nutrients because of an over-estimation of metabolic rate. This occurred because an allowance was made for pyrexia when the measured metabolic rate already included it, the measured metabolic rate was extrapolated from the acute phase to the recovery phase, and an erroneous belief was held that the catabolic response could be prevented with adequate nutrition (Elia 1995). Recently, the quantity of nutrients administered to critically-ill adults has declined.

The infant (particularly the pre-term infant) requires proportionately greater intakes of energy, fluid, protein and micro-nutrients than the older child or adult in order to support the greater demand arising from the determinants of energy requirements (Table 21.2). In malnutrition, lean body mass and particularly the mass of essential organs is greater. Basal energy expenditure may appear to be high, especially if body weight is used as the denominator. Conversely, acute severe starvation may result in reduced basal energy expenditure, justifying its measurement. The pre-term infant has a lower resting metabolic rate than the term infant when it is expressed per unit surface area, and lacks the ability to increase metabolic rate in response to cold stress due in part to a lack of brown fat. The clinical concept of the *thermo-neutral range*, the temperature range within which the infant should be nursed in order to minimize the metabolic energy cost for the infant, has arisen from these studies (Hey & Katz 1970).

Allowance for the metabolic cost of growth must be made, being between 20–30% of the energy value of the incorporated tissues (Micheli & Schutz 1987, Piero et al 1991). However, because of metabolic immaturity in the pre-term infant and in the first few days of life, renal thresholds may be readily exceeded and retention of water may occur as may sodium loss. Gastrointestinal absorption capacity may be exceeded. An additional factor to consider is the higher evaporative water loss from the skin in pre-term infants (Hammurland & Sedin 1979, Okken et al

Table 21.2 — Determinants of energy requirements

Growth (+ cost of protein synthesis)
Stress and temperature control
Basal
Obligate losses (e.g., urinary & faecal)
Repair
Immune system

1979). The hormonal adaptation to stress of the pre-term infant is sub-optimal (Lucas et al 1985). Extrapolation of adult data to predict the energy and nutrient requirements of ill infants must take into consideration the different body composition of the infant, with a higher body-water content and a greater proportion of metabolically-active tissues. Growth is sacrificed in favour of the other uses of energy if intake is insufficient for needs. Growth of essential organs, particularly the central nervous system, is sustained preferentially. Relevant studies in infants are less numerous than in adults. The nitrogen balance of pre-term infants over the first days of life is frequently negative using current feeding regimes (Mitton et al 1991). In newborn infants after surgery, negative nitrogen balance has been shown to last up to 96 h (Rickham 1957). However, it was not possible to show an increase in resting energy in 13 newborn infants undergoing surgery using an open circuit indirect calorimetry technique on the first, second, and seventh post-operative days (Shanbhogue & Lloyd 1992).

Antioxidant stress

Redox reactions in animal cells produce *oxidants* or *free radicals* (unstable molecules with unpaired electrons) either within or outside cells. Examples are H_2O_2, (hydrogen peroxide), OH–, (hydroxyl radical) and singlet oxygen (Table 21.3). Cytokine synthesis and immune activation result in increased production of these entities. H_2O_2 is an antibacterial weapon of the immune system. Free radicals react readily with double bonds, including those of polyunsaturated fatty acids in cell membranes, reducing fluidity and altering function (Table 21.4). Sulphur containing amino acids, nucleic acids and respiratory chain enzymes are also vulnerable to denaturing by free radicals. Prevention of free radical damage is achieved by many intracellular and extracellular substances (Table 21.5), including acute phase proteins synthesized by the liver (such as metalothionine) and intracellular catalase

Table 21.3 — Oxidants (free radicals)

Unstable compounds with unpaired electrons
From electron transport chain, immune activity, drugs etc.
Superoxide, H_2O_2, OH–, singlet O etc.
NO– intracellular or extracellular mediator
'Weapons' of the activated immune system
PG + LTr synthesis generate free radicals

PG = Prostaglandin, LTr = leukotreine

Table 21.4 — Targets of oxidant attack

Unsaturated bonds, especially in membrane lipids
Sulphate containing enzymes
Nucleic acids
Endothelial cells
Cells in inflammation

Table 21.5 — Antioxidants

Superoxide dismutases
Catalase, glutathione peroxidase
Metalothionine
Other Fe, Mn, Cu, Zn containing metaloenzymes
Vitamins C + E
Beta carotene
Taurine
Glutathione, cysteine, methionine
Uric acid, albumin, etc.
NAC, other drugs

and superoxide dismutase (which bind heavy metals). Sulphur containing molecules (such as cysteine, methionine, and glutathione): plasma urate and albumin are important. Nutritional substances including vitamins C and E, taurine, selenium and the drug N-acetyl cysteine have been used as treatment to protect against the effects of excess free radicals during severe illness, particularly sepsis. In very pre-term infants, however, total antioxidant activity has not been correlated with outcome yet (Drury et al 1998).

Benefits of intensive nutritional support

It may seem self-evident that maintaining growth during serious illness is a laudable aim, but data to support the relationship of nutrition and outcome has been slow to appear. Measures of nutritional outcome, including anthropometry and biochemical markers, and of immuno-competence may predict morbidity, mortality, duration of ventilation, duration of intensive care stay and time to discharge home (Wesley 1992). Much of the data in paediatric pratice relates to term and pre-term infants receiving neonatal intensive care support.

Effects on growth

A prospective randomized study in 125 sick newborn infants showed that aggressive nutritional support led to a better weight and length centile position in later infancy (Wilson et al 1997). The intervention group received an aggressive regime, including earlier introduction of major nutrients, a more rapid increase in administered amounts and a policy of increased reluctance to reduce administration in response of clinical symptoms. Studies on head circumference growth are less convincing as aggregated data in pre-term infants is confounded by changes in head shape with time and ventricular dilatation due to intraventricular haemorrhage. A study of 73 pre-term infants receiving intensive care in the newborn period showed that those who received < 85 kcal/kg/day for more than 4 weeks (if their weight at birth was appropriate for gestational age) or for only 2–3 weeks (if their weight at birth was small for gestational age) had head growth that achieved curves below minus 1 standard deviation (SD) on the growth chart, whereas other infants had mean growth above minus 1 SD (Georgieff et al 1985). The part played by micro-nutrients in successful growth is still not clear. In a recent study, supplementation of nutritional intake of small-for-gestational-age infants with nucleotides led to better catch-up growth (Cosgrove et al 1996).

Effects on tissue repair and inflammatory response

Nutritional status affects the lungs' ability to resist hyperoxic damage, effect repair, and resist infection (Fig. 21.1 and Table 21.6). It influences the development of chronic lung damage such as that found in bronchopulmonary dysplasia in surviving pre-term infants (Frank & Sosenko 1988). Nutrients such as polyunsaturated fatty acids (PUFA) (Fig. 21.2) have been shown to protect against free radical lung injury in animal models (Sosenko et al 1988). Supplementation of the intake of nucleotides in a population of children reduced diarrhoeal disease

Table 21.6 — Correlation of immune function and nutrition

Deficiencies may not parallel degree of malnutrition.
Immune recovery usually achieved with 90 days hyperalimentation.
Immune recovery does not necessarily correlate with nutritional recovery.
Immunological nutrients?

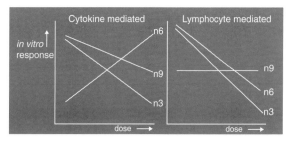

Figure 21.2 — Immune modulation by polyunsaturated fatty acids. Precursors: n3 = eicosapentaenoic, linolenic; n6 = arachidonic, linoleic; n9 = oleic, eicosatrienoic.

incidence significantly (Wilmore 1981), but the mechanism of this effect is not known. Glutamine has been shown to have beneficial effects on gut barrier function in adults and in neonatal pigs (Buirin et al 1994). A controlled trial in ill newborn infants showed a reduced length of time of administration of parenteral nutrition in very-low-birth-weight infants supplemented with glutamine (Lacey et al 1996). Inositol supplementation has been shown to produce significant improvements in short-term neonatal outcomes, but again by an unknown mechanism (Howlett & Ohlsson 1997).

Effects on long-term neuro-developmental outcome

The effects of increased nutritional intake during an early period of critical illness in pre-term infants on neuro-developmental outcome at 18 months was shown (Lucas et al 1990). Neuro-developmental outcome at 7 years of age was assessed in the same cohort and showed a correlation between weight at 9 months and later performance, particularly in verbal IQ scores and particularly in males (personal communication). Infants deprived of adequate nutrition for more than 4 weeks had developmental scores below the normal range by 1 year of corrected age. Relatively short periods of nutritional impairment on central nervous system growth may be incompletely

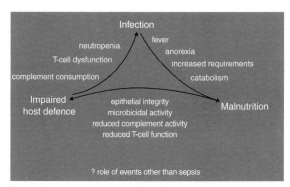

Figure 21.1 — Interaction of malnutrition and immune function.

recoverable (Georgieff et al 1985). Paradoxically, breast milk, despite its lower nutritional content, leads to better neuro-developmental outcome than formula milk (Lucas et al 1992), possibly due to the long-chain polyunsaturated fatty acid (LC-PUFA) content of breast milk. Recent studies have show better neurological function as measured by visual-evoked response times in infants given LC-PUFA (Carlson et al 1996).

Long-term priming/programming

There is no conclusive data yet on the long-term effects of periods of abnormal metabolism on subsequent metabolic responses. However the possibility of effects can be inferred from the relationships between growth in infancy and morbidity in middle age, which is known as the *Barker hypothesis* (Barker 1992). Although under-nutrition seems to predispose to later disease, bone mineralization in later childhood may paradoxically be better in infants with lower calcium and phosphate intakes in early infancy, suggesting long-term up-regulation of calcium and phosphate retention (Lucas 1998).

Practice and procedures

Assessing and measuring needs

On admission to intensive care, it is essential to undertake an assessment of pre-existing nutritional adequacy, whether *in utero* or post-natal. Knowledge of recent dietary management and clinical condition are essential in planning current intake. Anthropometric indices (particularly skin-fold thickness) and a comparison of indices with appropriate charts of normal values are important in establishing protein-calorie malnutrition. Weight, whilst valuable, is subject to fluid shifts and hydration status, typically under-estimating the severity of malnutrition. Other anthropometric indices that should be measured include occipito-frontal head circumference and lower-limb length by knemometry (Kaenipf 1998). Regular assessment provides information on lean

Table 21.7 — Growth assessment methods

Regular anthropometry, mnemometry
Photon absorptiometry
Dilution methods
Bioimpedance
Urine creatinine

versus fat, skeletal, and neurological growth (Table 21.7). Target rates for growth in pre-term infants should be the same as documented *in utero* growth rates for normal infants of the same sex and racial origin who are ultimately delivered at term and normal weight (Pereira & Barbosa 1986). Such data has been gathered by indirect methods such as ultrasound, and there may be significant errors for very small infants. However, these remain short-term yardsticks for success in nutritional intervention for sick pre-term infants. *Bioelectrical impedance*, a method suggested for assessing lean body mass, has not been evaluated sufficiently for current use in ill infants (Vettorazzi et al 1994).

These anthropometric indices can be supplemented by a basic set of biochemical indicators (Table 21.8). Because healthy growth is a process of accumulation of lean body mass, it is perhaps not surprising that plasma markers of nutritional status have not been shown to be valuable.

The requirement for dietary constituents can be approximated from the child's current size, current factors affecting metabolic rate (such as pyrexia and the clinical illness), and the need for catch-up growth. Macro-nutrient requirements are established within broad limits for term and pre-term infants, and are modified in the light of individual needs (Tsang et al 1993).

Table 21.8 — Biochemical indices of nutritional status

Protein	Plasma urea (should be > 2 mmol/L)
	Plasma albumin (should be > 35 g/L)
Carbohydrate	Blood glucose (should be > 2.6 mmol/L)
Lipid	Plasma triglycerides (should be > 0.3 mmol/L)
	Plasma cholesterol (should be > 1.5 mmol/L
Electrolytes	Urinary sodium (should be > 5 mmol/L)
	Serum calcium (should be > 1.8 mmol/L)
	Serum phosphate (should be > 1.5 mmol/L)
	Serum alkaline phosphatase (age dependent, low in zinc deficiency, high in phosphate deficiency)
	Serum zinc (should be > 9 µmol/L)
	Serum copper (should be > 3 µmol/L)

Pyrexia results in an increase in basal energy expenditure of 10% for each degree Celsius above 37. Historically Burns, head injury and organ failure have been associated with increased basal energy expenditure of up to 100%, but recognition of the problem and better management have reduced the extra requirement to 50% or less.

Once absorbed, nutrients may be metabolized to provide an immediate source of energy for obligate expenditure, the level of which may be normal, increased or decreased. In illness, substrates are also required to fuel the immune system and repair damaged tissues. If the nutritional and endocrine milieu is favourable, tissue growth may still be possible. Enterally-administered nutrition may be absorbed incompletely, and this needs to be considered. Methodology for estimating enteral losses and expenditure by the immune system and processes of repair remain in the realms of research. However, energy expenditure can be measured readily in even very sick infants. Indirect calorimeters such as the Deltatrac are highly sensitive and simple to use. Care is required, however, in excluding endotracheal gas leak in ventilated infants and in specifying the conditions under which measurements are made. Ignoring energy derived from protein oxidation results in an error of up to 4%.

The fate of dietary protein can be clarified using stable isotope labelled amino acids. These methods measure the flux of amino acids through the respective amino acid pools within the body. Unfortunately, different methods of assessing nitrogen turnover that use different labelled amino acids give different results because they measure flux in different pools (Pencharz et al 1989a, Pencharz et al 1989b). Stable isotope methods can also be used to assess the fate of dietary lipid. Rates of oxidation can be measured from the stable isotope content of exhaled gases. Oxidation of fat has been shown to be proportional to the severity of illness and inversely proportional to intake of carbohydrate (Letton et al 1996). Structural utilization versus adipose storage is more difficult to quantify. Infants undertake lipogenesis more readily than adults do. Plasma phospholipid and red-cell-membrance essential-fatty-acid content correlate with recent dietary intake rather than whole-body essential-fatty-acid status so that plasma studies do not clarify the fate of administered fatty acids (Rubin et al 1994). Occasional patients as well as those taking part in nutritional research may require assessment of the fate of absorbed nutritional components.

Feeding and administration

Requirements

The specific needs for macro-nutrients and minerals such as calcium and phosphorus are known, but achieving positive balance can be difficult. Fluid restriction, problems of tolerance including diarrhoea related to osmolarity or antibiotics, reduced gastric emptying particularly related to sedatives, failure of absorption, or glucose resistance during sepsis may result in targets being impossible to meet, even with combined parenteral and enteral feeding.

Some nutrients may be essential in non-physiological conditions (Cochran et al 1988). Pre-term infants (Table 21.9) have high requirements related to their body composition and high growth rates. They need supplementation to allow for poor renal retention, reduced vitamin D (Table 21.10) and other lipid interconversion, limited gastrointestinal absorptive capacity, and reduced stores of many nutrients including iron and trace elements. Taurine (Kendler 1989, Burger & Gobel 1992) carnitine and nucleotides may be conditionally essential during high growth rate periods (Table 21.11). Essential fatty acids, particularly the omega-6 and omega-3 series, may need to be supplemented to give ratios close to that found in human milk. The design of specialized and pre-term infant milks has been modified to take account of human milk content and perceived needs. Liver,

Table 21.9 — Energy requirements in low-birth-weight infants

Total	120–180 kcal/day
Basal	47–58
Activity	8–15
Growth**	25–60
Cold stress	0–8
Protein synthesis	0–5
Diet-induced etc. losses*	7–38

*greatest losses with greatest intakes. **weight gain 14–18 g/day.

Table 21.10 — Vitamins in pre-term infants

Low stores
Rapid growth and high requirement
Low absorption
Low intake (often)

Table 21.11 — Conditionally-essential nutrients

Cysteine (cystine)
Taurine
Arginine
Tyrosine
Glutamine
Choline
Nucleotides
Inositol
Carnitine

Table 21.12 — Enteral feed tolerance

Gastric emptying inferred from residuals
Diarrhoea
Distension and constipation
Glucose tolerance
Fluid and electrolyte balance
Amino acid and urea status

pancreatic, gastrointestinal and renal disease may be associated with failure of absorption, increased losses and increased requirements of macro-nutrients (particularly energy) and specific components (e.g., polyunsaturated fatty acids in liver disease).

Enteral administration

The enteral route has several advantages that make it the first choice. It promotes gastrointestinal growth, motility and adaptation, including that of the immune tissue preventing bacterial overgrowth and translocation. The absorbed nutritional substrates are presented first to the liver with less risk of metabolic derangement. Food in the gastrointestinal tract promotes bile flow and protects against parenteral nutrition (PN) cholestasis (q.v.). Thus, PN is associated with more septic complications, slower tolerance of enteral feeds subsequently, more biochemical disturbances and more liver disease. Intravenous lipid may reduce macrophage function and increase pulmonary blood pressure. PN currently costs approximately UK£80 per day compared with UK£10 per day for enteral nutrition (EN).

Even in surgical conditions such as gastroschesis, short-gut syndrome, Hirschprung's disease and necrotizing enterocolitis, EN has resulted in decreased morbidity (Wesley 1992). Advantages include early development to gastrointestinal function and immunology, including reduced bacterial translocation, the potential for greater calorie density with better growth, a lower rate of many of the complications associated with parenteral nutrition and reduced costs (Unger et al 1986).

Although non-nutritive sucking improves the weight gain of enterally-fed infants oral feeding is rarely possible in very sick infants. Swallowing is unco-ordinated in sick, sedated infants and tube feeding is usual. Most units prefer the tube to be passed orally in order to reduce nasal trauma and not to obstruct the

nasal airway, which is the preferred (if not obligate) air passage. Slow gastric emptying, and diarrhoea are practical issues. Issues affecting tolerance may hamper persisting with enteral feeding (Table 21.12). Accepting and replacing nasogastric aspirates (residuals) of up to 6–7 mL/kg before subsequent feeds, which are harmless, results in better intakes. There is no universal definition of diarrhoea. Six or more copious stools of watery consistency per day may not be pathological. So long as no gastrointestinal pathology is present, which may be worsened by enteral feeds, and no metabolic consequences result from osmotic fluid loss, the volume should be recorded and replaced if necessary and feeding continued. The risk of necrotizing enterocolitis is considered below.

Enteral feed can be administered via the stomach or duodenum. Benefits of the gastric route include ease of insertion of the feeding tube and a lower risk of intestinal perforation (Mandell & Finkelstein 1988). Disadvantages of gastric feeding focus on gastric dysmotility. Pre-term infants may manifest a type of pseudo-obstruction related to immaturity and growth retardation making gastric feeding impossible (Lamireau et al 1993). Gastro-oesophageal reflux may be associated with recurrent aspiration and chronic lung disease in a small proportion of infants. There is no difference between placement of gastric tubes by the nasal or the oral route with similar weight gain and episodes of bradycardia (Symington et al 1995).

Enteral feeding may be administered continuously, intermittently or by bolus. A well-designed study of continuous 24-h nasogastric versus intermittent 3-hourly bolus nasogastric feeding in 82 male infants between 27–34 weeks gestation showed no differences in retention of nitrogen, fat, total carbohydrate and lactose and no difference in complications (Silvestre et al 1996). Bolus feeding may be associated with more physiological endocrine function, in turn promoting more normal biliary kinetics. Tidal volume, minute volume ventilation and dynamic compliance decreased 28–44% in very-low-birth-weight neonates with respiratory distress given bolus feeds, showing that a slower rate of feeding is preferable in patients with respiratory instability (Blondheim et al 1993). Small decreases in cerebral blood flow velocity (about 10%) are seen 5–11 minutes after bolus feeding (Kraeft 1986). Open circuit calorimetry was used to compare diet induced thermogenesis in pre-term infants given either continuous nasogastric or bolus feeding over 5 minutes every 2–3 h. The order of feeding type was randomized. Peak energy expenditure was 15% higher in the bolus-fed group with a mean increase of 4%. Carers may tend not to replace nasogastric residuals so that bolus-fed infants may receive less feed than planned. Continuous gastric feeds appear preferable in unstable infants but should be replaced by bolus feeds as soon as conditions permit. Frequency of feeds is decreased according to gestational age and feed tolerance. Pulmonary aspiration of feed is seen in a few infants with severe gastro-oesophageal reflux. EN is contraindicated in those infants at high risk of necrotizing enterocolitis. Brief gastrointestinal rest after surgery may be indicated. The absence of a functioning gastrointestinal tract is the only consistent contraindication to its use. Perforation occasionally occurs.

Parenteral administration

Parenteral nutrition (PN) has been a major step forward in nutritional care of all very sick patients, especially pre-term and surgical neonates. It can provide growth nearly compatible with normal *in utero* rates in patients in whom enteral feeding is impossible. Many detailed regimes have been published in paediatric textbooks and handbooks; prescription issues are not addressed here.

PN may be administered through a peripheral intravenous line, through a percutaneously-placed long line, or through a surgically-placed long line. Peripheral lines should not be used for concentrations of glucose in excess of 12.5% because of the risk of skin necrosis if the line tissues. Particular care should be taken in the infant on restricted fluids, thereby getting concentrated infusions, with poor peripheral perfusion. Other factors contributing to tissue necrosis are the presence of inotropic drugs and calcium in the infusion. Ensuring that the end of the line is visible, hourly observation of the site, and attntion to alarms indicating increased resistance in the line reduce (but do not eliminate) the risk of damage. Ideally, avoiding pacing the tip of the line close to a joint is wise, but may not be possible. If a significant extravasation occurs and there are signs of dark discoloration of the overlying skin, irrigation with large volumes of saline by a plastic surgeon may help, but no controlled trial of this procedure has been carried out. Percutaneously-placed long lines help reduce the risk of these complications. Silastic lines may be threaded in until the tip is in the SVC or IVC. Surgically-placed lines are helpful in babies likely to require long-term PN, but meticulous care to reduce the risk of introduction of infection (by minimizing the number of line interventions, for example) is important, as there is a limited number of possible placement sites and running out of potential replacement sites may actually be life-threatening in the long term. In the newborn very-low-birth-weight infant (> 1000 g), placement of an umbilical venous line for the first few days is justified (despite its known but low risk of portal venous damage).

Complications

Although the benefits of adequate nutrition are clear, concerns focus on the complications of artificial methods of administration of nutritional needs. Complications are much more frequent for parenteral than for enteral feeding. Other concerns relate to the content of and deficiencies recognized in the feeding solutions.

Complications may be divided into those associated with the administration line (mechanical and infective); metabolic side effects including acidosis, respiratory, metabolic and electrolyte disturbance and glucose intolerance; and effects on the immune system, lungs, central nervous system, and liver.

Line complications

Although the proximate cause of infection in patients on PN is an ingress of an organism with adequate virulence, the aetiology is multifactorial. PN interferes with macrophage and complement function. The lack of gastrointestinal nutrition leads to intestinal barrier failure (Aranow & Fink 1996). Surveillance of 94 infants in a surgical unit that had a long-term rate of septicaemia of 7.3 episodes per 1000 days found that 15 of 24 episodes were due to translocation of enteral organisms occurring after 32–286 (median 58) days treatment. Organisms causing septicaemia were always present in the gastrointestinal tract, often at high concentration. *Candida* infection is particularly difficult to diagnose, but all cases are associated with thrombocytopenia, compared with about half of cases with Grain-negative septicaemia (McDonnell & Isaacs 1995). Nineteen percent of 82 pre-term infants became colonized with *Candida*, most often in the gastrointestinal tract. Five had *Candida* sepsis and one died. Prematurity, very low birth weight, previous colonization, prolonged antibiotic treatment, umbilical venous or arterial catheter insertion, intralipid and late feeding predisposed to clinical infection (Arisoy et al 1994, el Mohandes et al 1994).

Infective endocarditis is a recognized complication of positioning a central line. Coagulase-positive staphylococci are the most likely organisms (Brunvand & Fugelseth 1996). Colonization of PN catheters, connections and solutions was found on a total of 26 occasions from 52 central lines in a neonatal nursery, with a colonization rate of 36%. The major risk for colonization was the presence of the catheter *in situ* for > 3 weeks. Although removing central venous catheters may be the ideal way to manage catheter sepsis, it is not always possible. Seventy-seven episodes of catheter sepsis were evaluated in 61 children of whom 24 were neonates. Seventy-five percent of catheters had been used for multiple purposes including PN. Infective organisms included *staphylococcus epidermidis*, *Klebsiella* species, and *Streptococcus viridans*. *Pseudomonas* species were not seen in neonates. Thirty-five patients were treated without removal of the catheter. In 30, culture data permitted adjustment of treatment, and 26 responded within 5 days. Thirty-nine days of treatment was required in one case. The lack of response was associated with abscess formation, immune deficiency, and resistant organisms including *Pseudomonas* and *Candida*. Gentamicin and vancomycin were the best initial therapy. Line infection can be managed with antibiotics in the majority of cases, particularly when the infective organism is recognized early (Nahata et al 1988). The incidence of complications does not seem to be related to the type of catheter used for PN. When considered as infection rate per day of catheter life, umbilical artery and central venous routes have similar infection rates (1 in 224 versus 1 in 199). Aortic thrombosis was seen in one of the umbilical artery group, and tricuspid vegetation was seen in one of the central venous group (Kanarek et al 1991). Lipid emulsions in PN have been associated with high rates of bacterial infection in neonates. Tumour necrosis factor production is reduced in rat macrophages after 16 h exposure to 0.1% lipid emulsion (Vazquez et al 1994). Practical administrative aspects make PN more risky, but it can be monitored to achieve low risk (Pereira & Ziegler 1989).

Metabolic complications arise from an imbalance between administration of a nutrient and its metabolism by the patient. The number of potential complications is that of the number of nutrients administered or required. Common problems include hyponatraemia (especially in pre-term infants), hypophosphataemia and acidosis. Acidosis may be less likely if acetate is included in the intravenous fluid (Peters et al 1997). High plasma tyrosine, high manganese concentrations in brain and liver, accumulation of phytosterols, and high aluminium levels are al recognized to complicate PN, but their relationship to complications is unclear.

Cholestasis

Liver disease is a recognized complication of intravenous feeding, and it occurs most frequently in the smallest infants. Associated factors include surgical diagnosis (particularly intestinal atresias and malrotations with interruption of entero-hepatic circulation), bacterial translocation, low birth weight, duration of PN, delay in initiating enteral feeding, proven sepsis uncluding in intravenous lines, and the number of operations performed. Sixteen of 46 surgical neonates (35%) who received PN for more than 14 days developed evidence of cholestasis (Kubota et al 1988, Kanarek et al 1991). Incidence of jaundice was 57% of 77 neonates having PN following gastrointestinal surgery (Teitelbaum 1997). Mild and moderate cholestasis was found in 43 and 38% of historical controls in a study of cholecystokinin (CCK). CCK treatment reduced mild and moderate cholestasis to 24 and 9.5%, respectively. A suggested regimen for severe cholestasis consists of withdrawing PN when possible and CCK2. i.u. per kg for 3–5 days followed by 4 units per kg if necessary for a further 5 days. Seven of 8 infants treated by this regimen resolved jaundice and biliary sludge in 1–6 weeks. Phenobarbitone treatment does not seem to prevent PN cholestasis, but the role of ursodeoxycholic acid in prevention or treatment remains to be clarified.

The natural history of PN cholestasis has been studied by ultrasound. Sequential measurements comparing enterally- and parenterally-fed infants showed the latter to have larger gallbladders but no contractile response to feeding (Jawaheer et al 1995). Of 41 neonates, 18 developed evidence of sludge in the gallbladder on average 10 days of starting PN. Five progressed to develop 'sludge balls' and two developed gallstones, one of which resolved within 6 months (Matos et al 1987). Bile lipid concentration was measured before PN, curing the first 2 weeks of treatment and at 3–8 weeks. Before starting, bile acid concentration was low (below the critical micellar concentration), risking cholesterol precipitation. At 2 weeks, bile acid content had increased so that the risk of precipitation had disappeared. Bile acid levels had fallen again by 8 weeks, risking cholesterol precipitation and the development of biliary sludge. In rabbits on PN, bromsulphthalein excretion was reduced by 5 days, but showed no further deterioration after 15 days. Maximum bile flow response to ursodeoxycholic acid load was reduced by 15 days off PN, by which time the volume of the gallbladder and gallbladder bile acid concentration had increased. This model shows impairment of bile secretion, interruption of entero-hepatic circulation and conditions suitable for the development of galbladder sludge (Das et al 1993).

High plasma tyrosine, high manganese concentrations in brain and liver, accumulation of phytosterols and high aluminium levels are all recognized to complicate PN, but their relationship to clinical complications is unclear.

Special situations

The special considerations required for patients with liver disease and for neonatal patients are outlined.

Liver disease

The liver is the major nutritional homeostatic organ. The effects of liver dysfunction can be divided into those manifest in the gastrointestinal tract and those resulting from failure of liver homeostasis. The former result in reduced intraluminal bile acids with functional pancreatic insufficiency and consequent failure of absorption of lipids. Portal hypertension enteropathy may complicate liver disease, with a poorly-defined abnormality of motility and absorption and other secondary bacterial overgrowth. Failure of liver homeostasis may manifest as failed gluconeogenesis and impaired glycogen storage, particularly in skeletal muscle, so that a catabolic state with increased levels of intermediary metabolites can be seen after only 8 h of fasting compared with 48 h or more with normal liver function. Low insulin-like-growth factor-1 (IGF1) and low insulin-like-growth-factor binding proteins 3 (IGFBP3) and increased IGFBP1 are seen, further decreasing IGF1 bioavailability. Branch chain amino acid levels in plasma are decreased (Holt et al 1997).

Formula feeds to circumvent the defects of liver disease have been developed over 10 years or more. Typically, the lipids are up to 70% medium-chain triglyceride, avoiding the need for intraluminal bile for absorption. The carbohydrate is typically given as glucose polymer to reduce the osmolarity of the feed and reduce the

risk of diarrhoea. Protein is given at increased quantity compared with the normal diet, with an increased proportion of branch chain amino acids. The sodium content is low to reduce the likelihood of fluid retention; calcium and phosphate are at increased concentration in the hope of treating rickets. Two formulas based on these principles, Caprilon (Cow & Gate Nutrition) and Generaid + (SHS Nutricia), are marketed, and their efficacy has been demonstrated.

Neonatal patients

Lipids in neonatal nutrition
Polyunsaturated fatty acids are essential in humans for cell membrane and neurological growth because of the absence of desaturase enzymes. Three families, distinguished by the site of desaturation at omega 3, 6 and 9 respectively, are used in the body in proportion to their abundance in recent dietary intake. Each has a different effect, particularly on the immune system (see Fig. 21.2). Omega 6 fatty acids result in a pro-inflammatory cytokine profile, whereas omega 3 cytokines, generated particularly from fish oils, are anti-inflammatory. These effects may be employed to influence the immune system to reduce inflammation, a therapeutic modality called *nutritional pharmacology*. Although these effects are evident *in vitro*, in illness there are problems of absorption, preferential oxidation for energy, and uncertainty about dose.

Lipid is the preferred dietary calorie source because it has a greater energy density and low osmolarity and is a fuel source for most tissues with a lower respiratory quotient. A carbohydrate: lipid energy ratio of 2:1 is considered optimal for growth in well children. The optimal proportion of lipid for severely-ill children is less clear, in particular the proportion of lipids of different chain lengths and molecular conformations.

Essential fatty acids have an important role in visual function and normal learning. Higher retinal evoked potential thresholds at 57 weeks post-conception were shown in infants born at 30 weeks gestation if they had not received 18:3 omega 3 fatty acid supplementation or breast milk (Uauy Dagach et al 1994). Pre-term infants have a reduced capacity to lengthen carbon chains of omega 3 and 6 species (Van Aerde & Clandinin 1993), and a relatively higher requirement for essential fatty acids if neurological growth is to be maintained. Precise requirements remain unclear, and plasma and reb blood cell membrane levels probably reflect recent diet rather than whole-body status. Falls in plasma arachidonic and decosahexaenoic acids are seen during acute illness in PN or EN fed infants, suggesting preferential oxidation (Innis 1992). Intake of between 0.3–1.7% of energy or 0.8–4% of lipid is recommended (Innis 1992). Three percent may be insufficient to obtain normal profiles in sick infants (McClead et al 1985). Adequate simultaneous energy intake is required to prevent oxidation of lipid.

Carnitine is required to transport fatty acids across mitochondrial membranes to permit oxidation. PN is deficient in carnitine (Baruin 1995, Magnusson et al 1997). Supplementation increased plasma carnitine levels associated with improved ketogenesis, increased lipid tolerance shown as lower plasma triglyceride levels and improved weight gain in the first 2 weeks of life (Bonner et al 1995). Similar responses were seen in pre-term infants on PN with EN (Melegh et al 1986).

Protein in neonatal nutrition

Exact requirements of total protein for neonates and children with severe illness are not known, but there is evidence in terms of recovery and wound healing in burn patients that a higher protein intake than that required for normal growth may be beneficial. Protein status in 25 critically-ill malnourished infants correlated with plasma pre-albumin and retinol binding protein. However, these markers did not correlate with energy intake. Average protein intake > 2 g/kg/day was required to increase marker levels above baseline, with the response evident as early as 5–7 days (Innis 1992).

Protein, particularly from skeletal muscle, becomes a fuel during the stress of surgery or sepsis. Apart from providing energy by gluconeogenesis and amino acids as components for acute phase proteins, tissue repair and cell division of the immune system, groups of amino acids have specific importance. Branch chain amino acids, leucine, iso-leucine and valine provide a fuel for the immune system. Glutamine is also a fuel for the immune system and a precursor of nucleotides for dividing white cells. The gastrointestinal tract also consumes glutamine preferentially. Sulphydryl-containing amino acids are precursors of glutathione, supporting the antioxidant system. Arginine is a precursor of nitric oxide. However, it is not clear whether providing protein in superabundance prevents catabolism of muscle or other essential tissues. Excess dietary protein may be consumed by gluconeogenesis, but could result in excess ammonia, urea and aromatic amino acids, for example tyrosine. These phenomena are not seen in the child stressed by surgery or sepsis, but may complicate liver and kidney failure, suggesting that a high protein intake is well tolerated in certain illness.

Carbohydrate in neonatal nutrition

The process of birth transports the infant from an environment where glucose is supplied through the placenta from the mother to an environment where glucose must be produced from the infant's own resources. In the immediate post-natal period, glucose is provided by hepatic glycogen stores. In the case of infants where these stores are inadequate (which can be suspected from the assessment of prior nutritional adequacy), as is the case in infants who are small in weight for their gestational age, this mechanism may fail and hypoglycaemia may result. Over the first days of life, the changes in the hormonal environment induced by birth leads to a switching on of hepatic gluconeogenesis. In the case of ill infants, this mechanism may fail, and hypoglycaemia may result. In the newborn infant who is well, hypoglycaemia may be tolerated because of the use of ketone bodies, the production of which is increased under stress. However, in the ill infant, this mechanism may fail so that the consequences of hypoglycaemia for the brain may be exacerbated.

Discussion

The therapeutic role of nutritional management is becoming defined with important effects on prognosis. Short-term goals for nutritional success are defined as *in utero* anthropometric norms. It is not clear to what extent optimal nutrition can reverse the consequences of severe illness on short-term or long-term growth and development. Requirements of macro-nutrients in optimal care are known, but those of micro-nutrients and so-called conditionally-essential nutrients remain speculative. Methods for assessing individual patients beyond anthropometry, calorimetry and plasma levels of inorganic substances are not readily available and are of uncertain clinical value. Methods by which nutrition should be administered are clear as are their advantages and complications. Goals for the future should include better understanding of the fate of essential fatty acids, particularly with respect to the central nervous system; understanding of the preferred fuels of the immune system; recognition of the critical deficiencies that occur during the stress of neonatal intensive care management and of the associated complications; and identification of nutritional substances or growth factors that may protect the central nervous system, lungs and gastrointestinal tract. Also, complications may be reduced by greater training in proper feeding line management, the introduction of more feeding teams (Puntis et al 1991), and perhaps by novel therapies such as manipulation of the gastrointestinal pool of the organism by administration of live lactobacilli (Millar et al 1993).

References

Aranow, J.S., Fink, M.P. (1996) Determinants of intestinal barrier failure incritical illness. *Brit J Anaesth*, 77, 71–81.

Arisoy, E.S., Arisoy, A.E., Dwine, Jr. W.M. (1994) Clinical significance of fungi isolated from cerebrospinal fluid in children. *Pediatr Infect Dis J*, 13, 128–133.

Barker, D.J.P. (1992) Feta and infant origins of adult disease. *BMJ*.

Blondheim, O., Abbasi, S., Fox, W.W., Bhutani, V.K. (1993) Effect of enteral gavage feeding rate on pulmonary functions of very low birth weight infants. *J Pediatr*, 122, 751–755.

Bonner, C.M., DeBrie, K.L., Hug, G., Landrigan, E., Taylor, B.J. (1995) Effects of parenteral L-carnitine supplementation on fat metabolism and nutrition in premature neonates. *J Pediatr*, 126, 287–292.

Boruin, P.R. (1995) Carnitine in neonatal nutrition. *J Child Neurol*, 10(Suppl 2), S25–S31.

Brunvand, L., Fugelseth, D. (1996) Bacterial endocarditis in premature children. A complication caused by central venous catheters. *Tidsskr Nor Laegeforen*, 116, 1328–1330.

Buirin, D.G., Shulman, R.J., Langston, C., Storm, M.C. (1994) Supplemental alanylglutamine, organ growth, and nitrogen metabolism in neonatal pigs fed by total parenteral nutrition. *J Parent Enter Nutr*, 18, 313–319.

Burger, U., Gobel, R. (1992) Taurine requirement of premature infants in parenteral nutrition. *Monatsschr Kinderheilkd*, 140, 416–421.

Carlson, S.E., Werkman, S.H., Tolley, E.A. (1996) Effect of long-chain n-3 fatty acid supplementation on visual acuity and growth of preterm infants with and without bronchopulmonary dysplasia. *Am J Clin Nutr*, 63, 687–697.

Cochran, E.B., Phelps, S.J., Helms, R.A. (1988) Parenteral nutrition in pediatric patients. *Clin Pharm*, 7, 351–366.

Cosgrove, M., Davies, D.P., Jenkins, H.R. (1996) Nucleotide supplementation and the growth of ten small for gestational age infants. *Arch Dis Child*, 74, FI22–FI25.

Cuthbertson, D.P. (1931) Observations on the disturbance of metabolism produced by injury. *Q J Med*, 2, 233–246.

Das, J.B., Cosentino, C.M., Levy, M.F., Ansari, G.G., Raffensperger, J.G. (1993) Early hepatobiliary dysfunction during total parenteral nutrition: An experimental study. *J Pediatr Surg*, 28, 14–18.

Douglas, R.G., Shaw, J.H.F. (1989) Metabolic response to sepsis and trauma. *B J Surg*, 76, 115–122.

Drury, J.A., Nycyk, J.A., Baines, M., Cooke, R.W. (1998) Does total antioxidant status relate to outcome in very preterm infants? *Clin Sci*, 94, 197–201.

Elia, M. (1995) Changing concepts of nutrient requirements in disease: Implications for artificial nutritional support. *Lancet*, 345, 1279–1284.

El Mohandes, A.E., Johnson Robbins, L., Keiser, J.F., Simmens, S.J., Aure, M.V. (1994) Incidence of *Candida parapsilosis* colonization in an intensive care nursery population and its association with invasive fungal disease. *Pediatr Infect Dis J*, 13, 520–524.

Frank, L., Sosenko, I.R. (1988) Undernutrition as a major contributing factor in the pathogenesis of bronchopulmonary dysplasia. *Am Rev Respir Dis*, 138, 725–729.

Georgieff, M.K., Hoffinan, J.S., Pereira, G.R., Bembawn, J., Hoffman-Williamson, M. (1985) Effect of neonatal caloric deprivation on head growth and 1-year developmental status in preterm infants. *J Ped*, 107, 581–587.

Ginn Pease, M.E., Pantalos, D., King, D.R. (1985) TPN-associated hyperbilirubinemia: A common problem in newborn surgical patients. *J Pediatr Surg*, 20, 436–439.

Grant, J., Denne, S.C. (1991) Effect of intermittent versus continuous enteral feeding on energy expenditure in premature infants. *J Pediatr*, 118, 928–932.

Hammurland, K., Sedin, G. (1979) transepidermal water loss in newborn infants III. Relation to gestational age. *Acta Paediatrica Scandinavica*, 68, 795–801.

Hernandez Rastrollo, R., Agulla Rodino, E., Martinez Tallo, E.M., Espinosa Ruiz Cabal, J., Medicro Almendros, J. (1996) Prospective study of infective complications in newborns with fine silicone catheters used for parenteral nutrition infusion. *An Esp Pediatr*, 45, 626–630.

Hey, E.N., Katz, D.P. (1970) The optimum thermal environment for naked babies. *Arch Dis Child*, 45, 328–334.

Holt, R.I.G., Baker, A.J., Meill, J.P. (1997) The pathogenesis of growth failure in paediatric liver disease. *J Hepatol*, 27, 413–423.

Howlett, A., Ohlsson, A. (1997) *Inositol in Preterm Infants with RDS*. Cochrane Library.

Innis, S.M. (1992) n-3 fatty acid requirements of the newborn. *Lipids*, 27, 879–885.

Innis, S.M. (1992) Plasma and red blood cell fatty acid values as indexes of essential fatty acids in the developing organs of infants fed with milk or formulas. *J Pediatr*, 120, S78–86.

Jawaheer, G., Plei-ro, A., Lloyd, D.A., Shaw, N.J. (1995) Gall bladder contractility in neonates: Effects of parenteral and enteral feeding. *Arch Dis Child Fetal Neonatal Ed*, 72, F200–F202.

Kaenipf, D.E., Pfluger, M.S., Thiele, A.M., Hermanussen, M., Linderkamp, O. (1998) Influence of nutrition oil growth in premature infants: Assessment by knemometry. *Ann Hum Bio*, 25, 127–136.

Kanarek, K.S., Kuznicki, M.B., Blair, R.C. (1991) Infusion of total parenteral nutrition via the umbilical artery. *J Parenter Enteral Nutr*, IS, 15(1), 71–74.

Kendler, B.S. (1989) Taurine: An overview of its role in preventive medicine. *Prey Med*, 18, 79–100.

Kraeft, K., Roos, R., Mrozik, E. (1986) Influence of feeding tubes and gastrostomy on the colonization of the stomach in neonates. *Ann Istit Super Sanita*, 22, 899–903.

Kubota, A., Okada, A., Nezu, R., Kamata, S., Imura, K., Takagi, Y. (1988) Hyperbilirubinemia in neonates associated with total parenteral nutrition. *J Parenter Enteral Nutr*, 12, 602–606.

Lacey, J.M., Crouch, J-B., Benfell, K., et al. (1996) The effects of glutamine-supplemented parenteral nutrition in premature infants. *J Parent Enter Nutr*, 20, 74–80.

Lamireau, T., Millon, A., Sarlangue, J. et al. (1993) Transient intestinal pseudo-obstruction syndrome in premature infants. *Arch Fr Pediatr*, SO, 50(4), 301–306.

Letton, R.W., Chwals, W.J., Jamic, A., Charles, B. (1996) Neonatal lipid utilization increases with injury severity: Recombinant human growth hormone versus placebo. *J Pediatr Surg*, 31, 1068–1072.

Lucas, A. (1998) Programming by early nutrition: An experimental approach. *J Nutrition*, 128, 401S–406S.

Lucas, A., Bloom, S.R., Green, A.A. (1985) Gastrointestinal peptides and the adaptation to extrauterine nutrition. *Can J Physiol Pharmacol*, 63, 527–537.

Lucas, A., Morley, R., Cole, T.J. et al. (1990) Early diet in preterm babies and developmental status at 18 months. *Lancet*, 335, 1477–1481.

Lucas, A., Morley, R., Cole, T.J., Listei, G., Leeson-Payiie, C. (1992) Breast milk and subsequent intelligence quotient in children born preterm [see comments]. *Lancet*, 339, 261–264.

McClead, Jr. R.E., Meng, H.C., Gregory, S.A., Budde, C., Sloan, H.R. (1985) Comparison of the clinical and biochemical effect of increased alpha-linolenic acid in a safflower oil intravenous fat emulsion. *J Pediatr Gastroenterol Nutr*, 4, 234–239.

McDonnell, M., Isaacs, D. (1995) Neonatal systemic candidiasis. *J Paediatr Child Health*, 31, 490–492.

Magnusson, G., Boberg, M., Cederblad, G., Meurling, S. (1997) Plasma and tissue levels of lipids, fatty acids and plasma carnitine in neonates receiving a new fat emulsion. *Acta Paediatr*, 86, 638–644.

Mandell, G.A., Finkelstein, M. (1988) Gastric pneumatosis secondary to an intramural feeding catheter. *Pediatr Radiol*, 18, 418–420.

Matos, C., Avni, E.F., Van Gansbeke, D., Pardon, A., Struyven, J. (1987) Total parenteral nutrition (TPN) and gallbladder diseases in neonates. Sonographic assessment. *J Ultrasound Med*, 6, 243–248.

Melegh, B. Kemer, J., Sandor, A., Vinceller, M., Kispal, G. (1986) Oral L-carnitine supplementation in low-birth-weight newborns: A study on neonates requiring combined parenteral and enteral nutrition. *Acta Paediatr Hung*, 27, 253–258.

Micheli, J.L., Schutz, Y. (1987) Protein metabolism and postnatal growth in very low birthweight infants. *Biol Neonate*, 52(Suppl 1), 25–40.

Millar, M.R., Bacon, C., Smith, S.L., Wakker, V., Hall, N.M. (1993) Enteral feeding of premature infants with Lactobacillus GG. *Arch Dis Child*, 69, 483–487.

Mitton, S.G., Calder, A.G., Garlick, P.J. (1991) Protein turnover rates in sick, premature neonates during the first few days of life. *Pediatr Res*, 30, 418–422.

Nahata, M.C., King, D.R., Powell, D.A., Marx, S.M., Ginn Pease, M.E. (1988) Management of catheter-related infections in pediatric patients. *J Parenter Enteral Nutr*, 12, 58–59.

Okken, A., Jonxis, J.H.P., Rispens, P., Zijlstra, W.G. (1979) Insensible water loss and metabolic growth rate in low birth weight new-born babies. *Pediatric Research*, 13, 1072–1075.

Pencharz, P., Beesley, J., Sauer, P. et al. (1989a) Total-body protein turnover in parenterally fed neonates: Effects of energy source studied by using [15N]glycine and [1-13C]Ieucine. *Am J Clin Nutr*, 50(6), 1395–1400.

Pencharz, P., Beesley, J., Sauer, P. et al. (1989b) A comparison of the estimates of whole-body protein turnover in parenterally fed neonates obtained using three different end products. *Can J Physiol Pharmacol*, 67, 624–628.

Pereira, G.R., Barbosa, N.M. (1986) Controversies in neonatal nutrition. *Pediatr Clin North Am*, 33, 65–89.

Pereira, G.R., Ziegler, M.M. (1989) Nutritional care of the surgical neonate. *Clin Perinatol*, 16, 233–253.

Peters, O., Ryan, S., Matthew, L., Cheng, K., Lunn, J. (1997) Randomised controlled trial of acetate in preterm neonates receiving parenteral nutrition. *Arch Dis Child Fet Neonat Ed*, 77, F12–15.

Phillips, L.S., Unterman, T.G. (1984) Somatomedin activity in disorders of nutrition and metabolism. *Clin Endocrinol Metab*, 13, 145–189.

Piero, A., Carnielli, V., Filler, R.M., Kicak, L., Smith, J., Heim, T.F. (1991) Partition of energy metabolism in the surgical newborn. *J Pediatr Surg*, 26, 581–586.

Pierro, A., van Saene, H.K., Donnell, S.C. et al. (1996) Microbial translocation in neonates and infants receiving long-term parenteral nutrition. *Arch Surg*, 131, 176–179.

Puntis, J.W., Holden, C.E., Smaliman, S., Finkel, Y., George, R.E., Booth, I.W. (1991) Staff training: A key factor in reducing intravascular catheter sepsis. *Arch Dis Child*, 66, 335–337.

Rickham, P.P. (1957) *The Metabolic Response to Neonatal Surgery*. Cambridge: Harvard University Press.

Rintala, R.J., Lindah, H., Pohjavuori, M. (1995) Total parental nutrition-associated cholestasis in surgical neonates may be reversed by intravenous cholecystokinin: A preliminary report. *J Pediatr Surg*, 30, 827–830.

Ross, R.J.M., Buchanan, C.R. (1990) Growth hormone secretion: Its regulation and the influence of nutritional factors. *Nutr Research Rev*, 3, 143–162.

Ross, R.M.J., Meill, J.P., Freeman, E. et al. (1991) Critically ill patients — high basal growth hormone concentrations with attenuated oscillatory activity associated vath low concentration of insulin like growth factor 1. *Clin Endocrinol*, 35, 47–54.

Rubin, M., Moser, A., Naor, N., Merlob, P., Pakula, R., Sirota, L. (1994) Effect of three intravenously administered fat emulsions containing different concentrations of fatty acids on the plasma fatty acid composition of premature infants. *J Pediatr*, 125, 596–602.

Schmeling, D.J., Coran, A.G. (1991) Hormonal and metabolic response to operative stress in the neonate. *J Parent Enter Nutr*, 15, 215–238.

Scrimshaw, N.S. (1991) Rhoades Lecture. Effect of infection on nutrient requirements. *J Parent Enter Nutr*, 15, 589–600.

Shanbhogue, R.L., Lloyd, D.A. (1992) Absence of hypermetabolism after operation in the newborn infant. *J Parent Enter Nutr*, 16, 333–336.

Silvestre, M.A., Morbach, C.A., Brans, Y.W., Shankaran, S. (1996) A prospective randomized trial comparing continuous versus intermittent feeding methods in very low birth weight neonates. *J Pediatr*, 128, 748–752.

Sosenko, I.R., Innis, S.M., Frank, L. (1988) Polyunsaturated fatty acids and protection of newborn rats from oxygen toxicity. *J Pediatr*, 112, 630–635.

Symington, A., Ballantyne, M., Pinelli, J., Stevens, B. (1995) Indwelling versus intermittent feeding tubes in premature neonates. *J Obstet Gynecol Neonatal Nurs*, 24, 321–326.

Teitelbaum, D.H. (1997) Parenteral nutrition-associated cholestasis. *Curr Opin Pediatr*, 9, 270–275.

Tsang, R.S., Lucan, A., Uauy, R., Zlotkin, S. (1993) *Nutritional Needs of The Pre-term Infant*. Baltimore: Williams & Wilkins.

Uauy Dagach, R., Mena, P., Hoffinan, D.R. (1994) Essential fatty acid metabolism and requirements for LBW infants. *Acta Paediatr*, 405(Suppl), 78–85.

Unger, A., Goetzman, B.W., Chan, C., Lyons, A.B., 3rd, Miller, M.F. (1986) Nutritional practices and outcome of extremely premature infants. *Am J Dis Child*, 140, 1027–1033.

Van Aerde, J.E., Clandinin, M.T. (1993) Controversy in fatty acid balance. *Can J Physiol Pharmacol*, 71, 707–712.

Vazquez, W.D., Arya, G., Garcia, V.F. (1994) Long-chain predominant lipid emulsions inhibit in vitro macrophage tumor necrosis factor production. *J Parenter Enteral Nutr*, 18, 35–39.

Vettorazzi, C., Smits, E., Solomons, N.W. (1994) The interobserver reproducibility of bioelectrical impedance analysis measurements in infants and toddlers. *J Ped Gastroenterol Nutr*, 19, 277–282.

Wilmore, D.W. (1981) Glucose metabolism following severe injury. *J Trauma*, 21, 705–707.

Wilson, D.C., Cairns, P.A., Halliday, H.L. et al (1997) Randomised controlled trial of an aggressive nutritional regimen in sick very low birth weight infants. *Arch Dis Child*, 77, F4–F11.

Wesley, J.R. (1992) Efficacy and safety of total parenteral nutrition in pediatric patients,. *Mayo Clin Proc*, 67, 671–675.

22

Oral rehydration therapy: Guidelines for developed countries and the developing world

Caleb King and Christopher Duggan

Introduction

Diarrhoeal diseases are a major cause of paediatric morbidity and mortality worldwide, with 1 billion episodes and 3 million deaths of children under age 5 years estimated to occur annually (Bern et al 1992, Murray 1997). Even in countries with established market economies, diarrhoeal diseases account for a substantial portion of paediatric hospital admissions and remain a significant cause of mortality (Glass et al 1991).

The single most important medical achievement related to control of diarrhoea-induced mortality has been the demonstration of the safety and efficacy of oral rehydration solutions. Another major advance has been our increased knowledge about the appropriate dietary management of diarrhoea. The term *oral rehydration therapy* (ORT) is used to mean both the appropriate fluid and electrolyte management and dietary therapy. In this chapter, we review the scientific theory and clinical practice of ORT needed to manage successfully the clinical care of infants and children with acute diarrhoea.

Historical background

Early attempts at treating dehydration resulting from diarrhoea were first described in the medical literature in the 1830s during epidemics of *Vibrio cholerae* infections. It was not until 100 years later that the use of intravenous fluids became widespread. Accurate chemical analysis of diarrhoeal stools eventually permitted the formulation of physiologically-appropriate replacement solutions, leading to the successful treatment of cholera with intravenous fluids by the 1950s. Further research into intestinal electrolyte transport led to the development of oral solutions for rehydration. In 1971, these were put to the test in the field with the large-scale treatment of refugees from the Bangladesh war of independence (Hirschhorn & Greenough 1991). The remarkable success of oral solutions hastened the development of the World Health Organization [WHO] guidelines for ORT and production of standard packets of oral rehydration salts [ORS]. It may be argued that the initial application of ORT to cholera epidemics in the developing world hindered the acceptance of this therapy as a mainstay in the United States and Europe. With time, however, ORT has become accepted as the standard of care for clinically-efficacious and cost-effective management of acute diarrhoea (Duggan, Santosham, Glass 1992,

Santosham 1985, American Academy of Pediatrics 1996), although it remains under-utilized in settings where parenteral rehydration has been the established practice (Merrick et al 1996).

Practice and procedures

Physiological basis for the use of oral rehydration solutions

Basic scientific studies of intestinal solute transport mechanisms were crucial in designing ORT. Researchers delineated the molecular process of *co-transport*, in which the absorption of sodium ions is linked to that of glucose molecules at the intestinal brush border (Curran 1960). It was later shown that other organic molecules, such as amino acids, dipeptides, and tripeptides, could also participate in this co-transport phenomenon (Schultz 1964). Figure 22.1 provides a schematic of the co-transport process (reviewed in Acra & Ghishan 1996). Co-transport across the luminal membrane is facilitated by the protein sodium glucose cotransporter (SGLT1). Once in the enterocyte, the transport of glucose into the blood is facilitated by glucose transporter 2 (GLUT2) in the basolateral membrane. The Na^+-K^+ adenosinetriphosphatase (ATPase) provides the gradient that drives the process. Clinical studies have demonstrated that this mechanism remains intact in patients with severe cholera (Pierce 1968), and is responsible for the ability of oral solutions to effect rehydration.

In 1975, the WHO and the United Nations Children's Fund (UNICEF) agreed to promote a single solution (WHO-ORS) containing (in mmol/L): sodium 90, potassium 20, chloride 80, base 30, and glucose 111 (2%). This solution, representing a compromise between cholera and non-cholera stool sodium losses, was selected due to the realization that promotion of a single

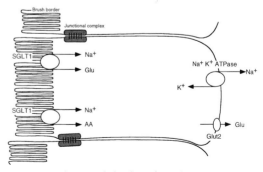

Figure 22.1 — Solute-coupled sodium absorption.

solution amongst populations with all levels of education in different countries would be simpler and more practical. Concern had been raised as to whether a solution designed for the treatment of a severe, secretory diarrhoea such as cholera would be appropriate for the management of less severe gastrointestinal infections. Clinical studies soon indicated that WHO-ORS was as effective in treating diarrhoea due to enterotoxigenic *E. coli* (Hirschhorn 1980) and rotavirus infection (Sack et al 1982) as it was in treating cholera.

Practice of oral rehydration therapy

Clinical assessment

Diarrhoea may be characterized by the passage of three or more loose, watery stools per day. In general, the consistency is more important than the frequency. The volume of fluid lost through the stools can vary from 5ml/kg/day (near normal) to 200ml/kg or more (WHO 1995). Infectious gastroenteritis is the most common cause of diarrhoea in infants and children. *Dehydration* (loss of body water) and electrolyte losses follow untreated diarrhoea, and cause the primary morbidity of acute gastroenteritis. Loose stools may also be amongst the presenting signs of non-gastrointestinal illnesses, including meningitis, bacterial sepsis, pneumonia, otitis media, and urinary tract infection. Vomiting alone can be the first symptom of metabolic disorders, congestive heart failure, toxic ingestions or trauma. In order to rule out other serious illnesses, a detailed history and physical examination should not be neglected in the diagnosis of acute gastroenteritis.

In addition, the overlap between diarrhoea and other concurrent conditions may have an important impact on the management of the patient. The WHO initiative for the integrated management of the sick child emphasizes the value of an integrated approach to caring for infants and children who may carry more than one diagnosis (WHO, Division of Diarrhoeal and Acute Respiratory Disease Control 1995). Treatment of diarrhoea may be complicated by concurrent conditions, in particular acute respiratory infections, measles, and malnutrition.

In addition to a complete physical examination, an accurate total body weight must be obtained. Auscultation for adequate bowel sounds is important before initiating oral therapy. Visual examination of the stool can confirm abnormal consistency and determine the presence of blood or mucus.

Signs and symptoms of dehydration are crucial in guiding therapy. Infants with acute diarrhoea are more prone to become dehydrated than are older children because they have a high body-surface:weight ratio, a higher metabolic rate, and are dependent on others for fluid. Although the most accurate assessment of fluid status is acute weight change, the patient's pre-morbid weight is often not known. The clinical signs and symptoms of dehydration are outlined in Table 22.1.

Assessment of the anterior fontanel is absent from Table 22.1 as numerous studies have shown that it may be an unreliable or misleading sign. In infants and children, a fall in blood pressure is a late sign that heralds shock and may correspond to fluid deficits greater than 10%. Increases in heart rate and slowed

Table 22.1 — Signs of dehydration

	Minimal or no dehydration	Mild-to-moderate dehydration	Severe dehydration
General condition	Well, alert	Restless, lethargic	Apathetic, unconscious
Thirst	Drinks normally	Thirsty, eager to drink	Drinks poorly, unable to drink
Skin fold	Instant recoil	< 2 s	> 2 s
Eyes	Normal	Slightly sunken	Deeply sunken
Tears	Present	Decreased	Absent
Mouth and tongue	Moist	Dry	Parched
Breathing	Normal	Fast	Deep
Pulse	Normal	Normal to tachycardic	Weak or thready
Extremities	Warm	Cool	Cold, cyanotic

peripheral perfusion may be more sensitive indicators of moderate dehydration, although both may be difficult to interpret as they may vary with degree of fever and capillary refill is affected by ambient temperature.

Supplementary laboratory studies in the assessment of the patient with acute diarrhoea are usually unnecessary, including serum electrolytes. Stool cultures are indicated in the case of *dysentery* (bloody diarrhoea), but are generally not indicated in the usual case of acute, watery diarrhoea in the immunocompetent patient.

Rehydration therapy based on degree of dehydration

Treatment should include two phases: rehydration and maintenance. In the *rehydration phase*, the fluid deficit is replaced and clinical hydration attained. In the *maintenance phase*, maintenance calories and fluids are given. In both phases, excess fluid losses from vomiting and diarrhoea are replaced in an ongoing manner.

Algorithms for treatment of watery diarrhoea have typically divided patients into sub-groups for mild (3–5% fluid deficit), moderate (6–9% fluid deficit), or severe dehydration (> 10%, shock or near shock). Recent studies have shown that it may be difficult to distinguish between mild and moderate dehydration based on clinical signs alone (Duggan et al 1996). For this reason, a revised treatment scheme, outlined in Table 22.2, that is consistent with the revised WHO classification may be more practical for the clinician.

Severe dehydration constitutes a medical emergency. Intravenous (iv) rehydration should begin immediately. Twenty mL/kg boluses of Ringer's lactate solution, normal saline or a similar solution should be given until pulse, perfusion and mental status return to normal. This may require two iv lines or even alternative access sites (e.g., intraosseous infusion, venous cutdown). As soon as the patient's level of consciousness returns to normal, therapy can often be changed to the oral route, with the patient taking by mouth the remaining estimated deficit. As with less-severely-ill patients, frequent re-assessment of hydration status should be performed to follow adequacy of replacement therapy.

For the mildly-to-moderately dehydrated patient, oral rehydration should commence with a fluid containing 50–90 meq/L of sodium. The amount of fluid administered should be 50–100 mL/kg and should be administered over 2–4 h. Using a teaspoon, syringe or medicine dropper, small volumes of fluid (e.g., 1 teaspoon) should be offered at first, with the amount gradually increased as tolerated. After 2–4 h, hydration status should be re-assessed. If the patient is rehydrated, treatment should progress to the maintenance phase of therapy (see below). If the patient is still dehydrated, the existing deficit should be re-estimated and rehydration therapy should continue.

If a child appears to want more than the estimated amount of ORS solution, and shows no sign of over-hydration, more can be offered. Oedema of the eyelids and extremities may indicate over-hydration. Diuretics

Table 22.2 — Treatment of acute diarrhoea

Degree of dehydration	Rehydration therapy	Replacement of stool losses	Maintenance therapy
Minimal or no dehydration	N/A	10 mL/kg or 4–8 oz ORS for each diarrhoeal stool	Continue diet★ Replace ongoing losses with ORS
Mild-to-moderate dehydration	ORS 50–100 mL/kg	same as above	same as above
Severe dehydration	Ringer's lactate or NS in 20 mL/kg iv boluses until mental status improves. Then give 50–100 mL/kg ORS	same as above	same as above

★Overly restricted diets should be avoided during acute diarrhoea. Breastfed infants should continue to nurse *ad libitum*. Full lactose formulas are generally well tolerated. If lactose malabsorption appears clinically significant, lactose-free formulas may be used. Reduced lactose or half-strength formula may be used where these are not available. Older children may safely resume normal diets, although tea, soft drinks, juices and high-fat foods may worsen diarrhoea. Complex carbohydrates, fresh fruits, lean meats, yoghurt, and vegetables are all recommended.
Abbreviations: N/A, Not Available; ORS, Oral Rehydration Salts; NS, Normal Saline.

should not be given. Once the oedema has subsided, maintenance therapy may continue.

For patients with acute diarrhoea but without signs of dehydration, the rehydration phase of therapy should be omitted and maintenance therapy begun immediately.

Replacement of ongoing losses

During both rehydration and maintenance therapy, ongoing stool and vomit losses must be replaced. If the patient is at a facility where such losses can be measured accurately, 1 mL of ORS should be given for each g of diarrhoeal stool. Alternatively, stool losses can be approximated by giving 10 mL/kg for each watery or loose stool passed, and 2 mL/kg of fluid should be given for each episode of emesis. Excess fluid losses during maintenance therapy may be replaced with either low sodium ORS (containing 40–60 meq/L of Na) or with ORS containing 75–90 meq/L of sodium. If the latter type of fluid is used, an additional source of low-sodium fluid is recommended (e.g., breast milk, formula or water).

Dietary therapy

Recommendations for maintenance dietary therapy depend on the age and diet history of the patient. Breastfed infants should continue nursing on demand. For bottle-fed infants, formula should be given immediately upon rehydration in amounts sufficient to satisfy energy and nutrient requirements. Lactose-free or reduced lactose formulas, when available, may help ensure that carbohydrate malabsorption does not complicate the clinical course. A meta-analysis of clinical trials shows no advantage of lactose-free formulas over lactose-containing formulas for most infants, although some infants with malnutrition or severe dehydration recover more quickly when given lactose-free formula (Brown et al 1994). Patients with true lactose intolerance have exacerbation of diarrhoea when a lactose-containing formula is introduced. The presence of low pH (< 6) or reducing substances (> 0.5%) in the absence of clinical symptoms is not diagnostic of lactose intolerance. Although medical practice has often favoured beginning feeds with diluted (e.g., half or quarter-strength) formula, there is insufficient evidence to justify this practice; in general, full caloric intake should be restored as soon as possible.

Older children receiving semi-solid or solid foods should continue to receive their usual diet during diarrhoea. Recommended foods include starches, cereals, yoghurt, fruits and vegetables. Foods high in simple sugars and fats should be avoided, given the possibility of steatorrhoea or osmotic diarrhoea complicating management.

Limitations of oral rehydration therapy

Although oral rehydration therapy is recommended for all age groups and for diarrhoea of any aetiology, some restrictions to its use do exist. In children presenting in shock, the administration of oral solutions may be contraindicated, as airway protective reflexes may be impaired. Likewise, patients with abdominal ileus should not be given oral fluids until bowel sounds are audible.

Stool output in excess of 10 mL/kg/h has been associated with a lower rate of success of oral rehydration (Sack et al 1980); however, no patient should be denied oral rehydration therapy simply because of a high purging rate, because most patients will respond well if given adequate replacement fluid.

A small proportion of infants with acute diarrhoea experience carbohydrate malabsorption, with a dramatic increase in stool output following the administration of ORS. The presence of stool-reducing substances alone is not sufficient to make the diagnosis because this is a common finding in patients with diarrhoea and does not in itself predict failure of oral therapy. Patients with true glucose malabsorption also show an immediate reduction in stool output when ORS is replaced with iv therapy. The incidence of clinically-significant glucose malabsorption during acute diarrhoea is approximately 1%, although rates as high as 8% have been reported in selected populations (Salazar-Lindo et al 1986).

Many patients with acute diarrhoea have concomitant vomiting. Most, however, can be successfully rehydrated with oral fluids if small volumes of ORS (5 mL) are given every five minutes, with a gradual increase in the amount consumed. Administration via a spoon or syringe with close supervision helps guarantee a gradual progression in the amount taken. In some cases, continuous, slow, nasogastric infusion of ORS via a feeding tube may be helpful. Often, correction of acidosis and dehydration lessens the frequency of vomiting.

Pharmacologic therapy

Apart from treatment of cholera and bloody diarrhoea, as discussed below, antimicrobial therapy of acute watery diarrhoea is not indicated. Because viral agents are the predominant cause of acute diarrhoea (Huilan et al 1991), the routine use of antimicrobial agents for the treatment of diarrhoea wastes resources and may lead to increased microbial resistance. Especially in the hospital setting, bacterial causes of diarrhoea are unusual. A survey of several years of stool cultures submitted to the microbiology laboratory at Children's Hospital in Boston, MA, USA, revealed such infrequent occurrence of bacterial infections that the practice of sending stool cultures in patients who develop diarrhoea while hospitalized has been curtailed. Hospitalized patients and patients with a history of recent antibiotic use are, however, at risk for infections with *C. difficile*. Infections with *C. difficile* documented by toxin assay should be treated with metronidazole 30 mg/kg divided t.i.d. given orally. Oral vancomycin is also effective, but should be reserved as a second-line agent given concerns over the possible emergence of vancomycin-resistant enterococcus.

The use of non-specific anti-diarrhoeal agents such as adsorbents (e.g., kaolin-pectin), anti-motility agents (e.g., loperamide), anti-secretory drugs, or toxin binders (e.g., cholestyramine) is a common practice. Few data are available to support their efficacy. Side effects of these drugs are well known, including opiate-induced ileus, drowsiness and nausea due to atropine effects, and binding of nutrients and other drugs. One report from Pakistan detailed 18 cases of severe abdominal distention in association with use of loperamide, including at least 6 deaths (Bhutta & Tahir 1990). Even in a controlled clinical setting, Motala et al (1990) reported that six of 28 patients given loperamide had side effects (ileus, drowsiness), necessitating discontinuation of therapy. Bismuth subsalicylate has shown some efficacy in traveller's diarrhoea and other causes of acute gastroenteritis in children (Gorbach 1990), and although side effects are less than anti-motility agents, some theoretical concerns over the potential toxicity of salicylate remain. A recent trial of the anti-secretory drug racecadotril should a significant reduction in stool output qmony peruvian boys with acute diarrhea (Salazar-Lindo et al 2000). In any event, reliance on anti-diarrhoeal agents shifts the therapeutic focus away from appropriate fluid, electrolyte and nutritional therapy, and adds unnecessarily to the economic cost of the illness.

Other clinical scenarios

Acute bloody diarrhoea (dysentery)

Bloody diarrhoea is defined as visible, red blood in the stool. This does not include occult blood (detected by guaiac card only), streaks of blood on the surface of formed stool or melena. The child with bloody diarrhoea is at higher risk as the infections may persist without adequate treatment and are often accompanied by significant anorexia. The malnourished child with bloody diarrhoea should be referred to the hospital, even without signs of severe dehydration.

Although a number of organisms, including *Salmonella*, *Shigella*, *Campylobacter jejuni* and enteroinvasive *E. Coli*, may cause bloody diarrhoea, studies have documented the importance of *Shigella* in both the developed and less-developed world (WHO 1994). As a result, empiric treatment with an antibiotic to which most local strains of *Shigella* are sensitive is recommended. When available, stool cultures with assays for drug sensitivity may help direct therapy. Amoebiasis is an unusual cause of bloody diarrhoea in young children (WHO 1995), so that treatment for amoebiasis should be reserved for those cases where trophozoites are detected on microscopic examination of the stools or when treatment with two different anti-microbials usually effective for *Shigella* has proved ineffective.

Ampicillin or Trimethoprim-Sulfamethoxazole may be used as first-line therapy for *Shigella*, except in those areas where resistance to these antibiotics is so extensive as to make their use generally ineffective. Nalidixic acid is a moderately-expensive, second-line agent. Ceftriaxone is generally effective, but very expensive. Metronidazole, streptomycin, tetracyclines, chloramphenicol, and sulfonamides are generally ineffective against *Shigella*.

Cholera

Management of cholera may be carried out using the methods for assessment of dehydration and treatment plans outlined above and summarized in Tables 22.1 and 22.2. The treatment differs from that of acute watery diarrhoea in that the health worker must be prepared to deliver prodigious quantities of fluid, either by ORS or intravenously, for replacement of voluminous stool losses. In addition, treatment with an antibiotic effective against *Vibrio cholerae* shortens the treatment course and reduces stool output. Traditional first-line agents are tetracycline, doxycycline, and Trimethoprim-Sulfamethoxazole. Alternatives include erythromycin and Furazolidone.

Persistent diarrhoea

Persistent diarrhoea may be defined as diarrhoea of acute onset that lasts more than 14 days. The approach to the patient with persistent diarrhoea should include assessing and treating diarrhoea as in the acute presentations. Concurrent illnesses (e.g., respiratory infections) should not be neglected and should also be treated. Attention to nutrition is crucial, with restoration of a nutritious diet and supplementation with vitamins and minerals to include at least two recommended daily allowances of folate, vitamin A, iron, zinc, magnesium and copper (WHO 1995).

Diarrhoea with severe malnutrition

Assessment of the malnourished child is difficult because many of the signs outlined in Table 22.1 may be unreliable. Skin turgor may appear poor, owing to the absence of subcutaneous fat. Eyes may be sunken from loss of periorbital fat. Irritability or apathy from malnutrition may complicate the assessment of mental status. When possible, malnourished children with diarrhoea should be referred to a hospital. A severely-malnourished child with signs of dehydration without a history of increased stool output should be treated for septic shock (WHO 1995).

Because iv therapy may cause over-hydration and heart failure in the severely-malnourished child, except for treatment of shock, slow oral rehydration is the treatment of choice. A nasogastric tube may be used for children who drink poorly. Rehydration should begin with 10 mL/kg over 2 h. This rate may be adjusted based on the child's thirst or ongoing stool losses. Increasing oedema is evidence of over-hydration.

Full strength WHO-ORS solution contains too much sodium and inadequate potassium for the severely-malnourished child. WHO guidelines (1995) recommend modified solutions, which contain 45 mmol/L sodium, 40 mmol/L potassium and 25 g/L sugar (Table 22.3). Resomal is an example of an ORS with lowered sodium and increased Potassium.

Feeding should begin as soon as possible once hydration has been achieved, and should continue every 2–3 h day and night. Malnourished children often exhibit anorexia and require coaxing to eat. The nutrition of the severely-malnourished child is covered in Chapter 2.

Home management of acute diarrhoea and instructions to parents

Ideally, management of acute diarrhoea should begin at home because earlier intervention may reduce complications such as dehydration and poor nutrition (Snyder et al 1990). In rural areas or poor urban neighbourhoods where access to health care may be delayed, this is particularly important; however in all areas, early administration of ORS may lead to fewer office or emergency room visits, hospitalizations or deaths. All families should be encouraged to have a supply of ORS in the home at all times, much in the same way that acetaminophen and syrup of ipecac are viewed as staples of the medicine chest. As soon as diarrhoea begins, one of the commercially-available products can be started at home. Alternatively, food-based fluids (e.g., soups or gruels) can be used to prevent dehydration. Regardless of the fluid used, an age-appropriate diet should be given as well. The most

Table 22.3 — ORS for the severely-malnourished child

Simple ORS for the severely-malnourished child	More effective ORS for the severely-malnourished child

Dilute 1 L WHO-ORS to make 2 L
Add 45 mL KCl solution from stock solution containing 100 g KCl/L
Add and dissolve 50 g sucrose
 	
Children given this solution should also receive:
 	
2 mL 50% $MgSO_4$ solution (4 meq Mg/mL) im once and zinc chloride solution (10 g/L) 1mL/kg/day until diarrhoea stops
	Dilute 1 L WHO-ORS to make 2 L
	Add the following salts:
	    3.6 g KCl
	    1.3 g K citrate
	    1.2 g MgCl
	    130 mg Zn acetate
	    22 mg $CuSO_4$
	    0.44 mg $NaSeO_4$
	    0.20 mg KI
	
	Add and dissolve 50 g sucrose

Based on WHO (1995).

crucial aspect underlying home management of diarrhoea is the need to give increased volumes of fluid as well as to maintain adequate caloric intake. Infants should be offered more frequent feeds at the breast or bottle, and children should also be given more fluids.

Availability of ORS solutions

Oral rehydration solutions may be distributed pre-mixed with water or as dry ingredients in packets. Packets are more common in developing countries, where low cost, long shelf life and ease of transport make them particularly suitable. The disadvantage of packets is the potential for mixing with inappropriate volumes of water, resulting in ORS that is either too diluted or too concentrated. When caretakers are asked to mix ORS from packets at home, detailed written and oral instructions should be given. Table 22.4 lists the components of several commercially-available formulations of pre-mixed ORS. For comparison, Table 22.4 also includes a number of fluids commonly used in treating diarrhoea, which do not contain physiologically-sound concentrations of carbohydrates and electrolytes. Interestingly, Merrick et al (1996) note that, in the United States, many physicians continue to recommend inappropriate oral rehydration fluids in spite of the availability of appropriate alternatives. An informal survey of numerous hospital web sites reveal recommendations for the treatment of diarrhoea that include non-standard fluids or recommendations for a 'BRAT' (bananas, rice, applesauce, toast) diet, which is more restrictive than necessary and too low in energy density to be a diet of choice.

Improved forms of oral rehydration solutions

Numerous attempts have been made to develop oral solutions with the capability of reducing stool water and electrolyte losses rather than merely replacing these losses in a physiological manner. These have generally included additional substrates for sodium co-transport (such as the amino acids glycine, alanine, and, glutamine) or substituting complex carbohydrates for the glucose (rice and other cereal-based ORS) to reduce osmolarity while preserving glucose-sodium co-transport. Given trials to date, the amino acid preparations do not appear more effective than traditional ORS and are more costly. Rice-based ORS seems superior to WHO-ORS for the treatment of cholera, but otherwise is comparable (Bhan et al 1994). Cereal-based ORS may be recommended where training is adequate and home preparation is preferable. Given the simplicity and safety of ORS packets in developing countries and commercially-available ORS in developed countries, these remain the first choice for most clinicians. Because numerous studies have shown that WHO-ORS can safely correct hyper- or hyponatraemia, WHO recommends the use of WHO-ORS for the treatment of diarrhoea in children and adults, regardless of the aetiology of the diarrhoea or initial serum sodium value. Recent studies have shown clinical results meeting or exceeding those of WHO-ORS using lower osmolar ORS (El-Mougi et al 1994). A recent multi-national, multi-centre trial has confirmed their efficacy and safety (CHOICE Study Group, 2001)

Table 22.4 — Composition of commercial oral rehydration solutions as well as frequently used oral solutions

Solution	CHO Osmolality (gm/L)	Na (mmol/L)	K (mmol/L)	Cl (mmol/L)	Base** (mmol/L)	Osmolarity (mosm/L)
WHO-ORS	20	90	20	80	30	310
Rehydralyte[1]	25	75	20	65	30	305
Infalyte[2]	30	50	25	45	10	200
Pedialyte[1]	25	45	20	35	30	250
Apple juice[3]	120	0.4	44	45	–	730
Coca Cola[4]	112	1.6	–	–	13.4	650
Gatorade[5]	46	23.5	2.5	17	3	330
Chicken broth[3]	8	260	0.5	260	–	450
Tea[3]	4	–	6	–	–	6

[1]Ross Laboratories, Columbus, OH; [2]Mead-Johnson Laboratories, Princeton, NJ; [3]USDA; [4]Coca-Cola Corporation, Atlanta, GA (Figures do not include electrolytes that may be present in local water used for bottling; base = phosphate); [5]The Gatorade Company, Chicago, IL; ** Actual or potential bicarbonate such as lactate, citrate or acetate.

Discussion

The treatment of acute diarrhoea has for many years been shown to rely upon the simple but overwhelmingly effective therapy of oral rehydration. More recently, the important co-principle in case management of early refeeding of children immediately upon rehydration has also gained wider acceptance (Duggan and Nurko 1997). The combination of oral rehydration and early nutritional support promises to guide a patient safely and effectively through a bout of diarrhoea. If the principles of therapy outlined above are accepted by all levels of the medical community, and if education of parents includes beginning oral rehydration therapy at home, numerous deaths and unnecessary hospitalizations can be avoided. Meanwhile, we await further technological breakthroughs (e.g., improved vaccines, superior rehydrating solutions) to better combat one of the most important public health problems today.

Acknowledgements

Supported in part by the Clinical Nutrition Research Centre at Harvard (National Institutes of Health Grant #P30-DK40561), by Applied Research on Child Health Project at Harvard University by means of a Co-operative Agreement with the US Agency for International Development, and NIH Training Grant # 5 T32DK07477-12.

References

Acra, S.A., Ghisan, F.K. (1996) Electrolyte fluxes in the gut and oral rehydration solutions. *Ped Clin N Amer*, 43, 433–448.

American Academy of Pediatrics, Provisional Committee on Quality Improvement, Subcommittee on Acute Gastroenteritis. (1996) Practice parameter: Management of acute gastroenteritis in young children. *Pediatr*, 97, 424–436.

Bern, C. et al (1992) The magnitude of the global problem of diarrhoeal disease: A ten-year update. *Bull WHO*, 70, 705–714.

Bhan, M.K. et al (1994) Clinical trials of improved oral rehydration salt formulations: A review. *Bull WHO*, 72, 945–955.

Bhutta, T.I., Tahir, K.I. (1990) Loperamide poisoning in children. *Lancet*, 335, 363.

Brown, K.H. et al (1994) Use of nonhuman milks in the dietary management of young children with acute diarrhea: A meta-analysis of clinical trials. *Pediatr*, 93, 17–27.

CHOICE Study Group (2001) Multicenter randomized double blind clinical trial to evaluate the efficacy and safety of a reduced osmolarity oral rehydration solution in children with acute watery diarrhoea. Paediatrics, in press.

Curran, P. (1960) NaCl and water transport by rat ileum in vitro. *J Gen Physiol*, 43, 1137–1148.

Duggan, C., Nurko, S. (1997) Feeding the gut: The scientific basis for continued enteral nutrition during acute diarrhea. *J. Pediatr* 131, 801–808.

Duggan, C. et al (1996) How valid are clinical signs of dehydration in infants? *J Pediatr Gastroenter Nutr*, 22, 56–61.

Duggan, C., Santosham, M., Glass, R.I. (1992) The management of acute diarrhea in children: Oral rehydration, maintenance, and nutritional therapy. *Morbidity and Mortality Weekly Report*, 41, RR–16.

El-Mougi, M. et al. (1994) Is a low-osmolarity ORS solution more efficacious than standard WHO-ORS solution? *J Ped Gastroenter Nutri*, 19, 83–86.

Glass, R.I. et al. (1991) Estimates of morbidity and mortality rates for diarrheal diseases in American children. *J Pediatr*, 118, S27–S33.

Gorbach, S.L. (1990) Bismuth therapy in gastrointestinal diseases. *Gastroenterol*, 99, 863–875.

Hirschhorn, N. (1980) The treatment of acute diarrhea in children. An historical and physiological perspective. *Am J Clin Nutr*, 33(3), 637–663.

Hirschhorn, N., Greenough, W. (1991) Progress in oral rehydration therapy. *Scientific American*, 264, 50–56.

Huilan, S. et al (1991) Etiology of acute diarrhoea among children in developing countries: A multicentre study in five countries. *Bull WHO*, 69, 549–555.

Merrick, N. et al. (1996) Treatment of Acute Gastroenteritis: Too much and too little care. *Clinical Pediatrics*, Sept., 429–435.

Murray, C.J. (1997) *Global Burden of Disease Study, Harvard School of Public Health and World Health Organization*. Cambridge, MA: Harvard Center for Population and Development Studies.

Pierce, N. et al (1968) Effect of intragastric glucose-electrolyte infusion upon water and electrolyte balance in Asiatic cholera. *Gastroenterology* 55, 333–342.

Pierce, N.F. et al. (1988) Effect of glucose electrolyte infusion upon water and electrolyte balance in Asiatic cholera. *Gastroenterol*, 55, 333–343.

Sack, D.A. et al. (1980) Oral therapy in children with cholera: A comparison of sucrose and glucose electrolyte solutions. *J Pediatr*, 96, 20–25.

Sack, D.A. et al. (1982) Carbohydrate malabsorption in infants with rotavirus diarrhea. *Amer J Clin Nutr*, 36, 1112.

Salazar-Lindo, E. et al. (1986) Bicarbonate versus citrate in oral rehydration therapy in infants with watery diarrhea: A controlled clinical trial. *J Pediatr*, 108, 55–60.

Salazar-Lindo, E. et al (2000) Racecadotril in the treatment of acute watery diarrhea in children. *New England Journal of Medicine* 343(7), 463–467.

Santosham, M. et al. (1985) Oral rehydration therapy for acute diarrhea in ambulatory children in the United States: A double blind comparison of four different solutions. *Pediatr*, 76, 159–166.

Schultz, S., R. Zalusky, (1964) Ion transport in isolated rabbit ileum. II The interaction between active sodium and active sugar transport. *J Gen Physiol*, 47, 1043–1059.

Snyder, J. et al. (1990) Home-based therapy for diarrhea. *J Ped Gastroenterol Nutr*, 11, 438–447.

World Health Organization. (1994) The management of bloody diarrhoea in young children. WHO/CDD/94.49.

World Health Organization. (1995) The treatment of diarrhoea. A manual for physicians and other senior health workers. WHO/CDR/95.3.

World Health Organization, Division of Diarrhoeal and Acute Respiratory Disease Control. (1995) Integrated management of the sick child. *Bull WHO*, 73, 735–740.

23

Food intolerance

Yoshikazu Ohtsuka, Ian R. Sanderson and Thomas T. MacDonald

Abbreviations

APC   antigen presenting cell
FCERI   high-affinity IgE receptor type I
IEL   intraepithelial lymphocyte
IFN   interferon
KGF   Keratinocyte growth factor
LT   leukotriene ,
MMP   matrix metalloproteinase
PP   Peyer's patches
TGF   transforming growth factor
IgA   Immunoglobulin A
IgE   Immunoglobulin E
IL   Interleukin
TNF   Tumour Necrosis Factor
IBD   Inflammatory bowel disease
G6PD   glucose-6-phosphate dehydrogenase
Th1   T helper cell type 1
MS   Multiple Sclerosis
MBP   Myelin Basic Protein
OVA   Ovalbumin
TCR   T cell receptor
MHC   Major Histocompatability Complex
CTLA-4   Cytotoxic T lymphocyte antigen-4
LT   Leukotriene
DSCG   Disodium chromoglycate
SRS-A   Slow reacting substance of anaphylaxis
mRNA   messenger RNA
LTB_4 leukotriene B_4
LTC_4 leukotriene C_4

Introduction

The physiological needs of nutrient absorption require that the gut has a large surface area, lined by a single layer of columnar epithelium. This means that the immune system of the gut is constantly bombarded by foreign proteins (food), while at the same time the immune system is specifically designed to react to the foreign proteins of pathogens. To get around this problem, the gut immune system has acquired mechanisms to avoid excessive reactions to foods, yet at the same time retain the ability to react to infectious agents. This system works efficiently in most individuals, but for an as yet undefined reason, some people react to food antigens as though they were pathogens, and because food antigens are needed for nutrition, disease persists until the offending antigen is identified and eliminated from the diet.

The clinical features of inappropriate responses to food include vomiting, malabsorption, diarrhoea, eczema and a protean range of other symptoms. The adverse reactions caused by ingested foods are defined as *food intolerance*. Intolerance can be divided into two categories, depending on whether they are immunologically mediated. This serves to exclude diseases where the pharmacological effects of foods or additives cause adverse reactions.

Table 23.1 shows the classification of food intolerance (Wright & Robertson 1987). Non-immunologically mediated food intolerance includes the pharmacological effect of foods containing caffeine, alcohol, and toxins. It also includes primary and secondary metabolic disorders. Lack of lactase due to the loss of microvilli during inflammation of the intestine is included here. Idiosyncratic reactions such as irritable bowel syndrome may also be included but the mechanism of intolerance, if present, is obscure.

There are cases where immunological reactions overlap with non-immunological processes, for instance, lactose intolerance in cow's milk allergy. When we consider treatments, therefore, we have to be aware that both mechanisms may coexist and exacerbate symptoms in a patient suffering from food intolerance.

Table 23.1 — Classification of food intolerance

Non-immunological reactions

Predictable reactions
> Pharmacological effects: Lectins, protease inhibitors, caffeine, salt, vasoactive amines, alcohol
> Bacterial effects: Enterotoxins and other toxins

Adverse food reactions associated with metabolic defects
> Hypolactasia: Primary and secondary (IBD, enterocolitis, food intolerance)
> Primary enzyme deficiencies: Sucrase-isomaltase, trehalase, trypsinogen, lipase, G6PD

Idiosyncratic reactions
> Irritable bowel syndrome, Non-IgE mast cell degranulation, etc.

Immunological reactions
> IgE-mediated reactions; Mast cells and eosinophils
> Antibody-dependent cytotoxic reactions
> Immune-complex mediated reactions
> Cell-mediated reactions
> Mixed-reactions

IBD   = Inflammatory bowel disease
IgE   = Immunoglobulin E
G6PD = glucose-6-phosphate dehydrogenase

Historical background

Adverse reactions to food were first reported more than 2000 years ago by Hippocrates. He had noted that gastric upset and urticaria could be induced by ingesting cow's milk. In modern times, Samuel Gee first described coeliac disease in 1888, although it was a further 65 years before Dicke discovered the disease was induced by gluten (Dicke et al 1953). Early in the nineteenth century, as the number of babies raised on formula milk increased, an increased incidence of eczema (Grulee & Sanford 1936) and mortality due to gastroenteritis and pneumonia (Woodbury 1922, Grulee et al 1934) was seen.

There is a need to prove that a certain food protein actually causes the adverse reactions, as opposed to another co-incident event. Thus, challenge tests were introduced in cow's-milk-intolerant patients by Goldman et al in 1963. This procedure of eliminating and giving suspected food protein directly to patients in a blind fashion allows accurate definition of the actual food antigen that introduces clinical symptoms. Similar criteria were also used in soya protein intolerance (Ament & Rubin 1972).

The discovery of immunoglobulin E (IgE) provided the mechanistic basis for immediate type hyper-sensitivity reactions to antigens, including foods (Ishizaka et al 1966). The subsequent discovery of the role of T cells in delayed type hypersensitivity gave another pathway by which the immune system could react to food antigens and cause disease, exemplified by the T-cell response to wheat, which causes coeliac disease.

Practice and procedures

The mucosal barrier in infants

Ingested foods are normally digested into peptides and amino acids by digestive enzymes before being absorbed by gut epithelial cells. Amino acids do not induce immunological reactions because they are too small to be recognized by antigen presenting cells (APC). However, some proteins are poorly digested in the intestinal lumen, and indeed intact macro-molecules can be detected in blood after feeding protein antigens. Immunological and non-immunological mechanisms control the penetration of these undigested proteins. For instance, mucus provides the intestinal epithelium with a mechanical (covering) and a chemical (washing) protection as well as an immunological protection involving secretory immunoglobulin IgA. IgA binds to antigens in the mucus layer. Despite this however, macro-molecules do cross the gut epithelium and can be recognized by the immune system.

In infants, non-specific defences in the gut may be compromised. First, both intracellular and paracellular transport of macro-molecules through epithelium is increased (Sanderson & Walker 1993). Second, insufficient secretion of digestive enzymes causes reduced digestion and increases the amounts of undigested proteins in the intestinal lumen. Third, the production and secretion of IgA is low. Fourth, infants often suffer gastrointestinal infections, which damage the epithelium and allow permeation of proteins into the lamina propria. Along these same lines, frequent infections activate mucosal immune cells, induce further reactions (such as induction of Th1-type cells) and enhance the expression of MHC class-II molecules on intestinal epithelial cells. Hence, food intolerance can be a feature of the post-enteritis syndrome.

Immunological mechanisms of food tolerance

T cells and cytokines play an important role in both preventing and regulating food intolerance. T cells can be classified into two types according to their cytokine pattern. Th1 cells produce IL-2, interfera-γ (IFN-γ) and TNF-α and mediate cell-mediated immunological reactions. Th2 cells produce IL-4, IL-5 and IL-13, which promote IgE production and eosinophilia, and generally boost antibody responses. In clinical studies, increased expression of IL-4 and IL-5 transcripts are observed in patients suffering from atopic asthma (Robinson et al 1992). In the context of gut disease, T-cell clones derived from coeliac disease patients are of a Th1 type with IFN-γ dominant pattern (Nilsen et al 1995). A rapid increase of IFN-γ transcripts was also seen in coeliac disease patients after gluten challenge (Kontakou et al 1995), but there is no elevation of IL-4 and IL-10 transcripts (Beckett et al 1996).

Tranforming growth factor-β (TGF-β) is an important cytokine that mediates active suppression against orally administered antigen. It is released by regulatory T (Th3) cells and macrophages. In studies of multiple sclerosis (MS) patients, feeding myelin basic protein (MBP) slightly ameliorated disease activity (Weiner et al 1993). Short-term cultures of blood lymphocytes from these patients showed an increased in frequency of MBP specific T cells that secreted TGF-β1 (Fukaura et al 1996).

There have been very many studies involving the T-cell responses to foods in humans. These have been reviewed by MacDonald (MacDonald 1995). Most of the studies examined blood T cells, not gut T cells, and there is good evidence that Th2 cells predominant in the blood of allergic patients. However, mechanistic studies are more advanced in rodent models. For example, the immunological mechanisms of food tolerance/intolerance are well studied in ovalbumin (OVA)-specific T-cell receptor (TCR) transgenic mice. Oral administration of OVA introduces tolerance in these mice. Feeding lower doses of OVA causes active suppression by inducing TGF-β, IL-4 and IL-10 producing T cells. At higher doses, clonal anergy occurs by deleting Th1 and Th2 cells by apoptosis, although TGF-β producing Th3 cells seem to be spared (Chen et al 1995). IFN-γ producing cells are also seen in Peyer's patches (PP), however this is transient. After feeding a high dose of OVA, systemic administrations of anti-IL-12 antibody inhibits IFN-γ production and enhances production of TGF-β in PP. IL-4 is not required for this TGF-β production, however it is able to enhance TGF-β production (Marth et al 1997). In addition, administration of OVA with anti-IL-12 antibody induced Fas-mediated apoptosis of antigen-specific T cells in local and systemic lymphoid tissue (Marth et al 1999). These studies demonstrate that orally administered food antigens can evoke TGF-β-producing T cells that can actively suppress immunological reactions, and inhibit antigen-specific Th1 cell responses in the PP. High doses of antigen also induce tolerance by clonal deletion of antigen-specific T cells via Fas-mediated apoptosis. These mechanisms are negatively regulated by IL-12 and IFN-γ.

Antigen-specific T-cell activation requires the engagement of the TCR with antigen/MHC complex as well as the engagement of appropriate co-stimulatory molecules. The most extensively characterized co-stimulatory molecules are CD28/CTLA-4 on T cells and their ligands, CD80 (B7-1)/CD86 (B7-2), on antigen-presenting cells. T-cell receptor activation in the absence of co-stimulation results in tolerance and T-cell anergy (Schwarz 1990, Harding et al 1992). Because intestinal epithelial cells express MHC class-II molecules on their surface (Mayer & Shlien 1987), but do not express co-stimulatory molecules in the normal state, lack of co-stimulatory molecules on the surface of epithelial cells may partially explain the unresponsiveness of T cells to foods in the epithelial compartment (Sanderson et al 1993).

Immunological food intolerance

Type I allergy — mast cells

There is an increase in the number of IgE-bearing mast cells in the intestinal mucosa and submucosa of food allergic patients (Rognum & Brandtzaeg 1992, Caffarelli et al 1998) and in mouse models (Ohtsuka et al 1999). The specific IgE bound to high-affinity IgE receptors on the surface of mast cells becomes cross-linked upon exposure to allergens and activates mast cells. These mast cells release mediators such as histamine, LTB$_4$, LTC$_4$, TNF-α, IL-4, and other cytokines. Significant elevation of serum histamine (Nolte et al 1989, Bengtsson et al 1997), LTB$_4$, LTC$_4$ (Ohtsuka et al 1999), and TNF-α (Heyman et al 1994, Majamaa et al 1996) concentrations are regularly observed after antigen challenge. It is likely that these mediators induce a local increase in vascular permeability (Jalonen 1991), lymph duct dilatation and increased mucus production. They also cause watery diarrhoea, resulting in blood hypocirculation and anaphylactic shock (Fig. 23.1).

Type I allergy — eosinophils

Eosinophils are also important in Type I allergy.

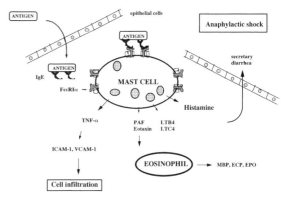

Figure 23.1 — Mechanisms of Type I allergy. Antigen and its specific IgE bound to high-affinity IgE receptors activates mast cells. Histamine, eotaxin, LTB$_4$, LTC$_4$, TNF-α, IL-4, and other chemical mediators are released and induce a local increase in vascular permeability and mucus production and elicit watery diarrhoea. Eosinophils migrate into the gut, responding to eosinophil chemotactic factors, such as eotaxin, platelet activating factor, histamine, and LTB$_4$. Eosinophils release major basic protein, eosinophil cationic protein (ECP), and eosinophil peroxidase (EPO), which are highly cytotoxic pro-inflammatory mediators that may disrupt the mucosal surface and contribute to the later phase of reactions. TNF-α released from mast cells enhances the expression of adhesion molecules on endothelial cells and leads to lymphocyte infiltration into the mucosa. This may promote further cell-mediated reactions against food antigen in the intestine.

Eosinophil migration into the mucosa is often seen in patients with food allergic colitis, and typically presents in children with an atopic family history before the age of 2 years. Eosinophils migrate into the gut, responding to eosinophil chemotactic factors, such as eotaxin, platelet activating factor, histamine, and LTB$_4$, mostly derived from mast cells. The eosinophils also participate in IgE-mediated inflammation directly because they have low-affinity receptors for IgE (Capron et al 1981). Eosinophils liberate an abundance of highly-cytotoxic and pro-inflammatory mediators, such as major basic protein, eosinophil cationic protein, and eosinophil peroxidase (Verge et al 1987, Bengtsson et al 1997). These mediators may disrupt mucosal surface and contribute to the later phase of reactions.

Type II and III allergies

Type II and III reactions very rarely cause allergic reactions in the intestine.

Type IV allergy — cell mediated reactions

Mucosal damage, such as villous atrophy and crypt hyperplasia, is seen in biopsy specimens taken from patients with food sensitive enteropathy, such as coeliac disease. Similar pathological findings are also seen in patients suffering from persistent diarrhoea, dehydration, malnutrition, and failure to thrive (Phillips et al 1979, Walker-Smith et al 1984). Because the mucosal infiltrate consists mainly of intraepithelial and lamina propria lymphocytes, but not of mast cells and eosinophils, lymphocyte-mediated responses are considered to be involved in mucosal damage in these patients. The relationship between cell-mediated reactions and their effects on intestinal morphology have been investigated in detail during graft-versus-host reactions (MacDonald & Ferguson 1976, 1977), which show a striking morphological similarity to the mucosal damage seen in food-sensitive enteropathy. Direct evidence for an important T-cell mediated process in the pathogenesis of the flat mucosal lesion has been shown in other *ex vivo* model systems (MacDonald & Spencer 1988). The same group also reported that as a result of an uncontrolled activation of T cells, increased synthesis of matrix metalloproteinases (MMP) (Pender et al 1997) and keratinocyte growth factor (KGF) (Bajaj-Elliott et al 1997) contribute to the gut damage. It is considered that MMPs and KGF may be directly involved in mucosal damage because they cause the degradation of mucosa and crypt hyperplasia by stimulating epithelial cell proliferation (Fig. 23.2).

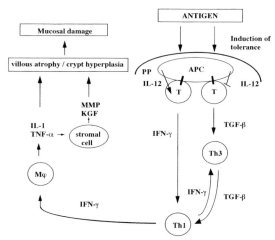

Figure 23.2 — Induction of tolerance and mucosal damage. In ovalbumin (OVA)-specific T-cell receptor (TCR) transgenic mice, orally-administered food antigen evokes TGF-β producing cells that can actively suppress immunological reactions and inhibit antigen-specific Th1 cell responses in the PP. This mechanism is negatively regulated by IL-12 and IFN-γ. As a result of an uncontrolled activation of Th1 cells, increased synthesis of Th1 cytokines stimulates macrophages and stromal cells. They may contribute to mucosal damage, such as villous atrophy and crypt hyperplasia, by releasing keratinocyte growth factor (KGF) and matrix metalloproteinases (MMP). PP = Peyer's patch

Mixed reactions

Could IgE-mediated reactions be involved in prolonged symptoms by chronic antigen exposure? This may be highly relevant to the clinical situation because even Type I allergic patients often suffer from frequent and prolonged allergic responses as a result of repeated antigen exposure. Hence, some investigators have shown that not only mast cells but also eosinophils and lymphocytes infiltrate into the intestinal mucosa upon chronic antigen exposure in antigen-specific IgE-mediated mouse models (Ohtsuka et al 1998). Cell adhesion molecule expression on endothelial cells is up-regulated as a result of continuous stimulation with chemical mediators derived from mast cells, especially TNF-α (Wershil et al 1996, Furuta et al 1997). This enhancement leads to increased infiltration of lymphocytes into the mucosa. These lymphocytes that have migrated, especially Th1 cells, produce IFN-γ and up-regulate antigen presentation by promoting MHC-class II molecule expression on APC in the intestine (Steinger et al 1989). This further promotes cell-mediated reactions against food antigen.

Symptoms

Although food antigens are encountered through the

gut, the symptoms of food intolerance are often seen in the skin and mucosa of the eyes, nose and respiratory system, causing eczema, erythema, itchiness, wheezing and respiratory distress. The common digestive symptoms of food intolerance are diarrhoea, vomiting and nausea. Oedema and ulceration of the oral cavity as well as constipation are seen in some cases (O'Farrelly et al 1991, Iacono et al 1998). Digestive symptoms are often severe in infants and young children. Respiratory and dermal symptoms are also seen but are more frequent in older children.

These symptoms, observed within minutes to 1 h after antigen ingestion, are due to antigen specific IgE-mediated reactions. These symptoms often start from the location where the antigen is encountered, and sometimes develop into severe systemic reactions. In the intestine, biopsy specimens reveal mucosal oedema and mast cell and eosinophil infiltration (Kosnai et al 1984). IgE-mediated reaction in the intestine causes secretary diarrhoea and bloody diarrhoea in patients with food allergic colitis. Diagnosis can be ascertained by the patient's past history, skin tests, the presence of food-specific serum IgE antibodies, and oral food challenge. Oral food challenge is necessary because the accuracy of antigen specific-IgE level and skin tests is generally unsatisfactory. However, challenge tests can be dangerous as they may induce shock. Therefore, they should be performed under intensive surveillance.

On the other hand, cell-mediated reactions are involved in prolonged symptoms, such as persistent diarrhoea, dehydration and failure to thrive. These symptoms are caused by mucosal damage, evident as villous atrophy and crypt hyperplasia (Phillips et al 1979, Walker-Smith et al 1984). Patients who suffer from cell-mediated reactions therefore show persistent diarrhoea with dehydration, malnutrition, and failure to thrive after antigen exposure. Prolonged exposure to an antigen may eventually result in anaemia, hypoproteinaemia and hypocirculation.

Treatment

Identification and elimination of the proteins that cause the adverse reaction improves the condition of these patients. In immunological food intolerance, hydrolysed cow's milk, soya, and gluten, are available. In Type I allergy, nutritional status and the level of hydration have to be considered. Elimination of the offending food from the diet should prevent further malnutrition and dehydration. Hypolactasia may be seen in prolonged diarrhoea with brush border damage,

so that substituting lactose with another sugar such as glucose is necessary.

Amongst several kinds of anti-allergic drugs, disodium cromoglycate (DSCG) has been frequently studied both in vitro and in vivo. Oral DSCG therapy has been reported to be effective in patients with food intolerance (Freier & Berger 1973). However, the pharmacological effects of DSCG are still obscure. DSCG is thought to stabilize mucosal-type mast cells and reduce the amount of chemical mediators released by antigen stimulation (Pearce et al 1984). DSCG also prevents antigen uptake from luminal surface into the mucosa (Falth-Magnusson et al 1984). Therefore, in cases in which dietary control is not well achieved, DSCG should be considered to prevent further antigen up-take from intestinal lumen. Another anti-allergic drug, keto-tifen, inhibits the release of histamine and SRS-A from mast cells, basophils and neutrophils. Both DSCG and ketotifen can be effective in reducing adverse reactions in patients with Type I allergy. However, the efficiency of these drugs in food intolerance is still unclear.

There are multiple steps that can be taken in intervention against immunological food intolerance. One potentially effective approach is to inhibit IgE-binding to the high-affinity IgE receptor (FcεRIα on mast cells to abrogate mast cell activation (Ra et al 1993). It has been demonstrated that the soluble form of human FcεRIα chain, suppresses the allergic response in passively-sensitized mice (Ohtsuka et al 1999). Allergic patients suffer from frequent IgE-mediated responses as a result of repeated antigen exposure, and these allergic reactions could be completely blocked by continuous administration of sFcεRIα because it can efficiently trap free IgE in the vicinity of mast cells before binding of the IgE to the cell surface FcεRIα. An alternative approach is to use a monoclonal anti-IgE antibody, which binds IgE on the mast cell membrane and blocks allergen-induced mast cell degranulation (Presta et al 1993).

Cytokine treatment may become an effective approach for treatment of food intolerance. As mentioned previously, an imbalance in the production of cytokines between IFN-γ, IL-12 and TGF-β is involved in the pathogenesis of food intolerance. Strategies may be developed to dampen tissue damaging responses by manipulation of cytokine production.

Discussion

Recent prospective studies suggest that cord-blood

T-cell cytokine responses for house-dust-mite allergen show a Th2 cell profile, producing IL-4, IL-6, IL-10 and IL-13 (Prescott et al 1999). As IFN-γ producing Th1 cells increase by 6 months of age, the cytokine profile moves towards Th1-type in non-atopic infants. Although cord-blood T cells produce relatively lower amounts of Th2 type cytokines in atopic infants, they maintain Th2 dominant cytokine synthesis with relatively slow increase in IFN-γ production. This study indicates that the immune system has a Th2 profile in the foetus, which develops into Th1 profile during infancy probably due to stimulation by infectious agents and the intestinal bacterial flora.

Animal data support the notion of a developmental regulation of Th1 versus Th2 response. Studies with brown Norwegian rats, which develop eosinophilic bronchial inflammation as well as airway hyper-sensitive reactions after Ag exposure, showed decreased allergic inflammation in aged animals (Ide et al 1999). The cells taken from aged rats expressed Th1 type cytokine mRNA, whereas those from young animals expressed Th2 dominant cytokines. It is suggested that decreased allergic inflammation in aged animals is attributable to age-dependent impairment of Th2 to Th1 generations in response to Ag.

Studies of the cytokine network leads to a deeper understanding of the mechanisms of food intolerance. By identifying the cells responsible for adverse reactions (e.g., mast cells, basophils, Th1 and Th2 cells), treatment will be easier and more efficient. It is hoped that these studies will give us an idea about how we can establish immunological tolerance in patients with food intolerance, thereby bypassing the need for eliminating certain food from diets.

References

Ament, M.E., Rubin, C.E. (1972) Soy protein–another cause of the flat intestinal lesion. *Gastroenterol*, 62, 227–234.

Bajaj-Elliott, M., Breese, E., Poulsom, R., Fairclough, P.D., MacDonald, T.T. (1997) Keratinocyte growth factor in inflammatory bowel disease. Increased mRNA transcripts in ulcerative colitis compared with Crohn's disease in biopsies and isolated mucosal myofibroblasts. *Am J Pathol*, 151, 1469–1476.

Beckett, C.G., Dell'Olio, D., Kontakou, M., Przemioslo, R.T., Rosen-Bronson, S., Ciclitira, P.J. (1996) Analysis of interleukin-4 and interleukin-10 and their association with lymphocytic infiltrate in the small intestine of patients with coeliac disease. *Gut*, 39, 818–823.

Bengtsson, U., Knutson, T.W., Knutson. L., Dannaeus, A.,

Hallgren, R., Ahlstedt, S. (1997) Eosinophil cationic protein and histamine after intestinal challenge in patients with cow's milk intolerance. *J Allergy Clin Immunol*, 100, 216–221.

Caffarelli, C., Romanini, E., Caruana, P., Street, M.E., de Angelis, G. (1998) Clinical food hypersensitivity: The relevance of duodenal immunoglobulin E-positive cells. *Pediatr Res*, 44, 485–490.

Capron, M., Capron, A., Dessaini, J., Torpier, G., Gunnar, S., Johannson, O., Prin, L. (1981) Fc receptors for IgE on human and rat eosinophils. *J Immunol*, 126, 2087–2092.

Chen, Y., Inobe, J., Marks, R., Gonnella, P., Kuchroo, V.K., Weiner, B.L. (1995) Peripheral deletion of antigen-reactive T cells in oral tolerance. *Nature*, 376, 177–180.

Dicke, W.K., Weijers, H.A., Vav De Kamer, J.H. (1953) The presence in wheat of a factor having a deleterious effect in cases of Coeliac disease. *Acta Paediatr*, 42, 34–42.

Falth-Magnusson, K., Kjellman, N.I., Magnusson, K.E., Sundqvist, T. (1984) Intestinal permeability in healthy and allergic children before and after sodium-cromoglycate treatment assessed with different-sized polyethyleneglycols (PEG 400 and PEG 1000), *Clin Allergy*, 14, 277–286.

Freier, S., Berger, H. (1973) Disodium cromoglycate in gastrointestinal protein intolerance. *Lancet*, 1, 913–915.

Fukaura, H., Kent, S.C., Pietrusewicz, M.J., Khoury, S.J., Weiner, B.L., Hafier, D.A. (1996) Induction of circulating myelin basic protein and proteolipid protein-specific transforming growth factor-beta1-secreting Th3 T cells by oral administration of myelin in multiple sclerosis patients. *J Clin Invest*, 98, 70–77.

Furuta, G.T., Schimidt-Choudhury, A., Wang, M.Y., Wang, Z.S., Lu, L., Furlano, R.I., Wershil, B.K. (1997) Mast cell-dependent tumor necrosis factor a production participates in allergic gastric inflammation in mice. *Gastroenterol*, 113, 1560–1569.

Goldman, A.S., Anderson, D.W., Sellers, W.A. et al. (1963) Milk allergy. Oral challenge with milk and isolated milk protein in allergic children. *Pediatrics*, 32, 425–430.

Grulee, C.G., Sanford, N.H. (1936) The influence of breast and artificial feeding on infantile eczema. *J Pediatr*, 8, 223–225.

Grulee, C.G., Sanford, N.H., Heron, P.H. (1934) Breast and artificial feeding. *JAMA*, 103, 735–737.

Harding, F.A., McArthur, J.G., Gross, J.A., Raulet, D.H., Allison, J.P. (1992) CD28-mediated signaling costimulates murine T cells and prevents induction of anergy in T-cell clones. *Nature*, 356, 607–609.

Heyman, M., Darmon, N., Dupont, C., Dugas, B., Hirribaren, A., Blaton, M.A., Desjeux, J.F. (1994) Mononuclear cells from infants allergic to cow's milk secret tumor necrosis factor alpha, altering intestinal function. *Gastroenterol*, 106, 1514–1523.

Iacono, G., Cavataio, F., Montalto, G., Florena, A., Tumminello, M., Soresi. M., Notarbartolo, A., Carroccio, A. (1998) Intolerance of cow's milk and chronic constipation in children. *N Engl J Med*, 339, 1100–1104.

Ide, K., Hayakawa, H., Yagi, T., Sato, A., Koide, Y., Yoshida, A., Uchijima, M., Suda, T., Chiba, K., Nakamura, H. (1999) Decreased expression of Th2 type cytokine MRNA contributes to the lack of allergic bronchial inflammation in aged rats. *J Immunol*, 163, 396–402.

Ishizaka, K., Ishizaka, T., Hornbrook, M.M. (1966) Physiochemical properties of human reaginic antibody. IV. Presence of a unique immunoglobulin as a carrier of reaginic activity. *J Immunol*, 97, 75–85.

Jalonen, T. (1991) Identical intestinal permeability changes in children with different clinical manifestations of cow's milk allergy. *J Allergy Clin Immunol*, 88, 737–742.

Kontakou, M., Przemioslo, R.T., Sturgess, R.P., Limb, G.A., Ellis, H.J., Day, P., Ciclitira, P.J. (1995) Cytokine MRNA expression in the mucosa of treated coeliac patients after wheat peptide challenge. *Gut*, 37, 52–57.

Kosnai, L., Kuitunen, P., Savilahti, E., Sipponen, P. (1984) Mast cells and eosinophils in the jejunal mucosa of patients with intestinal cow's milk allergy and celiac disease of childhood. *J Pediatr Gastroenterol Nutr*, 3, 368–372.

MacDonald, T.T. (1995) Evidence for cell-mediated hypersensitivity as an important pathogenetic mechanism in food intolerance. *Clin Allergy*, 25, 10–13.

MacDonald, T.T., Ferguson, A. (1976) Hypersensitivity reactions in the small intestine. 2. Effects of allograft rejection on mucosal architecture and lymphoid cell infiltrate. *Gut*, 17, 81–91.

MacDonald, T.T., Ferguson, A. (1977) Hypersensitivity reactions in the small intestine. 3. The effects of allograft rejection and graft-versus-host disease on epithelial cell kinetics. *Cell Tissue Kinet*, 10, 301–312.

MacDonald, T.T., Spencer, J. (1988) Evidence that activated mucosal T cells play a role in the pathogenesis of enteropathy in human small intestine. *J Exp Med*, 167, 1341–1349.

Majamaa, H., Ifiettinen, A., Laine, S., Isolauri, E. (1996) Intestinal inflammation in children with atopic eczema: Faecal eosinophil cationic protein and tumor necrosis factor-alpha as non-invasive indicators of food allergy. *Clin Exp Allergy*, 26, 181–187.

Marth, T., Strober, W., Seder, R.A., Kelsall, B.L. (1997) Regulation of transforming growth factor-beta production by interleukin-12. *Eur J Immunol*, 27, 1213–1220.

Marth, T., Zeitz, M., Ludviksson, B.R., Strober, W., Kelsall, B.L. (1999) Extinction of IL-12 signaling promotes Fas-mediated apoptosis of antigen-specific T cells. *J Immunol*, 162, 7233–7240.

Mayer, L., Shlien, R. (1987) Evidence for function of Ia molecules on gut epithelial cells in man. *J Exp Med*, 166, 1471–1483.

Nilsen, E.M., Lundin, K.E.A., Krajci, P., Scott, H., Sollid, L.M., Brandtzaeg, P. (1995) Gluten-specific, HLA-DQ restricted T cells from coeliac mucosa produce cytokines with Th1 or Th0 profile dominated by interferon-γ. *Gut*, 37, 766–776.

Nolte, H., Schiotz, P.O., Kruse, A., Stahl Skov, P. (1989) Comparison of intestinal mast cell and basophil histamine release in children with food allergic reactions. *Allergy*, 44, 554–565.

O'Farrelly, C., O'Mahony, C., Graeme-Cook, F., Feighery, C., McCartan, B.E., Weir, D.G. (1991) Gliadin antibodies identify gluten-sensitive oral ulceration in the absence of villous atrophy. *J Oral Pathol Med*, 20, 476–478.

Ohtsuka, Y., Naito, K., Yamashiro, Y., Yabuta, K., Okumura, K., Ra, C. (1999) Induction of anaphylaxis in mouse intestine by orally administered antigen and its prevention with soluble high affinity receptor for IgE. *Pediatr Res*, 45, 300–305.

Ohtsuka, Y., Suzuki, R., Nagata, S., Oguchi, S., Shimizu, T., Yamashiro, Y., Okumura, K., Ra, C. (1998) Chronic oral antigen exposure induces lymphocyte migration in anaphylactic mouse intestine. *Pediatr Res*, 44, 791–797.

Pearce, F.L., Befus, A.D., Bienenstock, J. (1984) Mucosal mast cells. 111. Effect of quercetin and other flavonoids on antigen-induced histamine secretion from rat intestinal mast cells. *J Allergy Clin Immunol*, 73, 819–823.

Pender, S.L., Tickle, S.P., Docherty, A.J., Howie, D., Wathen, N.C., MacDonald, T.T. (1997) A major role for matrix metalloproteinases in T cell injury in the gut. *J Immunol*, 158, 1582–1590.

Phillips, A.D., Rice, S.J., France, N.E., Walker-Smith, J.A. (1979) Small intestinal intraepithelial lymphocyte levels in cow's milk protein intolerance. *Gut*, 20, 509–512.

Prescott, S.L., Macaubas, C., Smallacombe, T., Holt, B.J., Sly, P.D., Holt, P.G. (1999) Development of allergen-specific T-cell memory in atopic and normal children. *Lancet*, 353, 196–200.

Presta, L.G., Lahr, S.J., Shields, R.L., Porter, J.P., Gorman, C.M., Fendly, B.M., Jardieu, P.M. (1993) Humanization of an antibody directed against IgE. *J Immunol*, 151, 2623–2632.

Ra, C., Kuromitsu, S., Hirose, T., Yasuda, S., Furuichi, K., Okumura, K. (1993) Soluble human high-affinity receptor for IgE abrogates the IgE-mediated allergic reaction. *Int Immunol*, 5, 47–54.

Robinson, D.S., Hamid, Q., Ying, S., Tsicopoulos, A., Barkans, J., Bentley, A.M., Corrigan, C., Durham, S.R., Kay, A.B. (1992) Predominant TH2-like bronchoalveolar T-Lymphocyte population in atopic asthma. *N Engl J Med*, 326, 298–304.

Rognum, T.O., Brandtzaeg, P. (1992) IgE-positive cells in human intestinal mucosa are mainly mast cells. *Int Arch Allergy Appl Immunol*, 89, 256–260.

Sanderson, I.R., Walker, W.A. (1993) Uptake and transport of macromolecules by the intestine: Possible role in clinical disorders (an update). *Gastroenterol*, 104, 622–639.

Sanderson, K., Ouellette, A.J., Carter, E.A., Walker, W.A., Harmatz, P.R. (1993) Differential regulation of B7 mRNA in enterocytes and lymphoid cells. *Immunol*, 79, 434–438.

Schwarz, R.H. (1990) A cell culture model for T lymphocyte clonal anergy. *Science*, 248, 1349–1356.

Steinger, B., Falk, P., Lohmuller, M., Van Der Meide, P.H. (1989) Class II MHC antigens in the rat digestive system. Normal distribution and induced expression after interferongamma treatment *in vivo. Immunol*, 68, 507–513.

Venge, P., Hakansson, L., Peterson, C.G. (1987) Eosinophil activation in allergic disease. *Int Archs Allergy Appl Immunol*, 82, 333–337.

Walker-Smith, J.A., Ford, R.P.K., Phillips, A.D. (1984) The spectrum of gastrointestinal allergies to food. *Ann Allergy*, 53, 629–636.

Weiner, B.L., Mackin, G.A., Matsui, M., Orav, E.J., Khoury, S.J., Dawson, D.M., Hafler, D.A. (1993) Double-blind pilot trial of oral tolerization with myelin antigens in multiple sclerosis. *Science*, 259, 1321–1324.

Wershil, B.K., Furuta, G.T., Wang, Z-S., Galli, S.J. (1996) Mast cell-dependent neutrophil and mononuclear cell recruitment in immunoglobulin E-induced gastric reactions in mice. *Gastroenterol*, 10, 1482–1490.

Woodbury, R.M. (1922) The relation between artificial feeding and infant mortality. *M J Hyg*, 2, 668–672.

Wright, R., Robertson, D. (1987) Non-immune Damage to The Gut. In: Brostoff, J., Challacombe, S.J. (eds.) *Food Allergy And Intolerance*. London: Baillière Tindall. pp. 248–254.

24

Low-fat diets in children

Jitka Vobecky

Abbreviations

AAP   The American Academy of Pediatrics
CHD   coronary heart disease
HDL-C   high-density lipoprotein cholesterol
LDL-C   low-density lipoprotein cholesterol
PUFA   polyunsaturated fatty acid
SFA   saturated fatty acid

Introduction

Diet is considered an important factor in the aetiology of arteriosclerosis. The consumption of a low-fat diet is advocated for its prevention. When this regimen is implemented during childhood, it should, however, satisfy the child's increased needs for energy, vitamins and other micro-nutrients, which are necessary for growth and development. A controversy still exists about whether a fat intake that is below 30% of total dietary calories can maintain optimal growth and supply a suitable quantity of nutrients.

Historical background

Clinical and experimental evidence confirm the important association between diet and the beginning of arteriosclerosis in early life (Glueck 1986, Nicklas et al 1988, Wynder et al 1989). Atherogenesis is an evolving process that is influenced by environmental factors, and it is related to the development of coronary heart disease (CHD) (Kleinman et al 1996). This knowledge is based mostly on studies in adults, as pointed out by Zlotkin (1996), Newman et al (1990), Resnicow et al (1991) and others. A decrease in fat consumption is recommended as an effective step for reducing cardiovascular morbidity and mortality (Wynder et al 1989). In spite of almost general agreement about fat reduction for adults, the amount for children is still not clearly defined. According to the National Research Council (1989) and Dietary Guidelines Advisory Committee (1995), 30–40% of calories provided by fat may assure adequate growth and development. An intake of total fat that is not higher than 30% of calories and of saturated fatty acid (SFA) that does not exceed 10% is generally recommended for adults. Although this diet may appear to be without adverse effects in infants and children, some harmful consequences such as impaired myelinization of nerves, increased requirements of vitamin E and slow growth have been reported (Lifshitz & Moses 1989).

Nicklas et al (1992) also expressed concern that low fat intake may have deleterious effects on growth and development because it may be deficient in total calories and essential nutrients. In order to prevent the adverse effects of reduced fat intake, McPherson et al (1996) and Smith-Schneider et al (1992) underlined the importance of consuming a wide variety of food as well as appropriate caloric intake.

The National Nutrition Monitoring and Related Research Program (1996) in the United States indicate that the intakes of total fat and SFA remain above recommended levels for a large proportion of the population. Less than 20% of 6–11-year-old children and adolescents, only 21% of adult males and 25% of females consumed diets containing levels of total fat that were < 30% of calories in 1989–1991. Also, the median intakes for most adults, adolescents and children older than 2 years were above recommended values (i.e., for total fat < 30% and for SFA < 10% of calories).

Infants and young children

The primary goal for paediatric nutrition is to provide nutrients for optimal growth and development. Over the recent years, increasing attention has been also directed towards developing nutritional intervention that may lower the risk of chronic disease later in life. Kleinman et al (1996) gave the credit for this to the widely-applied nutritional recommendations for decreasing the total and saturated fat content in the diet of children and adolescents. This dietary fat reduction obviously contributed to the decrease in the mean serum cholesterol level of the population as a whole. They also believe that children can safely eat a low-fat diet in which fat yields 30% and SFA < 10% of total energy.

This briefly-quoted evidence was criticized by Zlotkin (1996), particularly, for three reasons:

1. The studies on dietary intervention in children were of short duration and measured a very small percentage (< 5%) of increased or decreased values (Puska et al 1982, Walter et al 1988);

2. The presented data did not demonstrate the persistence of reduction (Newman et al 1990, Resnicow et al 1991);

3. No controlled studies evaluating the efficacy of a low-fat diet were available (Kwiterowich 1989, Kaplan & Toshima 1992, Lifshitz 1992).

Prescription of a low-fat diet

The recommendation of a low-fat diet for children

is not unanimously accepted. The American Heart Association (1992) and the National Cholesterol Education Program strongly considered the recommendations as an effective way to prevent CHD. Several experts justified such an approach because excessive fat intake may lead to known health hazards. The positions of the American Academy of Pediatrics (AAP) (1992) and, namely, of the Dietary Guidelines Advisory Committee (1995) were more cautious.

Kaplan & Toshima (1992) reviewed the available evidence about the detrimental consequences related to dietary fat restriction. Some studies on secular trends, migration and on vegetarianism reported minor effects upon growth. It seems that only children exposed to severe dietary restriction experience growth stunting. The existing controversies on dietary fat restriction for children were analysed by Lifshitz & Tarim (1996) also. They did not find any data demonstrating the beneficial effects of starting such diets in childhood for all children, including those with normal serum cholesterol levels. According to this review, dietary restrictions in early life may not necessarily induce a long-lasting decrease in blood cholesterol levels (i.e., that persists into adulthood) and/or reduce disease incidence. Such diets also may result in sub-optimal growth and development. Furthermore, low-fat diets may lower high-density lipoprotein cholesterol (HDL-C) levels and not specifically low-density lipoprotein cholesterol (LDL-C).

Fat intake and somatic growth

Increased attention has been drawn to the association between short stature and/or nutritional status and deficiencies in intrauterine and early life with coronary artery disease in adulthood (Barker et al 1993).

Boulton & Magarey (1995) and Boulton et al (1995) analysed dietary energy and nutrient intake in relation to somatic growth measured from infancy to 8 years in the Adelaide Nutrition Cohort Study. No clinically-significant differences were observed in height, weight or skin-fold thickness according to the percentage of energy provided by fat. Obviously, children exposed to a low-fat diet had a greater proportion of energy supplied by sugar and/or starch. The authors concluded that a lower-fat diet eaten in family surroundings is unlikely to have deleterious effects on growth caused by inadequate nutrient intake, if the family eating patterns meet good food guidelines. On the contrary, in another cohort study (Vobecky et al 1991), a not negligible percentage of children having a low-fat intake repeatedly during the pre-school years had not attained the

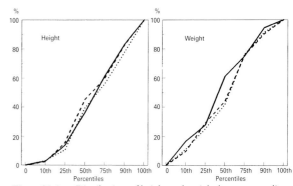

Figure 24.1 — Distribution of height and weight by age according to the Canadian reference values (in percentiles*) (both sexes at the age of 6 years). Children with % of calories provided by fat < 30%: Solid line, twice and +; broken line, dotted line, neurs. *(Gibson 1991).

50th centile for body weight by age (Fig. 24.1). At 6 years, the risk was significantly higher for girls (p = 0.016) and for both sexes together (p = 0.047).

Misapplication of dietary recommendations

Some overzealous individuals may believe that a largely reduced-fat intake is a key factor for ensuring optimal nutritional strategy. This misinterpretation of dietary guidelines risks inappropriate eating patterns, namely during childhood and adolescence (Lifshitz & Moses 1989). During this age, special, almost individual, attention is required to assure an adequate intake of energy and essential nutrients when diets with reduced fat are consumed. The failure to satisfy such a requirement can be seen by delayed growth and retarded puberty (Pugliese et al 1987).

Lowering fat intake for intervention reason

The aim of the Dietary Intervention Study in Children (DISC 1995) was to assess the efficacy and safety of lowering dietary intake of total fat, SFA and cholesterol to decrease LDL-C levels in sick children. The well-prepared and continuously-controlled behavioural, nutritionally-balanced, intervention focused on the promotion of adherence to a diet providing 28% of energy from total fat, < 8% from SFA, up to 9% from polyunsaturated fatty acid (PUFA), and less than 75 mg/4200 kJ (1000 kcal) per day of cholesterol (not to exceed 150 mg/d). This dietary intervention achieved modest lowering of LDL-C levels over 3 years while maintaining adequate growth, iron stores and psychological well being during the critical growth period of adolescence.

Practice and procedures

Low-fat diet and calories

A low-fat diet can be associated with diminished energy intake. Therefore, this energy shortage should be replaced by other energy sources, most often by complex carbohydrates. Obviously, this source is bulky and has a smaller energetic density. In practice, the child exposed to this kind of diet must eat more in order to consume enough energy. Again, careful attention is needed to warrant what kind of food should be used to maintain adequate nutrient intake (Vobecky et al 1988, Stephen & Deneer 1990, Vobecky et al 1995, Lifshitz & Tarim 1996).

To determine whether a moderately-reduced fat diet affects the stature or growth of healthy pre-school children, Shea et al (1993) studied a predominantly Hispanic group of 215 children aged 3–4 years at baseline of a cohort study with a mean of 25 months follow-up in a primary care paediatrics' practice at a large urban medical centre. Total fat provided 27.1% of calories in the lowest quintile as compared with 38.4% in the highest quintile of intake. These findings were consistent across two methods of diet assessment. Children who consumed a smaller percentage of total calories from fat received significantly less total calories, SFA, cholesterol, calcium and phosphorus, but more carbohydrates, iron, thiamin, niacin, vitamins A and C. These data suggest that a diet moderately reduced in fat can be safe for healthy pre-school children.

Low-fat diet and vitamins

The adequacy of energy and nutrient intakes of children consuming a low-fat diet is of some concern. It is questioned whether this intake covers the increased needs of fat-soluble vitamins and of other nutrients (Vobecky et al 1995). In a cohort of pre-school children studied by this group, the mean daily intake of vitamins A, D and E was always lower in those consuming < 30% of calories from fat (Fig. 24.2). As expected, the water-soluble vitamins showed a different less-consistent relationship, and for some of them the trend was opposite that of the fat-soluble vitamins (Figs. 24.3 and 24.4). However, the serum level for vitamin C was significantly higher in those with a low-fat diet. The risk of sub-optimal values expressed as odds ratio and of 95% confidence interval is shown in Table 24.1. Then, the crucial question of whether a low-fat intake is associated with vitamin inadequacy warrants a thorough examination.

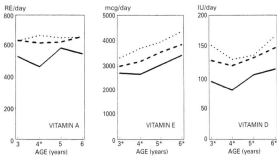

Figure 24.2 — Mean daily dietary intake of fat-soluble vitamins. Children with % of calories provided by fat: Solid line, < 30%; broken line, 30–40%; dotted line, > 40%. ★p(F) < 0.05 for this age.

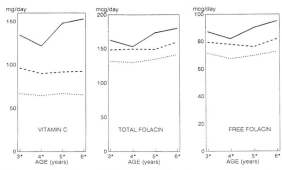

Figure 24.3 — Mean daily dietary intake of water-soluble vitamins – I. Solid line, < 30%; broken line, 30–40%; dotted line, > 40%. ★p(F) < 0.05 for this age.

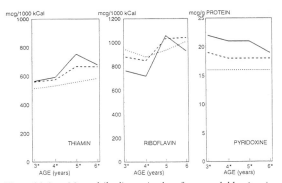

Figure 24.4 — Mean daily dietary intake of water-soluble vitamins – II. Soline line, < 30%; broken line, 30–40%; dotted line, > 40%. ★p(F) < 0.05 for this age.

Vegetarian diet

In recent years, the problems with vegetarian diets and with other unusual food habits (Van Dusseldorp et al 1996) have become more frequent, especially in some groups of the population. The popularity of healthy food whether for maintaining good health or for maintaining one's body is steadily increasing. A considerable amount of literature deals with this kind

Table 24.1 — Risk of sub-optimal intake of fat- and water-soluble vitamins according to hte proportion of calories provided by fat: Comparison between the proportions below and above 30% of calories.

Vitamin	Limits	Age in years							
		3		4		5		6	
		OR	p	OR	p	OR	p	OR	p
A	< 20 ER/kg	1.87	NS	2.52	0.010	2.13	NS	0.84	NS
D	< 100 IU/day	2.25	0.001	5.40	0.001	3.91	0.001	2.10	NS
E	< 50% RNI	1.57	NS	2.85	0.001	1.75	NS	2.75	0.0.27
Folacin:									
total	< 90 mg/day	1.28	NS	1.77	NS	1.36	NS	1.92	NS
free	< 40 mg/day	1.50	NS	2.83	0.022	0.48	NS	2.21	NS
C	< 25 mg/day	0.71	NS	0.72	NS	–	–	–	–
B1	< 400 mg/1000 kcal	2.19	0.080	0.54	NS	–	–	–	–
B2	< 550 mg/1000 kcal	3.09	0.008	4.26	0.006	2.93	NS	3.92	NS
B6	< 15 mcg/g Protein	0.16	NS	0.21	NS	0.11	NS	0.33	NS

–, non-calculable; NS, not significant; OR, odds ratio.

of nutrition (Dwyer 1986). According to Jacobs & Dwyer (1988) an appropriate vegetarian diet can provide all the necessary nutrients for growth.

On the other hand, under a vegan-like diet, it is impossible for a child to obtain all the needed nutrients for growth unless special care is ensured. The most common nutrient deficiencies encountered in vegan diets are not only lack of calories and essential amino acids but also of vitamin B12, D, calcium, iron and zinc.

Familial environment

The effects of implementing a low-fat diet during childhood and development remain to be further investigated. The problem of associated psychological consequences, family conflicts and costs should not be ignored (Barker et al 1993). This diet may be imposed on children by parents without any supervision and could result in an impaired nutritional status. Furthermore, eating habits developed by childhood can influence life-time practices. From this point of view, the child population is an extremely important target for prevention (Vobecky et al 1995).

The Finnish study on cardiovascular risk in young Finns (Laitinen et al 1995) shows that fat intake is related to the familial socio-economic status. Children of families with a higher socio-economic status consumed more fruit, low-fat milk, and soft margarine and less high-fat milk, butter, rye products and coffee. The main differences were observed in fat, vitamins D and C, and SFA; only minor differences were observed in energy intake and mineral density.

In another study (Vobecky et al 1991) based on an apparently healthy homogenous child population mostly from French-speaking families of good socio-economic standing, it was found that children from families with a higher socio-economic status had also a significantly-higher intake of iron, vitamins A and E, riboflavin, folate and cobalamin. No differences were observed for intake of energy, protein and vitamin C. Furthermore, maternal education was an important positive factor related to food selection.

In order to maintain a low, but acceptable, level of total fat, SFA and cholesterol intakes, healthy children should be encouraged to share good food choices with their family. Obviously, to succeed families should adhere to a healthy lifestyle and include the appropriate food guidelines.

Recommendations for infants and young child

In early age, infants should be preferably breastfed. If not, then the fatty acid composition of infant formulas should correspond to the amount and proportion of fatty acids contained in breast milk. During weaning and at least until 2 years of age, a child's diet should contain 30–40% of energy from fat and provide similar levels of essential fatty acids as are found in breast milk (Joint Working Group 1995). Gaull et al (1995) pointed out that the 1992 AAP policy of dietary fat and cholesterol restrictions in all children over 2 years of age was based on incomplete evidence. A low-fat diet has never been demonstrated to be beneficial for pre-pubescent healthy children, and the un-guided rapid implementation of any guidelines could lead to ill effects. This cautious approach does not imply that 30% of dietary fat is necessarily unhealthy for children, but it does apprehend the need for greater nutritional guidance for parents. In the absence of good nutritional education, a low-fat regimen might not achieve an adequate nutrient intake to assure optimal growth and development, especially in young children.

It should be noted that the current changes of lifestyle result in less parental supervision in all spheres of behaviour, making closer dietary direction less likely (Vobecky et al 1995).

Nutritional policy making

The Joint Working Group of the Canadian Paediatric Society and Health Canada (1993) and several other working groups around the world examined the available information on the nutritional needs for growth and development in relation to the risk of the onset of chronic diseases later in adulthood. Special attention was paid to efficacy and safety. Nevertheless, the efficacy of the recommended diet cannot be presumed. There is no evidence that implementation of a diet providing < 30% of energy as fat and < 10% of energy as SFA in children would reduce illness in later life.

With respect to safety, some children consuming a low-fat diet may have inadequate energy intake and food patterns, compromising nutritional density. The feasibility of an adequate low-fat diet for children was demonstrated. However, food costs associated with this type of diet appear to be high. It is important to acquire good dietary habits in children and to establish sound eating patterns in the whole family. Obviously, children with special conditions such as hyper-lipidaemia, who require dietary interventions, need particular and continuous attention by a physician and dietitian.

Discussion

A potentially-beneficial low-fat intake can be compromised when it is imposed without any dietary counselling, supervision or consideration of real needs, and it can result in an impaired nutritional status.

Knowledge of the nutritional profile of children is very important in order to establish a sound basis for preventive intervention into nutritional habits. As stated by Beal (1980) nutrient intake is a major determinant of the child's health. A well-nourished child is more likely to reach genetic potential in physical growth, physiological function and mental capacity.

If the impact of a prudent low-fat diet with < 30% of calories provided by fat was analysed in children, then the data demonstrated a significantly-decreased intake of fat-soluble vitamins. Considering this observation, it should be emphasized that vitamins have a role as antioxidants, and are powerful risk factors for serious CVD and malignant diseases of adulthood. However, as quoted by Glinsmann et al (1966) and in agreement with many others, nutrition priority during infancy and childhood should reflect the promotion of growth and development, rather than the prevention of degenerative disease in later life. The appropriate dietary counselling should be easily accessible. It should be emphasized again that the synthesis of individual recommendations for a single disease into complex and coherent requirements of vitamins and other nutrients is needed for preventive nutrition at the population level.

References

American Academy of Pediatrics, Committee on Nutrition. (1992) Statement on cholesterol. *Pediatrics*, 90, 469–473.

American Heart Association, Medical/Scientific Statement. (1992) Integrated cardiovascular health promotion in childhood. *Circulation*, 85, 1638–1650.

Anderson, S.A., Waters, J.H. (1996) Executive Summary from the Third Nutrition Monitoring in the United States. *J Nutr*, 126, 1907S–1936S.

Barker, D.J.P., Gluckman, P.D., Godfrey, K.M., Harding, J.E., Owens, J.A., Robinson, J.S. (1993) Fetal nutrition and cardiovascular disease in adult life. *Lancet*, 341, 938–941.

Beal, V.A. (1980) *Nutrition in The Life Span*. New York: John Wiley and Sons.

Boulton, T.J., Magarey, A.M. (1995) Effects of differences in dietary fat on growth, energy and nutrient intake from infancy to eight years of age. *Acta Paediatr*, 84, 146–150.

Boulton, T.J., Magarey, A.M., Cockington, R.A. (1995) Serum lipids and apolipoproteins from 1 to 15 years: Changes with age and puberty, and relationships with diet, parental cholesterol and family history of ischaemic heart disease. *Acta Paediatr*, 84, 1113–1118.

Dietary Guidelines Advisory Committee. (1995) *Report of*

The Dietary Guidelines Advisory Committee on The Dietary Guidelines for Americans, to the Secretary of Health and Human Services. Washington, DC.

DISC Collaborative Research Group. (1993) Dietary intervention study in children (DISC) with elevated low-density-lipoprotein cholesterol. Design and baseline characteristics. *Ann Epidemiol*, 4, 393–402.

Dwyer, J. (1986) Promoting good nutrition for the year 2000. *Pediatr Clinic N Am*, 33, 799.

Gaull, G.E., Glombetti, T., Woo, R.W. (1995) Pediatric dietary lipid guidelines: A policy analysis. *J Am Coll Nutr*, 14, 411–418.

Gibson, R.S. (1990) *Principles of Nutritional Assessment.* New York: Oxford University Press.

Glinsmann, W.H., Bartholmey, S.J., Coletta, F. (1966) Dietary guidelines for infants: A timely reminder. *Nutr Rev*, 54, 50–57.

Glueck, C.J. (1986) Pediatric primary prevention of atherosclerosis. *N Engl J Med*, 14, 175–176.

Jacobs, C., Dwyer, J. (1988) Vegetarian children appropriate and inappropriate diet. *Am J Clin Nutr*, 48, 811–818.

Kaplan, R.M., Toshima, M.T. (1992) Does a reduced fat diet cause retardation in child growth? *Prev Med*, 21, 33–52.

Kleinman, R.E., Finberg, L.F., Klish, W.J., Lauer, R.N. (1996) Dietary guidelines for children: U.S. Recommendations. *J Nutr*, 126, 1028S–1030S.

Kwiterowich, P.O. (1986) Biochemical, clinical, epidemiologic, genetic and pathologic data in the pediatric age group relevant to the cholesterol hypothesis. *Pediatrics*, 78, 349–362.

Laitinen, S., Räsänen, L., Viikari, J., Akerblom, H.K. (1995) Diet in Finnish children in relation to the family's socio-economic status. *Scand J Soc Med*, 23, 88–94.

Lifshitz, F. (1992) Children on adult diets: Is it harmful? Is it healthful? *J Am Coll Nutr*, 11(suppl), 894S–90S.

Lifshitz, F., Moses, N. (1989) Growth failure. A complication of dietary treatment of hypercholesterolemia. *Am J Dis Child*, 143, 537–542.

Lifshitz, F., Tarim, O. (1996) Considerations about dietary fat restrictions for children. *J Nutr*, 26, 1031S–1041S.

McPherson, R.S., Nichaman, M.Z., Kohl, H.W., Reed, D.B., Labarth, D.R. (1990) Intake and food sources of dietary fat among school children in Woodland, Texas. *Pediatr*, 86, 520–526.

National Cholesterol Education Program. (1992) Report of the expert panel on blood cholesterol levels in children and adolescents. Overview and summary. *Pediatrics*, 89, 525–527.

National Research Council. (1989) Diet and Health: *Implications for Reducing Chronic Disease Risk. Committee on*

Diet and Health, Food and Nutritional Board. Commission on Life Sciences National Research Council. Washington: National Academy Press.

Newman, T.B., Browner, W.S., Hulley, S.B. (1990) The case against childhood cholesterol screening. *J Am Med Assoc*, 264, 3039–3043.

Nicklas, T.A., Farris, R.P., Smoak, C.G., Srinivasan, S.R., Webber, L.S., Berenson, G.S. (1988) Dietary factors relate to cardiovascular risk factors in early life: Bogalusa Heart Study. *Arteriosclerosis*, 8, 193–199.

Nicklas, T.A., Webber, L.S., Koschak, M., Berenson, G.S. (1992) Nutrient adequacy of low fat intakes for children: The Bogalusa Heart Study. *Pediatr*, 89, 221–228.

Report of the Joint Working Group of the Canadian Paediatric Society and Health Canada. (1993) Nutrition Recommendations Update. Dietary Fat and Children. Ottawa.

Pugliese, M.T., Weyman-Daum, M., Moses, N., Lipshitz, F. (1987) Parental health beliefs as a cause of non-organic failure to thrive. *Pediatrics*, 80, 175–182.

Puska, O., Vartiainen, E., Pallonen, U., Salonen, J.T., Poyhia, P., Koskela, K., McAlister, A. (1982) The North Karelia Youth Project: Evaluation of two years of intervention on health behavior and CVD risk factors among 13- to 15-year-old children. *Prev Med*, 11, 550–570.

Resnicow, K., Berenson, G., Shea, S., Srinivasan, S., Strong, W., Wynder, E.L. (1991) The case against childhood cholesterol screening. *J Am Med Assoc*, 265, 3003–3005.

Shea, S., Basch, C.E., Stein, A.D., Contento, I.R., Irigoyen, M., Zybert, P. (1993) Is there a relationship between dietary fat and stature or growth in children three to five years of age? *Pediatr*, 92, 579–586.

Smith-Schneider, L.M., Sigman-Grant, M.J., Kris-Etherton, P.M. (1992) Dietary fat reduction strategies. *J Am Diet Assoc*, 92, 34–38.

Stephen, A.M., Deneer, M.J. (1990) The effect of dietary fat reduction on intake of major nutrients and fat soluble vitamins. *J Can Diet Assoc*, 51, 281–285.

Van Dusseldorp, M., Arts, I.C.W., Bergsma, J.S., De Jong, N., Dagnelie, P.C., Van Staveren, W.A. (1996) Catch-up growth in children fed a macrobiotic diet in early childhood. *J Nutr*, 126, 2977–2983.

Vobecky, J.S., David, P., Vobecky, J. (1988) Dietary habits in relation to tracking of cholesterol level in young adolescents: A 9-year follow-up. *Ann Nutr Metab*, 32, 312–323.

Vobecky, J.S., Grant, A.M., Laplante, P., David, P., Vobecky, J. (1993) Hypercholesterolemia in childhood: Repercussion in adulthood. *Eur J Clin Nutr*, 47(suppl 1), S47–S56.

Vobecky, J.S., Vobecky, J., Marquis, L. (1991) *Nutritional*

Inadequacy in Children with Low Fat Intake. Heidelberg: Proc 4th Int Symp Clin Nutr.

Vobecky, J.S., Vobecky, J., Normand, L. (1995) Risk and benefit of low fat intake in childhood. *Ann Nutr Metab*, 39, 124–133.

Walter, H.J., Hofman, A., Vaughan, R.D., Wynder, E.L. (1988) Modification of risk factors for coronary heart disease: Five-year results of a school-based intervention trial. *N Engl J Med*, 318, 1093–1100.

The Writing Group for the DISC Collaborative Research Group. (1995) Efficacy and safety of lowering dietary intake of fat and cholesterol in children with elevated low-density lipoprotein cholesterol. *JAMA*, 273, 1429–1435.

Wynder, E.L., Berenson, G.G., Strong, W.B., Williams, C. (eds.) (1989) Coronary artery disease prevention: Cholesterol, a pediatric perspective. *Prev Med*, 18, 323–409.

Zlotkin, S.H. (1996) A review of the Canadian Nutrition Recommendations Update: Dietary Fat and Children. *J Nutr*, 126, 1022S–1027S.

25

Nutrition in the child
with disabilities

Richard D. Stevenson and Robin Meyers

Introduction

Nutrition is an important aspect of the health management of children with disabilities. In fact, nutritional status can have a significant influence on a child's disability. The National Center for Medical Rehabilitation Research (NCMRR) of the U.S. National Institutes of Health has developed a framework to describe the multiple dimensions of disability for both adults and children. Five dimensions of disability are recognized: pathophysiology (tissue and cellular effects of disease or injury), impairments (organ systems' dysfunction), functional limitations (dysfunction of whole body or segmental activities), disability (effects on role functions and quality of life), and societal limitations (barriers in the community and environment). For example, a child with cerebral palsy may have sustained hypoxic ischaemic injury to the brain, leading to periventricular encephalomalacia (pathophysiology), which has resulted in poor motor control, weakness, spasticity and contractures (impairments). These resulting impairments can lead to functional limitations such as difficulty sitting upright, awkward use of utensils, and difficulty with eating. If not compensated in some way, these impairments may interfere with the child's ability to sit at the dinner table with the rest of his/her family or eat in the cafeteria with his/her schoolmates (functional disability). Societal limitations can worsen the situation if his/her insurance refuses to pay for his/her wheelchair, that would assist his/her ability to eat at the table, or if the school lunchroom cannot accommodate his/her wheelchair and his need for physical assistance. Thus, the multiple dimensions of the child's disability impact on eating, nutrition and the important social role eating plays in his life. Conversely, malnutrition resulting from these problems negatively affects the child's disability at multiple levels.

The provision of nutrition services and the treatment of under-nutrition have been deemed essential aspects of care to individuals with developmental disabilities and special health needs. A deficit in self-feeding leading to malnutrition is one of the most common predictors of early death amongst persons with severe disabilities (Eyman et al 1990). In a position paper, the American Dietetic Association stated that 'nutrition services are an essential component of comprehensive care for children with special health needs (Kozlowski & Powell 1995)'. In a separate position paper, the same organization stated that 'program planning for persons with developmental disabilities should include comprehensive nutrition services as part of health care, vocational and educational programs (Lucas & Blyler 1997)'. The Nutrition Committee of the Canadian Paediatric Society stated, in their clinical practice guidelines, that 'it is unacceptable not to treat under-nutrition associated with neurodevelopmental disability,' and that restoration of nutrition in these children should be regarded as an important part of their clinical management (Nutrition Committee 1994). After reviewing the literature, they concluded that children with developmental disabilities who are receiving adequate nourishment are generally calmer, appear more normal and have increased functional status (Nutrition Committee 1994).

Children with disabilities are at high risk for nutritional problems. This chapter discusses nutritional issues related to children with developmental disabilities. As a model for discussion, the chapter focuses on the child with cerebral palsy. Nutritional problems, particularly malnutrition, can complicate the overall status of a child with disabilities across all five dimensions of the NCMRR framework. Fortunately, these problems can be often anticipated, sometimes prevented, and usually treated successfully.

Historical background

Causes of malnutrition

Specific factors that contribute to feeding disorders and malnutrition in children with disabilities are outlined in Table 25.1. Anatomical problems such as cleft palate, choanal atresia, or tracheo-oesophageal fistula often manifest themselves in the first few days of life. These problems affect feeding and swallowing and interfere with the child's learning of normal feeding behaviours. Sensory-perceptual abnormalities, whilst difficult to quantify, most likely play a role amongst disabled children as well. These can be manifested as either hypersensitivity, such as a child who gags at the slightest touch on his tongue, or hyposensitivity, such as a child who requires a large bolus size to initiate swallowing. Hypersensitivity may be acquired and caused, or exacerbated, by medical procedures or treatments. For example, prolonged nasogastric tube feeding may lead to oral hypersensitivity that worsens feeding difficulties.

Motor dysfunction leads to various difficulties that can affect feeding. First, many children with motor impairment have poor head and trunk control (gross motor problems) and are unable to sit upright for eating.

Table 25.1 — Factors contributing to feeding problems, malnutrition, and poor linear growth in children with disabilities

Contributors to malnutrition	Contributors to poor linear growth
Anatomical defects (micrognathia, cleft palate, etc.)	Nutritional stunting
Poor posture due to motor deficits	Nutritional or Vitamin D deficiency rickets
Dependent feeding due to motor deficits	Decreased blood flow to affected extremities
Oral motor dysfunction and dysphagia	Disuse of limbs
Oral hypersensitivity	Lack of weight-bearing
Poor dentition	Growth hormone deficiency
Gastro-oesophageal reflux	Direct neural effects
Constipation	
Chronic lung disease/aspiration	
Uncontrolled seizures	

Second, fine-motor impairment, coupled with limited mobility, may make it difficult for children to bring foodstuffs to their mouths. Not only does this impair the physical act of feeding, but it also may secondarily exacerbate sensory abnormalities by decreasing oral experience and contributing to oral hypersensitivity. Gross and fine motor impairments often combine to render a child dependent upon others for feeding. This necessitates communication between the child and caregiver to convey hunger, satiety and food preferences. Thus, motor dysfunction hampers the child's ability to learn how to eat because it hampers his/her ability to attain and consume food.

Often children with motor dysfunction also have specific dysfunction of their oral motor mechanisms. These children may have pathological oral reflexes. One such reflex is the *tonic bite reflex*, which causes a child to bite down on the spoon without being able to let go. Another such reflex is the *tongue thrust*, which pushes food out of the mouth. The child with oral motor dysfunction may be unable to keep foodstuffs in the mouth due to tongue thrust or poor mouth closure. Such a child may also have difficulty organizing a swallow or may spill oral contents posteriorly into the pharynx before initiating a swallow. Additionally, the child with disabilities may have poor pharyngeal clearance of a bolus, leading to pharyngeal pooling. Thus, oral motor dysfunction can lead to drooling, spillage of foodstuffs, prolonged feeding times (because each mouthful may be painstakingly slow), pharyngeal pooling, laryngeal penetration and aspiration. In this way, oral-motor dysfunction can be one of the most important factors contributing to feeding difficulties, respiratory symptoms and malnutrition.

Co-morbid medical problems often have a large impact on feeding through their effects on appetite, energy needs and oral-motor function. These problems are very important to identify because treatment is often straightforward and helpful. Constipation is probably the most common medical problem in children with disabilities. It negatively affects the appetite, may slow gastric emptying and exacerbates gastro-oesophageal reflux (Lewis et al 1994). Chronic lung disease increases energy needs and complicates the co-ordination of feeding and breathing, particularly in young infants (Wolf & Glass 1992). Malnutrition itself, whilst generally a result of feeding problems, can also contribute to the perpetuation of the problem through its negative effects on appetite, generalized weakness and behavioural apathy. Gastro-oesophageal reflux is another common problem that causes the loss of nutrients from vomiting and can cause anorexia. It can lead to oesophagitis, which may cause pain upon swallowing and may eventually lead to oesophageal stricture. Other medical problems that must be assessed include seizures, chronic infections and congenital heart disease.

From a behavioural standpoint, a child's temperament can contribute to feeding problems. Fussy, irritable babies can be very difficult to feed. In addition, some children learn food aversion. For example, a child with chronic lung disease who spends his first year of life in the hospital and requires frequent intubation and suctioning may learn that oral sensations are unpleasant. This child may become averse to any kind of stimulation around the mouth, including food. This can lead to feeding refusal. These children are very difficult to treat at times. And finally, specific attachment or interactional disorders can play an important role in feeding problems. This can occur due to chronic hospitalization and separation of the child from the mother or primary caregiver. Emotional difficulties of the parent may contribute as well.

Significance of nutritional problems in children with disabilities

Malnutrition is an important co-morbidity of children who have developmental disabilities. Malnutrition has many deleterious effects on development and health and so is worthy of considerable attention. Table 25.2 summarizes the complications of malnutrition commonly seen in children with disabilities. Malnutrition has a well documented impact on growth that, when prolonged during childhood, leads to permanent stunting of stature. This effect on linear growth may, or may not, have any deleterious effect on the child's disability. In fact, having a smaller body size may be advantageous to children with severe disabilities, but this has not been clearly established. However, the other complications of malnutrition have significant negative effects on disability. For example, malnutrition leads to weakness that may decrease mobility and increase the risk of decubitus ulcers. This weakness also lessens the effectiveness of the cough reflex, thus making aspiration and pneumonia more likely (Sullivan 1992). In addition, malnutrition decreases peripheral circulation. Malnutrition seems to increase gastro-oesophageal reflux, as nutritional rehabilitation has been associated with resolution of reflux (Lewis et al 1994). Malnutrition has a further negative impact on wound healing and immunity, contributing to increased risk of complication perioperatively. Children with pre-operative nutritional deficiencies have a greater risk of post-operative complications following surgery for fundoplication (Weber 1995) and scoliosis (Jevsevar & Karlin 1993). Finally, malnutrition decreases the energy available for discretionary activity, which then decreases social interaction,

Table 25.2 — Complications of malnutrition

Growth: nutritional stunting

Immune function poor

Wound healing poor

Skin integrity: poor circulation (cool extremities), risk for decubitus ulcers

Muscle weakness: decreased mobility, cough; increased disability

Behaviour/learning: irritability, apathy, less social interaction

Decreased quality of life

increases apathy and negatively affects learning and quality of life.

Practice and procedures

Clinical assessment of growth and nutrition

An important part of routine health care maintenance for all children is the surveillance of growth and nutritional status. Normal growth is a marker for health, whilst abnormal growth is a red flag that the child may be ill or that something may be awry in his environment. Although in principle this is also true for children with disabilities, two problems exist that make the interpretation of routine growth measurements difficult. The first problem is that obtaining reliable measures of growth may be impossible, and the second is that generally accepted reference standards may not be appropriate.

The measurement of weight is generally straightforward using standard infant and paediatric/adult scales. Larger children with disabilities may be difficult to weigh if they are too large for the infant scale and are unable to stand independently for a standard scale. Our institution uses a bed scale for these children. Unfortunately, most paediatric offices do not have such a scale. The least expensive, but still reliable method for many children is to have the caregiver hold the child and weigh them together, and then subtract the weight of the caregiver. Once children get too large for this method, paediatricians or dietitians cannot obtain an accurate weight in their offices. Weight may need to be obtained at a local hospital on a bed scale.

Reliable measures of height or length in children with cerebral palsy or other motor impairment are often impossible to obtain due to fixed joint contractures, involuntary muscle spasms and poor co-operation due to associated cognitive deficits (Tobis et al 1961, Spender et al 1989). Alternatives to height or length, namely the segmental measures of upper-arm length and lower-leg length and knee height, have been investigated for use in children with cerebral palsy (Davies et al 1989, Spender et al 1989) and have been recommended for children and adults with various disabilities (Chumlea et al 1994, Stevenson 1996). Formulas for estimating stature from the segmental measures of upper-arm length, tibial length, and knee height have been developed for children with cerebral palsy (Stevenson 1995) and children and adults with disabilities (Chumlea et al 1994). Once a reliable measure of weight and a direct measure or estimation of stature are obtained, the interpretation of the data, and the diagnosis of malnutrition, in children with disabilities is often unclear. Standards for height and weight are based on studies of normally-active children (Hamill et al 1979). The application of these standards, particularly the weight-for-height norms, to children with less muscle mass and bone density due to physical inactivity may not be appropriate (Patrick & Gisel 1990, Samson-Fang & Stevenson 1998). Weight-for-height, which is typically used as a screening tool for malnutrition, is a poor predictor of low fat stores in children with cerebral palsy (unpublished data 1998). Specialized growth charts have been developed for many populations of children with developmental disabilities, including Down's syndrome, Prader-Willi syndrome, Williams syndrome, and DeLang syndrome (Cronk et al 1988, Butler & Meaney 1991, Pankau et al 1992, Kline et al 1993), but adequate growth standards for children with cerebral palsy have not been developed (Table 25.3).

Thus, although the standard nutritional screening of children involves only weight and a measure of stature, this may not be adequate for children with disabilities because of poor reference standards. Other measures that can be extremely useful are triceps and subscapular skinfolds (Patrick et al 1986, Davies et al 1989). Standard techniques for skinfolds are well established and can be used for children with disabilities (Cameron 1986, Lohman et al 1988). The single best screening tool for the assessment of nutritional status in children with cerebral palsy is triceps skinfold (unpublished data 1998). See Chapter 4 for more

detailed information about the nutritional assessment of children with disabilities.

Management of malnutrition

Once children are identified as being malnourished or at risk of malnutrition, treatment is straightforward, although it may be difficult. Figure 25.1 presents a proposed algorithm for the management of malnutrition in children with disabilities. The first step is to interpret the child's nutritional status, based on the history, physical examination, diet history and anthropometry. The history and physical examination is necessary to identify factors that may be contributing to the feeding difficulties and that may be amenable to intervention. Physiotherapists, occupational therapists and feeding

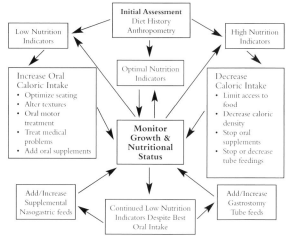

Figure 25.1 — Algorithm for assessment and management of nutritional status in children with disabilities.

Table 25.3 — Nutrition and growth: Methods of assessment in children with developmental disabilities

	Estimate of height	Nutritional status	Reference data
Cerebral Palsy	Knee height Tibial length Upper-arm length	Weight Triceps and subscapular skinfolds	Diagnosis-specific data not available
Meningomyelocele	Upper-arm length	Weight Triceps and subscapular skinfolds	Diagnosis-specific data not available
Mental Retardation syndromes (without motor impairment)	Standing height or recumbent length	Weight Triceps and subscapular skinfolds	Some diagnosis-specific data available[1]

[1]Cronk et al 1988, Butler & Meaney 1991, Pankau et al 1992, Kline et al 1993.

specialists can be very helpful with the evaluation and management. A dietary history is generally more useful to obtain qualitative data regarding intake rather than quantitative data. Stallings et al (1995) showed that careful quantitative assessment of oral intake in children with quadriplegic cerebral palsy was greatly overestimated.

It is useful to determine a target weight or, perhaps, a target skinfold thickness to work towards. With this as a goal, one then works to maximize the child's oral intake. This may involve adjusting textures, altering postural supports, treating medical problems (such as constipation and gastro-oesophageal reflux) and adding oral supplements. One then carefully monitors the response to treatment.

To guide nutritional management, it is important to estimate the child's caloric needs. Estimating caloric needs in this population is difficult. Table 25.4 summarizes the various methods that can be used. Regardless of what calorie level is estimated, the intake of the child must be increased or decreased to support optimal growth. The World Health Organization equations (Table 25.5) for predicting basal metabolic rate from body weight (Joint FAO/WHO/UNU Expert Consultation 1985) are simple to use and appear to estimate closely resting energy expenditure in children with cerebral palsy (Bandini et al 1991, Stallings et al 1996). This is especially true in children with cerebral palsy who have adequate fat stores. In children with cerebral palsy

Table 25.4 — Methods for the estimation of caloric needs in non-ambulatory and ambulatory children with developmental disabilities

Non-ambulatory children	Ambulatory children
WHO estimate of BMR[1]	WHO estimate of BMR
RDA for age[2]	× activity factor
Krick Method[3]	Activity factor = 1.6 – 2.1[4]
BMR × Tone factor × activity + growth factor	RDA for age
BMR = BSA × standard metabolic rate × 24 h	Krick Method

Abbreviations: WHO, World Health Organization; BMR, Basal Metabolic Rate; RDA, Recommended Dietary Allowances; BSA, Body surface area. [1]World Health Organization, basal metabolic rate estimate based on weight; [2]Recommended Dietary Allowances. National Research Council (USA), 10th Edn, 1989; [3]Krick et al 1992; [4]Bandini 1991.

Table 25.5 — World Health Organization equations for predicting basal metabolic rate from body weight

Age range (years)	kcal/day	Mjoules/day
Boys		
0–3	60.9 W − 54	0.255 W − 0.23
3–10	22.7 W + 495	0.095 W + 2.07
10–18	17.5 W + 651	0.073 W + 2.72
Girls		
0–3	61.0 W − 51	0.255 W − 0.21
3–10	22.5 W + 499	0.094 W + 2.09
10–18	12.2 W + 746	0.051 W + 3.12

Abbreviations: W, body weight in kilograms. Adapted from World Health Organization (1985).

and low fat stores, this method may underestimate calorie needs. The Krick method (Krick et al 1992) also appears to be an accurate predictor of calorie needs, but it is more involved and may be difficult to use in some settings. The United States Recommended Dietary Allowances (National Research Council 1989) are used frequently by dieticians in the United States, but they seem to overestimate caloric needs (Stallings et al 1996). These recommendations are currently being revised and may be of limited usefulness outside the United States. Regardless of the method used to estimate the caloric needs of the child, the response to treatment is the marker of success or failure. The treatment must be adjusted accordingly.

Once calorie needs have been calculated, the problem is how to get the calories into the child. If a child is taking only oral feedings several things can be tried to increase calorie intake. Parents and caretakers are encouraged to add fats to food, to add dry milk powder or cream to foods, and to offer oral supplements. Many acceptable, nutritionally-balanced commercial supplements are available, both in a juice or milk base. One of the most important aspects of recommending an oral supplement is taste. If the child will not drink the supplement, the formulation of the product does not matter. Once a specific dietary plan is instituted, children should be followed closely for weight gain and change in skinfolds.

If the child's nutritional status remains poor despite the best oral intake and medical management, then supplemental tube feedings are necessary. Tube feedings have become an accepted standard of care for children with severe disabilities (Sullivan 1992, Eltumi & Sullivan 1997). Tube feedings can be nasogastric (short-term supplementation) or via gastrostomy (long-term supplementation). For example, a child whose seizures are out of control may require supplemental tube feedings for a limited time until new treatments become effective. However, frequently, children with motor disabilities require long-term tube-feedings. The decision to place a gastrostomy tube is often a difficult one for families and requires preparation, education, and discussion. This is discussed in Chapters 7–10.

Initially, a child may be given 100% of her estimated calories by tube and allowed to continue to eat by mouth. Alternatively, some children may be given 50–75% of their calorie and fluid needs by tube. This is usually determined by how malnourished a child is at the time the tube is placed. To minimize the likelihood of vomiting, it is prudent to begin with small amounts and to advance gradually, as tolerated. Feedings can be given by continuous drip, bolus feedings or a combination of both. Tolerance and family schedule determine the specific mode of delivery and timing.

Once children are re-nourished, their calorie needs are not as high, so follow-up to monitor growth and adjustment of feedings is important. In the clinical management of children with cerebral palsy and malnutrition, often their caloric intake must be cut back once they become adequately nourished. Failure to decrease the dietary prescription at this point leads to obesity.

When a child is totally tube fed, formula selection is important. Again, feedings can be given as boluses or continuous drip, depending on tolerance and daily schedule. The formula should be age appropriate to provide adequate nutrients. If a blended tube feeding is given, a recipe should be written and followed to insure that all nutrients are provided. Again follow-up is important to ensure growth and adequate intake of vitamins and nutrients. This becomes challenging if the children become overweight and calories need to be drastically reduced to control weight gain. When calories are reduced so are protein, calcium, vitamin D and other nutrients. These must be replaced by vitamin and mineral supplements to ensure optimal growth and health. Because there is little specific information for children with disabilities, we utilize recommended daily allowances of the USDA (National Research Council 1989).

Discussion

Children with cerebral palsy and other developmental disabilities frequently grow poorly. Sometimes the poor growth is simply a manifestation of the underlying disability, or its root cause, and therefore does not require intervention. However, often the poor growth is a manifestation of malnutrition, and malnutrition has many well-documented, adverse effects. The consensus among clinicians and researchers is that malnutrition in children with disabilities warrants treatment. This statement may seem quite obvious; however, there is limited scientific data to support the hypothesis that well-nourished children with disabilities are truly better off than malnourished children with disabilities are. Prudence, clinical judgement and results of scientific studies dictate that malnutrition should be treated; however, more data to support this stance are needed. Currently malnutrition is defined quantitatively using body measurements, without correlation with functional status. So, the specific body measurements that lead to optimal functioning are unknown. The body habitus that is adequate or 'just right' has not been defined yet. Herein lies the critical need for future research. If our goal is to optimize functioning and quality of life for our clients with disabilities, then investigators must determine the range of nutritional measurements that leads to optimal functioning.

Acknowledgements

This work was supported, in part, by the Kluge Research Fund of the University of Virginia, the Genentech Foundation for Growth and Development, and the National Center for Medical Rehabilitation Research (1 R01 HD35739-01). The authors would like to thank Audrey Kocher for her review of the manuscript.

References

Bandini, L.G., Schoeller, D.A., Fukagawa, N.K., Wykes, L.J., Dietz, W.H. (1991) Body composition and energy expenditure in adolescents with cerebral palsy or myelodysplasia. *Pediatr Res*, 29, 70–77.

Butler, M.G., Meaney, F.J. (1991) Standards for selected anthropometric measurements in Prader-Willi syndrome. *Pediatrics*, 88, 853–860.

Cameron, N. (1986) The Methods of Auxological Anthropology. In: Falkner, F., Tanner, J.M. (eds.) *Human Growth: A Comprehensive Treatise*, 2nd edn. Vol. 3. New York: Plenum Press.

Chumlea, W.C., Guo, S.S., Steinbaugh, M.L. (1994) Prediction of stature from knee height for black and white adults and children with application to mobility-impaired or handicapped persons. *J Am Diet Assoc*, 94, 1385–1388.

Cronk, C., Crocker, A.C., Pueschel, S.M., Shea, A.M., Zackal, E., Pickens, G., Reed, R.B. (1988) Growth charts for children with Down Syndrome: 1 month to 18 years of age. *Pediatrics*, 81, 102–110.

Davies, J.C., Antonucci, D.L., Charney, E.B., Stallings, V.A. (1989) Use of upper-arm length and per cent body fat for nutritional assessment of children with cerebral palsy. *Dev Med Child Neurol*, 31(supp), 39–40.

Eltumi, M., Sullivan, P.B. (1997) Nutritional management of the disabled child: The role of percutaneous endoscopic gastrostomy. *Dev Med Child Neurol*, 39, 66–68.

Eyman, R.K., Grossman, H.J., Chaney, R.H., Call, T.L. (1990) The life expectancy of profoundly handicapped people with mental retardation. *N Engl J Med*, 323, 584–589.

Hamill, P.V.V., Drizd, T.A., Johnson, C.L., Reed, R.B., Roche, A.F., Moore, W.M. (1979) Physical growth: National center for health statistics percentiles. *Am J Clin Nutr*, 32, 607–629.

Jevsevar, D.S., Karlin, L.I. (1993) The relationship between preoperative nutritional status and complications after an operation for scoliosis in patients who have cerebral palsy [published erratum appears in J Bone Joint Surg Am 1993 Aug;75(8):1256]. *Journal of Bone & Joint Surgery — American Volume*, 75, 880–884.

Joint FAO/WHO/UNU Expert Consultation. (1985) *Energy and Protein Requirements*. Geneva: World Health Organization.

Kline, A.D., Barr, M., Jackson, L.G. (1993) Growth manifestations in the Brachmann-de Lange syndrome. *Am J Med Genet*, 47, 1042–1049.

Kozlowski, B.W., Powell, J.A. (1995) Position of the American Dietetic Association: Nutrition services for children with special health needs. *J Am Diet Assoc*, 95, 809–812.

Krick, J., Murphy, P.E., Markham, J.F.B., Shapiro, B.K. (1992) A proposed formula for calculating energy needs of children with cerebral palsy. *Dev Med Child Neurol*, 34, 481–487.

Lewis, D., Khoshoo, V., Pencharz, P.B., Golladay, E.S. (1994) Impact of nutritional rehabilitation on gastroesophageal reflux in neurologically impaired children. *J Pediatr Surg*, 29, 167–170.

Lohman, T.G., Roche, A.F., Martorell, R. (1988) *Anthropometric standardization reference manual*. Champaign: Human Kinetics Books.

Lucas, B.L., Blyler, E. (1997) Position of the American Dietetic Association: Nutrition in comprehensive program planning for persons with developmental disabilities. *J Am Diet Assoc*, 97, 189–193.

National Research Council. (1989) *Recommended dietary allowances*, 10th edn. Washington, DC: National Academy of Science.

Nutrition Committee, C.P. (1994) Undernutrition in children with a neurodevelopmental disability. *Canadian Medical Association Journal*, 151, 753–759.

Pankau, R., Partsch, C.-J., Gosch, A., Oppermann, H.C., Wessel, A. (1992) Statural growth in Williams-Beuren syndrome. *Eur J Pediatr*, 151, 751–755.

Patrick, J., Boland, M., Stoski, D., Murray, G.E. (1986) Rapid correction of wasting in children with cerebral palsy. *JDMCN*, 28, 734–739.

Patrick, J., Gisel, E. (1990) Nutrition for the feeding impaired child. *J Neuro Rehab*, 4, 115–119.

Samson-Fang, L.J., Stevenson, R.D. (1998) The use of NCHS weight for height standards in children with cerebral palsy. *Dev Med Child Neurol* (Abstract).

Spender, Q.W., Cronk, C.E., Charney, E.B., Stallings, V.A. (1989) Assessment of linear growth of children in cerebral palsy: Use of alternative measures to height or length. *Dev Med Child Neurol*, 31, 206–214.

Stallings, V.A., Cronk, C.E., Zemel, B.S., Charney, E.B. (1995) Body composition in children with spastic quadriplegic cerebral palsy. *Journal of Pediatrics*, 126, 833–839.

Stallings, V.A., Zemel, B.S., Davies, J.C., Cronk, C.E., Charney, E.B. (1996) Energy expenditure of children and adolescents with severe disabilities: A cerebral palsy model. *Am J Clin Nutr*, 64, 627–634.

Stevenson, R.D. (1995) Use of segmental measures to estimate stature in children with cerebral palsy. *Arch Pediatr Adolesc Med*, 149, 658–662.

Stevenson, R.D. (1996) Measurement of growth in children with developmental disabilities. *Dev Med Child Neurol*, 38, 855–860.

Sullivan, P.B. (1992) Gastrostomy and the disabled child. *Dev Med Child Neurol*, 34, 547–555.

Tobis, J.S., Saturen, P., Larios, G., Posniak, A.O. (1961) Study of growth patterns in cerebral palsy. *Arch Phys Med Rehabil*, 42, 475–481.

Weber, T.R. (1995) A prospective analysis of factors influencing outcome after fundoplication. *J Pediatr Surg*, 30, 1061–1064.

Wolf, L.S., Glass, R.P. (1992) *Feeding and Swallowing Disorders in Infancy: Assessment and Management*. Tucson, Arizona: Therapy Skill Builders.

26

Nutritional abnormalities due to Munchausen's syndrome by proxy

Howard I. Baron

Introduction

Munchausen's syndrome by proxy (MSP) is a term used to describe a parent who systematically fabricates illness in his/her child or intentionally makes his/her child ill. Although this term can be applied to any caregiver, the overwhelming majority of cases have been reported in families in which the mother is the perpetrator of the falsified condition in one or more child victims. The person fabricating the illness intentionally feigns or produces symptoms of an illness in the victim for psychological reasons and not for obvious external incentives such as drugs or money.

The most common modes of symptom inducement in MSP involve seizures, apnoea, failure to thrive, vomiting and diarrhoea, asthma/allergies and infections (Schreier & Libow 1994). For this reason, many nutritional disorders in infants and children can result from this potentially fatal form of child abuse. Thus, it is imperative that a complete discussion of nutrition in the paediatric age group includes a discussion of this perplexing and often unrecognized form of child mal-treatment.

Historical background

The term *Munchausen's syndrome* was first used to describe self-induced or fabricated illness by an adult in order to gain medical attention (Asher 1951). The name was taken from an eighteenth century military mercenary, Baron Hieronymus Karl Friedrich Freiherr Von Munchausen, who was known for telling fantastical stories of his exploits. Although the term *Munchausen's by proxy* was first used to describe a case of psycho-social dwarfism in 1975 (Money 1976), the first clinical description of the disorder is credited to a British paediatrician, Roy Meadow (Meadow 1977). Dr. Meadow described several cases of children who were repeatedly hospitalized, tested and treated for a variety of medical conditions ultimately found to be fabricated by their mothers.

Since 1977, over 300 professional papers have been published describing many of the manifestations of this bizarre syndrome. In a survey of paediatric gastroenterologists and neurologists (two of the most commonly involved subspecialties in these cases), Schreier & Libow (1993a) found that there were a total of 465 probable cases of MSP amongst 316 of these sub-specialists. As well, 82% of paediatric gastroenterologists responding to the survey reported contact with MSP.

Probably the most difficult aspect of MSP cases is the conscious violation of social norms on the part of the perpetrator, making it all too easy to dupe the physician into willing participation in the actual abuse. Physicians and associated health care workers are trained to take detailed histories from parents, told to believe what mothers report and taught to use this information in arriving at a diagnostic and treatment plan. Health care workers are never taught to suspect that a person who appears to be a deeply-caring parent can in fact be an individual attempting, in a perverse but well-organized way, to cause harm to their child and secondarily to gain a relationship with the health care worker whom the parent sees as a powerful, sought-after parental figure (Schreier & Libow 1994). Mothers with MSP are so good at their charade that a group that arranges surreptitious video recording in a hospital in England recommends not disclosing the plans for video surveillance to the family doctor because he or she may be under the sway of the mother and likely to warn her (Samuels et al 1992).

It is for this very reason (i.e., the inability to see the mother as perpetrator), that it takes a mean of 14.9 months in these cases to unravel the true cause of the child's illness (Rosenberg 1987). It is also why MSP is considered one of the most lethal forms of child abuse, with a reported mortality rate of over 9% (Rosenberg 1987, Schreier & Libow 1993b). Rosenberg (1987) characterized the syndrome using the four defining features in Table 26.1.

Practice and procedures

Although the main obstacle to identifying and treating MSP appears to be the physician's inability to recognize when he is being fooled, the innumerable ways in which MSP can present also create a huge obstacle to

Table 26.1 — Defining features of Munchausen's syndrome by proxy

- Illness in a child that is simulated (faked) or produced by a parent or someone in loco parentis;
- Persistent presentation of the child for medical assessment and care that often results in multiple medical procedures;
- Denial by the parent of knowledge about the cause of the illness;
- Abatement of acute symptoms when the child is separated from the parent.

Table 26.2 — Presenting complaint in cases of Munchausen's syndrome by proxy

Bleeding	44%
Seizures	42%
Central nervous system depression	19%
Apnoea	15%
Diarrhoea	11%
Vomiting	10%
Fever	10%
Rash	9%

From Rosenberg (1987).

rapid identification and treatment. Rosenberg (1987) categorized the cases by presenting complaint (Table 26.2).

In the sense that any and all of these symptoms can be fabricated or induced, it stands to reason why they are the most commonly-reported symptoms in cases of MSP. It can also be inferred from this list that a multitude of nutritional imbalances can be induced, both acutely and chronically, by a person who appears to be an exemplary mother. Nutritionally-relevant signs and symptoms include: abuse dwarfism (Patton & Gardner 1962, Silver & Finkelstein 1967, Money 1976); anorexia (Rogers et al 1976, Fleisher & Ament 1977, Sugar et al 1991); central venous catheter sepsis (Frederick et al 1990, Boros & Brubaker 1992); cystic fibrosis (Orenstein & Wasserman 1986, Single & Henry 1991); dehydration (Ackerman & Strobel 1981, Bauman & Yalow 1981, Chan et al 1986, Alexander et al 1990); diarrhoea (Ackerman & Strobel 1981, Bauman & Yalow 1981, Baugh et al 1983, Chan et al 1986); feculent vomiting (Meadow 1982); failure to thrive (Fenton et al 1988, Sutphen & Saulsbury 1988, Sullivan et al 1991, Lyall et al 1992); feeding difficulties (Stevenson & Alexander 1990, Sullivan et al 1991); food allergy (Meadow 1984, Warner & Hathaway 1984, Kahan & Yorker 1991); glucosuria (Hvizdala & Gellady 1978, Verity et al 1979, Meadow 1982, Nading & Duval-Arnould 1984); hyper-/hypo-natraemia (Rogers et al 1976, Meadow 1977, Chan et al 1986); hypoglycaemia (Pickering 1968, Bauman & Yalow 1981, Mayefsky et al 1982); hypokalaemia (Rogers et al 1976, Chan et al 1986); hypotonia (Berkner et al 1988, Johnson et al 1991); hypochromic microcytic anaemia (Ernst & Philip 1986); lethargy (Bauman & Yalow 1981, Baugh et al 1983, Greene et al 1983); polydipsia (Hvizdala & Gellady 1978, Verity et al 1979); polyphagia (Hvizdala & Gellady 1978); polyuria (Hvizdala & Gellady 1978, Verity et al

1979, Nicol & Eccles 1985, Chan et al 1986); rash (Meadow 1982, Jones 1983); weakness (Rogers et al 1976); and vomiting (Bauman & Yalow 1981, Chan et al 1986, Berkner et al 1988, Colletti & Wasserman 1989, Alexander et al 1990, Baron et al 1995).

In review of the literature on this topic, there is a tendency toward the submission of case reports which are the most bizarre, or in which a specific elucidative test helped differentiate true disease from fictitiously-induced symptoms. In practice, however, there is rarely a 'smoking gun' or single diagnostic clue that confirms the suspicion of fictitiously-induced illness or symptoms. Despite the plethora of these cases, in order to examine specific nutritional abnormalities, it is helpful to separate these cases into four categories. These include: electrolyte disturbances/dehydration; failure to thrive; induced or factitious nutrient losses in stool/urine; and poisonings. Many of the cases in the existing literature cross over more than one of these categories, as the forthcoming case examples demonstrate.

Case one (Meadow 1977)

The third child of healthy parents had recurrent illnesses associated with hypernatraemia since the age of 6 weeks. The attacks came on suddenly, with vomiting and drowsiness, and on arrival to the hospital he had plasma sodium concentrations in the range of 160–175 mmol/L. Urinary sodium was also excessive. The attacks seemed to occur as often as every month, and between attacks he was healthy and developing normally. Extensive investigations in three different centres included radiological, biochemical and other pathological procedures during several hospital admissions. No abnormalities were measured between attacks, and endocrine and renal evaluations were normal. When given a salt load, he excreted it efficiently. The attacks became more frequent and severe, and by the age of 14 months it became clear that they only occurred at home. During a prolonged hospitalization in which the mother was deliberately excluded, they did not happen until the weekend that she was allowed to visit. Investigation proved that the illness must be caused by exogenous salt administration, and the temporal association between attacks and the mother's presence were clearly incriminating. The mother had been a nurse and was presumably experienced in the use of gastric feeding tubes and suppositories.

Unfortunately, while the medical team was planning

arrangements for this child, he arrived at the hospital one night, collapsed with extreme hypernatraemia, and died. Necropsy disclosed mild gastric erosions 'as if a chemical had been ingested'. The mother wrote thanking the doctors for their care and then attempted suicide. The mother was viewed as very caring by the medical staff, whereas her husband was described as undemonstrative. As a student, she had been labelled hysterical, and during one hospital admission, she had been thought to be interfering with the healing of a wound.

This case report appeared in Meadow's defining paper on MSP (1977). It is one of several cases in the literature of fictitiously-induced hypernatraemia, either from administration of exogenous salt or as a result of free-water deprivation (Pickel et al 1970). Meadow (1993) went on to describe the clinical features of 12 children who incurred non-accidental salt poisoning. The children usually presented to the hospital in the first 6 months of life with unexplained hypernatraemia. In four of the children, the serum sodium concentrations were above 200 mmol/L. Seven children had incurred other fabricated illness, drug ingestion, physical abuse and failure to thrive/neglect. Two of these children died and the other 10 remained healthy in alternative care.

There are two main reasons why salt poisoining is primarily a problem in infants and young children (Meadow 1993). First, the immature kidney has limited ability to excrete an excess sodium load. Second, an infant or young pre-ambulatory child can be denied access to water fairly easily.

Short-term signs and symptoms associated with hypernatraemia include irritability, hyper-reflexia, seizures and coma. When infants have died as a result of salt poisoning, necropsy has revealed extensive haemorrhages involving the brain (Walter & Maresch 1987). This has been presumed due to changes in cell volume, tissue shrinkage and tearing of blood vessels. Children who withstand repeated salt poisoning may have an adaptive response, making these haemorrhagic changes in the brain less likely to occur (Meadow 1993). Meadow outlined how to calculate the quantity of salt needed to cause a specific level of hypernatraemia, as well as useful data for diagnosing salt poisoning (Table 26.3).

Case two

The patient presented as a 9-year-old male with chronic diarrhoea and failure to thrive. His parents had

Table 26.3 — Useful calculations in the diagnosis of salt poisoning

1 g of sodium chloride contains 17 mmol of sodium.

One level 5 ml tsp of table salt holds nearly 6 g of salt, that is approximately 100 mmol of sodium.

One level 10 ml dessert spoon holds nearly 12 g of salt, that is approximately 200 mmol of sodium.

The quantity of salt needed to cause a specific level of hypernatraemia can be calculated as follows:
Given an infant weighing 10 kg with a serum sodium of 216 mmol/L, that represents an excess of 216–140 = 76 mmol/L. A 10 kg infant has appoximately 6 L of total body water of which 2.5 L is extracellular fluid. Therefore, the excess sodium is represented by: 76 × 2.5 = 190 mmol; 190 mmol is contained in 190/17 = 11 g of salt (just under 2 tsp).

The usual urine sodium: potassium ratio is 2.8 (range 1.4–5.2).

The usual urine sodium:creatinine ratio is 39.

Gastric aspirate usually contains 50–60 mmol/L of sodium. If concentrations over 200 mmol/L are identified, it is highly suggestive of salt ingestion.

From Meadow (1993).

sought medical attention for him in two other states before presenting to a large teaching hospital in California. The patient reportedly had diarrhoea since infancy, with inability to tolerate most foods. Interestingly, his parents espoused strange stories of his ability to tolerate only certain foods, such as a single brand of canned ham or a particular brand of cookies. They reported that their son could digest foods from a certain hotel breakfast buffet, but short of these restrictions, he had massive diarrhoea whenever he attempted to eat other brands of the same foods or in places other than those specified by his parents.

At 9 years of age, this patient was well below the third centile for height and weight, and weight-for-height was also < the third centile. Sketchy records from the two previous locations were available at the time of presentation, but they indicated extensive testing to uncover the exact aetiology of the diarrhoea and growth failure had been performed, all without an identifying cause. In addition to the growth failure, the child was non-ambulatory (wheelchair bound) and not able to control his bowel movements, consigning him to nappies at the age of 9 years.

Although there was strong suspicion of MSP from the time of initial presentation to our institution, this child had several signs of chronic malnutrition including poor wound healing of cutaneous lesions, cheilosis, coarse but fragile hair, microcytic hypochromic anaemia, and abnormal growth parameters as presented above.

Our immediate plan was to hospitalize this patient for nutritional resuscitation and for further examination for an underlying reason for his chronic diarrhoea and failure to thrive. The family was given a container in which to obtain a quantitative stool collection, which they submitted directly to the attending physician. The stool was checked for reducing substances, quantity of fat, occult blood, and for phenolphthalein as well as magnesium concentration. When the magnesium concentration was found to be substantially-elevated above normal, the suspicion of MSP escalated and the child was placed in protective custody while hospitalization continued.

While hospitalized, the family was limited to supervised visits only, yet the child's diarrhoea persisted. Endoscopic evaluation of the upper and lower digestive tract led to the findings of non-specific colitis with melanosis coli (Fig. 26.1). This is a finding commonly seen in patients with chronic laxative use (Walker et al 1988). Despite a low-residue and then elemental diet, the patient continued to have more than two L of stool output per day, and subsequently required total parenteral nutrition with bowel rest in order to facilitate nutritional repletion and growth. The patient was treated with anti-inflammatory agents including prednisone and sulfasalazine, as well as with immunomodulatory agents such as 6-mercaptopurine and cyclosporine, but his stool output persisted at least two to three times the normal output (greater than 20 g/kg/day) for his weight.

During the prolonged (over three-month) hospitalization, the patient gained weight (over 4 kg) and began to demonstrate some linear growth. Bone age X-rays revealed significantly-delayed skeletal maturation indicative of chronic malnutrition. The patient had marked improvement in his skin and hair texture, began

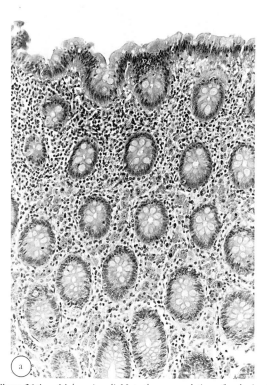
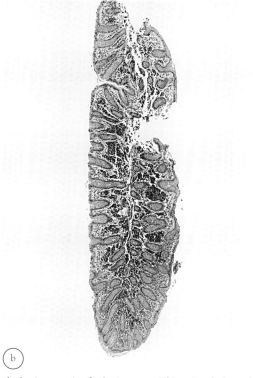

Figure 26.1 — Melanosis coli. Note the accumulation of melanin pigment in the lamina propria of colonic mucosa. This patient had a multi-year history of laxative abuse, both with magnesium-based cathartics and authraquinones.

to ambulate without assistance and was successfully toilet trained during the span of his hospitalization, which was prolonged largely due to legal proceedings and resolution of custody issues. At last notification, this patient continued to thrive in foster care, with accelerated weight and linear growth and improvement in gross motor and some cognitive delays.

This case demonstrates that chronic diarrhoea can be induced, leading to chronic malnutrition and failure to thrive. It also demonstrates that simple separation of the victim from the alleged perpetrators does not always alleviate the symptoms, especially when the abuse has been perpetrated over an extended period of time. In this case, the laxative ingestion led to findings consistent with chronic over-exposure to laxatives and chronic changes in the colonic mucosa, where most of the sodium and water re-absorption occurs. This led to a largely irreversible secretory diarrhoea (evidenced by continued high output from the colon even when the patient was restricted from all food and liquid, and supported only with intravenous nutrition).

Fine et al (1991) established a method for diagnosing magnesium-induced diarrhoea using quantitative faecal analysis for soluble magnesium. The upper limits of faecal output of soluble magnesium and faecal magnesium concentration in normal adult subjects were 14.6 mmol/day and 45.2 mmol/L, respectively. When normal subjects had diarrhoea due to the ingestion of magnesium hydroxide alone or in combination with phenolpthalein, faecal magnesium output was always abnormally high. For each mmol increase in faecal magnesium output, faecal weight increased by approximately 7.3 g. The faecal magnesium concentration was very high when magnesium was the only cause of diarrhoea, but only moderately elevated when diarrhoea was induced by magnesium hydroxide plus phenolpthalein. Thus, stool magnesium quantification can play an important role in the evaluation of chronic diarrhoea of unclear aetiology.

In our patient, the nutritional abnormalities found that could be directly caused by induction of chronic diarrhoea included: hypoproteinaemia; zinc deficiency; selenium deficiency; iron deficiency; and fat-soluble vitamin deficiency (specifically vitamin E and vitamin A were measurably low, with indirect evidence of Vitamin K deficiency noted with prolonged prothrombin time and partial thromboplastin times prior to initiation of parenteral vitamin supplementation). All of these abnormalities were corrected by the time of hospital discharge.

Many other authors have reported cases of MSP in which induction of chronic diarrhoea and subsequent failure to thrive was noted (Fleisher & Ament 1977, Ackerman & Strobel 1981, Sugar et al 1991, Gray & Bentovim 1996). Most of these reports include the findings of phenolphthalein in the stool. Gray & Bentovim (1996) reviewed an extensive group of cases in which the patients failed to thrive, largely due to purposeful withholding of food (ten children) or due to alleged food allergies to many different food stuffs (five children). In these cases, it becomes imperative to hospitalize the patient and perform feeding challenges under close scrutiny, without any interference from the parent. The authors point to a case from their series in which a mother was actually caught on video surveillance disposing of her child's hospital meals, later causing the consultant to puzzle over how the patient could be failing to thrive with adequate caloric intake.

These examples illustrate that failure to thrive may be factitiously induced by administration of cathartics (or even appetite suppressants), emetogenic agents (see *Case four*) or simply by purposefully-withholding food.

Case three (Orenstein & Wasserman 1986)

One of the ways in which a parent can fabricate medical illness in a child is by tampering with specimens of urine/stool/sputum or any body effluent, as this case demonstrates.

This is a case of a 5.5-year-old boy first seen in a cystic fibrosis (CF) centre at the insistence of his mother, who claimed to be a nurse. The mother reported that the child had been diagnosed at 5 months of age with CF when a sweat chloride concentration was said to be 95 mEq/L (normal < 40 mEq/L). The patient presented at age 5.5 years due to reported coughing spells with apnoea and choking on thick mucous. Despite repeated attempts, medical records from other institutions were not obtained.

The patient's physical findings initially included a non-productive cough, mild increase in anterior-posterior diameter of the chest, moderate digital clubbing, and weight and height both well below the third centile. A chest X-ray revealed moderate hyper-inflation and right lower lobe atelectasis. The mother would not permit a repeat sweat chloride test, and the physicians agreed to treat the child 'as though he had CF'.

Multiple hospitalizations ensued with the mother

typically at bedside 24 h a day, often taking responsibility for administering the child's medications. During one hospitalization an attempt at obtaining a fully-supervised sweat sample resulted in the mother suddenly announcing that the child had to go to the bathroom. Sputum samples obtained from this child typically revealed normal flora, although on one occasion, *Pseudomonas aeruginosa*, a typical CF-associated pathogen grew from the child's sputum. Bronchoscopy was performed after about 20 months of care, revealing essentially normal findings with only *Haemophilus influenzae* sensitive to ampicillin retrieved. When confronted with these findings, the mother quickly began experiencing her own set of symptoms including vertigo and vomiting. She warned her son's physicians that discharge home without parenteral antibiotics would result in rapid recurrence of illness. Sure enough, repeat admission for persistent cough and post-tussive emesis occurred within 2 days of hospital discharge.

In the meantime, the hospital bacteriology lab received a phone call from a woman claiming to be a medical student who had been in the laboratory the preceding week with a classmate who she said switched this child's culture plates (which she said had shown *Haemophilus*, *Klebsiella*, and *Pseudomonas*) with plates he had in his pocket. She espoused that she had heard the boy was being re-admitted and therefore called because 'it might make a difference' in his care.

Upon re-admission, the mother questioned the continued use of oral antibiotics alone, and submitted a 72-h stool collection for fat, which showed 22 g of fat/24 h (normal = 7 g/24 h).

The mother was then said to have called the local CF foundation, falsely identifying herself as a mother of a hospitalized infant with newly-diagnosed CF who wanted the names of other families, so she could learn more about the disease. She then contacted one of these families and set up a meeting with a teenager with CF in the hospital parking lot, stating that she was a pharmacy student who needed a sputum sample for research.

The medical team was tipped off by the CF foundation when they found that the address and the phone number left by the woman was non-existent and that no newly diagnosed infant with CF existed in the hospital at that time. The Department of Human Services was contacted and a court order was obtained to place the child in protective custody after the mother submitted the sputum specimen of the teenager

with CF as if it came from her own son and after the CF-afflicted teenager accurately identified the patient's mother as being the 'pharmacy student' to whom he had submitted his sputum sample.

Upon elimination of the mother from the hospital, all medications were stopped and vomiting ceased within hours. Repeat sweat chloride samples showed normal concentrations of 13 and 14 mEq/L. Stool collection for fat quantification was also normal at 3.5 g/24 h, and the patient began to gain weight at an accelerated pace. After a 6-month foster-care placement in his grandparents' home, the child (against medical advice) was returned to the parents, who subsequently moved and could no longer be located by the Department of Human Services.

This case demonstrates the tenacious ability of an MSP mother to falsify laboratory samples in order to make the biochemical results consistent with a particular disease. The mother surreptitiously made her child appear to have chronic fat malabsorption, recurrent bacterial pneumonia with organisms typically seen in CF patients, and failure to thrive allegedly due to poor eating/vomiting/malabsorption, but later found to be due to withholding of food and falsification of stool samples. The child's body habitus, by the time he presented to the authors at age 5.5 years, was consistent with CF, but in fact was due to a completely different problem.

Although specific nutritional deficiencies were not outlined by the authors in this case, it can be inferred that some did exist given the growth parameters and chronic under-feeding that this child experienced. In sharp contrast to this case is a report from Single & Henry (1991) of an 11-year-old boy who was brought to a CF clinic at the insistence of his father, with a history compatible with CF but an exam revealing a surprisingly healthy boy. A third case report (Conway & Pond 1995) describes a girl who was mistakenly diagnosed with CF at 2 years of age, at the insistence of her mother. This child later grew up to become an adult with Munchausen's syndrome, no longer dependent on her mother to present her for unnecessary medical tests and intervention. Although specific nutritional deficiencies are not outlined in either of these reports, the latter (like the patient presented in case three) had poor weight gain except when under the care of someone other than her mother.

Other ways in which bodily fluids have been altered in order to simulate disease include: the injection of faeces and foodstuffs into the bladder in order to contaminate the urine (Reich et al 1977, Lyall et al 1992); covertly submitting glucose-containing urine in place of a child's urine, thus simulating diabetes mellitus (Nading & Duval-Arnould 1984); and addition of blood or other materials to the stool or nappy of an infant or child (Fleisher & Ament 1977).

Case four (Schneider et al 1996)

In addition to salt-poisoning, failure to thrive, and covert tampering with laboratory specimens, parents with MSP can induce specific nutritional deficiencies and dysfunction by chronically poisoning their children covertly, as is demonstrated in this case.

An almost 4-year-old boy was admitted with a 3-week history of vomiting and diarrhoea occurring 4–8 times daily. The past medical history was notable for extensive medical attention for a variety of reported problems since birth, the most significant of which was vomiting. This had prompted contrast radiography, endoscopy, and at least six hospital admissions between 6 months and 2 years of age. Eventually, a nasojejunal feeding tube was placed, followed by a percutaneous gastro-jejunal feeding tube for feedings, yet the vomiting persisted.

Other evaluations included endocrine and orthopaedic consultations for leg pains, legs 'giving out,' and lethargy. Although several medical staff members noted discrepancies in the mother's history and more than one consultant suggested a non-organic basis for this child's problems, the problems persisted up to this admission.

During the admission, the patient underwent initial intravenous rehydration, then gradual re-introduction of enteral feedings, as well as parenteral nutritional support. On the fifth hospital day, the patient became tachypnic, tachycardic and hypotensive. While resuscitative efforts were instituted, the QRS complex widened on the cardiac rhythm tracing with a gradual drop in heart rate from 180 bpm to 55 bpm. Resuscitative efforts continued, but the patient died.

Necropsy revealed an emaciated boy with weight of only 30 pounds and length of 39.5 inches. Internal organs were normal except the heart, which had a globoid configuration due to biventricular dilatation. Light microscopy of the cardiac muscle revealed focal areas of myofibrillar degeneration, and electron microscopy revealed changes in the myocardium characteristic of emetine toxicity. A post-mortem blood sample revealed an emetine level of 845 ng/ml

and a cephaeline level of 1200 ng/ml. The mother subsequently admitted to administration of ipecac when confronted by the authorities after the post-mortem examination.

This case again represents the high potential for morbidity and mortality in MSP. In a review of the epidemiology of MSP, McClure et al (1996) found 44 children poisoned with a total of 38 different agents over a 2-year prospective study. Anticonvulsants were the most commonly employed poisons in their review.

The cascade of events in this case included the recognition of under-nutrition with poor growth parameters, but never the underlying cause. Because ipecac constituents accumulate in the kidneys, their detection in the urine is facilitated weeks after the administration of the drug, a time when serum samples may be negative (Day et al 1989). Complicating the detection of this problem even further is the fact that most laboratories do not systematically evaluate serum or urine samples for ipecac alkaloids as part of their standard toxicology screens. Thus, the ordering physician must already have a suspicion of ipecac poisoning so that he can indicate specific testing for these substances.

Because of the chronic vomiting induced by this form of poisoning, electrolyte disturbances such as hypokalaemia and metabolic alkolosis are possible findings. However, the emetine component of ipecac induces diarrhoea by increasing peristalsis and is felt to be primarily responsible for cardiac and neuromuscular toxicity (Johnson et al 1991). The recurrent diarrhoea in patients like the one presented in case four make them subject to potential deficiencies in trace minerals (e.g., Zinc, Selenium) and essential fatty acids, as well as to hypoproteinaemia due to an induced protein-losing enteropathy. Because of chronic bicarbonate loss in the stool, metabolic acidosis is possible but when vomiting and diarrhoea are present, the serum pH may be remarkably normal. Haemorrhagic colitis and pseudomelanosis coli has also been described in chronic ipecac poisoning (Johnson et al 1991).

In reversing the nutritional deficiencies caused by MSP, the first rule of thumb is to simply suspect the diagnosis. This should then allow for a systematic approach to diagnosis and treatment. In that a larger percentage of patients suffering at the hands of a parent with MSP improve their symptoms when separated from the perpetrator, an effort should be made to arrange this separation, which may require legal intervention.

Once the separation has been established, initial efforts at nutritional repletion should take place, either enterally with oral or tube feeding or parenterally if initial symptoms exist that preclude use of the digestive tract. For example, in a patient with a reported history of chronic intestinal pseudo-obstruction that resulted in central venous catheter placement for parenteral nutrition, full micro- and macronutrient support should begin intravenously, followed by rapid transition to enteral nutrition as soon as tolerated in a supervised setting (Baron et al 1995). Once enteral nutrition is fully provided, removal of unnecessary routes of nutrition support (e.g., central venous catheter, gastrostomy tube) should quickly follow. Sufficient time in the confines of the supervised setting must be allowed in order to demonstrate both consistent tolerance of feeding and accelerated weight gain. Despite the usual absence of laboratory proof of induced malnutrition in most cases, demonstration of ability to tolerate feedings previously reported by the parent as intolerable and appropriate or even supra-normal weight gain in a supervised hospital setting are usually required to effect legal separation of the child victim from the perpetrating parent.

Specific deficiencies in visceral protein, trace elements, and vitamins should be documented immediately upon presentation, and follow-up measurement of these substances should document normalization within the expected time frame. For example, hypo-albuminaemia secondary to factitiously-induced diarrhoea may take several weeks to correct with appropriate nutritional support, and thus it would not be expected that an initially low serum albumin level be completely normalized during the course of a 1–2 week hospitalization.

It should be noted that, as in case two, separation from the suspected perpetrator and appropriate treatment do not always completely reverse the chronic effects of the abuse. This patient continued to have excessive stool volume (albeit improved) beyond the point of hospital discharge to foster care. Continued medical therapy as well as nutritional support may be required beyond the confines of the hospital.

Discussion

In the cases summarized above, examples of four types of presentations of MSP have been presented. These have been separated into electrolyte disturbances, failure to thrive, body fluid specimen alteration, and

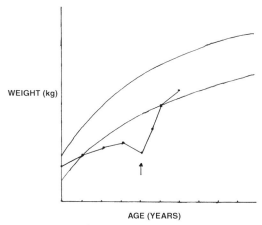

Figure 26.2 — Growth curve in a patient with failure to thrive due to Munchausen's syndrome by proxy. This composite represents a typical pattern in MSP, with gradual drop off of weight percentile, then rapid weight acceleration upon separation (arrow) of the child from the perpetrating parent.

poisoning, because the more than 300 case reports on this subject lend themselves to classification in at least one of these four categories. However, similarities between these cases quickly blur any discrete boundaries between this system of classification. For example, the primary nutritional deficiencies reported in cases two, three and four were simply failure to thrive. Similarly, while case four was chosen as a classic example of poisoning, cases one and two can be highlighted as examples of poisoning as well. Thus, the distinction between 'types' of cases is at best meant to be a convenient way in which to discuss nutritional deficiencies in MSP. Because this disorder has been classically documented in case reports only, specific nutritional deficiencies are usually not documented due to limitations in space afforded by peer-reviewed journals for these types of articles. Future reports, such as that of Johnson et al (1991) should be prospective, with more time spent on the specific morbidity incurred in these children.

A misconception that physicians and especially the judiciary and child protective service workers maintain is the concept that a 'smoking gun' must be found in order to implicate the perpetrator. The cases presented here all have the common thread of a specific laboratory study that confirmed the diagnosis (two unfortunately post-mortem). However, this is generally not the case in medical practice, and most other MSP cases are not resolved medically or legally by such concrete and conclusive evidence (Schreier & Libow 1993b).

Figure 26.2 represents a composite growth curve, which could be representative of a multitude of MSP cases, including cases two, three, and four presented above. Of specific import is the discrepant weight-for-age, weight-for-height, and subsequent accelerated weight gain upon removal of the patient from the custody of the perpetrator.

In summary, MSP represents a bizarre form of child abuse. It often leads to failure to thrive and nutritional deficiencies, which directly result from withholding of appropriate nutrition or willful poisoning of the child by a parent (usually the mother) suffering from a psychiatric disturbance. Since its initial description 20 years ago, much has been learned as to the characteristics of the disorder, yet it continues to be a very lethal form of child abuse. Its prevention depends on further education of health care professionals and judicial authorities as to its nature and potentially devastating effects.

Acknowledgements

I would like to thank Dr. Edith Marley, Chief of Paediatric Pathology at Sunrise Children's Hospital, for providing the example of melanosis coli. Special thanks to Ms. Cecelia Hendricks for her assistance in the preparation of this manuscript, and to Dr. Marvin Ament for mentoring me in many cases involving this compelling diagnosis.

References

Ackerman, N.B., Strobel, C.T. (1981) Polle syndrome: Chronic diarrhea in Munchausen's child. *Gastro*, 81, 1140–1142.

Alexander, R., Smith, W., Stevenson, R. (1990) Serial Munchausen syndrome by proxy. *Pediatrics*, 86, 581–584.

Asher, R. (1951) Munchausen's syndrome. *Lancet*, i, 339–341.

Baron, H.I., Beck, D.C., Vargas, J.H., Ament, M.E. (1995) Over-interpretation of gastroduodenal motility studies: Two cases involving Munchausen syndrome by proxy. *J Pediatr*, 126, 397–400.

Baugh, J.R., Krug, E.F., Meir, M.R. (1983) Punishment by salt poisoning. *Southern Med J*, 76, 540–541.

Bauman, W.A., Yalow, R.S. (1981) Child abuse: Parenteral insulin administration. *J Pediatr*, 99, 588–591.

Berkner, P., Kastner, T., Skolnick, L. (1988) Chronic ipecac poisoning in infancy: A case report. *Pediatrics*, 82, 384–386.

Boros, S.J., Brubaker, L.C. (1992) Munchausen syndrome by proxy case accounts. *FBI Law Enforcement Bullletin*, 61, 16–20.

Chan, D.A., Salcedo, J.R., Atkins, D.M., Ruley, E.J. (1986) Munchausen syndrome by proxy: A review and case study. *J Pediatr Psychol*, 11, 71–80.

Colletti, R.B., Wasserman, R.C. (1989) Recurrent infantile vomiting due to intentional ipecac poisoning. *J Ped Gastro Nut*, 8, 394–396.

Conway, S.P., Pond, M.N. (1995) Munchausen syndrome by proxy abuse: A foundation for adult Munchausen syndrome. *Aust NZJ Psych*, 29, 504–507.

Day, L., Kelly, C., Reed, G., Andersen, J.M., Keljo, J.M. (1989) Fatal cardiomyopathy: Suspected child abuse by chronic ipecac administration. *Vet Hum Toxicol*, 31, 255–257.

Ernst, T.N., Philip, M. (1986) Severe iron deficiency anemia. An example of covert child abuse (Munchausen by proxy). *Western J Med*, 144, 358–359.

Fenton, A.C., Wailoo, M.P., Tanner, M.S. (1988) Severe failure to thrive and diarrhea caused by laxative abuse. *Arch Dis Child*, 63, 978–979.

Fine, K.D., Santa Ana, C.A., Fordtran, J.S. (1991) Diagnosis of magnesium-induced diarrhea. *N Engl J Med*, 324, 1012–1017.

Fleisher, D., Ament, M.E. (1977) Diarrhea, red diapers, and child abuse. *Clin Pediatr*, 17, 820–824.

Frederick, V., Luedtke, G.S., Barrett, F.F., Hixson, S.D., Burch, K. (1990) Munchausen syndrome by proxy: Recurrent central catheter sepsis. *Ped Inf Dis J*, 9, 440–442.

Gray, J., Bentovim, A. (1996) Illness induction syndrome: Paper I-A series of 41 children from 37 families identified at the Great Ormond Street Hospital for Children NHS Trust. *Child Abuse Negl*, 20, 655–673.

Greene, J.W., Craft, L.T., Ghishan, F. (1983) Acetaminophen poisoning in infancy. *Am J Dis Child*, 137, 386–387.

Hvizdala, E.V., Gellady, A.M. (1978) Intentional poisoning of two siblings by prescription drugs. *Clin Pediatr*, 17, 480–482.

Johnson, J.E., Carpenter, B.L.M., Benton, J., Cross, R., Eaton, L.A., Rhoads, J.M. (1991) Hemorrhagic colitis and pseudomelanosis coli in ipecac ingestion by proxy. *J Ped Gastro Nut*, 12, 501–506.

Jones, D.P.H. (1983) Dermatitis artefacta in mother and baby as child abuse. *Br J Psych*, 143, 199–200.

Kahan, B.B., Yorker, B.C. (1991) Munchausen syndrome by proxy: Clinical review and legal issues. *Behavioral Sciences and the Law*, 9, 73–83.

Lyall, E.G., Stirling, H.F., Crofton, P.M., Kelnar, C.J. (1992)

Albuminuria growth failure. A case of Munchausen syndrome by proxy. *Acta Paediatrica*, 81, 373–376.

McClure, R.J., Davis, P.M., Meadow, S.R., Sibert, J.R. (1996) Epidemiology of Munchausen syndrome by proxy, non-accidental poisoning, and non-accidental suffocation. *Arch Dis Child*, 75, 57–61.

Mayefsky, J.H., Sarnaik, A.P., Postellon, D.C. (1982) Factitious hypoglycemia. *Pediatrics*, 69, 804–805.

Meadow, R. (1977) Munchausen syndrome by proxy: The hinterland of child abuse. *Lancet*, ii, 343–345.

Meadow, R. (1982) Munchausen syndrome by proxy. *Arch Dis Child*, 57, 92–98.

Meadow, R. (1984) Fictitious epilepsy. *Lancet*, ii, 25–28.

Meadow, R. (1993) Non-accidental salt poisoning. *Arch Dis Child*, 68, 448–452.

Money, J. (1976) The syndrome of abuse dwarfism (psycho-social dwarfism or reversible hyposomatotropism). *Am J Dis Child*, 131, 508–513.

Nading, J.H., Duval-Arnould, B. (1984) Factitious diabetes mellitus confirmed by ascorbic acid. *Arch Dis Child*, 59, 166–167.

Nicol, A.R., Eccles, M. (1985) Psychotherapy for Munchausen syndrome by proxy. *Arch Dis Child*, 60, 344–348.

Orenstein, D.M., Wasserman, A.L. (1986) Munchausen syndrome by proxy simulating cystic fibrosis. *Pediatrics*, 78, 621–624.

Patton, R.G., Gardner, L.I. (1962) Influence of family environment on growth: The syndrome of 'maternal deprivation'. *Pediatrics*, 70, 957–962.

Pickel, S., Anderson, C., Holliday, M.A. (1970) Thirsting and hypernatremic dehydration – a form of child abuse. *Pediatrics*, 45, 54–59.

Pickering, D. (1968) Neonatal hypoglycemia due to salicylate poisoning. *Proceeding of the Royal Society of Medicine*, 61, 1256.

Reich, P., Lazarus, J.M., Kelly, M.J., Rogers, M.P. (1977) Factitious feculent urine in an adolescent boy. *JAMA*, 238, 420–421.

Rogers, D., Tripp, J., Bentovim, A., Robinson, A., Berry, D., Goulding, R. (1976) Non-accidental poisoning: An extended syndrome of child abuse. *Br Med J*, 1, 793–796.

Rosenberg, D. (1987) Web of deceit: A literature review of Munchausen syndrome by proxy. *Child Abuse Negl*, 11, 547–563.

Samuels, M.P., McClaughlin, W., Jacobson, R.R., Poets, C.F., Southall, D.P. (1992) Fourteen cases of imposed upper airway obstruction. *Arch Dis Child*, 67, 162–170.

Schneider, D.S., Perez, A., Knilans, T.E., Daniels, S.R., Bove, K.E., Bonnell, H. (1996) Clinical and pathological aspects of cardiomyopathy from ipecac administration in Munchausen's syndrome by proxy. *Pediatrics*, 97, 902–906.

Schreier, H.A., Libow, J.A. (1993a) Munchausen syndrome by proxy: Diagnosis and prevalence. *Am J Orthopsychiatry*, 63, 318–321.

Schreier, H.A., Libow, J.A. (1993b) Hurting for Love: Munchausen by proxy syndrome. New York: The Guilford Press.

Schreier, H.A., Libow, J.A. (1994) Munchausen by proxy syndrome: A modern pediatric challenge. *J Pediatr*, 125, S110–115.

Silver, H.K., Finkelstein, M. (1967) Deprivation dwarfism. *J Pediatr*, 70, 317–324.

Single, T., Henry, R.L. (1991) An unusual case of Munchausen syndrome by proxy. *Aust N Z J Psych*, 25, 422–425.

Stevenson, R., Alexander, R. (1990) Munchausen syndrome by proxy presenting as developmental disability. *J Developmental and Behavioral Pediatr*, 11, 262–264.

Sugar, J.A., Belfer, M., Isreal, E., Herzog, D.B. (1991) A 3-year-old boy's chronic diarrhea and unexplained death. *J Am Acad Child Adol Psych*, 30, 1015–1021.

Sullivan, C.A., Francis, G.L., Bain, M.W., Hartz, J. (1991) Munchausen syndrome by proxy: 1990. A portent for problems? *Clin Pediatr*, 30, 112–116.

Sutphen, J.L., Saulsbury, F. (1988) Intentional ipecac poisoning: Munchausen syndrome by proxy. *Pediatrics*, 82, 453–456.

Verity, C.M., Winckworth, C., Burman, D. (1979) Polle syndrome: Children of Munchausen. *Br Med J*, 2, 422–423.

Walker, N.I., Bennett, R.E., Axelsen, R.A. (1988) Melanosis coli: A consequence of anthraquinone-induced apoptosis of colonic epithelia cells. *Am J Pathol*, 131, 465–476.

Walter, G.F., Maresch, W. (1987) Accidental saline poisoning in newborn infants. Morphologic findings and pathogenetic discussion. *Klin Padiatr*, 199, 269–273.

Warner, J.O., Hathaway, M.J. (1984) Allergic form of Meadow's syndrome (Munchausen by proxy). *Arch Dis Child*, 59, 151–156.

27

Nutrition after small intestinal transplantation

Philip E. Putnam and Samuel A. Kocoshis

Introduction

Small intestinal transplantation has become a reality for adults and children with irreversible intestinal failure. More than 25 centres internationally have developed programmes for intestinal replacement over the past decade, and have transplanted more than 200 individuals. Tacrolimus, an immunosuppressive agent 100 times more potent than its predecessor, cyclosporine A, has contributed greatly to the success of these programmes. A 1-year survival of 75% and a 5-year survival of 50% can now be expected.

Intestinal failure implies total parenteral nutrition (TPN) dependence due to the inability of the small intestine to digest and absorb sufficient nutrients to support the individual. To qualify for intestinal transplantation, candidates must have irreversible intestinal failure and at least one serious complication of its management, such as TPN-induced liver failure or impending loss of central venous access due to multiple thromboses or repeated infection. Many children referred for transplantation suffer from short-gut syndrome because of disorders such as necrotizing enterocolitis or midgut volvulus, which have resulted in massive bowel resection. Other paediatric patients who experience intestinal failure caused by disorders such as microvillous inclusion disease or chronic intestinal pseudo-obstruction also may require intestinal transplantation. In contrast, the principal cause of intestinal failure in adults referred for transplantation has been short-bowel syndrome after resection for vascular accidents, thromboses or Crohn's disease.

Intestinal transplantation can only be considered successful if it permits the initiation or restoration of enteral feeding and sustenance of the individual via the oral route, suspension of the need for central venous access and TPN, and recovery of full digestive function of the allograft. These goals are achievable, but numerous impediments after transplantation can frustrate their accomplishment.

Although animal studies have rigorously characterized intestinal function following transplantation, few human studies have been published to date. The animal studies have been useful in predicting human intestinal recovery, but have been done in a highly-controlled fashion (e.g., auto-transplantation or with isolated loops not contributing to the nutritional support of the subject) that may eliminate clinically-relevant phenomena such as rejection. This chapter examines current concepts of post-transplant nutrition and intestinal function from a clinical perspective.

Variables affecting intestinal function

Many variables affect post-transplant intestinal function. Amongst these are pre-transplant intestinal injury caused by donor illness or haemodynamic compromise; time of assessment from transplantation; concurrent medication used during assessment; presence and severity of rejection; preservation of intestinal motility; and the recovery and integrity of enterocytes, extrinsic innervation and intestinal lymphatics after transplantation.

Transplantation

Removing the intestine from the donor necessarily disrupts the blood supply, extrinsic nerves and intestinal lymphatics. The allograft may then be subjected to ischaemia and cold for several hours before placement within the recipient. Cold ischaemia and reperfusion injury might be expected to affect sensitive aspects of allograft mucosal function. Transient changes in water and electrolyte absorption have been described in animals, but no significant permanent deficits in either of these have been demonstrated to date (Sigalet et al 1992, Teitelbaum et al 1993, Oishi & Sarr 1995). At the same time, the metabolic needs of an intestine undergoing cold ischaemia are substantial and glutamine metabolism may be increased for weeks following transplantation. A stressed, marginally-nourished organ recipient might theoretically be unable to mobilize glutamine in satisfactory quantities to keep up with metabolic demands (Nemoto et al 1996). At the same time, allograft mucosal disaccharidase levels appear to be unaffected by transplantation (Sarr et al 1996).

The blood supply to the allograft is restored by anastomosis with the recipient vascular system at transplantation, but there is no surgical reconnection of neurons or lymphatics. The gut's complex intrinsic nervous system affords primary control over many intestinal functions, and integration of intestinal activity into the needs of the normal individual is modulated by the central nervous system via the parasympathetic and sympathetic nerves (the extrinsic innervation). The absence of extrinsic innervation affects, but does not ablate, primary functions such as absorption and motility (Sigalet et al 1992, Sarr et al 1994, Oishi & Sarr 1995, Behrns et al 1996). Changes in gut function may also result from alterations in neurohormonal mediators such as neuropeptide Y, which is decreased after sympathectomy (Sarr et al

1996). Post-transplant re-innervation of the gut has been demonstrated, although the degree to which it affords resumption of normal function is unknown (Liu et al 1992, Kiyochi et al 1994).

Lymphatics are required to transport fat in the form of chylomicrons from the intestine to the systemic circulation. In addition, extravascular fluid and lymphocytes return to the circulation within intestinal lymphatics. Surgical division of the lymphatics at transplantation leads to only transient steatorrhoea and protein loss, as their recovery and in-growth does seem to occur within weeks to months of transplantation (Liu et al 1992). Notably, processing of bacteria that have translocated across the mucosal barrier is compromised until lymphatic regeneration has restored continuity with mesenteric lymph nodes. The risk for sepsis and endotoxaemia is then heightened.

Rejection

Rejection of the allograft has many potential implications for nutrition. Severe exfoliative rejection leaves the allograft totally denuded of its absorptive epithelium. Enteral nutrition then must be avoided and TPN is resumed, sometimes for extended periods. Mucosal recovery can occur after exfoliative rejection, but with a very high cost (Sigurdsson et al 1996). Although TPN supports the nutritional needs of the patient, the need for continued central venous access mimics pre-transplant challenges. The risks of bacterial sepsis or opportunistic fungal or viral infections are increased due to the intense immunosuppression required to manage the rejection.

Despite the ability of exfoliated bowel to regenerate epithelium, subepithelial fibrosis appears to be long lived, leading to severe hypomotility and resultant bacterial overgrowth syndrome with its concomitant carbohydrate malabsorption, steatorrhoea and creatorrhoea.

Lesser degrees of rejection may not prohibit use of the allograft, but abdominal pain, anorexia, or ileus diminish oral intake. Rapid transit and epithelial injury impair digestion and absorption of nutrients, and lead to diarrhoea.

Motility

Rapid transit frequently develops after SBTx. The allograft usually retains inherent phasic fasting motor activity, but co-ordination of contractions with the native stomach and duodenum across the proximal anastomosis is unusual. Isolated intestinal allografts often do not develop a 'fed' pattern in the post-prandial state (Mousa et al 1998). Migrating myoelectric complexes commonly persist throughout the post-prandial period. Subsequent rapid transit contributes to diarrhoea and malabsorption, and may be managed with loperamide, opiates, or clonidine, with variable efficacy.

Infection

Intestinal infections are common after small intestinal transplantation as a consequence of immunosuppression. Viruses (e.g., cytomegalovirus, Epstein-Barr virus, adenovirus, rotavirus, etc.), bacteria or parasites can infect the allograft, residual native bowel, or both. Fever, diarrhoea, vomiting, gastrointestinal bleeding and abdominal pain can indicate infection, but clinicians should recognize these are also signs and symptoms of rejection. Suspension or alteration of enteral nutrition may be required during acute infectious illnesses until the infection-induced ileus or enteritis resolves.

Practice and procedures

Providing nutrition after small intestinal transplantation

The transition from TPN dependence to complete enteral nutrition varies from patient to patient, and the patient's overall nutritional state is affected by host variables in addition to the allograft factors discussed above. For example, nutrient intake is influenced by time to recover from surgery, appetite, lingering effects of abnormal pre-transplant feeding behaviour, and the presence of intercurrent illness.

All patients continue to receive TPN in the immediate post-transplant period until sufficient recovery from the surgery is achieved. At the time of transplantation, a gastrostomy and/or jejunostomy tube is placed. Tube feedings are usually required, and are begun when there is evidence for anastomotic integrity and resumption of graft motility (16 $\pm$ 10 days) (Abu-Elmagd et al 1994). Weaning from TPN is initiated when approximately 50% of calories can be tolerated by means of enteral infusion (Nour et al 1994). TPN is weaned as tube feeding is increased commensurate with patient tolerance. The time required to discontinue TPN has varied from 18–210 days (Abu-Elmagd et al 1994).

A low-fat elemental formula containing glutamine (e.g., Pediatric Vivonex, Sandoz Nutrition Corp, Minneapolis, MN) is often used as the initial enteral feeding source because of the recently-transplanted allograft's increased metabolic needs and preferential glutamine uptake and utilization. Another advantage of Pediatric Vivonex is its low-fat content, which circumvents the impaired fat transport from the bowel engendered by the disruption of lymphatics at the time of transplant. However, patients without a functioning colon may develop diarrhoea with rapid infusions, as the osmolarity of this formula is quite high. After a few weeks, when the lymphatic connections have been established, an isotonic enteral formula containing partially-hydrolysed protein and medium chain triglycerides (e.g., Peptamen, Clintec Nutrition Co., Deerfield, IL) is commonly employed.

Oral intake is permitted, but its acceptance is highly variable. Some children with extreme short-gut syndrome who never received substantive oral intake pre-operatively refuse to feed orally for extended periods after transplant and require formal behaviour modification therapy to attain more normal oral feeding (Cohen et al 1992). An oral diet appropriate for age is offered, with modifications made depending on patient tolerance and graft function.

An ileostomy is created in virtually all patients at transplantation, which facilitates endoscopy with biopsy for gross and histological monitoring of allograft health. The ileostomy also allows careful monitoring of stool outputs. Unfortunately, bypassing the colon and its efficient water and electrolyte absorptive capability permits large quantities of obligate electrolyte and fluid losses seen in other patients with an end ileostomy. The clinician should be cognisant that in the early post-operative weeks, losses of not only sodium and potassium but also calcium, magnesium, and trace elements such as zinc, are copious. Fluid and electrolyte balance is maintained with enteral (i.e., via tube) or intravenous solutions on an individual basis. These supplements are usually temporary, and become unnecessary when intestinal continuity is restored by closure of the ileostomy, which occurs several months after transplantation when the need for frequent endoscopic monitoring dwindles.

In addition, bypassing the colon prevents colonocyte recovery of energy derived from fermentation of malabsorbed carbohydrate to short-chain fatty acids. Butyrate, and to a lesser extent acetate and propionate, are used preferentially as an energy source by colonic epithelium, and their reclamation is important in

the efficient utilization of calories by the intestine (Roediger 1980).

Monitoring of nutritional status

Intake of specific dietary components including fat, carbohydrate, protein, fluid and electrolytes, can be measured as for other patients. Traditional anthropometric parameters such as height, weight, weight-for-height, body-mass index, triceps-skin-fold thickness, and mid-arm muscle circumference must be followed after small intestinal transplantation. Measurement of albumin and other serum proteins such as pre-albumin and retinol binding protein reflect protein nutriture. It must be recognized, however, that decreased serum proteins may reflect loss from the intestine (e.g., prior to lymphatic recovery or during rejection) rather than poor intake. In selected cases, nitrogen balance studies may be helpful as is determination of basal metabolic rate by means of the metabolic cart. More sophisticated techniques such as bioelectric impedance have not been employed routinely by most large transplant centres.

Monitoring of small intestinal function by non-invasive means is possible if somewhat difficult. D–xylose absorption provides basic information regarding mucosal integrity, but is influenced by a number of variables. Normally, the test is performed by delivering a standardized dose of D–xylose to the stomach with subsequent measurement of peripheral blood D–xylose level. After transplantation, the peak serum level may be missed if gastric emptying is abnormal or intestinal transit is accelerated. Frequent assays (e.g., at 20 minute intervals) or 5-h urine recovery may provide more information.

Mucosal disaccharidase activity can be assayed from biopsy material obtained at endoscopy. Enzyme levels should correlate with allograft carbohydrate absorptive function, and may provide evidence for mucosal recovery after severe exfoliative rejection (Kaufman et al 1996a, 1996b).

Fat balance as measured by comparison of 72-h faecal fat excretion with oral intake may be technically feasible in continent older patients and those with ileostomies, but diarrhoea in nappies usually results in failure to collect the total stool output, limiting the utility of this test in toddlers whose stoma has been closed. Multiple variables affect fat balance, including intestinal transit, lymphatic integrity, exocrine pancreatic function and rejection. Because most patients are receiving a mixture of long- and medium-chain triglycerides, to obtain the most reliable measure of fat balance in the laboratory the Jeejeebhoy method for measurement of faecal fat must be employed rather than the Van de Kamer assay (Caliari et al 1996). The solvent system employed in the Van de Kamer method fails to extract efficiently medium-chain triglycerides, leading to under-estimation of their excretion, whereas the Jeejeebhoy method extracts and detects both long- and medium-chain triglycerides.

Outcome of intestinal transplantation

Intestinal transplantation offers recipients the opportunity to resume oral intake, and to avoid further complications of TPN. Digestion and absorption by the allograft can be affected transiently by infection, abnormal motility, rejection and infection. Nutritional management is individualized to account for these factors, but total enteral nutrition by a combination of oral and tube feedings is successful in the vast majority of survivors of intestinal transplantation.

At our institution, 78% of adults who had survived transplantation for 1 year were on full oral feedings. However, 33% still required some intravenous fluid and electrolyte supplementation. These patients generally had no remaining native or allograft colon to aid in water salvage. Paediatric outcomes are slightly better, with > 90% of children on oral feedings. Nutritional status of children is unquestionably improved following transplant beyond what it had been while on TPN. Data from the university of Pittsburgh (Rovera et al 1998) displayed in Figures 27.1 and 27.2 summarize our observations. Mean weight-for-height of survivors is lower, but mid-arm muscle circumference is improved by the end of the first transplant year. Just as importantly, linear growth

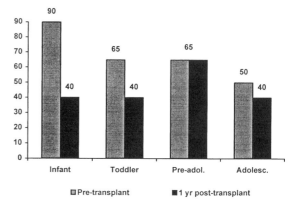

Figure 27.2 — Weight/Height percentile normative standard.

velocity improves following intestinal transplantation across the entire age spectrum of paediatric recipients despite the generous administration of glucocorticoids for control of rejection. Thus, children surviving small bowel transplantation can be expected to grow and thrive despite the many impediments to optimal nutrition that they face.

Discussion

The typical patient being considered for small intestinal transplantation is customarily bound to TPN due to profoundly-disordered gastrointestinal physiology. The underlying cause of intestinal dysfunction or TPN itself renders that patient at significant risk for death. Most patients experience one or more adverse nutritional consequences of their primary disease or their TPN therapy. Although the risks of intestinal transplantation are significant, and although the post-operative course may be stormy, the patient under-going small intestinal transplantation can look forward to a favourable nutritional outcome if the minefield of technical problems, infection, and rejection can be successfully negotiated.

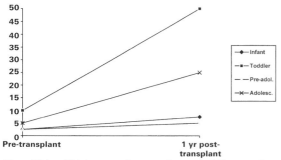

Figure 27.1 — Height percentile normative standard. Pre-transplant and 1 year post-transplant.

References

Abu-Elmagd, K., Todo, S., Tzakis, A., Reyes, J., Nour, B., Furukawa, H., Fung, J.J., Demetris, A., Starzl, T.E. (1994) Three years clinical experience with intestinal transplantation. *J Am Coll Surg*, 179, 385–400.

Behrns, K.E., Sarr, M.G., Hanson, R.B., Zinmeister, A.R. (1996) Jejunoileal transplantation: Effects on characteristics of canine jejunal motor activity *in vivo*. *Dig Dis Sci*, 41, 884–893.

Caliari, S., Vantini, I., Sembenini, C., Gregori, B., Carnielli, V., Benini, L. (1996) Fecal fat measurement in the presence of long- and medium-chain triglycerides and fatty acids. *Scand J Gastroenterol*, 31, 863–867.

Cohen, W.I., Zamberlan, K.E., Underwood, J., Quast, A., Quirk, P., Smith, A. (1992) Developmental issues in childhood small bowel transplantation: Eating and elimination. *Transpl Proc*, 24, 1246.

Kaufman, S., Dhawan, A., Iverson, A., Snell, L., Brown, C., Davis, C., Fox, I., Heffron, T., Sudan, D., Pillen, T., Vanderhoof, J., Langnas, A. (1996) Digestive function following intestinal transplantation (abstract). *J Pediatr Gastroenterol Nutr*, 23, 374.

Kaufman, S., Dhawan, A., Vanderhoof, J., Wisecarver, J., Radio, S., Markin, R., Fox, I., Heffron, T., Sudan, D., Pillen, T., Langnas, A. (1996) Correlation of mucosal disaccharidase activities with histology in evaluation of rejection following intestinal transplantation (abstract). *J Pediatr Gastroenterol Nutr*, 23, 374.

Kiyochi, H., Ono, A., Shimahara, Y., Kobayashi, N. (1994) Extrinsic reinnervation after intestinal transplantation in rats. *Transpl Proc*, 26, 951–952.

Liu, H., Teraoka, S., Nozawa, M., Fujita, S., Fuchinoue, S., Takahashi, K. (1992) Successful lymphangiographic investigation of mesenteric lymphatic regeneration after orthotopic intestinal transplantation in rat. *Transpl Proc*, 24, 1113–1114.

Mousa, H., Bueno, J., Griffith, J.G., Todo, S., Reyes, J., Kocoshis, S., DiLorenzo, C. (1998) Intestinal motility in children after small bowel transplantation. *Transpl Proc*, 30, 2535–2536.

Nemoto, A., Krajack, A., Suzuki, T., Takeyoshi, I., Hamada, N., Nomoto, M., Zhang, S., Shu, Y., Starzl, T.E., Todo, S. (1996) Glutamine metabolism of intestine grafts: Influence of mucosal injury by prolonged preservation and transplantation. *Transpl Proc*, 28, 2545–2546.

Nour, B., Reyes, J., Tzakis, A., Kocoshis, S., Abu-Elmagd, K., Furukawa, H., Kadry, Z., Fung, J. (1994) Intestinal transplantation with or without other abdominal organs: Nutritional and dietary management of 50 patients. *Transpl Proc*, 26, 1432–1433.

Oishi, A.J., Sarr, M.G. (1995) Intestinal transplantation: Effects on ileal enteric absorptive physiology. *Surgery*, 117, 545–553.

Roediger, W.E. (1980) Role of anaerobic bacteria in metabolic welfare of the colonic mucosa in man. *Gut*, 21, 793–798.

Rovera, G.M., Strohm, S., Bveno, J., Kocoshis, J. (1998) Nutritional monitoring of pediatric intestinal transplant recipients. *Transpl Proc* 30, 2519–2520.

Sarr, M.B., Siadati, M.R., Bailey, J., Lucas, D.L., Roddy, D.R., Duenes, J.A. (1996) Neural isolation of the jejunoileum: Effect on tissue morphometry, mucosal disaccharidase activity, and tissue peptide content. *J Surg Res*, 61, 416–424.

Sarr, M.G., Walters, A.M., Benson, J.T., Zinsmeister, A.R. (1994) Absorption of simple nutrients from the *in vivo* neurally isolated canine jejunum and ileum. *Surgery*, 115, 578–587.

Sigalet, D.L., Kneteman, N.M., Fedorak, R.N., Kizilisik, A.T., Thomson, A.B.R. (1992) Intestinal function following allogeneic small intestinal transplantation in the rat. *Transplantation*, 53, 264–271.

Sigurdsson, L., Kocoshis, S., Todo, S., Putnam, P., Reyes, J. (1996) Severe exfoliative rejection after intestinal transplantation in children. *Transpl Proc*, 28, 2783–2784.

Teitelbaum, D.H., Sonnino, R.E., Dunaway, D.J., Stellin, G., Harmel, R.P. (1993) Rat jejunal absorptive function after intestinal transplantation: Effects of extrinsic denervation. *Dig Dis Sci*, 38, 1099–1104.

28

Nutritional requirements and treatment regimens after gastrointestinal resection

Marcel JIJ Albers and Dick Tibboel

Introduction

When one or more segments of the intestine dysfunction and are not expected to resume their normal function, resection of the dysfunctioning segment or segments is usually indicated. Resection allows the remainder of the intestine to resume its function. However, after resection the total absorptive surface is lower than before, and segments that absorb specific nutrients or secrete important hormones may have been resected or by-passed. Important segmental functions are summarized in Table 28.1. Gut motility may be affected and gastrointestinal transit further impaired by a difference in diameter between re-anastomosed bowel loops. Faster intestinal transit may also result from resection. The overall result depends on the type and extent of resection, and may vary from transient-mild to persistent-severe or life-threatening symptoms. Based on the procedure performed, three categories of resection are discerned:

1. *Resections resulting in an enterostomy*: the colon is by-passed either permanently or temporarily. Resection of (part of) the small and large intestine can result in a permanent end-enterostomy or a temporary enterostomy in combination with a colonic mucus fistula or a blind colon loop. A double-barrel enterostomy is the result of resection of a segment of the small intestine or used to by-pass a sick part of the intestine without resecting it.

2. *Resections leaving the remainder of the small intestine in continuity with the (remainder of the) colon*: as a result of a direct end-to-end anastomosis or after re-anastomosis in a separate procedure. Usually performed after previous resection of parts of both small and large intestine including the ileocaecal valve.

3. *Resection of part of the colon*: in combination with a direct end-to-end anastomosis or a colostomy.

Resection of the stomach is so extremely rare in infancy as not to be discussed in this chapter.

Not every gastrointestinal resection calls for specific nutritional interventions. Frequently, the management centres on direct post-operative maintenance of fluid and electrolyte homeostasis. Parenteral nutrition is used to bridge the period of post-operative paralytic ileus and then tapered as enteral feedings are advanced. General rules of parenteral nutrition support apply here. Enteral feedings can often be started within a couple of days and advanced to full strength within 1 week.

Specific nutritional interventions are needed when gastrointestinal transit is seriously impaired or when the intestine has been resected or by-passed to the extent that malabsorption occurs.

Impaired gastrointestinal transit

Impairment of gastrointestinal transit can be primarily mechanical, as in the atresias, or functional due to interruption of peristaltic complexes (after every resection) or hypomotility (e.g., in gastroschisis). *Intestinal atresias* (i.e., absence of a gut lumen in one or more segments of the intestine) are surgically treated by primary (side-to-side) anastomosis without resection (duodenal atresia) or resection and re-anastomosis (jejunal, ileal and colon atresias). As a rule, the proximal

Tabel 28.1 — Segmental intestinal function

	Duodenum and Jejunum	Ileum	Colon
absorption	fluids carbohydrates proteins fat iron, calcium, magnesium, copper, zinc most vitamins	water fat (iron, calcium, magnesium, copper, zinc) B12, ascorbic acid, vitamin K bile salts	water (fermented carbohydrates)
secretion	water, sodium cholecystokinin, secretin	enteroglucagon, peptide YY	
other		feedback gastric emptying	

Brackets indicate functions after adaptation following gastrointestinal resection.

intestine is dilated and the distal intestine has a very small diameter (micro-intestine). Initially, intestinal transit may be remarkably impaired both by the difference in diameter of proximal and distal intestine (cul-de-sac phenomenon) and by the inability of the micro-intestine to accommodate significant volumes of chyme. The aim of nutritional management is to allow the intestine time to accommodate significant volumes. Drip or frequent small volume enteral feedings can usually be started within days after surgery. Depending on the type of atresia, advancing to full volume enteral feedings may take anywhere between a week and several months. Complementary parenteral nutrition is used to bridge this period. Generally, the intestine's digestive potential is adequate and the infant can be fed breast milk or a normal infant formula. Occasionally, a substantial length of small intestine is atretic or multiple small intestinal atresias exist that call for a two-stage procedure. The first stage is a type I resection resulting in a temporary enterostomy. In these cases, the small intestinal digestive potential is permanently or temporarily compromised. In effect, the nutritional management then becomes the management of short-bowel syndrome.

Short-bowel syndrome

When resection of part of the intestine results in malabsorption, the ensuing clinical picture is referred to as *short-bowel syndrome* (SBS). A number of factors determine whether malabsorption follows resection:

- *Residual small intestinal length*: the importance of residual small intestinal length as a major determinant of prognosis is self-evident. Indeed, SBS used to be defined—and sometimes still is defined—as an arbitrary absolute or percentual upper limit of small intestinal length remaining after resection. These anatomical definitions however have two major flaws. First, the length of the small intestine is extremely variable and difficult to measure. Second, these definitions incorrectly suggest that other factors do not play a role.
- *Quality of intestine remaining*: the absorptive potential of previously over-distended or ischaemic bowel segments often remains compromised. Cystic fibrosis can be the underlying cause of meconium peritonitis and, if present, aggravates malabsorption after resection.
- *Part or parts resected*: resection of the jejunum is tolerated better than resection of the ileum due to the greater potential of the ileum to adapt. The

distal ileum is essential for the absorption of vitamin B12 and bile salts. Resection of the ileocaecal valve can result in malabsorption both as a result of faster intestinal transit and as a result of backflow and bacterial overgrowth in the small intestine.
- *Colon in continuity*: the colon salvages large quantities of water and sodium that have not been absorbed more proximally. Unabsorbed carbohydrates are fermented by colonic bacteria to short-chain fatty acids that are used as a fuel and absorbed by the mucosa. The anorectal sphincter slows intestinal transit when compared to an enterostomy.
- *Age at presentation*: based on the substantial difference in small bowel length measured at autopsy in premature versus term infants, it has been suggested that any segment of small bowel in a premature infant may grow and function as well as a longer segment in a term infant.

Causes of SBS in children

SBS in children usually presents at or shortly after birth as the result of a congenital anomaly or a neonatally-acquired condition. In the past decades, with increasing numbers of immature and premature infants surviving, necrotizing enterocolitis seems to have taken the place of intestinal atresia, midgut volvulus and gastroschisis as the single most frequent cause of gastrointestinal resection and SBS in infants. Occasionally, SBS arises later in childhood. Sporadically late presentation of a congenital anomaly leads to SBS later in life.

Causes of SBS in children are summarized in Table 28.2.

Clinical course of SBS

Within a few days after resection, structural changes can be seen to occur in the intestine both distally and proximally of the resection. Crypt depth, villus height, muscle layer thickness and bowel circumference increase. The intestinal villi become hyperplastic. Whether bowel length changes is a matter of contention. The net result is an increase in functional capacity of the remaining intestine. In the majority of cases, this process of adaptation takes weeks to months, but occasionally it may take years before completion. Schematically, the clinical course can be divided into three phases:

- *Acute phase*: starts as post-operative ileus and is characterized by excessive loss of fluids and electrolytes resulting from massive diarrhoea that starts or persists after the ileus has subsided and

Table 28.2 — Causes of short-bowel syndrome in children

Necrotizing enterocolitis
Intestinal atresia
Midgut volvulus
Gastroschisis
Omphalocele†
Intestinal aganglionosis † (only if extensive small bowel involvement)
Meconium ileus/peritonitis
Intussusception★
Trauma★
Inflammatory bowel disease★
Vascular anomalies★
Adhesions after intra-abdominal surgery★
Neoplasias★
Connective tissue diseases (Ehlers-Danlos, Marfan's)★†
Radiation enteritis★

†sporadically
★(usually) in older children

Table 28.3 — Complications of short-bowel syndrome in infancy

Dehydration
Malnutrition
Growth failure
Electrolyte depletion (acute or chronic)
Micro-nutrient deficiencies
Carnitine deficiency
Rachitis/osteomalacia
Gastric hyperacidity
Cholelithiasis
Cholecystitis
Pancreatitis
Liver dysfunction
Sepsis
Venous thrombosis
Oxalate renal stone formation, hyperoxaluria
Bacterial overgrowth
D-lactic acidosis
Feeding refusal

wears off in the course of 1 to several weeks. Patients are fed parenterally.

- *Adaptive phase*: as a result of the adaptive changes in the intestine the patient tolerates increasing amounts of enteral nutrition. The adaptive phase can last anywhere between 1 month and 2 years.
- *Chronic phase*: adaptation is maximal. Many patients can be maintained on enteral nutrition only; some still need parenteral supplements or remain dependent on parenteral nutrition. The equilibrium is easily upset by intercurrent diseases.

The core of early SBS symptomatology is loss of water and macro- and micro-nutrients from the body. Later in the course of SBS, the clinical picture may be dominated by the long-term sequelae of SBS or by the complications of treatment, summarized in Table 28.3 and 28.5.

After the clinical introduction of parenteral nutrition late in the 1960s, malnutrition ceased to be a determinant of long-term outcome in SBS. Mortality in SBS, particularly in infants, is now mainly caused by parenteral-nutrition-associated liver failure and to a lesser extent by (catheter-related) sepsis.

Practice and procedures

Nutritional management

The primary goal of nutritional management in SBS is to meet both qualitative and quantitative demands so that the patient may thrive. In SBS, nutritional interventions may also aim to prevent or treat complications and support the adaptive process in the gut.

Beginning with total parenteral nutrition in the acute phase, the hope is to end on a normal diet. Going through the clinical phases described earlier, the nutritional regimen needs to be tailored to the individual patient's needs again and again, usually through trial and error.

Absolute or age-related weight and height are poor markers of the succes of the nutritional regimen. Weight and height gain, measured over 1 or more weeks, are essential; the levelling off of weight and height gain serves as an alarm. In this context, it should be emphasized that many infants suffering from SBS are behind in weight and height in the first year of life, but have made up by the end of the second year, seemingly without having suffered any adverse effects. Similarly, when assessing the digestive capacity of the intestine, it should be remembered that some degree of malabsorption (and therefore abnormal test results) is to be expected and does not in itself imply that the nutritional regimen is inadequate. Assessment of digestive function in the face of absent or marginal weight gain on the other hand may be very helpful, particularly when tests that were performed when weight gain was satisfactory are available. A second word of caution is with respect to the timing of digestive function tests: imminent or recent sepsis very much affects the digestive and absorptive potential.

Pharmacological interventions may be useful in support of nutritional management. When conservative strategies are to no avail, surgical techniques may yet offer some hope of enhancing intestinal function.

Acute phase

The first concern in the early post-operative phase after gastrointestinal resection is to maintain fluid and electrolyte balance. Fluid losses from a nasogastric tube, gastrostomy or one or more enterostomies may be large and vary considerably with time. Initially, fluids need to be replaced every 1–2 h. Gradually, these losses decrease and replacement intervals may safely be extended. When the consistency of the stomal output or faeces becomes less watery, replacement may correspondingly decrease and finally stop.

The electrolyte content of gastric and enterostomy fluids can be estimated from clinical experience or measured (Table 28.4). Any replacement solution should have a comparable electrolyte content. Sodium losses invariably are large. Acidosis resulting from bicarbonate loss occurs frequently. Deficiencies of calcium, magnesium, phosphorus and occasionally zinc and copper may occur. Potassium deficiency may arise secondary to sodium or magnesium deficiency.

The authors generally start compensation of losses with Ringer's lactate and add extra sodium or other electrolytes, guided by serum electrolyte and bicarbonate concentrations (initially measured several times a day), urine production, body weight and fluid balance. In the acute phase, patients are fed parenterally. Standard rules of total parenteral nutrition apply, but extra care should be taken not to overfeed the patient. Overfeeding is one of the factors that has

been associated with parenteral-nutrition-associated liver dysfunction. The aim should not be to avoid all weight loss. Indeed, all patients loose some weight in the peri-operative period.

Enteral feeding is usually withheld or administered in very small amounts as it tends to increase diarrhoeal losses. Recently, the concept of 'minimal enteral feeding' emerged. This states that minimal amounts of enteral feeding should be given as early as possible, preferably within a day after surgery, not because of the nutritional value but because it prevents the breakdown of intestinal integrity (villus atrophy) that normally follows upon a few days of bowel starvation.

Adaptive phase

The transition from parenteral to enteral nutrition is a gradual process that may take months or even years. In some patients, the transition is never complete; they remain dependent on parenteral supplements or parenteral nutrition. It is important to provide enough calories and avoid deficiencies of fluids, electrolytes, trace elements and vitamins throughout the adaptive process.

Particularly when starting enteral nutrition, formulas with high osmolality should not be given because they increase the secretion of fluids and sodium into the proximal gut lumen and thus augment enterostomy production or diarrhoea. Concentrating the enteral formula is not recommended for the same reason. Diluting the formula on the other hand creates the potential problem of fluid overloading without delivering an adequate amount of calories. As a rule, an elemental or chemically-defined formula is used when initiating enteral feedings in infants. A protein hydrolysate, a mixture of medium- and long-chain fats, and a carbohydrate polymer or a mixture of polymers and disaccharides are the main constituents. The relative content of proteins, fats and carbohydrate should be within the normal range for age and weight. Initially,

Table 28.4 — Electrolyte content of body fluids (in mmol/L)

	Na	K	CI	HCO$_3$$^-$
Gastric secretions	20–80	5–20	100–150	–
Pancreatic secretions	120–140	5–15	90–120	115
Small intestinal secretions	100–140	5–15	90–130	30
Bile	120–140	5–15	80–120	35
Ileostomy fluids	45–135	3–15	20–115	
Diarrhoea	10–90	10–80	10–110	

the formula is given as a continuous enteral drip. This technique makes optimal use of the functional capacity of the intestine. Moreover, energy requirements are lower when compared to bolus feedings, and gastric distension and emesis are minimized. On the other hand, feeding the infant small boluses or solid foods a few times a day may help prevent food refusal later on.

Enteral feeding is started at a drip rate equivalent to 5–10 ml/kg bodyweight/day. Initially, the drip rate is increased every day by the equivalent of 5–10 ml per/kg bodyweight/24 h. The interval between advancements is extended to several days or even weeks when the limit of intestinal absorptive capacity has been reached. An increase in stool volume of more than 50% or a total stool volume of more than 40–50 ml/kg/day indicates that feedings should not be advanced further. Also indicative are a slowing down of weight gain or outright weight loss. Simultaneously with the advancement of the formula, the parenteral infusion is decreased in an isocaloric fashion, keeping in mind that calories provided via the enteral route have a lower bio-availibility than calories delivered parenterally. One way to compensate for the difference is to only start weaning the patient off parenteral nutrition when at least 20% of calories can be given via the enteral route. Also, the enterally-administered volume may be increased to as much as 200 mL/kg/day, bearing in mind however, that concomitant high protein intake may result in protein overloading.

When the infant's weight gain is satisfactory on enteral feeds, the next step is to go from drip to portions and then gradually lower the frequency of feedings. The last step then is to replace the elemental formula by a normal formula and introduce solid foods.

When to introduce breast milk, if available, is controversial. In extreme SBS, the uncertainty about its caloric content often prevails its use in earlier stages, but there are theoretical arguments to introduce breast milk early in the course of the adaptive phase. Unsatisfactory weight gain is the result of one of several potential problems. Usually the amount given enterally exceeds the absorptive capacity. Alternatively, the capacity to digest and absorb either carbohydrates or fats has not been taken full advantage of. In patients with an end-enterostomy, increasing the amount of calories given as fat usually does not change the percentage of fat absorbed so that more calories are absorbed. The capacity to digest and absorb carbohydrates on the other hand is easily exceeded.

Infants who have a colon in continuity may profit from a higher carbohydrate content, as unabsorbed carbohydrates are fermented by colonic bacteria to short-chain fatty acids that are used as a fuel and absorbed by the colonic mucosa. Unabsorbed fats (long-chain fatty acids) on the other hand inhibit resorption of water, and short-chain fatty acids (through a toxic effect on colonic flora) cause steatorrhoea and calcium and magnesium deficiency (through saponification) as well as promote renal oxalate stone formation (because oxalates not bound to calcium are resorbed as sodium salt). The down side of increasing carbohydrate intake in infants with a colon incontinuity is that malabsorbed carbohydrates cause osmotic diarrhoea and may give rise to episodes of D-lactic acidosis (see below). Malabsorption of carbohydrates is suspected when the stool pH is below 5.5, when the stools contain large amounts of reducing substances or when an H_2-breath test performed with the diet as provoking substance is strongly positive. Small amounts of reducing substances or a mildly-positive breath test are to be expected when one aims for bacterial fermentation to aid intestinal function. One way of increasing the fat or carbohydrate content is to add 1–2% medium chain triglyceride (MCT)-emulsion or 2–4% polymeric carbohydrate to the continuous enteral infusion. An alternative is to use a modular feed. Increasing the fat or carbohydrate content is an option to consider at any time during adaptive phase.

Fluid and electrolyte deficiencies present more insidiously than in the acute phase. Chronic sodium depletion may present as failure to gain weight, is characterized by abnormally-low urinary sodium excretion (below 10 mmol/L) often in the face of a normal serum sodium, and is treated with (preferably enteral) sodium supplements (oral NaCl starting dose 75–100 mg/kg/day, divided over 4–6 doses). It is frequently encountered in end-enterostomy patients, but very rare if the colon is in continuity.

Calcium (and phosphorus) deficiency is seen most frequently in patients with a proximal jejunostomy or in patients with the colon in continuity secondary to formation of calcium soaps. Treatment with calcium and phosphorus supplements (and vitamin D) may be difficult due to low solubility in total parenteral nutrition and low bioavailability when enterally administered. Zinc deficiency is seen in patients with a jejunostomy and as a complication of severe fat malabsorption. If severe, it leads to the typical clinical picture of 'acrodermatitis enteropathica,' characterized by growth arrest, irritability, lethargy, alopecia, acute dermatitis or chronic hyperkeratotic plaques close to body orifices and at the extremities. Magnesium, selenium, copper and iron deficiencies are seen in end-jejunostomy patients in particular. Water-soluble vitamin deficiencies are occasionally seen after extensive jejunal resection. Deficiencies of the fat-soluble vitamins and of vitamin B12 are seen after ileal resection. Carnitine deficiency frequently occurs and tends to escape notice.

Reinfusion of enterostomy output into the distal enterostomy loop or mucus fistula augments absorptive capacity in patients with a long segment of defunctioned bowel. It is however a cumbersome procedure and not always tolerated well.

Chronic phase

Considering that adaptation can take more than a year, an infant can only have entered the chronic phase when thriving on a more or less normal nutritional regimen. The diet should be normal with the possible exception of a supranormal intake that compensates for lower bioavailability due to malabsorption. The problems encountered are deficiencies of minerals, trace elements, vitamins and carnitine, often subclinical, and the temporary setbacks as a result of intermittent infections that have a tendency to unveil the limited reserve of the gut. Such setbacks may cause a relapse with renewed dependency on parenteral nutrition.

Parenteral-nutrition-associated liver dysfunction

Parenteral-nutrition-associated liver dysfunction is a potentially life-threatening complication in infants with SBS. It usually presents as cholestatic jaundice with slightly-elevated liver enzymes, but over time may turn into liver fibrosis or cirrhosis and liver failure. In one form or another it is diagnosed in 8–80% of infants on long-term parenteral nutrition. It is the single most important cause of death in infants with SBS. Its origin is multifactorial. Both prevention and treatment include trying to wean the infant off total parenteral nutrition: which means starting and advancing enteral feeding as soon as possible, using a balanced substrate, avoiding overfeeding (particularly of dextrose), and trying to eliminate other causes of liver dysfunction with special emphasis on sepsis or bacteriaemia.

Other complications of SBS

Diarrhoea is one of the cardinal symptoms of SBS and as such may be provoked by a change in the nutritional regimen. It may also be the presenting symptom of selective overgrowth of bacteria in the small intestine. Bacterial overgrowth usually presents as disturbed gut motility with a longer transit time. The diagnosis is made if overgrowth is shown in cultures or indirectly by an acid faeces pH ($<$ 5.5), a (further) elevation of H_2-breath test values or urinary indicans. Temporary cessation of enteral nutrient delivery is a fundamental aspect of treatment.

Resection of the distal ileum inevitably results in bile salt depletion, in spite of enhanced liver synthesis. Bile salt depletion causes fat malabsorption and predisposes to cholelithiasis and oxalate renal stone formation, complications seldomly seen in the first year of life. Although the altered metabolism of cholesterol (together with disturbed gallbladder emptying and altered bilirubin metabolism) may be instrumental in cholelithiasis in SBS, the role of nutrition in preventing this complication is unclear. Malabsorbed bile salts increase the permeability of the colon for sodium oxalate that is present because the calcium that normally precipitates with oxalates is saponified with malabsorbed long-chain fatty acids. This complication is only encountered if the colon is in continuity. The nutrional preventive and therapeutic strategy consists of a diet low in oxalates and fat in combination with calcium and magnesium supplements.

A rare complication of SBS seen in patients with a colon in continuity is recurrent D-lactic acidosis. Symptoms include headache, drowsiness, stupor, confusion, ataxia, ophthalmoplegia, blurred vision and impaired gut motility sometimes resembling paralytic (sub)ileus. D-lactate is formed when carbohydrates are fermented by acid-resistant anaerobes like lactobacilli. Symptoms result from formation of excessive quantities of D-lactate and subsequent systemic absorption and seem to be aggravated by thiamine deficiency. The diagnosis depends on the presence of metabolic acidosis with an anion gap consistent with serum D-lactate levels and demonstration of selective overgrowth of anaerobes capable of producing D-lactate in the stools. Lowering the amount of (oligomeric) carbohydrates supposedly prevents the episodes. In the authors' experience, however, only long-term oral antibiotic prophylaxis has been successful. Withholding all enteral nutrition, particularly carbohydrates, is usually necessary when treating an episode. A similar clinical picture has been associated with the presence of a yeast (*Torulopsis glabrata*) in the proximal small intestine.

Gut adaptation

The presence of nutrients in the gut lumen is by far

Table 28.5 — Characteristics of short bowel syndrome in infancy

	Acute Phase	Adaptive Phase	Chronic Phase
Weight gain	absent – slight	subnormal – normal	normal
Calories route	parenteral	parenteral → enteral	enteral
		drip → normal to high frequency	(high-)normal frequency
Amount	avoid overfeeding	normal to high	id.
Type	balanced	elemental → normal	normal
	avoid high carbohydrate	enterostomy: high fat	
		colon i.c.: high carbohydrate	
Depletion			
Electrolytes			
–Na	+++	enterostomy: ++	id.
		colon i.c.: –	id.
–HCO_3^-	++	+	–
–K	++	+	–
–Ca, P, Mg, Zn	++	+	+
Trace elements	+	++	±
Vitamins			
–water-soluble	– (provided with TPN)	jejunostomy: +	id.
–fat-soluble	– (provided with TPN)	++	+
–B12		distal ileum resected: +	distal ileum resected: +
Carnitine	– (provided with TPN)	++	+
Complications			
PN-associated	cholestasis, sepsis	cholestasis, liver failure, sepsis, thrombosis	(resolving cholestasis)
Other	hypergastrinaemia	bacterial overgrowth	bacterial overgrowth
	gastric hyperacidity		
		(cholelithiasis)	
		colon i.c.: hyeroxaluria; (D-lactic acidosis)	

Abbreviations: –, never or hardly ever; +, occasionally; ++, regularly; +++, frequently; i.c., in continuity; (T)EN, (T)PN, (total) enteral nutrition, (total) parenteral nutrition.

the most important stimulus for gut adaptation. Several nutrients have been tested for their specific potential to stimulate gut adaptation. This research has largely been conducted in laboratory animals and has so far not led to recommendations about nutritional strategies. In the near future, an exception should possibly be made for parenteral glutamine. Glutamine has been shown to be safe and to prevent mucosal atrophy in adult surgical patients when added to total parenteral nutrition in doses approximating 25–50% of daily protein intake. In bone marrow transplant recipients it lowered the number of infections and the length of hospital stay. Whether SBS infants may profit from parenteral glutamine remains to be shown. Addition of glutamine to enteral nutrition has so far not proved to be beneficial. Currently growth hormone and other hormones, growth factors and regulatory peptides are also being tested for their potential to stimulate gut adaptation.

Pharmacological management

Proper and timely use of certain drugs may support nutritional management. Many of the drugs used do, however, have side effects that are of particular importance in SBS. H_2-antagonists counteract the hyperacidity that follows hypergastrinaemia in the early phase after resection, especially in patients with a very short bowel without colon in continuity, but increase the risk of bacterial overgrowth. Loperamide, codeine and phenoxylate by slowing intestinal transit have the same side effect. The somatostatine analogue octreotide inhibits intestinal motility and reduces gastrointestinal secretions, but may impair adaptation.

Cholestyramine binds bile salts, but by doing so further depletes the bile salt pool and impairs fat absorption. Cholestyramine is part of the treatment of oxalate renal stone formation. Its long-term use has recently been questioned because of its suspected carcinogenic potential. Antibiotics probably are of use when treating bacterial overgrowth, but induce microbial selection and resistance. Cholecystokinin has been used to treat gallbladder dysfunction. A more detailed discussion of pharmacological support is outside the scope of this chapter. The authors are rather hesitant with respect to pharmacological support in SBS. The authors think it is good policy to test at intervals what effect, if any, discontinuation of a drug once deemed necessary has.

Surgical management

Re-anastomosing the colon or distal small intestine to the proximal small intestine (i.e., turning a category I into a category II resection) greatly augments absorptive capacity. Cholecystectomy is indicated in symptomatic cholelithiasis, but questionable as a prophylactic measure.

Other surgical interventions are seldom performed in infancy, as adaptive capacity has not reached it limits. However, life-threatening complications of parenteral nutrition may force the physician to try and accelerate adaptation surgically. Surgical techniques aim to slow intestinal transit, improve the function of the existing small intestine or increase its length. As an ultimate measure, intestinal transplantation, often combined with liver transplantation, may be considered. Recent results are encouraging.

29

Nutritional requirements and support in HIV/AIDS

Robin A. Henderson and Arlene M. Butz

Abbreviations

HIV	human immunodeficiency virus
AIDS	acquired immunodeficiency syndrome
REE	resting energy expenditure
RDA	recommended dietary allowances
NCHS	National Center for Health Statistics
WHO	World Health Organization
AZT	azidothymidine
PCR	polymerase chain reaction
TNF	tumour necrosis factor

Introduction

The World Health Organization (WHO) currently estimates that there are 21 million adults and 800,000 children infected with HIV worldwide (Joint United Nations Programme on HIV/AIDS 1996a). The human immunodeficiency virus (HIV), the aetiologic agent of acquired immunodeficiency syndrome (AIDS), results in destruction and progressive loss of circulating $CD4^+$ lymphocytes, causing global immuno-suppression and increased susceptibility to neoplasms and both common and opportunistic infections. HIV is transmitted by blood and body secretions. Infection by contaminated blood products is now rare, and the primary route of infection in infants is perinatal transmission from an HIV-infected mother. Casual or family-type contact is not considered to be a source of transmission.

The psycho-social and financial consequences of HIV are staggering for individuals, families and society. Therapies for HIV-infected patients are aimed at inhibiting viral replication, treating or preventing opportunistic infection, and restoring or compensating for the immune deficit caused by HIV. Malnutrition is a hallmark of HIV disease, and efforts to prevent or treat malnutrition can have a positive impact on the course and severity of HIV disease. This chapter discusses the current knowledge regarding the metabolic changes caused by HIV and the practical aspects of nutritional care of children born to HIV-infected mothers, with a particular emphasis on children who are themselves HIV-infected.

Historical background

Optimal outcomes for infants and children with HIV infection rely on early diagnosis. Perinatal transmission of HIV may occur *in utero*, at delivery or in the post-partum period, and affects between 15–40% of infants born to HIV-infected women. However, azidothymidine (AZT) therapy for the mother during the ante-partum and intra-partum periods and for the newborn post-natally reduces perinatal transmission by approximately two-thirds (from 24.9% to 7.8%) (Connor et al 1994). Therefore, perinatal prophylaxis with AZT is recommended for all HIV-infected women, as is treating the newborn with AZT, regardless if the mother was treated. A definitive diagnosis can be made by 4–6 months of age using HIV culture or polymerase chain reaction (PCR) for HIV DNA. For children who are not identified during infancy, several clinical signs and symptoms may suggest HIV infection and warrant HIV testing, including failure to thrive, generalized lymphadenopathy, recurrent bacterial infections, chronic diarrhoea, hepatosplenomegaly, developmental delay, recurrent oral candidiasis and radiographic evidence of persistent diffuse lung disease (Pizzo & Wilfert 1994). Standard HIV antibody tests are adequate to diagnose HIV infection in children over 2 years of age.

For the majority of perinatally-acquired HIV-infected children, the mean age of survival has increased to 9 years. Shorter survival is associated with early onset of opportunistic infections, growth retardation, recurrent oral candidiasis and encephalopathy (Oleske 1994). Two patterns of disease progression have been described, and each has different survival times (Table 29.1). Some perinatally-infected children can remain asymptomatic or mildly symptomatic through adolescence (Wilfert et al 1994).

The immunological changes and the resultant opportunistic infections that occur with protein-energy malnutrition are similar to those seen during HIV infection. The reason that some children remain asymptomatic for long periods, whereas others progress rapidly to AIDS is unclear. Growth failure often precedes the diagnosis of AIDS, and a decrease in $CD4^+$ lymphocyte number is a predictor of disease progression (Brettler et al 1990) and is associated with significantly shorter survival time (McKinney & Wilfert 1994). Further research is needed to determine whether preventing growth failure and optimizing nutritional status affect immune function, morbidity and survival.

Practice and procedures

Nutritional status assessment

The nutritional evaluation should include routine

Table 29.1 — Early and late symptomatic onset of HIV infection in children

Early Onset (< 2 year old) (10–25% of infected children)	Late Onset (> 4 years old) (75–90% infected children)
Survival < 6 years old	Survival > 8 years old
Severe failure to thrive	Growth failure (mild-moderate)
Developmental delay	Chronic multi-system disease
Progressive encephalopathy	Persistent generalized lymphadenopathy
Severe Candidiasis (oral-oesophageal infection)	Lymphoid interstitial pneumonitis (LIP)
Pneumocystis carinii pneumonia	Malabsorption syndrome
Severe, life-threatening bacterial infections	Malignancies

Adapted from Pizzo (1994).

assessments of growth; dietary, social, and medical histories; and laboratory evaluation (Table 29.2). Routine nutritional follow-up allows timely implementation of appropriate nutritional interventions. Infants born to HIV-infected mothers are often at nutritional risk initially whether or not they are themselves HIV-infected, and careful monitoring of the growth and diet of all infants is recommended during early infancy. HIV-infected infants require more intensive nutritional monitoring.

Growth and body composition

Growth is a highly sensitive indicator of nutritional status in children. Alterations in physical growth have been well described in children with HIV, even in children with relatively few other physical symptoms of HIV infection (McKinney & Robertson 1993, Saavedra et al 1995, Moye et al 1996). However, secondary HIV-related morbidity may adversely affect growth in children over 1 year of age (European Collaborative Study 1995).

At birth, children born to HIV-infected mothers in developing countries have been demonstrated to be smaller in weight, length, and head circumference than children born to HIV-seronegative mothers (Bulterys et al 1994, Henderson et al 1996). This was true even after controlling for potential confounders such as cigarette smoking, maternal age, parity, and history of sexually transmitted diseases (Bulterys et al 1994). However, studies in developed countries have not reported a difference at birth related to maternal HIV serostatus in women with similar risk-taking profiles (Butz et al 1991, Ross et al 1995), but infants have been demonstrated to be smaller than those born to HIV seronegative women who do not abuse illicit drugs (Ross et al 1995) and when compared to the

National Center for Health Statistics (NCHS) median (Saavedra et al 1995). Pre-natal factors (excluding drug abuse) associated with reduced intrauterine growth in HIV-infected mothers, including the impact of maternal nutritional status, remain to be determined.

Post-natal growth of children born to HIV-infected mothers is affected by infant HIV serostatus. Although HIV-uninfected infants have been demonstrated to 'catch-up' to children born to seronegative mothers, HIV-infected children remain small for both height and weight-for-age (European collaborative study 1995, Saavedra et al 1995, Henderson et al 1996, Moye et al 1996). Children in the United States have been demonstrated to become stunted, with proportional decreases in weight and length-for-age. Wasting, or decreased weight-for-height, occurs less frequently, suggesting chronic under-nutrition rather than acute starvation (McKinney & Robertson 1993, Saavedra et al 1995). This does not appear to be the case in developing countries, where weight appears to be affected earlier and more severely than length (Henderson et al 1996). These differences may be related to the availability of more intensive nutritional support and anti-retroviral therapies and other treatment modalities.

Alterations in body composition associated with wasting in HIV-infected adults include a loss of body weight and fat stores with a disproportionately greater loss of body cell mass (Kotler et al 1985). Reduced body cell mass has been demonstrated in asymptomatic adults, prior to changes in body weight and body mass index (Ott et al 1993), suggesting that weight and body mass index may not be valid indicators of nutritional status, especially in the early stages of HIV infection. Miller et al (1993) suggested that lean body mass is also decreased in the early stages of HIV

Table 29.2 — Nutritional assessment of infants and children born to HIV-infected mothers

Anthropometric assessment

Accurate measurement of height, weight, and head circumference at each visit. Standardized technique and appropriate pediatric equipment is essential.

Plot growth charts at each visit, including attention to weight-for-height.

Body composition: body circumference and skinfold thickness measurements can be readily compared to available standards for age and gender,[1] and are useful to track individual trends over time. Bioelectrical impedance analysis is a promising new technique under study for quick, non-invasive measurement of body composition.

Diet and social history

Infants: timing and length of each feeding, and the amount of formula consumed. Feeding problems or concerns and development of age appropriate feeding skills.

Older children: Pattern of food intake, food and beverage preferences, dietary practices, supplements.

All children: Feeding practices, maternal-child feeding interactions. Estimate current caloric intake by 24-h dietary recall or diet record if possible.

Environmental factors, such as the availability of electricity, adequate refrigeration, cooking and measuring utensils to mix formula or prepare foods, ability to procure foods or supplements.

Impairment of the child's primary caretaker due to illness or substance abuse.

Medical history

Identify children at greatest risk for malnutrition and metabolic derangements due to acute or chronic illnesses.

GI symptoms: 1) Stool exam: occult blood, polymorphonuclear leukocytes, viral, bacterial and parasitic enteropathogens; reducing sugars (Clinitest) and pH for children receiving lactose or glucose. Watery stools with reducing sugars and a low pH (< 5.5) suggests carbohydrate malabsorption. Glucose polymers have a lower reducing power and sucrose is not a reducing sugar, so malabsorption of these sugars cannot be detected by this test; 2) Lactose and sucrose malabsorption, and small bowel bacterial overgrowth, can be identified by elevation of hydrogen concentration in expired air (breath); 3) 72-h faecal fat analysis for the presence of steatorrhoea; 4) Urinary excretion of D-xylose suggests loss of mucosal integrity and associated malabsorption; 5) Upper and lower endoscopy with biopsies to establish the presence and aetiology of gastrointestinal disease should be considered in consultation with a gastroenterologist.

Endocrine function in children with growth failure.

Neurological and developmental functioning.

Current medications and their potential side effects or benefits, drug-nutrient interactions.

Laboratory assessment

Individualize laboratory examinations on an individual basis following medical history review. Haemoglobin and haematocrit establish the occurrence of anaemia and may suggest a nutritional aetiology. In symptomatic children, it may be necessary to assess fluid and electrolyte status, total protein and albumin to determine visceral protein status, and pre-albumin to determine response to nutritional therapy. The micro-nutrient status of children with malnutrition or chronic diarrhoea should be assessed periodically, including zinc, copper, selenium, vitamins A, D, and E, and prothrombin time to assess vitamin K, particularly when there is evidence of hepatobiliary disease. Elevated amylase and lipase may suggest pancreatitis. Bilirubin, liver enzymes and alkaline phosphatase abnormalities. Immunological and virological measurements such as $CD4^+$ lymphocyte number and the quantitation of plasma HIV RNA may help to identify children at risk of disease progression and alterations in nutritional status.

[1]Frisancho (1993)

infection in children. However, the authors found that HIV-infected children without acute illness had significantly-reduced mean fat mass compared to HIV-uninfected children. They did not observe a selective reduction of lean body mass with a relative sparing of fat mass (Henderson et al 1998). Inadequate accretion of lean body mass due to mild chronic malnutrition or recurrent illness may negatively impact growth over time.

Several factors are thought to be responsible for the alterations in growth and body composition that are observed, including reduced food intake, gastrointestinal dysfunction, metabolic disturbances resulting in reduced nutrient utilization, and neuroendocrine dysfunction. Usually there are a combination of factors unique to an individual child that vary over time.

Dietary and social history

Thorough dietary and social histories are necessary to evaluate the adequacy of present food intake to meet nutritional goals and the ability of caretakers to provide adequately appropriate food choices in a nurturing environment. Mean energy intakes of HIV-infected children have been found to be similar to uninfected children and to the RDA (Zuin 1994, Alfaro 1995, Henderson et al in press). Although the specific nutrient requirements of HIV-infected children have not been determined, it is generally accepted that they are greater than those of uninfected children. Thus, the oral intake demonstrated thus far in HIV-infected children may be insufficient for optimal growth and nutritional status. Many practitioners recommend as much as 150% of the RDA to achieve normal growth and nutritional status. The authors generally begin with standard guidelines for age, with additional energy and protein as necessary to allow for normal or catch-up growth or to account for additional requirements according to HIV-associated symptoms.

Reduced food intake may occur for a variety of reasons. Anorexia may be related to acute infection, drug therapy or depression. Dysphagia and odynophagia can result from infection and other inflammatory processes affecting the oral cavity, pharynx and oesophageal tract. Dysphagia may also result from central nervous system dysfunction, leading both to reduced food intake and increased risk for aspiration. Upper and lower gastrointestinal symptoms such as nausea, vomiting, early satiety, abdominal pain and diarrhoea can also impair food intake.

The role of environmental factors such as decreased food availability and the ability of caretakers to provide appropriate foods consistently deserves further investigation. Several factors identified in caregivers of infants experiencing failure to thrive are prevalent amongst mothers with HIV-related illness, including ongoing social stress, maternal perceptions of lack of support and unresolved issues about their health status (Altemeier et al 1985). Maternal-child interactions may also be important, because some children may be more difficult to feed and have more difficulty engaging caregivers and some parents may fail to create an environment in which children consume sufficient calories. HIV disease is unique compared to other chronic childhood illnesses in that both the

caregiver and child are chronically ill. The HIV-infected mother alone is reportedly the most common primary caretaker of her children, with half of these mothers caring for more than one child (Schable et al 1995). In Schable et al (1995), only 30% of mothers knew about assistance services in their community and only 8% used these services. Mothers of HIV-infected children are likely to be of low socio-economic status and either themselves or their partners may be struggling with drug addiction. Functional status is impaired in HIV-infected adults, with 30% of adults with AIDS and 15% of asymptomatic adults reporting dependency on others for activities of daily living such as cooking, shopping, and taking medicine (Stanton et al 1994). Thus, the ability of caregivers to adequately care for HIV-infected children and the identification of appropriate support systems must be assessed and fostered.

Medical history

The medical history provides information regarding risk factors and mechanisms of malnutrition and poor growth. HIV-infected children suffer from both chronic infection with HIV and intermittent acute infections. Increased metabolic demands can place them at particular risk for insufficient accumulation of lean tissue and growth retardation. Increased resting energy expenditure (REE) may occur at all stages of HIV disease in adults (Melchior et al 1993), but total energy expenditure may be unchanged (Macallan et al 1995a). A study of 9 HIV-infected children suggested that they were not hyper-metabolic compared to standard prediction equations (Alfaro et al 1995). The authors have evaluated REE in 29 HIV-infected children compared with 9 HIV-uninfected children who were afebrile and free of obvious acute illness (Henderson et al 1998). Mean REE per kg body weight was 12% higher in HIV-infected children with normal growth, and 16% higher in HIV-infected children with growth retardation. Although not statistically significant, these findings may be clinically relevant given that growth represents only a small proportion of total energy requirements.

Both increased and decreased rates of protein turnover have been reported in HIV-infected adults. Stein et al (1990) demonstrated decreased protein turnover in men with AIDS compared to seronegative controls, suggesting a starvation-type response to under-nutrition. Macallan et al (1995b) demonstrated that the rate of protein turnover was significantly increased in HIV-infected patients with stage IV, but not stage II disease, compared to seronegative controls. HIV-infected patients with symptomatic illness had significantly greater rates of protein turnover than those who were asymptomatic. The authors found the mean rate of whole body protein turnover was 40% greater in HIV-infected children with growth retardation, and 20% greater in HIV-infected children with normal growth compared to HIV-uninfected children, although these changes were not statistically significant (Henderson et al submitted). This study also demonstrated that children with the greatest degree of growth retardation had the highest rates of protein turnover, as evidenced by a significant correlation between protein turnover and weight and height-for-age Z-scores.

Hommes et al (1991) demonstrated increased fat oxidation and unchanged carbohydrate oxidation, suggesting a hyper-metabolic state. Aspects of lipid metabolism and other metabolic regulatory activities are modulated by cytokines, including tumour necrosis factor (TNF), interferon-alpha and interleukin-1. Cytokine levels have been found to be elevated in children with symptomatic HIV infection, but this was not associated with cachexia (Arditi et al 1991).

The gastrointestinal tract is a common target organ for complications associated with HIV infection. A number of gastrointestinal, pancreatic, and hepatobiliary conditions can result in intestinal malabsorption and reduce nutrient availability. Diarrhoea is the most common gastrointestinal problem in HIV-infected patients, and may be acute, chronic, or intermittent in nature. HIV-infected infants have been shown to have more frequent and prolonged episodes of diarrhoea than uninfected infants (Kotloff et al 1994). Most gastrointestinal disturbances result from infection, associated malabsorption, bacterial overgrowth, or as a side effect of medications such as antibiotics. Intestinal nutrient malabsorption has been demonstrated in both adults and children with HIV infection, but may not be clinically evidenced by diarrhoea or growth failure nor associated with the presence of enteric pathogens or degree of immune dysfunction (Italian Paediatric Intestinal/HIV Study Group 1993). Lactose malabsorption has been found to be more prevalent in HIV infected children with diarrhoea (Yolken 1991). Hypochlorhydria can increase the risk for bacterial contamination of the small bowel, and decrease folate and iron absorption.

Neuroendocrine dysfunction has been documented in children with HIV infection, including thyroid abnormalities (Hirschfeld et al 1996); decreased somatomedin-C (Schwartz et al 1991); and *in vitro*

resistance to the growth promoting actions of IGF-1, growth hormone, and insulin, particularly in children with more advanced symptoms of HIV (Geffner et al 1993). Endocrine abnormalities may contribute to growth failure in some children and should be considered when evaluating the growth and nutritional status of children with HIV.

HIV-infected children often require the chronic intake of multiple medications to treat HIV or other infections, each with potential side effects that can cause nutritional disturbances. Some of the most commonly used medications and their side effects are listed in Table 29.3. At present, combination anti-retroviral therapy using AZT in combination with didanosine (DDI) or lamivudine are the drugs of choice for *initial* treatment of HIV infection in infants and children. Additional medications or new combinations are used according to guidelines based on results from AIDS clinical trials group protocols.

Laboratory monitoring of nutritional status

The most common haematological problem associated with paediatric HIV infection is anaemia. The aetiology of anaemia is multifactorial and is related to severity of HIV disease, anti-retroviral therapy, and age. Unlike adults, where anaemia is typically normochromic and normocytic, the anaemia observed in HIV-infected children is microcytic and hypochromic. Characteristics of the anaemia seen in HIV-infected children include: 1) normal or elevated serum ferritin; 2) normal or decreased iron binding capacity; 3) red cell indexes usually normal; and 4) low serum iron, transferrin saturation, and haemoglobin. Treatment of iron deficiency anaemia with ferrous sulphate (6 mg/kg/day) produces reticulocytosis after 1–2 weeks and a low haemoglobin corrects over 4–8 weeks. Chronic anaemia may require transfusions with packed red blood cells to achieve haemoglobin above 8 g/dL. Severe anaemia in children taking AZT may necessitate a dose reduction or a change in anti-retroviral therapy (Pizzo & Wilfert 1994).

Multiple micro-nutrient deficiencies have been described, even during asymptomatic HIV infection (Bogden et al 1990, Beach et al 1992a). Zinc deficiency has been reported in 26% of men with asymptomatic HIV infection (Beach et al 1992a), and reduced serum zinc has been correlated with progression to AIDS (Graham et al 1991). Selenium deficiency has been reported in 15% of adults with asymptomatic HIV infection (Mantiero-Atienza et al 1991), and may be associated with AIDS cardiomyopathy (Kavanaugh-

Table 29.3 — Drug therapies for HIV-infected infants and children

Drug name	Description	Major toxicities
Zidovudine (AZT) Trade name: Retrovir	Slows HIV reproduction. Associated with improved activity, growth, neurological and cognitive functioning.	Anaemia, neutropaenia, headache, nausea, abdominal pain, hepatic transaminitis.
Didanosine (DDI) Trade name: Videx	Slows HIV reproduction. Empty stomach required.	Pancreatitis, peripheral neuropathy, hypocalcaemia, transient rise in serum amylase and triglyceride, headache, nausea, diarrhoea.
Zalcitabine (DDC)	Slows HIV reproduction. Use in children is limited.	Peripheral neuropathy, pancreatitis, mouth sores, rash, nausea.
Lamivudine (3TC) Trade Name: Epivir	Slows HIV reproduction. Associated with improved growth and sense of well being.	Fatigue, diarrhoea, insomnia, rash, neutropenia, anaemia.
Niverapine	Non-nucleoside reverse transcriptase inhibitor.	Mild headache, rash.
Protease inhibitors Ritonavir (Noravir) Nelfinavir (Viracept)	Prevent cleavage of protein precursors essential for new cell infection and viral replication.	*Ritonavir*: nausea, vomiting, diarrhoea, altered taste, elevated serum triglycerides, cholesterol, hepatic transaminase. *Nelfinavir*: diarrhoea, nausea, flatulence, abdominal pain, rash.
Trimethoprim-sulfamethoxizole (Bactrim, Septra)	Treat and prevent *Pneumocystis carinii* pneumonia (PCP).	Nausea, vomiting, neutropaenia, liver damage.

McHugh et al 1991). Vitamin A deficiency was found in 15% of HIV-infected adults and was associated with a decreased CD4 cell number and increased mortality (Semba 1993), and may also contribute to increased risk of maternal-child transmission of HIV infection (Semba et al 1994). Vitamin A supplementation has also been demonstrated to reduce morbidity in HIV-infected infants (Coutsoudis et al 1995). Vitamin B6 deficiency may impair peripheral blood lymphocyte response to mitogens and reduced natural killer cell cytotoxicity (Baum 1991). Vitamin B12 deficiency has been associated with cognitive impairment (Beach et al 1992b), and patients with decreased serum vitamin B12 levels may be more susceptible to the development of anaemia during AZT therapy (Richman et al 1987). Hypoalbuminaemia has been demonstrated in mal-nourished (Kotler et al 1985) but not well-nourished (McCorkindale et al 1990) adults with AIDS, and was associated with decreased survival (Guenter et al 1993).

Plasma and serum of HIV-infected children without acute infection were compared to seronegative controls for the following: total protein, albumin, pre-albumin, vitamin A, zinc and selenium (Henderson et al in press). No statistically-significant differences in mean levels of albumin, pre-albumin, zinc or selenium were found between groups. Mean serum vitamin A was significantly higher in HIV-infected children with growth retardation, and the significance of this finding is unclear. There were no significant differences between groups in the frequency of deficiency for any nutrient studied. Serum total protein was significantly higher in HIV seropositive children than seronegative children, presumably due to HIV-induced hyper-gammaglobulinaemia. Given that abnormal serum or plasma protein or micro-nutrient levels were uncommon, routine monitoring of these proteins and micro-nutrients is unnecessary in the absence of specific clinical risk factors for deficiency.

Nutritional management

The nutritional management of children born to HIV-infected mothers necessitates a continuum of care beginning as soon as possible after birth. Early monitoring and counselling help to assure appropriate feeding practices and establish an adequate growth rate. Nutritional care is often complicated by a variety of medical and social factors, and an interdisciplinary team of physicians, nurses, dietitians and social workers is optimal.

Asymptomatic children with normal growth should receive an adequate, well-balanced oral diet. The risks and benefits of micro-nutrient supplementation to prevent deficiencies and slow HIV disease progression remains to be determined. Thus, a daily multi-vitamin and mineral supplement providing approximately one times the RDA is recommended, but additional micro-nutrient supplementation should be based on clinical indication of deficiency. Special fad diets, medicinal herbs and mega-doses of vitamins and minerals can cause adverse effects, can be very expensive and should be discouraged. Periodic review of proper handling and storage of food is important because HIV-infected persons are more susceptible to food-borne illnesses and developing bacteraemia from these infections. Raw eggs and shellfish should be avoided, and meat products should be fully cooked. There is no evidence to support using 'sterile', or 'low bacteria' diets.

Infants

Breastfeeding provides a number of benefits for both mother and infant. For the infant, human milk is of optimal nutritional quality, confers immunologic protection against infection and provides many psycho-social benefits. Of the many maternal health benefits of breastfeeding, maternal suppression of ovulation is critical for child spacing for many women. However, breastfeeding has been demonstrated to be a potential source of HIV transmission from mother to infant (Ruff 1994), although the extent of risk associated with breastfeeding in women pre-natally infected with HIV may be low (Guay et al 1996). In an interim statement regarding HIV and infant feeding, the Joint United Nations Programme on HIV/AIDS (1996b) has emphasized the right to informed choice regarding the best feeding method for each child and family. Infants who can be assured uninterrupted access to nutritionally adequate breast-milk substitutes that can be prepared and fed safely are at less risk of illness and death if they are not breastfed. However, when these conditions cannot be fulfilled, in particular in environments where infectious diseases and mal-nutrition are the primary causes of death during infancy, artificial feeding substantially increases the child's risk of illness and death. Further research is needed to determine whether factors such as anti-retroviral therapy or vitamin A may reduce the risks of HIV transmission from breastfeeding while allowing the benefits of breastfeeding to HIV-exposed infants.

Unless clinically contraindicated, formula-fed infants should receive a standard milk-based formula. There is presently no evidence to support altering the formula composition of infants born to HIV-infected mothers, although supplementation at the earliest possible time is of theoretical benefit to HIV-infected children.

The majority of HIV-infected infants can and should progress to solid feedings and transition from bottle to cup feedings at the normal recommended ages. Neurological dysfunction from HIV infection may manifest as feeding problems such as difficulty with sucking or swallowing. It is essential that caregivers receive reassurance regarding the difficulties involved with feeding these infants. Experimenting with different feeding positions or thickening formula may be helpful. For infants experiencing difficulty with solid foods, changing the type of spoon or the texture or consistency of the food may be helpful.

For infants with growth failure or gastrointestinal symptoms, several options can be considered. Increasing the caloric density of formula may be helpful. However, this can increase renal solute load or cause gastro-intestinal intolerance, and should be increased slowly with close monitoring of potential side effects. Concentration can be increased either by using less dilute infant formula or with the addition of glucose polymers, sucrose, or fat as medium-chain triglycerides or vegetable oil. Convenience of preparation is important to consider when formulating such recipes for home use.

Older children

Several methods of increasing oral nutrient intake are available when weight gain or growth is inadequate (Table 29.4). Efforts to increase nutrient intake are more successful if they can be extended to daycare and school. Packing lunches or snacks may be necessary, and instructing children on appropriate food choices may be helpful. More frequent meals and snacks using nutrient dense and favourite foods can be helpful. Beverages such as milk or fruit shakes taken between meals can provide additional calories and nutrients. For children with gastrointestinal symptoms, juices and beverages containing large amounts of sucrose and fructose may worsen diarrhoea. For persons with difficulty swallowing due to pain or neurological complications, modifying the consistency, texture or

Table 29.4 — Suggestions for increasing oral nutrient intake

Use cream, whole, evaporated whole, or sweetened condensed milk instead of water for baking whenever possible. Add skim milk powder (2–4 Tbsp/cup) or instant breakfast powder to regular whole milk for use as a beverage. Make milkshakes with ice cream.

Use liberal portions of butter, margarine, oil, and cheeses on vegetables, breads, and in soups and hot cereals. Use gravies or sauces on meats and starches.

Add sugar, jelly, or honey to toast and cereals. Use fruits canned in heavy syrup, or sweeten fresh fruits with added sugar. Serve dried fruits like raisins or apricots.

Use peanut butter or cheese on fruit or crackers, make finger sandwiches for meals or snacks.

Use mayonnaise or salad dressings liberally on sandwiches, and salads, or as a dip for vegetables.

Make sour cream or cream cheese dips for chips or fruits.

---

temperature of liquids and solid foods may be necessary. Using a straw can be helpful for patients with mouth pain. The assistance of a speech pathologist or feeding therapist may be useful to facilitate safe oral feeding.

Various pharmacological agents have been used in HIV-infected individuals to improve dietary intake and nutritional status. Adults receiving Megestrol acetate increased their caloric intake, had an improved sense of well being, and had a significant increase in body weight (Oster et al 1994, Von Roenn et al 1994). However, only one of the studies demonstrated a significant improvement in lean body mass (Von Roenn et al 1994). Children treated with Megestrol acetate for 6 months demonstrated significant weight gain (Clarick et al 1997). Further studies are necessary to evaluate the long-term effectiveness on dietary intake and growth. Dronabinol, a marijuana derivative, may also be effective in stimulating appetite and weight gain (Beal et al 1995).

Specialized nutrition support

When growth faltering or poor oral intake continues despite routine dietary manipulations, supplementation with medical nutritionals either orally or by tube feedings is indicated. Most are packaged in convenient, single-serving sizes, but can be costly if needed on a daily basis. Early intervention is thought to be critical, as reversing growth deficits may be difficult, particularly as children become more symptomatic (Henderson et al 1994, Miller et al 1995). In addition, higher CD4 cell number and lower weight-for-height predicted a positive response to tube feedings, and children who responded favourably had a lower mortality risk (Miller et al 1995).

Enteral formula selection

Many enteral formulas are available. Two studies have suggested that altering formula composition may result in improved nutritional status compared to standard formulas in HIV-infected adults (Chlebowski et al 1993, Suttmann et al 1996). No data exists regarding the optimal nutrient composition for children with HIV. It is helpful to consider the source of macronutrients, fibre content and caloric density when selecting an enteral formula for oral or tube feeding (Table 29.5). In general, milk-based formulas are appropriate for children without symptoms of gastrointestinal dysfunction. Modification of formula composition may help to improve growth and minimize gastrointestinal distress. Diarrhoea due to nutrient malabsorption worsens with feedings, whereas secretory diarrhoea improves very little while nothing by mouth (NPO) and rarely responds to dietary manipulation.

Enteral tube feedings

Tube feeding is indicated when oral intake is unsafe or inadequate to meet nutrient requirements. Although tube feedings increase the effort of care, they often greatly improve quality of life by reducing the pressure on family and child to further increase oral intake or consume unpalatable formula and by decreasing gastrointestinal symptoms due to delayed gastric emptying or diarrhoea. Tube feedings can be used as a supplement to oral intake when weight gain is poor despite oral dietary interventions or as the sole source of nutrient intake when oral feeding is precluded due to odynophagia or dysfunctional swallowing, which poses a safety risk due to direct aspiration and pulmonary complications. Routes and modes of delivering tube feedings are summarized in Table 29.6. Optimizing the feeding schedule minimizes symptoms such as regurgitation, vomiting, abdominal distention or discomfort and diarrhoea. The feeding schedule should be determined following consideration of the family's lifestyle needs. Home tube feeding can offer a safe and cost-effective alternative to hospitalization or confinement to a chronic care facility. Patient selection criteria include the child's clinical status, ability to achieve nutritional goals, the abilities and wishes of the family members, the home environment, resources for obtaining supplies and equipment, financial resources and quality of life issues.

Table 29.5 — Considerations for enteral formula selection

Formula component	Uses	Comment
Protein		
Whole (casein or soy)	Children without evidence of malabsorption	Most palatable Low osmolality useful for children with delayed gastric emptying
Peptides or free amino acids	Children with diarrhoea or malabsorption	Less palatable Require less digestion Higher osmolality may delay gastric emptying Expensive
Carbohydrate		
Lactose	Children without evidence of lactose intolerance	Most enteral formulas do not contain lactose
Glucose polymers/corn syrup solids	Carbohydrate malabsorption	
Glucose	Severe malabsorption, intolerance to other sugars	Readily absorbed Higher osmolality may delay gastric emptying
Sucrose	Carbohydrate malabsorption	As part of total CHO content, helps diversify route of CHO digestion and absorption
Fat		
Long-chain triglycerides	Children without steatorrhoea	
Medium-chain triglycerides	Children with steatorrhoea	May increase fat absorption, decrease GI symptoms. Children with steatorrhoea at risk for essential fatty acid and fat soluble vitamin deficiency on formulas with very low levels of LCT
Fibre (soy polysaccharide)	Children with diarrhoea	Facilitates care of perianal inflammation and excoriation helps older children control bowel movements Increased abdominal distension due to gas from fibre fermentation may result, particularly when there is uncontrolled bacterial overgrowth
Increased caloric density	Volume sensitivity Reduce nocturnal awakenings due to urination	Standard density is 1 kcal/mL. Commercially available formulas are available up to 2 kcal/mL, or additional fat and/or CHO may be added

Abbreviations: CHO, carbohydrate, GI, gastrointestinal; LCT, long chair, triglycerides

Table 29.6 — Enteral tube feedings: methods for administration

Route	Indications	Complications
Nasogastric	Short-term use	May cause or exacerbate sinusitis or otitis Frequent need for replacement may deter compliance
Gastric	Long-term use Facilitates medication delivery	Primary infectious complication is ostomy site infection, may be ameliorated with meticulous maintenance of a clean tube and ostomy site
Jejunal	Severe impairment of gastric emptying To minimize risk of pulmonary aspiration A tube with both gastric and jejunal ports allows gastric decompression while administering feedings	Small opening(s) at the distal tip prone to occlusion
Mode of delivery		
Bolus	For children without significant diarrhoea or vomiting May be least restrictive and easy to administer	May interfere with oral intake
Continuous Drip	Overnight supplement to oral feedings To improve absorption and reduce GI discomfort	Sleep disturbance due to feedings or the need to urinate or defecate Need to interrupt feedings for medications requiring an empty stomach, such as dideoxyinosine

Parenteral nutrition

Parenteral nutrition may be necessary if adequate enteral feeding becomes impossible due to persistent feeding intolerance or poor nutritional response to enteral feedings. Parenteral nutrition resulted in improved weight and body cell mass and improved well-being in adults with AIDS (Melchior et al 1996). In our experience, significant improvement in comfort and well being can be achieved with parenteral feedings, in addition to nutritional rehabilitation or maintenance. Administration through a peripheral intravenous catheter is useful for short-term support (less than 2–3 weeks) during an acute complication, but central venous catheter are during requiring long-term support. Portable intravenous pumps facilitate home care, and cycling the infusion to allow time off during the day should be considered when possible to enhance the child's mobility. When considering home parenteral nutrition support, the risks, benefits and burden must be considered carefully by the family. Procurement of additional caregivers and home nursing care may be required to administer and monitor home parenteral feedings.

Complications associated with parenteral nutrition include infectious, metabolic and mechanical problems.

The majority of central venous catheters placed in HIV-infected adults were found to be free of complications, and could be used safely and effectively with an acceptable infection rate (Sweed et al 1995). Metabolic complications include fluid and electrolyte disturbances and glucose or lipid intolerance. Frequent monitoring and manipulation of the parental solution may be necessary under these circumstances. Maintaining the maximal amount of enteral feedings tolerated is important to maintain gastrointestinal tract integrity and reduce the risk of cholestasis. Mechanical problems with central intravenous catheters include occlusion, damage and accidental removal of the catheter.

References

Alfaro, M.P., Siegel, R.M., Baker, R.C., Heubi, J.E. (1995) Resting energy expenditure and body composition in pediatric HIV infection. *Pediatr AIDS HIV infect*, 6, 276–280.

Altemeier, W.A., O'Connor, S.M., Sherrod, K.B., Vietze, P.M. (1985) Prospective study of antecedants for nonorganic failure to thrive. *J Pediatr*, 106, 360–365.

Arditi, M., Kabat, W., Yogev, R. (1991) Serum tumor necrosis factor alpha, interleukin 1-beta, p24 antigen concentrations, and CD4$^+$ cells at various stages of human immunodeficiency virus 1 in children. *Pediatr Inf Dis J*, 10, 450–455.

Baum, M.K., Mantero-Atienza, E., Shor-Posner, G., et al. (1991) Association of vitamin B6 status with parameters of immune function in early HIV-1 infection *J AIDS*, 4, 1122–1132.

Beach, R.S., Mantero-Atienza, E., Shor-Posner, G., Javier, J.J., Szapocznik, J., Morgan, R., Sauberlich, H.E., Cornwell, P.E., Eisdorfer, C., Baum, M.K. (1992a) Specific nutrient abnormalities in asymptomatic individuals. *Acquir Immunodefic Syndr*, 6, 701–708.

Beach, R.S., Morgan, R., Wilkie, F. et al. (1992b) Plasma vitamin B12 level as a potential co-factor in studies of human immunodeficiency virus type-1 related cognitive changes. *Arch Neurol*, 49, 501–506.

Beal, J.E., Olson, R., Laubenstein, L. et al. (1995) Dronabinol as a treatment for anorexia associated with weight loss in patients with AIDS. *J Pain Symptom Manage*, 10, 89–97.

Bogden, J.D., Baker, H., Frank, O. (1990) Micronutrient status and human immunodeficiency virus (HIV) infection. *Ann NY Acad Sci*, 587, 189–195.

Brettler, D.B., Forsberg, A., Bolivar, E., Brewster, F., Sullivan, J. (1990) Growth failure as a prognostic indicator for progression to acquired immunodeficiency syndrome in children with hemophilia. *J Pediatr*, 117, 584–588.

Bulterys, M. et al. (1994) Maternal human immunodeficiency virus 1 infection and intrauterine growth: A prospective cohort study in Butare, Rwanda. *Pediatr Inf Dis J*, 13, 94–100.

Butz, A., Hutton, N., Larson, E. (1991) Immunoglobulins and growth parameters at birth of infants born to HIV seropositive and seronegative women. *Am J Pub Health*, 81, 1323–1326.

Chlebowski, R.T., Beall, G., Grosvenor, M. et al. (1993) Long-term effects of early nutritional support with new enterotropic peptide-based formula vs. standard enteral formula in HIV-infected patients: Randomized prospective trial. *Nutrition*, 9, 507–512.

Clarick, R.H., Hanekom, W.A., Yogev, R., Chadwick, E.G. (1997) Megestrol acetate treatment of growth failure in children infected with human immunodeficiency virus. *Pediatr*, 99, 354–357.

Connor, E.M., Sperling, R.S., Gelber, R. et al. (1994) Reduction of maternal-infant transmission of human immunodeficiency virus type 1 with zidovudine treatment. *N Engl J Med*, 331, 1173–1180.

Coutsoudis, A., Bobat, R.A., Coovakia, H.M., Kuhn, L., Tsai, W.Y., Stein, Z.A. (1995) The effects of vitamin A supplementation on the morbidity of children born to HIV-infected women. *Am J Pub Health*, 85, 1076–1081.

European Collaborative Study. (1995) Weight, height and human immunodeficiency virus infection in young children of infected mothers. *Pediatr Inf Dis J*, 14, 685–690.

Frisancho, A.R. (1993) *Anthropometic Standards for The Assessment of Growth And Nutritional Status*. Ann Arbor: University of Michigan Press.

Geffner, M.E., Yeh, D.Y., Landaw, E.M. et al. (1993) In Vitro insulin-like growth factor-1, growth hormone, and insulin resistance occurs in symptomatic human immunodeficiency virus-1-infected children. *Pediatr Res*, 34, 66–72.

Geunter, P., Muurahainin, N., Simons, G., Kosok, A., Cohan, G.R., Rudenstein, R., Turner, J.L. (1993) Relationships among nutritional status, disease progression, and survival in HIV infection. *J Acquir Immune Defic Syndr*, 6, 1130–1138.

Graham, N.M.H., Sorensen, D., Odaka, N., Brookmeyer, R., Chan, D., Willett, W.C., Morris, J.S., Saah, A.J. (1991) Relationship of serum copper and zinc levels to HIV-1 seropositivity and progression to AIDS. *J Acq Immune Defic Syndr*, 4, 976–980.

Guay, L.A. et al. (1996) Detection of human innumodeficiency virus type 1 (HIV-1) DNA and p24 antigen in breast milk of HIV-1 infected Ugandan women and bertical transmission. *Pediatr*, 98, 438–444.

Henderson, R.A., Miotti, P.G., Saavedra, J.M. et al. (1996) Longitudinal growth during the first 2 years of life in children born to HIV-infected mothers in Malawi, Africa. *Pediatr AIDS and HIV infect*, 7, 91–97.

Henderson, R.A., Saavedra, J.M., Perman, J.A., Hutton, N., Livingston, R.A., Yolken, R.H. (1994) Effect of Enteral tube feeding on growth of children with symptomatic human immunodeficiency virus infection. *J Pediatr Gastroenterol Nutr*, 18, 429–434.

Henderson, R.A., Talusan, K., Hutton, N., Yolken, R.H., Caballero, B. (1999) Whole body protein turnover in children with HIV infection. *Nutrition* 15, 189–194.

Henderson, R.A., Talusan, K., Hutton, N., Yolken, R.H., Caballero, B. (1997) Serum and plasma markers of nutritional status in children with HIV infection. *J Am Diet Assn.* 97, 1377–1381.

Henderson, R.A., Talusan, K., Hutton, N., Yolken, R.H., Caballero, B. (1998) Resting energy expenditure and body composition in asymptomatic children with HIV infection. *J AIDS*, 19, 150–157.

Hirschfeld, S., Laue, L., Cutler, G.B., Pizzo, P.A. (1996) Thyroid abnormalities in children infected with human immunodeficiency virus. *J Pediatr*, 128, 70–74.

Italian Paediatric Intestinal/HIV Study Group. (1993) Intestinal malabsorption of HIV-infected children: Relationship to diarrhoea, failure to thrive, enteric micro-organisms and immune impairment. *Acquir Immunodefic Syndr*, 7, 1435–1440.

Joint United Nations programme on HIV/AIDS (UNAIDS). (1996a) The HIV/AIDS situation in mid 1996: Global and regional highlights. Fact sheet. Geneva, Switzerland: World Health Organization, 71, 205–212.

Joint United Nations programme on HIV/AIDS (UNAIDS). (1996b) HIV and infant feeding: An interim statement. Geneva, Switzerland: World Health Organization, 71, 289–296.

Kavanaugh-McHugh, A.L., Ruff, A., Perlman, E., Hutton, N., Modlin, J., Rowe, S. (1991) Selenium deficiency and cardiomyopathy in acquired immunodeficiency syndrome. *J Parenter Enteral Nutr*, 15, 347–349.

Kotler, D.P., Wang, J., Pierson, R.N. (1985) Body composition studies in patients with the acquired immunodeficiency syndrome. *Am J Clin Nutr*, 42, 1255–1265.

Kotloff, K.L., Johnson, J.P., Nair, P. et al. (1994) Diarrheal morbidity during the first 2 years of life among HIV-infected infants. *JAMA*, 271, 448–452.

Macallan, D.C., Noble, C., Baldwin, C. et al. (1995a) Energy expenditure and wasting in human immunodeficiency virus infection. *N Engl J Med*, 333, 83–88.

Macallan, D.C., McNurlan, M.A., Milne, E., Calder, A.G., Garlick, P.J., Griffin, G.E. (1995b) Whole-body protein turnover from leucine kinetics and the response to nutrition in human immunodeficiency virus infection. *Am J Clin Nutr*, 61, 818–826.

McCorkindale, C., Dybevik, K., Coulston, A.M., Sucher, K.P. (1990) Nutritional status of HIV-infected patients during the early disease stages. *J Am Diet Assoc*, 90, 1236–1241.

McKinney, R.E., Robertson, J.W.R. (1993) Duke Pediatric AIDS Clinical Trials Unit. Effect of human immunodeficiency virus infection on the growth of young children. *J Pediatr*, 123, 579–582.

McKinney, R.E., Wilfert, C. (1994) AIDS Clinical Trials Group Protocol 043 Study Group. Growth as a prognostic indicator in children with human immunodeficiency virus infection treated with zidovudine. *J Pediatr*, 125, 728–733.

Mantero-Atienza, E., Beach, R.S., Gavancho, M.C., Morgan, R., Shor-Posner, G., Fordyce-Baum, M.K. (1991) Selenium status of HIV-1 infected individuals. *J Parenter Enter Nutr*, 15, 693–694.

Melchior, J.C., Chastang, C., Gelas, P. et al. (1996) Efficacy of 2-month total parenteral nutrition in AIDS patients: A controlled randomized prospective trial. *Acquir Immunodef Syndr*, 10, 379–384.

Melchior, J.C., Raguin, G., Boulier, A. et al. (1993) Resting energy expenditure in human immunodeficiency virus-infected patients: Comparison between patients with and without secondary infections. *Am J Clin Nutr*, 57, 614–619.

Miller, T.L., Awnetwant, E.L., Evans, S., Morris, V.M., Vazquez, I.M., McIntosh, K. (1995) Gastrostomy tube supplementation for HIV-infected children. *Pediatr*, 96, 696–702.

Miller, T.L., Evans, S.J., Orav, E.J. et al. (1993) Growth and body composition in children infected with the human immunodeficiency virus-1. *Am J Clin Nutr*, 57, 588–592.

Moye, J., Rich, K.C., Kalish, L.A., Sheon, A.R., Diaz, C., Cooper, E.E.R., Pitt, J., Handelsman, E. (1996) Women and infants transmission study group. Natural history of somatic growth in infants born to women infected by human immunodeficiency virus. *J Pediatr*, 128, 58–69.

Oleske, J.M. (1994) The many needs of the HIV-infected child. *Hospital Practice*, 29, 81–87.

Oster, M.H., Enders, S.R., Samuels, S.J. et al. (1994) Megesterol acetate in patients with AIDS and cachexia. *Ann Int Med*, 121, 400–408.

Ott, M., Lembcke, B., Fischer, H. et al. (1993) Early changes of body composition in human immunodeficiency virus-infected patients: Tetrapolar body impedance analysis indicates significant malnutrition. *Am J Clin Nutr*, 57, 15–19.

Pizzo, P.A., Wilfert, C.M. (1994) *Pediatric AIDS: The Challenge of HIV Infection in Infants, Children and Adolescents*, 2nd edn. Baltimore: Williams & Wilkens.

Richman, D.D., Fischl, N.A., Grieco, M.H. et al. (1987) The toxicity of Azidothymidine (AZT) in the treatment of patients with AIDS and AIDS-related complex. *N Engl J Med*, 317, 192–197.

Ross, A., Raab, G.M., Mok, J. et al. (1995) Maternal HIV infection, drug use, and growth of uninfected children in their first 3 years. *Arch Dis Child*, 73, 490–495.

Ruff, A.J. (1994) Breastmilk, breastfeeding, and transmission of viruses to the neonate. *Seminars in Perinatol*, 18, 510–516.

Saavedra, J.M., Henderson, R.A., Perman, J.A., Hutton, N., Livingston, R.A., Yolken, R.H. (1995) Longitudinal assessment of growth in children born to mothers with human immunodeficiency virus infection. *Arch Pediatr Adolesc Med*, 149, 497–502.

Schable, B., Diaz, T., Chu, S.Y., Caldwell, M.B., Conti, L., Alston, O.M., Sorvillo, F., Checko, P.J., Hermann, P., Davidson, A.J., Boyd, D., Fann, S.A., Herr, M., Frederick, M. (1995) Who are the primary caretakers of children born to HIV-infected mothers? Results from a multistate surveillance project. *Pediatr*, 95, 511–515.

Schwartz. L.J., St Louis, Y., Wu, R., Wiznia, A., Rubenstein, A., Saenger, P. (1991) Endocrine function in children with human immunodeficiency virus infection. *Am J Dis Child*, 145, 330–333.

Semba, R.D., Graham, N.M.H., Caiaffa, W.T., Margolick, J.B., Clement, L., Vlahov, D. (1993) Increased mortality with vitamin A deficiency during human immunodeficiency virus type 1 infection. *Arch Int Med*, 153, 2149–2154.

Semba, R.D., Miotti, P.G., Chiphangwi, J.D., Saah, A.J., Canner, J.K., Dallabetta, G.A., Hoover, D.R. (1994) Maternal vitamin A deficiency and mother-to-child transmission of HIV-1. *Lancet*, 343, 1593–1597.

Stanton, D.L., Wu, A.W., Moore, R.D., Rucker, S.C., Piazza, M.P., Abrams, J.E., Chaisson, R.E. (1994) Functional status of persons with HIV infection in an ambulatory setting. *J Acquir Immune Defic*, 7, 1050–1056.

Stein, T.P., Nutinsky, D.C., Condoluci, D. et al. (1990) Protein and energy substrate metabolism in AIDS patients. *Metabolism*, 39, 876–881.

Suttmann, U., Ockenga, J., Schneider, H. et al. (1996) Weight gain and increased concentrations of receptor proteins for tumor necrosis factor after patients with symptomatic HIV infection received fortified nutrition support. *J Am Diet Assn*, 96, 565–569.

Sweed, M., Guenter, P., Lucente, K., Turner, J.L., Weingarten, M.S. (1995) Long-term central venous catheters in patients with acquired immunodeficiency syndrome. *Am J Infect Control*, 23, 194–199.

Von Roenn, J.H., Armstrong, D., Kotler, D.P. et al. (1994) Megesterol acetate in patients with AIDS-related cachexia. *Ann Int Med*, 121, 393–399.

Wilfert, C.M., Wilson, C., Luzuriaga, K. et al. (1994) Pathogenesis of pediatric human immunodeficiency virus type-1 infection. *J Infect Dis*, 170, 286–292.

Yolken, R.H., Hart, W., Oung, I. et al. (1991) Gastrointestinal dysfunction and disaccharide intolerance in children infected with human immunodeficiency virus. *J Pediatr*, 118, 359–363.

Zuin, G., Comi, D., Fontana, M., Tornaghi, R., Brugnani, M., Fadini, S., Principi, N. (1994) Energy and nutrient intakes in HIV-infected children. *Pediatr AIDS and HIV Infect*, 5, 159–161.

30

Nutritional requirements and support in liver disease

Susan M. Protheroe and Deirdre A. Kelly

Abbreviations

AA	Amino acid
AAA	Aromatic amino acid
BCAA	Branched chain amino acid
DHA	Docosahexaenoic acid
EAR	Estimated average requirements
EFA	Essential fatty acid
EHBA	Extrahepatic biliary atresia
EPA	Eicosapentaenoic acid
IGF1	Insulin like growth factor1
IGFBP3	Insulin like growth factor binding protein3
LCPUFA	Long-chain polyunsaturated fatty acid
LCT	Long-chain triglyceride
LT	Liver transplantation
MAC	Mid-arm circumference
MCT	Medium-chain triglyceride
PEM	protein energy malnutrition
PN	Parenteral nutrition
PUFA	Polyunsaturated fatty acid
TSF	Triceps skinfold

Introduction

Protein energy malnutrition (PEM) is an inevitable consequence of chronic liver disease, particularly in the developing infant. Severe malnutrition (weight and/or height < 2 standard deviations below the mean) with loss of fat stores and muscle wasting affects 60% of infants with liver disease (Beath et al 1993a). Both morbidity and mortality post liver transplantation are related to the degree of pre-transplant malnutrition, and thus nutritional status is an important risk factor for survival (Moukarzel et al 1990, Beath et al 1994).

Although the pathophysiology is not fully understood, there are many different mechanisms leading to malnutrition. Reduced energy intake secondary to anorexia and vomiting, fat malabsorption, disordered metabolism of carbohydrate and protein, increased energy requirements and vitamin and mineral deficiencies all contribute towards growth failure. As the severity of the absorptive and metabolic defects may vary, each child should be assessed to determine both content and method of nutritional support, which may range from increased enteral supplementation to parenteral nutrition (PN). Accurate nutritional assessment combined with early intervention and prevention of malnutrition is essential and may increase survival as well as improve the quality of life and the outcome of liver transplantation (Moukarzel et al 1990, Chin et al 1992).

Historical background

Pathophysiology of malnutrition in liver disease

Reduced energy intake

Anorexia is common and may be due to ascites and hepatosplenomegaly or dietary manipulations such as fluid restriction or prescription of unpalatable feeds.

Fat malabsorption

At least 50% of long-chain triglycerides (LCT), along with fat-soluble vitamins and the essential polyunsaturated fatty acids (PUFA) may be malabsorbed due to reduced intraluminal bile concentration (Beath et al 1993b).

Portal hypertension, leading to congested gastric and intestinal mucosa, combined with small-bowel overgrowth (in the presence of a Roux en Y 'blind' loop created in a Kasai portoenterostomy) may furthur exacerbate malabsorption, as may Cholestyramine (which is used to reduce pruritus) by binding bile salts. Pancreatic function is usually intact (Beath et al 1993b), except for children with Alagilles syndrome in whom pancreatic lipase may be low (Chong et al 1989). Fat malabsorption produces steatorrhoea, reduction in body fat stores leading to wasting and stunting, and fat-soluble vitamin (vitamins A, D, E and K) deficiency. Essential fatty acid (EFA) deficiency may lead to skin rash and hair loss.

Hepatic metabolism

Reduced hepatic and muscle glycogen stores lead to early recruitment of fat and increased reliance on amino acids as alternative fuels (McCullough et al 1989). These metabolic changes result in muscle wasting, hyperammonaemia, hypoproteinaemia, hypoglycaemia, hyperlipaemia and reduced circulating triglycerides (due to increased fat oxidation). Low branched chain amino acids (BCAA) and raised aromatic amino acids (AAA) and methionine reflect abnormal protein utilization (Weisdorf et al 1987). Growth failure may be compounded by the impaired response to growth hormone (Quirk et al 1994, Holt et al 1996), since insulin like growth factor1 (IGF1) and its major circulating binding protein, insulin like growth factor binding protein3 (IGFBP3), are derived from the liver.

Increased energy expenditure

Energy requirements are increased up to 140%

(Pierro et al 1989, McKiernan et al 1994) by different mechanisms, including porto-systemic shunting and ascites, abnormal intermediary metabolism and the energy demands of complications such as sepsis and variceal haemorrhage.

Practice and procedures

Assessment of malnutrition

Assessment and monitoring of patients involves clinical assessment (Table 30.1) and anthropometric, laboratory and radiological tests.

Anthropometry

Growth failure may precede the clinical signs of liver disease such as ascites or splenomegaly. Measurements of body weight and linear growth detect acute malnutrition (decreased weight for height) and chronic malnutrition (decreased height for age) (Waterlow 1973). The ratio between head circumference and mid-arm circumference (MAC) indicatates malnutrition in children under the age of 5 (normal > 0.3). Triceps skinfold (TSF) and mid-arm circumference are useful indicators of body fat and protein reserves and allow the calculation of mid-arm muscle area, which reflects body muscle mass. Serial anthropometric recordings of TSF may demonstrate early loss of fat stores before weight and height changes become obvious (Frisancho 1981, Sann et al 1988, Sokal & Stall 1990). For comparison, data is expressed as standard deviation scores (or 'Z' scores) related to the median value for the child's age and sex, where a Z score of zero equals the fiftieth percentile.

Practical difficulties when monitoring infants with liver disease

The need for nutritional support in infants with liver disease is often underestimated due to abnormal body composition. Body weight is a useful index of nutrition in most children, but is unreliable in patients with liver disease with ascites and/or organomegaly. Linear growth may be more sensitive but is a late sign of growth failure in infancy, particularly as stunting (or negative height velocity) may not be apparent until 1 year of age (Beath et al 1993c). Serial measurements of MAC and TSF, taken in combination with changing trends in height or weight are the most sensitive indicators for the instigation of nutritional support.

Table 30.1 — Clinical manifestations of malnutrition in liver disease

Aetiology	Clinical manifestations
Protein energy malnutrition	Growth failure
Protein catabolism	Muscle wasting, motor development delay
Fat malabsorption	Steatorrhoea
EFA deficiency	Peeling skin rash
Vitamin A deficiency	Conjunctival and corneal drying, abnormal retinal function, night blindness
Vitamin E deficiency	Peripheral neuropathy, ophthalmoplegia, ataxia, haemolysis
Vitamin D deficiency	Osteopenia, rickets, fractures
Vitamin K deficiency	Bruising, epistaxis, coagulopathy
Zinc deficiency	Acrodermatitis, anorexia, poor growth
Hypercholesterolaemia	Xanthomata
Impaired gastrointestinal function, hypochlorhydria, reduced mucosal function	Diarrhoea
Immunosuppression secondary to reduced cell mediated immunity	Systemic infections

Selecting patients for nutritional support

Patients at particular risk of development of malnutrition

- Under 2 years of age;
- Severe cholestasis (serum bilirubin > 70 mmol/L; > 50% conjugated);
- Progressive liver disease such as biliary atresia, severe neonatal hepatitis;
- Patients awaiting liver transplantation.

Growth failure should be anticipated and prevented by frequent anthropometric assessment. Urgent support is required if the MAC and TSF are more than 2 standard deviations below the mean.

Nutritional requirements and strategies for nutritional support

Nutritional intervention should attempt to compensate for anorexia, increased energy requirements, mal-absorption and abnormal hepatic metabolism (Fig. 30.1).

Components of nutritional support

Lipids

The energy value of dietary lipids is 8–9 kcal/g. They are the major energy source for infants. Increasing fat intake, despite increasing steatorrhoea, may increase the overall amount of fat absorbed (Beath et al 1993b).

Medium-chain triglycerides

Medium-chain triglycerides (MCT) are well absorbed in cholestatic infants. Therefore, the addition of 30–50% MCT is a useful substrate, reducing steatorrhoea (Burke & Danks 1966, Cohen & Gartner 1971) with subsequent nutritional improvement (Beath et al 1993b).

Essential fatty acids

Although the exact requirements for infants are not known, clinical deficiency symptoms may occur at PUFA intakes below 1% of energy (Crawford et al 1978). Mature human milk contains 11% wt/wt essential fatty acids. The minimal intake of linoleic acid recommended for young infants is 2.7–4.5% of energy and a ratio of linoleic:linolenic acid of 5:1.

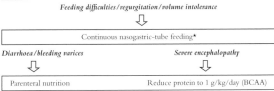

Figure 30.1 — Nutritional support for infants with liver disease. ★ – +/– energy supplement eg Maxijul Liquigen Gastrostomy feeding is not recommended due to potential formation of gastric varices and ascites secondary to portal hypertension.

Fat-soluble vitamins (see Fig. 30.1)

Proprietary oral multivitamin preparations, such as Ketovite liquid and tablets (Paines & Byrne), may be inadequate for infants with cholestasis, and it is best to prescribe these vitamins separately. Generous oral doses may be required to produce therapeutic plasma concentrations. Occasionally, intramuscular vitamin D is required.

Carbohydrate

Complex carbohydrates such as maltodextrin or glucose polymer (Maxijul, Scientific Hospital Supplies (SHS)) restrict the osmolality of the feed while maintaing a high energy density (> 1 kcal/mL) allowing fluid restriction. Additions are made slowly to establish intestinal tolerance.

Protein

There may be a reluctance to increase protein intake beyond the estimated requirement for normal children because low protein diets were previously prescribed to prevent encephalopathy. Increasing the calorie density of proprietary infant formulae with carbohydrate and fat supplements may result in decreased protein concentration. It is now recognized that infants with advanced liver disease may tolerate up to 4 g/kg/day protein without encephalopathy or an increase in plasma amino acid abnormalities (Charlton et al 1992). In practice, 3–4 g/kg/day of a whole protein, which is more palatable, is preferred. Modified amino acid formulations designed to improve the balance of AAA and BCAA in plasma may be of nutritional benefit and are under evaluation.

Mineral supplementation

Zinc deficiency secondary to chronic malabsorption may contribute to anorexia and poor linear growth. Plasma zinc concentration may not reflect total body zinc status, but supplementation may be helpful if deficiency is suspected because of persistent poor growth.

Modular feeds

If ascites or encephalopathy develop, fluid and salt restriction may make commercial feeds impractical. The use of calorie-dense supplements in a modular feed allows individual prescription of protein, energy, sodium and water intake to produce a feed of high-energy density (> 1 kcal/mL). Calogen and Liquigen emulsions (Scientific Hospital Supplies, UK, Ltd) supply a mixture of LCT and MCT. Super Soluble Maxipro, a low salt whey protein (SHS) and Maxijul (SHS), a complex carbohydrate polymer, provide protein and carbohydrate components respectively. Vitamin and mineral requirements are added (e.g., Paedatric Seravit, SHS) as well as sodium (not < 1 mmol/kg/day for growth) and potassium (as molar solutions).

Mode of delivery

Enteral feeds

A soft silastic nasogastric tube is well accepted in infants. It is not, by itself, likely to provoke bleeding from oesophageal varices, and it allows reliable delivery of medications. It is essential to prepare infants with play therapy and to train parents carefully. The success of home enteral feeding depends on a dedicated

multi-disciplinary team including dietician, liaison nurse, clinician and community support. Intensive enteral feeding is highly effective in reversing PEM in infants with liver disease. It may induce a transformation in the child's affect and even increase voluntary intake (Moreno et al 1991, Charlton et al 1992, Beath et al 1994).

Behavioural problems

Behavioural feeding problems are common and are secondary to long-term tube feeding, unpalatable feeds or medications. These infants may miss their developmental milestones for chewing, swallowing and perhaps speech. The pre-transplant emphasis on intensive nutritional support often creates parental anxiety about feeding. It is not surprising that behavioural feeding problems may become manifest pre and post transplantation and contribute towards persistent growth failure. Strategies to prevent this include daytime feeding to provide oral stimulation, particularly if nocturnal nasogastric feeding is undertaken. A multi-disciplinary approach, involving participation of clinician, nurse specialist, clinical psychologist and play therapist is required to prevent or treat these difficult problems.

Post liver transplantation

Parenteral nutrition (PN) is commenced on post-operative day 1 for infants with pre-transplant mal-nutrition, if feeding is to be delayed. In most cases, oral feeding is started as soon as post-operative ileus has resolved. Nutritional support provides an energy intake of around 120% of EAR as a modular feed or as a high energy or follow-on formula prior to discharge. Additional supplements of fat and carbohydrate may be required for some time to maintain growth while establishing normal oral intake. In 10% of infants, nocturnal enteral feeding is required for up to 1–2 years. Osteopenia often persists after successful liver transplantation (LT), and it may take many months of vitamin D and adequate nutrition to correct (Argao et al 1994).

Parenteral nutrition

PN is rarely necessary unless there is persistent diarrhoea or feed intolerance. If there is severe PEM or malabsorption, PN may be helpful. Short-term PN is essential during complications such as intra-abdominal sepsis, variceal bleeding and liver failure, which are associated with marked catabolism and weight loss.

Despite perceived reluctance to use PN in children with chronic liver disease because of the association with hepato-biliary dysfunction (Puntis et al 1987, Sax & Bower 1988), short-term PN does not increase cholestasis, and standard amino acid mixtures (e.g., Vaminolact) are safe. Patients need careful biochemical monitoring and attention to fluid and electrolyte balance, including concurrent intravenous infusion therapy.

Delivery of PN

Central venous catheterization with double or triple lumen catheter offers convenient and reliable venous access if the duration of feeding is more than a week.

Laboratory parameters

Serial monitoring of laboratory parameters may detect malnutrition in time to allow nutritional intervention. Proteins, such as albumin or retinol-binding protein may assess recent or long-term adequacy of protein and calorie intake, but are non-specific as serum protein concentrations may vary due to protein loss, distribution, vitamin and mineral status and hepatic disease.

Laboratory monitoring of calcium, phosphate and magnesium levels reflects vitamin D intake and metabolism. Plasma concentrations of vitamins A and E demonstrate therapeutic levels and stores. Coagulation tests reflect both hepatic synthetic function and vitamin K supplementation. Zinc may be depleted in patients with persistent anorexia or poor growth. Elevated serum copper reflects disturbed biliary copper excretion, but treatment is seldom necessary measurement of triglyceride and cholesterol may assess the balance of the energy providing fuels in the feed, while plasma amino acids may assess protein metabolism in the face of progressive liver dysfunction.

Radiology

Wrist and knee X-rays are performed to detect osteopenia and rickets if alkaline phosphatase is elevated (> 1000 IU).

Future developments

Long-chain polyunsaturated fatty acids (LCPUFA)

LCPUFAs such as aracidonic acid and docosahexaenoic acid (DHA) are emerging as essential nutrients in infancy. LCPUFAs have been reported to affect the development of visual acuity and mental development in the first year of life, and DHA plays an important role in the development of the nervous system, particularly the retina and visual pathway (Makrides et al 1995). Neonatal DHA is supplied trans-placentally, but after birth the major source is dietary. Aracidonic acid, which is formed from linoleic acid, may be important for normal growth, at least in pre-term infants (Carlson et al 1992).

Infants with cholestatic liver disease are at risk of DHA deficiency secondary to malabsorption of long-chain triglycerides (LCT), prescription of diets rich in MCT and inadequate liver desaturase enzyme activity. Low red cell phospholipid percentage of DHA has been documented in cholestatic infants and may be associated with impaired visual development. Deficiency arises between 3 and 12 months of age when maternally-derived DHA is exhausted (Spray et al 1995). This suggests that infants with cholestatic liver disease may benefit from DHA supplements.

Branched Chain Amino Acids (BCAA)

Leucine, valine and isoleucine have several properties of potential benefit to malnourished infants with liver disease (Weisdorf 1989). BCAA, especially leucine, may be an energy substrate, promote muscle protein synthesis, and inhibit muscle protein breakdown through the formation of its ketoanalogue, alpha-ketoisocaproate (Tischler 1982, Garlick & Grant 1988). A trial conducted in children awaiting liver transplantation (Chin et al 1992) suggests that supplementation with 32% BCAA is associated with improved lean body mass.

The effect of a modified amino acid supplement (50% BCAA) in a modular feed was compared to an isonitrogenous formula (22% BCAA) on protein kinetics (measured by whole body protein turnover) and plasma amino acid profile in infants with liver disease (Protheroe et al 1996). The BCAA supplemented feed normalized the plasma amino acid profile and improved protein retention by suppressing endogenous protein catabolism. The effects of BCAA are under evaluation, and until the results of randomized trials are available, BCAA are reserved for those patients with demonstrated protein intolerance.

Structured lipids

Triglycerides that contain both long- and medium-chain fatty acids bound to the same glycerol molecule are absorbed directly like MCT. Clinical studies of these modified lipids (to increase the absorption of long-chain fatty acids) are currently in preliminary stages (Carnielli et al 1996).

Discussion

An understanding of the pathophysiological mechanisms contributing towards malnutrition in infants with liver disease is essential when planning therapeutic strategies. Growth failure should be anticipated by serial anthropometric assessment. This includes the estimation of fat and muscle stores by measurement of MAC and TSF as estimates of body composition. Patients at particular risk of development of malnutrition are those with severe cholestasis, progressive liver disease and those awaiting liver transplantation.

The first step in nutritional support for infants with liver disease includes increased calorie intake, generous oral fat soluble vitamin supplementation and nasogastric tube feeding. It is vital to increase the energy intake to 140–200% of EAR, depending on the needs of the infant. This is achieved by supplementing feeds with extra fat (up to 8 g/kg/day) and carbohydrate (up to 15–20 g/kg/day) to produce a feed with a high-energy density (1 kcal/mL) and with an intake of 3–4 g/kg/day protein. Nocturnal enteral feeding may circumvent the abnormal homeostatic control of carbohydrate and protein metabolism and avoid vomiting due to the small capacity of the stomach. A modular feed system permits flexibility in infants with end-stage liver disease when fluid or salt restriction for management of ascites may make commercially-available nutritionally-complete feeds impractical.

Future advances include BCAA and DHA supplementation and the use of structured lipids. The key to providing successful nutritional support is involvement of a multi-disciplinary team including paediatric dietician, liaison nurse, feeding pyschologist and clinician.

Acknowledgements

We are grateful for the insight and support provided by the members of the Paediatric Liver Unit and department of Dietetics at Birmingham Children's Hospital NHS Trust, especially Gill Brook, Graham Gordon, Jaswant Sira, Rosie Jones, Sara Janes and Anne Daly. We gratefully acknowledge the generous support provided by Action Research and The Children's Liver Disease Foundation for supporting some of the research advances described.

References

Argao, E.A., Balistreri, W.F., Hollis, B.W. et al (1994) Effect of orthotopic liver transplantation on bone mineral content and serum vitamin D metabolites in infants and children with chronic cholestasis. *Hepatology*, 20, 598–603.

Beath, S., Pearmain, G., Kelly, D., McMaster, P., Mayer, A., Buckels, J. (1993a) Liver transplantation in babies and children with extra hepatic biliary atresia: Pre-operative condition, complications, survival and outcome. *J Pediatr Surg*, 28, 1044–1047.

Beath, S., Hooley, I., Willis, K., Johnson, S., Kelly, D., Booth, I. (1993b) Long chain triacyglycerol malabsorption and pancreatic function in children with protein energy malnutrition complicating severe liver disease. *Proc Nutr Soc*, 52, 252A.

Beath, S.V., Booth, I.W., Kelly, D.A. (1993c) Nutritional support in liver disease. *Arch Dis Child*, 69, 545–549.

Beath, S., Brook, G., Kelly, D., McMaster, P., Mayer, D., Buckels, J. (1994) Improving outcome of liver transplantation in babies less than 1 year. *Transpl Proc*, 26, 180–182.

Burke, V., Danks, D.M. (1966) Medium chain triglyceride diet: Its use in treatment of liver disease. *BMJ*, 2, 1050–1051.

Carlson, S.E., Cooke, R.J., Werkman, S.H., Tolley, E.A. (1992) First year growth of preterm infants fed standard compared to marine oil n-3 supplemented formula. *Lipids*, 27, 901–907.

Carnielli, V.P., Luijendijk, I.H.T., Van Goudoever, J.B. et al (1996) Structural position and amount of palmitic acid in infant formulas: Effects on fat, fatty acid and mineral balance. *JPGN*, 23, 553–560.

Charlton, C.P.J., Buchanan, E., Holden, C.E., Preece, M.A., Green, A., Booth, I.W., Tarlow, M.J. (1992) Intensive enteral feeding in advanced cirrhosis: Reversal of malnutrition without precipatation of hepatic encephalopathy. *Arch Dis Child*, 67, 603–607.

Chin, S.E., Shepherd, R.W., Thomas, B.J., Cleghorn, G.J., Patrick, M.K., Wilcox, J.A., Hin Ong, T., Lynch, S.V., Strong, R. (1992) Nutritional support in children with end-stage liver disease: A randomised crossover trial of a branched-chain amino acid supplement. *Am J Clin Nut*, 56, 158–163.

Chong, S.K.F., Lindridge, J., Moniz, C., Mowat, A. (1989) Exocrine pancreatic insufficiency in syndromic paucity of interlobular bile ducts. *JPGN*, 9, 445–449.

Cohen, M.I., Gartner, L.M. (1971) The use of medium-chain triglycerides in the management of biliary atresia. *J Pediatr*, 79, 379–384.

Crawford, M.A., Hassam, A.G., Rivers, J.P.W. (1978) Essential fattty acid requirements in infancy. *Am J Clin Nutr*, 31, 2181–2185.

ESPGAN Committee on Nutrition (1991) Committee report. Comment on the content and composition of lipids in infant formulas. *Acta Paediatr Scan*, 80, 887–896.

Frisancho, A.R. (1981) New norms of upper limb fat and muscle areas for assessment of nutritional status. *Am J Clin Nut*, 34, 2540–2545.

Garlick, P.J., Grant, I. (1988) Amino acid infusion increases the sensitivity of muscle protein synthesis in vivo to insulin. *Biochem J*, 254, 579–584.

Holt, R.I., Jones, J.S., Stone, N.M. et al (1996) Sequential changes in insulin-like growth factor (IGF-1) and IGF-binding proteins in children with end-stage liver disease before and after successful orthotopic liver transplantation. *J Clin Endocrin Metabol*, 81, 160–168.

McCullough, A.J., Mullen, K.D., Smanik, E.J. et al (1989) Nutritional therapy and liver disease. *Gastroenter Clin N Amer*, 18, 619–643.

McKiernan, P.J., Magnay, A.R., Booth, I.W., Kelly, D.A. (1994) Determinants of resting energy expenditure in childhood liver disease. *J Paediatr Gastro Nutr* 19, 337.

Makrides, M., Neuman, M., Simmer, K. et al (1995) Are long-chain polyunsaturated fatty acids essential nutrients in infancy? *Lancet*, 345, 1463–1468.

Moreno, L.A., Gottrand, F., Hoden, S. et al (1991) Improvement of nutritional status in cholestatic children with supplemental nocturnal enteral nutrition. *J Ped Gastroenterol Nutr*, 12, 213–216.

Moukarzel, A.A., Najm, I., Vargas, J. et al (1990) Effect of nutritional status on outcome of orthotopic liver transplantation in pediatric patients. *Transpl Proc*, 22, 1560–1563.

Pierro, A., Koletzko, B., Carnielli, V. et al (1989) Resting energy expenditure is increased in infants with extra hepatic biliary atresia and cirrhosis. *J Ped Surg*, 24, 534–538.

Protheroe, S., McNurlan, M., Garlick, P. et al (1996a) Failure to suppress protein breakdown contributes towards malnutrition in infants with liver disease. *Hepatology*, 24, 141A.

Puntis, J.W.L., Ball, P.A., Booth, I.W. (1987) Complications of neonatal parenteral nutrition. *Int Ther Clin Mon*, 8, 48–56.

Quirk, P., Owens, P., Moyse, K. et al (1994) Insulin-like growth factors I and II are reduced in plasma from growth retarded children with chronic liver disease. *Growth Regulation*, 4, 35–38.

Sann, L., Durand, M., Picard, J. et al (1988) Arm fat and muscle areas in infancy. *Arch Dis Child*, 63, 256–260.

Sax, H.C., Bower, R.H. (1988) Hepatic complications of Total Parenteral Nutrition. *J Parent Enter Nutr*, 12, 615–618.

Sokal, R.J., Stall, C. (1990) Anthropometric evaluation of children with chronic liver disease. *Am J Clin Nutr*, 52, 203–208.

Spray, C.H., Beath, S.V., Willis, K.D. et al (1995) Docosahexaenoic acid (DHA) and visual function in infants with fat malabsorption secondary to liver disease. *Proceed Nutr Soc*, 54, 108A.

Tischler, M.E. (1982) Does leucine, leucyl-RNA or some metabolite of leucine regulate protein synthesis and degradation in skeletal and cardiac muscle? *J Biol Chem*, 257, 1613–1621.

Waterlow, J.C. (1973) Note on the assessment and classification of protein energy malnutrition in children. *Lancet*, 2, 87–89.

Weisdorf, S.A. (1989) Nutrition in Liver Disease. In: Lebenthal, E. (ed.) *Textbook of Gastroenterology and Nutrition in Infancy*, 52, pp. 665–676, 2nd Edn. New York: Raven Press.

Weisdorf, S.A., Freese, D.K., Fath, J.J. et al (1987) Amino acid abnormalities in infants with extrahepatic biliary atresia and cirrhosis. *J Ped Gastroenterol Nutr*, 6, 860–864.

31

Nutritional management of diabetes mellitus

Ruth M. Ayling

Historical background

Diabetes mellitus is the most common metabolic disease occurring in childhood. It is a chronic metabolic disorder characterized by disturbance of carbohydrate, fat and protein metabolism due to lack of insulin, resistance to its actions or a combination of these. The earliest descriptions of diabetes were about 1500 BC. In the first century AD, the disease was described as a 'melting down of the flesh and limbs into the urine,' and it was named diabetes from the Greek word for syphon. Later the urine from patients with diabetes was noted to taste sweet (mellitus in Latin), hence the name diabetes mellitus. In the late nineteenth century, it was noted in animals that pancreatectomy resulted in diabetes mellitus. In 1921, insulin was successfully extracted and became available for use in treatment for the first time.

Management of diabetes is directed in the short term towards control of the blood–glucose concentration and in the long term towards the prevention of complications such as nephropathy, retinopathy, neuropathy and cardiovascular disease.

There are several different types of diabetes mellitus occurring in children, but about 95% of children affected have type1 or insulin-dependent diabetes mellitus (IDDM). The discussion of nutritional principles in this chapter is therefore targeted towards the management of this group. In the United Kingdom, the incidence of IDDM has risen in the last 20 years, and is now $15–19/10^5$/year up to age 14 years (Watkins 1998), with a prevalence of 1 in 800. There is marked geographical variation in incidence, varying from $> 30/10^5$/year in Finland to $< 1/10^5$/year in Japan (Laron 1995). IDDM is thought to be the result of environmental factors, for example viruses and genetic factors acting together to trigger destruction of pancreatic β-cells. The IDDM1 locus is the most important single locus underlying genetic susceptibility in the United Kingdom. It is located on chromosome 6 and encompasses the major histocompatibility complex (MHC), the strongest association with IDDM within the MHC being with class II DQ alleles (Gough 1996). Other much rarer variants of childhood diabetes include maturity onset diabetes of the young (MODY 2) due to abnormalities of glucokinase, Wolfram's (DIDMOAD) syndrome and Rabson-Mendenhall syndrome caused by mutations in the insulin receptor.

Practice and procedures

Nutrition in the development of diabetes

Certain nutritional practices have been implicated in the development of diabetes mellitus. Malnutrition-related diabetes has been described but is rare. Over-nutrition and obesity have a well-established causative relationship with type2 diabetes, but nutritional influences in the development of type1 diabetes are less well identified.

In Iceland, seasonal variation in the incidence of diabetes has been linked to consumption of smoked and cured foods. These foods contain nitrosamines which are similar to streptozotocin—an agent well known to cause damage to β-cells (Helgasson & Jonason 1981). An increased risk of type1 diabetes has been associated with early dietary exposure to cow's milk and short duration of breast feeding (Verge et al 1994). A difference in T-lymphocyte proliferation to β-casein has been observed in patients with recently-diagnosed IDDM compared with normal controls and those with autoimmune disease (Cavallo et al 1996). A primary prevention trial whereby the early introduction of cow's milk protein into the diet is avoided in a group of genetically-susceptible individuals and included in the diet of a genetically-similar control group is currently in progress in Finland (Akerblom 1996).

Dietary recommendations for children with diabetes mellitus

Although the treatment of diabetes mellitus in children almost always requires insulin, dietary modification also has an important role in the management of the condition. Education of both patient and parents is vital, and ensuring understanding of recommended dietary practices is dependent on input from a specialist dietitian. The aims of the dietary management of diabetes are shown in Table 31.1.

Prior to the introduction of insulin a 'starvation diet' was the only available treatment for diabetes mellitus. The recommendations for the most suitable diet have changed since the introduction of insulin. It used to be considered necessary to restrict the percentage of the diet taken as carbohydrate and to provide 70% of

Table 31.1 — Aims of dietary management of diabetes mellitus

To abolish symptoms
To maintain normal blood glucose concentrations
To avoid hypoglycaemia
To achieve normal growth and development
To reduce the risk of long-term complications

Table 31.2 — Recommended dietary allowances

Food	Recommended amount (% of calories)
Complex carbohydrates	48–50
Sugars	10–12
Protein	7–13
ratio of animal to vegetable protein	< 1
Total fat	30%
saturated	< 10
monounsaturated	10–15
polyunsaturated	7–10

energy as fat. Now it is recommended that only 30% of daily calories should be from fat and that children with diabetes mellitus should have essentially the same nutritional intake as other children. As well, dietary recommendations should involve healthy eating practices for the whole family. Recommended dietary allowances (Bonnici 1998) are shown in Table 31.2.

As insulin is given intermittently and at fixed times, the timing of meals should not be widely varied and snacks should be eaten mid-morning, mid-afternoon and before bed to minimize extremes of blood glucose. There is no role for a 'diabetic diet,' and standard diet-sheets should not be used. The old fashioned practice of dividing carbohydrate into 10 g portions or exchanges is no longer recommended, but a similar approach may be useful to help the patient and parents to understand basic dietary principles and to assess food intake during intercurrent illness. Proprietary 'diabetic foods' are readily available but are not recommended. The insulin requirements of each child should be considered individually based on assessment of energy requirements, level of activity, social and ethnic circumstances and daily routines. An insulin regimen should be chosen whenever possible to coincide with family lifestyle and with preferred eating patterns. These factors need continual review throughout childhood and adolescence. For example, a pre-pubertal child may require 150 g of carbohydrate per day and a growing adolescent 280 g. The height and weight of patients should be plotted on centile charts at clinic visits to ensure that adequate growth is being achieved and that weight remains appropriate.

Carbohydrate

The total amount of carbohydrate in the diet is now held to be more important than the type (American Diabetes Association 1994). Studies have shown that few adults with diabetes actually achieve an ideal carbohydrate content in their diets (Close et al 1992, Humphreys et al 1994), and the same is no doubt true in children. It used to be thought that optimal control would be achieved by maximal limitation of simple sugars. In fact, sucrose produces a similar glycaemic effect to bread and potatoes (Hollenbeck et al 1985) and has not been found to be detrimental to glycaemic control. An isocaloric amount of fructose results in less increase in plasma glucose than sucrose (Bantle et al 1986). However, the beneficial use of fructose as a sweetener is offset by the fact that it may raise low-density lipoprotein (LDL) cholesterol (Crapo et al 1986). Saccharin, aspartame and acesulfame K may be more suitable as sweetening agents. These can be useful to sweeten drinks and can be added to food. The recommended daily intake of saccharin is < 5 mg/kg/day but aspartame and acesulfane K have no restriction. Aspartame has been proposed as the preferred sweetener for children with diabetes (Brink 1987). Artificial sweeteners may be damaged by heat and are best added to food after cooking where feasible. Sugar alcohols such as sorbitol provoke a low glycaemic response but may have a laxative effect. Sugar-free soft drinks are to be recommended. Some foods, such as fruit juice, are labelled as containing 'no added sugar' but care should be taken as they may have a high intrinsic sugar content.

Protein

The recommended protein intake for patients with diabetes is similar to that for the general population, and it is recommended that after the first year of life 7–13% of calories as protein is adequate. Reduction of dietary protein intake and the preferential intake of vegetable protein has been postulated to decrease both proteinuria and progression of diabetic nephropathy (Cohen et al 1987, Evanoff et al 1987, Kupin et al 1987, Walker et al 1989); it has been suggested that children with a duration of diabetes mellitus for > 5 years, or with microalbuminuria, should eat a low-protein diet. However, children have greater protein requirements to sustain growth. Protein restriction has not been found to improve glycaemia (Mooradian & Morley 1987).

Fat

The most recent dietary recommendations suggest a lower proportion of calories from fat. Perhaps a more important issue is the type of fat consumed, and even in childhood attempts should be made to minimize its atherogenic potential. Even in the absence of dyslipidaemia, diabetes is a risk factor for coronary heart disease (CHD) (Reaven 1992). Epidemiological studies have shown that non-diabetic adults resident in countries with a low intake of saturated fatty acids have a lower incidence of CHD than those with a high saturated fatty acid intake. Monounsaturated fats are less susceptible to oxidation than polyunsaturated fats and also lead to decreased triglyceride and increased high-density lipoprotein (HDL) concentrations. These factors are associated with a decreased risk of CHD (Ferro-Luzzi & Sette 1989). Whilst these observations have principally been made in adults, it would seem sensible to base the fat content of the diet of diabetic children on these principles. It is therefore recommended that < 30% of caloric intake should be as fat, with < 10% as saturated, 10–15% as monounsaturated, and 7–10% as polyunsaturated. Associations have been described between the proportion of long-chain polyunsaturated fats in cell membranes and insulin sensitivity and the percentage of saturated fatty acids and insulin resistance (Borkman et al 1993, Pan et al 1995). This may be important in the development of long-term complications in IDDM (Ruiz-Gutierrez et al 1993).

Fibre

It is suggested that people with diabetes should consume a diet that is high in dietary fibre. Dietary fibre comprises a number of substances that are partially digested within the gastrointestinal tract but that are not absorbed. These include cellulose, hemicellulose, pectin and lignin. High-carbohydrate, high-fibre diets can lower both blood glucose and lipid concentrations (Crapo 1986). Viscous water-soluble fibres found in fresh fruit and vegetables, such as guar and pectins, are the fibres that result in the lowest glycaemic responses (Jenkins et al 1978). Fibre intake should be limited to about 35 g/day (less in younger children) as it may interfere with trace element absorption.

Sodium

Diabetes has no effect on sodium requirements, recommended intake being 1.5–1.8 g/day (Bonnici 1998). However, as sodium intake has been linked to hypertension—an independent risk factor for CHD—excessive salt intake should be avoided.

Calcium, phosphate and magnesium

Increased urinary excretion of calcium, phosphate and magnesium has been observed in patients with type1 diabetes, without nephropathy, together with decreased plasma concentrations of ionized calcium and magnesium (Malone et al 1987). This, together with a proneness to acidosis and insulin deficiency, may contribute to a decrease in bone mineral density. A diet adequate in calcium, phosphate and magnesium should therefore be assured. Magnesium deficiency has also been reported to be a risk factor for ischaemic heart disease and severe retinopathy. However, magnesium supplements have not been shown to affect glycaemic control, lipids or blood pressure (Ericksson & Kohvakka 1995).

Trace elements and vitamins

Whilst the diet of people with diabetes should contain at least the recommended amounts of trace elements and vitamins, certain modifications to these amounts have been suggested. Trace element deficiency may occur due to decreased absorption secondary to dietary fibre and to increased urinary loss if there is persistent glycosuria. Zinc deficiency can exacerbate glucose intolerance. Vanadium is reported to have an insulin-like effect, and chromium not only increases tissue sensitivity to insulin but tends to raise HDL and the HDL:LDL ratio (Tuvemo & Gebre-Medhin 83–1985, Fantus et al 1995). However, deficiency of these elements is unlikely whilst consuming a normal diet. Elevated selenium concentrations have been found in children with diabetes (Cser et al 1993). Selenium has an important role in the defence against degradation products associated with LDL and very-low-density lipoprotein. In healthy children, serum selenium concentrations are related to LDL, but this has been found not to be the case in diabetic children (Gebre-Medhin et al 1988) and the raised selenium concentrations may be a response to altered lipid metabolism. If poor glycaemic control results in glycosuria, loss of water-soluble vitamins may occur. Especially in infants, vitamin supplementation may be indicated for a greater time than is usual in healthy children. Nicotinamide, a soluble B-group vitamin and precursor of nicotinamide adenine dinucleotide (NAD), may protect pancreatic β-cells from immune-mediated damage, and it is being evaluated in the primary prevention of IDDM in those with a genetic predisposition (Gale 1996).

Anti-nutrients

Lectins, phytates and tannins are anti-nutrients (i.e., natural enzyme inhibitors), which are contained in such foods as leguminous seeds. They reduce the rates of both carbohydrate digestion and absorption.

Practical aspects of dietary management of diabetes mellitus in childhood

Whilst the nutritional aims are essentially the same in all children with diabetes, children of different ages pose specific problems in both the choice of optimal insulin regimens and in the application of suitable food intake. In order to achieve a reasonable degree of glycaemic control and yet not compromise the emotional well being of children and adolescents, it may be necessary for compromises to be made by both the patients and those responsible for their medical care.

Infancy

Diabetes is rare in very young children but when it does occur it provides particular dietary challenges. Regular frequent feeds are necessary in all infants and this is of use in minimizing the risk of hypoglycaemia. There is no contraindication to breastfeeding, which should be encouraged. Weaning can be started from the age of 3 months, according to current recommendations.

Young children

In young children, aims are to establish a diet containing unrefined carbohydrate and having a relatively-low fat content. However, skimmed milk is not recommended for children under the age of 5 years because its fat content is too low and, in particular, it lacks the essential fatty acids which are necessary for continued brain growth and development (Committee on Medical Aspects of Food Policy 1988). Erratic eating habits such as food refusal, fads and large variations in day-to-day dietary intake provide particular management problems in children of this age. An adaptable insulin regimen may help to deal with these factors, but the habit of administering chocolate and other forms of refined carbohydrate on days of seemingly-low food intake should be avoided as it is open to the possibility of manipulation by the child and encourages unsound dietary habits.

Junior-school-age children

As children reach school age, compliance with a dietary regimen may well be relatively easier than at other times. Children of this age tend to be co-operative and are encouraged by praise. It is also a good time to educate the child, rather than the parents, in nutritional principles. Managing unpredictable amounts of exercise is one of the major dietary problems in this age group. Extra carbohydrate is required and can easily be given as a 'chocolate treat' before predicted exercise; when exercise has been taken during the afternoon, an increased bedtime snack may be required. School meals are usually supervised at this age and their adequacy can be assured by communication between dietitians and the school. The need for mid-morning and afternoon snacks should also be made clear. Likewise, adequate liaison is essential before school outings. Activities such as birthday parties are an important part of school life. Light over-indulgence at tea time is usually offset by the increased exercise occasioned by such events.

Senior-school-age children

Rapid changes in both physical and emotional maturity at this age brings difficulties of diabetic management. Aspects of eating behaviour in adolescents that complicate dietary compliance have been summarized by Truswell (1981). These include a tendency to miss meals, to enjoy snacks and fast food, and to eat an unbalanced diet. Specific eating disorders such as anorexia nervosa or bulimia occur in diabetes and are complicated by the ability to manipulate insulin. Energy requirements increase enormously at the time of puberty, and relative insulin resistance at this age may also necessitate large increases in insulin dose. There should be education about the use of alcohol and general guidelines given regarding limits of acceptable consumption. Adolescents should be advised to avoid the possible hypoglycaemic effect of alcohol by ensuring concurrent food intake. Sweet wines and liqueurs are best avoided, dry wines being more suitable. Beers and lagers are high in sugar and the carbohydrate they contain should be counted as part of the diet. Low-alcohol beers also tend to have a high carbohydrate content and sugar-free beers tend to be high in both calories and alcohol.

Particularly in this age group, advice must be sensitive

Table 31.3 — Key points

Nutrition may have a role in the aetiology of diabetes.
Children with diabetes have essentially the same nutritional requirements as other children.
Dietary recommendations should include healthy eating practices for the whole family, considering its particular habits and customs.
Frequent review should take place to take account of alteration of dietary requirements and habits with age.
About 60% of the calorific content of the diet should be taken as carbohydrate, 7–13% as protein and the remainder as fat.
Specific requirements for vitamins and trace elements may be altered in diabetes.

to individual lifestyles as ownership of dietary management passes gradually from parents to child at a time when peer pressure to conform is at its greatest.

Discussion

There is some evidence that nutritional factors are involved in the development of diabetes mellitus, but the major role of dietary management in diabetes is in the treatment of those who already have established disease. The principles of nutrition for children with diabetes does not differ markedly from that of other children apart from a certain rigidity in the timing of meals and the necessity for intervening snacks. However, problems with compliance are almost inevitable and need to be minimized by good diabetes education and flexibility to accommodate individual preferences, cultures and social activities.

Key points are summarized in Table 31.3.

References

Akerblom, H.K. (1996) Diabetes and cow's milk. *Lancet*, 348, 1656–1657.

American Diabetes Association. (1994) Nutritional recommendations and principles for people with diabetes mellitus. *Diabetes Care*, 17, 519–522.

Bantle, J.P., Laine, C.W., Thomas, J.W. (1986) Metabolic effects of dietary fructose in types 1 and 2 diabetic subjects. *JAMA*, 256, 32411–3246.

Bonnici, F. (1998) Workshop 2: Diet. *Acta Paediatr Suppl*, 425, 48–49.

Borkman, M., Storlien, L.H., Pan, D.A., Jenkins, A.B., Chisholm, D.J., Campbell, L.V. (1993) The relation between insulin sensitivity and fatty-acid composition of skeletal-muscle phospholipids. *N Engl J Med*, 328, 238–244.

Brink, S.J. (1987) *Pediatric and Adolescent Diabetes Mellitus*. Chicago Yearbook Pub 283.

Cavallo, M.G., Fava, D., Monetini, L., Barone, F., Pozilli, P. (1996) Cell-mediated immune response to beta casein in recent-onset insulin-dependent diabetes: Implications for disease pathogenesis. *Lancet*, 348, 926–928.

Close, E.J., Wiles, P.M., Lockton, J.A., Walmsley, D., Oldham, J., Wales, J.K. (1992) Diabetic diets and nutritional recommendations: What happens in real life. *Diabet Med*, 9, 181–188.

Cohen, D., Dodds, R., Viberti, G. (1987) Effect of protein restriction in insulin dependent diabetics at risk of nephropathy. *Br Med J*, 294, 795–798.

Committee on Medical Aspects of Food Policy. (1988) *Present Day Practice in Infant Feeding: Third Report. Report of A Working Party on Child Nutrition. Report on Health and Social Subjects No 32*. London: HMSO.

Crapo, P.A. (1986) Carbohydrate in the diabetic diet. *J Am Coll Nutr*, 5, 31–43.

Crapo, P.A., Kolterman, O.G., Henry, R.R. (1986) Metabolic consequences of two-week fructose feeding in diabetic subjects. *Diabetes Care*, 9, 111–119.

Cser, A., Sziklai-Laszio, I., Menzel, H., Lombeck, I. (1993) Selenium status and lipoproteins in healthy and diabetic children. *J Trace Elem Electrolytes Health Dis*, 7, 205–210.

Ericksson, J., Kohvakka, A. (1995) Magnesium and ascorbic acid supplementation in diabetes. *Am Nutr Metab*, 39, 217–223.

Evanoff, G.V., Thompson, C.S., Brown, J., Weinman, E.J. (1987) The effect of dietary protein restriction on the progression of diabetic nephropathy. A 12-month follow-up. *Arch Intern Med*, 147, 492–495.

Fantus, I.G., Deragon, G., Lai, R., Tang, S. (1995) Modulation of insulin action by vanadate: Evidence of a role for phosphotyrosine phosphatase activity to alter cellular signalling. *Mol Cell Biochem*, 153, 103–112.

Ferro-Luzzi, A., Sette, S. (1989) Mediterranean diet: An attempt to define its present and past composition. *Eur Clin Nut*, 43 (Suppl 2), 13–29.

Gale, E.A.M. (1996) Theory and practice of nicotinamide trials in pre-type 1 diabetes. *J Pediatr Endocrinol Metab*, 9, 375–379.

Gebre-Medhin, M., Ewauld, U., Tuveno, T. (1988) Serum selenium is related to low-density lipoproteins in healthy children but not in children with diabetes. *Ups J Med Sci*, 93, 57–62.

Gough, S.C.L. (1996) Genetics of insulin-dependent diabetes mellitus. *Ballières Clin Paediatr*, 4, 593–608.

Helgasson, T., Jonason, M.R. (1981) Evidence for a food additive as a cause of ketosis-prone diabetes. *Lancet*, ii, 716–720.

Hollenbeck, C.B., Coulston, A.M., Donner, C.C., Williams, R.A., Reaven, G.M. (1985) The effects of variations in percent of naturally occurring complex and simple carbohydrate on plasma glucose and insulin response in individuals with non-insulin dependent diabetes mellitus. *Diabetes*, 34, 151–155.

Humphreys, M., Cronin, C.C., Barry, D.G., Ferris, J.B. (1994) Are the nutritional recommendations for insulin-dependent diabetic patients being achieved? *Diabet Med*, 11, 79–84.

Jenkins, D.J., Wolever, T.M., Leeds, A.R., Gassull, M.A., Haisman, P., Dilawari, J., Goff, D.V., Metz, G.L., Alberti, K.G. (1978) Dietary fibres, fibre analogues and glucose tolerance: Importance of viscosity. *Br Med J*, 27, 1392–1394.

Kupin, W.L., Cortes, P., Dumler, F., Feldkamp, C.S., Kilates, M.C., Levin, N.W. (1987) Effect on renal function of change from high to moderate protein intake in Type I diabetic patients. *Diabetes*, 36, 73–79.

Laron, Z., Ballabriga, A., Brunser et al (1995) Diabetes in Childhood and Adolescence: The Role of Nutrition. *Clinical Nutrition of the Young Child*. United States, Raven Press vol 2, 31, 603–619.

Malone, J.I., Lowitt, S., Duncan, J.A., Shah, S.C. (1987) Hematuria and hypercalcaemia in children with diabetes. *Pediatrics*, 79, 756–759.

Mooradian, A.D., Morley, J.E. (1987) Micronutrient status in diabetes mellitus. *Am J Clin Nut*, 45, 877–895.

Pan, A.D., Lilloja, S., Milner, M.R., Kriketos, A.D., Baur, L.A., Bogardus, C., Storlein, L.H. (1995) Skeletal muscle membrane lipid composition is related to adiposity and insulin action. *J Clin Invest*, 96, 2802–2808.

Reaven, G.M. (1992) The role of insulin resistance and hyperinsulinism in coronary heart disease. *Metabolism*, 41, 16–19.

Ruiz-Gutierrez, V., Stiefel, P., Villar, J., Garcia-Donas, M.A., Acosta, D., Carneado, J. (1993) Cell-membrane fatty acid composition in Type 1 (insulin-dependent) diabetic patients: Relationship with sodium transport abnormalities and metabolic control. *Diabetologia*, 36, 850–856.

Truswell, A.S., Darnton-Hill, I. (1981) Food habits of adolescents. *Nutr Rev*, 39, 73–88.

Tuvemo, T, Gebre-Medhin, M. (1983–1985) The role of trace elements in juvenile diabetes. *Pediatrician*, 12, 213–219.

Verge, C.F., Howard, N.J., Irwig, L., Simpson, J.M., Mackerras, D., Silink, M. (1994) Environmental factors in childhood IDDM. A population-based, case-control study. *Diabetes Care*, 17, 1381–1389.

Walker, J.D., Bending, J.J., Dodds, R.A., Mattock, M.B., Murrells, T.J., Keen, H., Viberti, G.C. (1989) Restriction of dietary protein and progression of renal failure in diabetic nephropathy. *Lancet*, ii, 1411–1415.

Watkins, P.J. (1998) *ABC of Diabetes*, 4th edn. BMJ Publishing Group. London.

32

Nutritional support in Crohn's disease

R.M. Beattie

Introduction

Crohn's disease is an inflammatory disorder that can affect any part of the gastrointestinal tract from the mouth to the anus. The histology is characteristic. The disease is mostly seen in adults, but 10–15% of cases present in childhood, usually in adolescence. The important paediatric dimension is growth, and the aims of treatment are to induce remission and allow normal growth and development to occur.

The clinical manifestations are varied and diagnosis is often delayed. Characteristic symptomatology includes abdominal pain, diarrhoea and weight loss, although atypical presentations are common. The clinical features at diagnosis in 54 children referred to the paediatric inflammatory bowel disease clinic at St Bartholomew's Hospital are listed in Table 32.1. Useful screening investigations in children with chronic gastrointestinal symptoms include a full blood count, erythrocyte sedimentation rate (ESR) and C-reactive protein; the C-reactive protein is raised in most children with Crohn's disease at diagnosis (Beattie et al 1995). Diagnosis is by barium radiology and colonoscopy with biopsy (Chong et al 1982, Chong et al 1985). The most common disease site is the terminal ileum.

Therapeutic options include enteral nutrition, corticosteroid therapy and surgery (Table 32.2). The surgical option is effective and often necessary for local disease complications. Corticosteroid therapy induces a clinical remission and is as effective as enteral nutrition. However, side effects are common and as a consequence enteral nutrition as primary therapy is used increasingly.

Historical background

Growth failure nutritional impairment in Crohn's disease

Growth failure is present in up to 50% of children and adolescents with Crohn's disease at presentation and up to 90% are underweight (Brain & Savage 1994, Seidmann 1997). The growth failure seen is characterized by delayed linear growth with delayed skeletal maturation and delayed onset of puberty (Fig. 32.1). This means that children with Crohn's disease, once in remission, have the potential to grow into early adult life and that disease remission, particularly during the adolescent years, is of crucial importance in order to achieve the best final adult height (Markowitz et al 1993).

Table 32.1 — Incidence (as %) of clinical features at diagnosis in 54 children with Crohn's disease

Symptom	
Diarrhoea	72
Rectal bleeding	28
Abdominal pain	85
Urgency	25
Anorexia	75
Weight loss	78
Lethargy	75
Tenesmus	25
Nausea/Vomiting	22
Delayed growth	43
Perianal symptoms	25
Fever	22
Constipation	20
Skin rash	15
Joint pains	10
Mouth ulcers	8
Physical sign	
No significant abnormality	10
Weight loss	52
Pallor	32
Tender abdomen	34
Growth retardation	46
Abdominal distension	32
Mouth lesions	8
Perianal abnormality	46
Jaundice	0
Toxic dilatation	0
Rectal prolapse	0
Abdominal mass	6
Finger clubbing	8
Erythema nodosum	6
Peripheral oedema	6
Uveitis	4

Reproduced from Chong et al (1982), with permission.

Table 32.2 — Crohn's disease: Therapeutic options

Enteral Nutrition
polymeric
elemental or semi-elemental
Drugs
5 ASA derivatives
Corticosteroids
Azathioprine
Others, e.g., Cyclosporin
Surgery

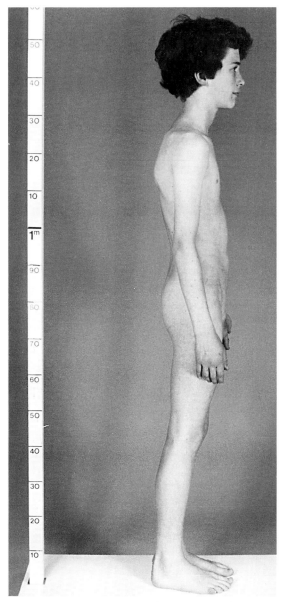

Figure 32.1 — 16-year-old boy with long-standing Crohn's disease. Note the short stature and lack of secondary sexual characteristics.

The growth failure is multifactorial and poorly understood. Poor dietary intake is a major factor. Thomas et al (1993a) showed that mean energy intake in children with Crohn's disease in relapse was lower than in age and height matched controls. The appetite is reduced as a consequence of systemic inflammatory activity, and the symptoms are provoked by eating large amounts of food. Many studies have shown that nutritional therapy corrects nutritional impairment and in doing so promotes linear growth. In short children who undergo surgical resection, catch up growth occurs (Davies et al 1990). Some authors think that this occurs both as a result of improved nutrition following disease remission and as a consequence of the removal of the inflammatory mass, which reduces systemic levels of pro-inflammatory and inflammatory cytokines including tumour necrosis factor which may inhibit growth directly (Murch et al 1991). There is also an endocrine disturbance: insulin like growth factor 1 (which is the peripheral mediator of growth hormone) levels are low when disease is active and normalize as disease control is achieved (Thomas et al 1998, Beattie et al 1993b).

A further factor is corticosteroid therapy. Many children with Crohn's disease require long-term corticosteroid therapy. Side effects are common including the suppression of linear growth (Friedmann & Strang 1966), which can lead to short stature in adult life (Markowitz et al 1993). There are other side effects and these include inappropriate weight gain, acne, bruising, striae, mood disturbance and osteopenia.

Nutritional therapy in Crohn's disease

Many studies have shown the energy intake to be reduced in children with Crohn's disease and to improve following treatment (Kirschener et al 1981, Thomas 1993). Kirschener et al reported 7 children with moderately-active Crohn's disease, all of whom had significant growth retardation. All responded to aggressive nutritional supplementation with improved well being and an increase in height velocity. The use of enteral nutrition as primary therapy to induce remission in Crohn's disease was first described in adult series by Axelsson & Jarnum in 1977 and by O'Morain et al in 1980. O'Morain et al in 1983 reported 15 children and adolescents who received the elemental diet Vivonex (Eaton laboratories) for 4 weeks followed by a four-week period of food re-introduction. After 1–2 weeks of therapy, all of the patients felt clinically better. Significant improvements were seen in haemoglobin, ESR, serum albumin and weight. By the end of the 3-month follow-up period, six patients had crossed the centiles for weight and three had crossed centiles for height. One of the patients (aged 19 years) with delayed puberty short stature achieved a striking increase in his height and weight.

Sanderson et al (1987) compared the peptide-based,

semi-elemental formula Flexical (Mead Johnson) with more conventional corticosteroid therapy and showed equal efficacy in the induction of remission. The diet was given for 6 weeks by nasogastric tube. New foods were introduced every 2 days for a 2-month period after that. No adverse effects were seen associated with the introduction of any particular food. Linear growth as assessed by height velocity over 6 months was significantly greater in the group treated with elemental diet than the group treated with steroids.

There have been a number of other paediatric studies. Thomas et al (1993) compared the elemental formula EO28 (Scientific Hospital Supplies) with steroids in a group of 29 and found equal efficacy in both groups. Height velocity was better in the group treated by diet, despite the fact that energy intake was higher in the group treated with steroids. In this study, elemental diet was well tolerated by mouth. Papadopoulou et al (1995) in a retrospective analysis found elemental diet (EO28, Scientific Hospital Supplies) to be as effective as steroid therapy and better for the treatment of proximal disease.

More recent interest has been in the use of cheaper and more palatable polymeric formulae. The author reported seven children, all new patients with small-bowel Crohn's disease treated with the polymeric formula feed AL110 (Nestle-Clintec), who entered a full clinical remission by 8 weeks. In all children, the C-reactive protein that was initially high normalized by 2 weeks (Fig. 32.2). Initial and follow-up ileal histology was obtained and showed good evidence of mucosal healing in six out of seven, implying healing had occurred as a consequence of nutritional therapy (Beattie et al 1994). Ruuska et al (1994) reported a

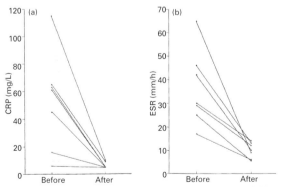

Figure 32.2 — C-reactive protein (a) and ESR (b) in seven children with newly-diagnosed small-bowel Crohn's disease before and 8 weeks after enteral nutrition. From Beattie et al (1994), with permission.

randomized controlled trial comparing Nutrison Standard (Nutricia), which is a whole protein feed, with corticosteroid therapy. Nutritional treatment was for 8 weeks followed by food re-introduction over a 3-week period. Corticosteroid therapy was with prednisolone initially at high dose (1.5 mg/kg/day, maximum 60 mg), tapered according to clinical response. Response was assessed clinically and by biochemical parameters including C-reactive protein. Response to therapy was equal in both groups and equal whether disease was in the small or large bowel or both. The relapse rate was lower in the group treated with diet.

The main argument for using enteral nutrition over corticosteroid therapy in childhood is that if both are equally efficacious then the avoidance of side effects, particularly suppression of growth, is desirable. Most of the paediatric studies are small and do not convey the impression of many paediatric gastroenterologists that nutritional therapy is more effective particularly in highly-motivated new patients with proximal disease. It is also an essential part of the treatment plan in more refractory patients with long-standing recurrent relapsing disease.

Many adults series have compared steroids with enteral diets, and for a period a number of centres advocated enteral nutrition as primary therapy. However, compliance is very poor and most of the studies have a higher drop out rate. Gorard et al (1993) compared the elemental diet E028 (Scientific Hospital Supplies) with prednisolone. The drop out rate of the elemental diet group was 41%. This was quoted in the paper as being due to unpalatability and the need for a nasogastric tube. When tolerated, elemental diet was reported as being as effective as steroids in the short term but with a higher relapse rate. Rigaud et al (1991) compared elemental and polymeric diets in an adult group with both small and large intestinal disease. Diets were given exclusively for 4–6 weeks, dependent upon clinical response, after which food was introduced over a 5-day period. Seventy percent of the patients responded in both groups. Response was assessed clinically and by repeat endoscopic assessment. There have been many other studies. Raouf et al (1991) found polymeric to be as effective as elemental formula and postulated that one of the beneficial effects of enteral nutrition may be its low residue. Giaffer et al (1990) found elemental diets to be more effective. Mansfield et al (1995) compared an oligopeptide-based diet with an elemental diet and found both to be equally efficacious in terms of the induction of remission and time to relapse. These studies are beset with difficulty. Crohn's disease is a heterogeneous condition and most studies are small. Large numbers would need to be recruited in order to achieve statistically valid comparisons. Fernandez-Banares et al (1995) published a meta-analysis of studies comparing enteral nutrition (polymeric, oligopeptide and elemental) with steroids that suggested that steroids were more efficacious in the induction of remission. Only one paediatric study was included. Toxicity was not considered and many of the studies included in the analysis were flawed by poor compliance. Therefore, it would be wrong to extrapolate from this analysis conclusions that would influence paediatric therapy. However, it does perhaps reinforce the importance of larger and therefore presumably multi-centre work being done. A second meta-analysis published by Griffiths et al in 1995 drew similar conclusions, again looking principally at adult studies. This second meta-analysis suggested that there was no difference between polymeric and elemental diets in terms of efficacy and favoured steroid therapy as initial therapy in adults with Crohn's disease.

Practice and procedures

Patient assessment

Prior to starting enteral nutrition, it is essential that the patient is fully assessed with regard to nutritional status, disease extent and severity in order to plan therapy. Particular attention needs to be paid to growth and pubertal status. The full assessment is listed in Table 32.3. Barium radiology and endoscopy are

Table 32.3 — Nutritional therapy: Patient assessment

Symptoms and signs
Weight and weight standard deviation score
Skin-fold thickness
Height and height standard deviation score
Height velocity
Pubertal status
Bone age
Haemoglobin
ESR
Serum albumin
C-reactive protein
Barium radiology
Endoscopy

indicated in new cases and in long-standing cases where complications (e.g., stricture formation) are suspected or where disease is resistant to medical therapy.

Which diet should be used?

Different diets used as enteral therapy include elemental, semi-elemental (oligopeptide) and polymeric. Different centres have allegiance to different feeds: the most commonly prescribed is E028 (Scientific Hospital Supplies), which is an elemental feed. This comes in 'user friendly' 250 ml packs. The feed has a calorie content of 0.86 kcal/mL. Palatability, which is partially a function of the whole protein content of a feed, is a problem. This is helped by the various flavours that are marketed including grapefruit, summer fruits, and orange and pineapple. Polymeric feeds are more palatable because of their whole protein content. The most commonly used polymeric feeds are Nutrison (Nutricia) and AL110 (Nestle). Feeds such as Flexical (Mead Johnson) and Peptamen (Nestle) are semi-elemental or oligopeptide based. Whether these different feeds are equally efficacious in children has not been resolved in a large trial. Whether the actual feed used matters is unclear, and other constituents such as calorie density, glutamine, fat and carbohydrate content may be relevant (van der Hulst et al 1993, Fernandez-Banares et al 1994). Cost is certainly a factor as elemental feeds are very much more expensive than polymeric formulae.

How much feed should be given?

This is very much patient dependent, and depends on disease severity, patient tolerance and the degree of nutritional impairment at the onset of therapy. One hundred to one hundred and twenty percent of the recommended daily allowance should be used. Standard reference tables are available to calculate this. Most feeds are between 0.7–1 kcal/mL. Around 2000 kcal per day is required for a 10-year-old and 2500 kcal for a 14–16-year-old. This means that the volume of feed required per 24 h is large.

Method of administration

This is crucial. The compliance of dietary therapy, particularly in adult series, is poor. This is a consequence of feed unpalatability and patients finding it difficult to drink the large amounts required. Compliance in paediatric studies is higher. In children, the feed is usually administered either wholly or in part by nasogastric tube. This does not mean that palatable formulae cannot be drunk. A number of children prefer the whole feed to be administered by nasogastric tube, whereas others drink it all and some prefer a combination. Most children who drink the feeds prefer them chilled. Use of flavoured formula feeds that have been frozen as ice lollies, particularly in the summer, is very popular.

Regimen

Enteral feeding needs to be for 4–8 weeks. During that period, no other foodstuffs should be taken, although water can be drunk. The amount of feed should be increased gradually in quantity and strength over a number of days in order to ensure that it is well tolerated and to avoid the common side effects of nausea and bloating. This is best done with the child as an inpatient. Prior to starting, a severely-affected child may require a short period on intravenous fluid to correct electrolyte disturbance. The precise regimen used is very much a matter for the individual patient. If the child chooses to drink the feed, then a careful watch needs to be made to ensure an adequate amount is taken. If the nasogastric route is used at least initially, then it is best to infuse the feed continuously for the first few days, after which a more suitable regimen can be established. Alternatives include regular bolus feeding, bolus feeding plus overnight continuous feeding and continuous feeding. Some health care workers prefer some daytime boluses to be included in the regimen in order to avoid daytime hunger. In addition, daytime feeding is more physiological and avoids some of the problems that occur with giving large volumes of feed overnight, including nocturnal enuresis and diarrhoea.

It is useful to teach the child to pass a nasogastric tube if they are happy to learn. Some children insert the tube at night for overnight feeding, remove it in the morning prior to school attendance, and take a midday bolus by mouth at lunch time.

There is no clear consensus on how long dietary therapy should be given. The main paediatric series have used between 6–8 weeks (Sanderson et al 1987, Thomas et al 1993a, Ruuska et al 1994). A preferred regimen is to establish a child on enteral nutrition and persist with this therapy for a minimum of 8 weeks as sole therapy (Beattie et al 1994). It is important that any therapy is continued for long enough to induce a remission of disease symptoms. Additional attention needs to be paid to inflammatory indices, which represent the systemic response to disease, and to whether endoscopic and histological remission occurs. This means treatment should be continued for longer than the period taken to make the child feel better. It is likely that this increases the time to first relapse (Beattie et al 1994).

Monitoring

The child usually feels better within days of starting treatment, and the resulting improved well being provides a powerful incentive to continue. All patients should be monitored twice weekly. At each review, general progress should be assessed. The weight should be checked. One would expect, particularly in children who are underweight at onset, continuous weight gain with therapy. If not, feed volume may need to be increased. Inflammatory indices such as the C-reactive protein should also be checked. These should improve as treatment progresses (see Fig. 32.2), but the failure of this to occur is an early indicator of problems. Psychological support is necessary. The community nurse and paediatric dietician are particularly helpful in this regard.

Failure of response

This may be as a consequence of poor compliance, an inadequate amount of calories being given or poor tolerance of the feed. Alternatively, the disease may be resistant to enteral nutrition. Risk factors for this include colonic disease, disease of long duration and disease in which surgical complications such as stricture have arisen. Twenty to thirty percent fail to respond. Wilschanski et al (1996) reported 65 patients treated over 7 years with enteral nutrition and found an overall remission rate of 72%. However, there was a much higher remission rate in small-bowel and ileo-colonic disease when compared with isolated colonic disease (p < 0.03). Seidman et al (1993) reported in the Canadian Multicentre trial of exclusive enteral semi-elemental diet (Vital HN, Abbots Laboratories) that new patients did better that those with established disease. It is important that failure to respond to enteral nutrition does not necessarily mean that it needs to be discontinued; in the nutritionally-impaired child, particularly if surgery is indicated, it is important to maintain adequate nutrition in the pre-operative period.

Food re-introduction

A period of food re-introduction should follow

Table 32.4 — Protocol for the re-introduction of food following a period of dietary exclusion

Each new food is introduced into the diet 2 days after the previous food

Potatoes
Lamb
Chicken
Yeast
Wheat (spaghetti)
Bread
Cabbage
Rice
Apple
Carrot
Beef
Milk
Butter
Cheese
Eggs

A free diet is allowed once these foods have been re-introduced.

dietary restriction. In general, food should be re-introduced over a 4–8 week period according to a schedule such as that in Table 32.4. In most patients, this is straightforward.

Much has been written about food intolerance in Crohn's disease. Care must be taken not to over-emphasize this in children where an adequate calorie intake is the first priority and a restricted diet, particularly in a child who is not keen on eating, may put the child at high risk of being calorie deficient. Initial problems with food re-introduction may represent a general rather than a specific intolerance. Studies in children have failed to isolate specific foods that consistently provoke symptoms on food re-introduction following a period of dietary exclusion. However, in particular patients, specific foodstuffs can be found to exacerbate symptoms (Beattie & Walker-Smith 1994).

Pearson et al 1993 reported food intolerance in 20 out of 28 adults treated with 4 weeks of enteral nutrition on food re-introduction. These intolerances were to many different foodstuffs, and were mostly seen during the first few weeks of food re-introduction. The commonest offending items were milk (5) and peanuts (5). Interestingly, only three were confirmed on double-blind challenge. Riordan et al 1993 reported a high

incidence of intolerance following 2 weeks of enteral nutrition. Offending foodstuffs in order of frequency included corn, milk, yeast, egg, potatoes, rye, tea, coffee, apples, mushrooms, oats and chocolate. Double-blind challenge was not used.

Maintainence therapy

Crohn's disease has a high frequency of relapse and once disease remission has been induced maintenance therapy needs to be considered. 5' ASA derivatives are the most widely used therapy and should be continued for at least 2 years after the last relapse (Murch & Walker-Smith 1994). There are many preparations available such as Salazopyrin (Sulphalazine), which comes in tablet form and as a syrup, and Asocol (Mesalazine). Maintenance therapy with prednisolone is occasionally required in severe cases.

Continued nutritional supplementation is often required. Belli et al 1988 reported eight children aged between 10 and 14 years all of whom had Crohn's disease associated with severe growth failure. They were given an elemental diet (Vivonex, Norwich Eaton) for 1 out of each 4 months. All achieved catch-up growth during the subsequent 12 months, and corticosteroid requirements fell and disease activity improved during the same period. More recently, the same group (Seidmann et al 1996) showed in a multi-centred randomized controlled study that cyclical elemental diet (Vital HN, Ross Products, Abbots Laboratories) was better than low-dose alternate steroids in prolonging the time to relapse in children with Crohn's disease. As well, patients had a statistically-significant improvement in height velocity. Similar results have been found using cyclical enteral nutrition by Polk et al (1992). It is unclear whether the maintenance therapy needs to be cyclical or whether the beneficial effect is a consequence of the period on oligoantigenic therapy or of the maintenance of good nutritional status. Wilschanski et al 1996 reported in a retrospective series a longer time to first relapse and better long-term growth in children who elected to continue nutritional support after the induction of remission with enteral therapy. Imes et al (1988) looked at 137 adults in a prospective randomized controlled trial and showed that dietary advice and support was associated with a significant decrease in the Crohn's disease activity index, prolonged remission, reduced need for mediation and reduced absence from work when compared to control patients who were seen for regular follow-up but not offered dietary counselling.

An appropriate approach based on this data is the close follow-up of patients with close attention paid to nutritional intake and nutritional status, including height velocity with aggressive supplementation where appropriate and the early treatment of disease relapse.

Long-term nutritional supplementation is sometimes given by nasogastric tube. This can be uncomfortable, particularly if prolonged, and embarrassing for the self-conscious child or adolescent if left *in situ*. Percutaneous endoscopic gastrostomy (PEG) tube feeding is an appropriate alternative that can be considered in this instance. Cosgrove & Jenkins (1997) reported ten children with Crohn's disease who had PEG tubes sited. No complications were seen, and in all children the method of administration was preferred to the nasogastric tube that they had previously.

Relapse

Crohn's disease is characterized by recurrent relapses. The relapse rate following either enteral nutrition or corticosteroid therapy is between 50–90% by 12 months. The published relapse rates are variable for several reasons. First, many of the published series do not follow up all the patients for a full 12 months. Second, the definition of relapse varies and can be purely a symptomatic one, based on raised inflammatory indices or on changes at endoscopy. There have been several studies that have shown in patients who were clinically well following therapy with either corticosteroids or enteral nutrition that inflammatory change was still present at repeat endoscopy (Rigaud et al 1991, Modigliani et al 1991, Beattie et al 1994). The significance of this is uncertain but suggests that conventional therapy dampens down the disease process rather than puts it into a 'true' remission.

Alternative therapeutic options

The efficacy of corticosteroids in the induction of remission in Crohn's disease is well established. In many patients, corticosteroid therapy is more acceptable and compliance better. Two recent meta-analyses of adult studies comparing enteral nutrition as therapy with steroids suggest that steroids are more effective in symptom control. This work cannot automatically be extrapolated to children. In paediatric studies, compliance is much higher and alternative therapies such as coricosteroids have unacceptably high side effects, particularly on growth. In addition, the studies do not distinguish between newly-diagnosed patients

and those with established disease. In childhood, a higher proportion of new patients is likely to improve outcome following enteral nutrition. Undoubtedly, in disease that is resistant to enteral nutrition, corticosteroid therapy is appropriate. If used, courses should be for a limited period and maintenance doses avoided where possible. Prednisolone is the most widely used corticosteroid. The initial dose is 2 mg/kg (maximum 40 mg). The initial high dose is used to induce a remission. The dose should then be tapered slowly over the subsequent weeks. A number of children become steroid dependent (i.e., they are unwell unless on steroid therapy) or steroid resistant (i.e., they are unwell even if on steroids). Azathioprine helps a proportion, reducing steroid dependency and inducing disease remission, and is being used early in children with difficult disease. Surgery is best reserved for refractory cases.

Budesonide has recently been shown to be as effective as prednisolone in the induction of remission in proximal disease with less toxicity, although its use is not yet widespread. Other therapies for steroid dependant or resistant cases include Cyclosporin, tumour necrosis factor antibody and other immuno-supressives mostly used in adult practice. This subject is reviewed elsewhere (Beattie 2000).

Surgery is not a disaster in the child with Crohn's disease. It is required in up to 50% within 5 years in historical cohorts (Sedgewick et al 1991), although probably less now with the widespread use of enteral nutrition and Azathioprine. McLain et al (1990) reported 17 children who underwent bowel resections over a 16-year period, during which 72 patients were seen. Failure of medical treatment was the indication for surgery in six. The others were: stricture (6), perforation (1), mass (1), diagnosis (2) and peri-anal sepsis (1). Of the 17 children, 13 had evidence of retardation of linear growth at surgery and 12 exhibited catch-up growth afterwards, crossing at least one centile band. Catch-up growth can occur if surgery is instituted before epiphyseal closure. This can be late in children with Crohn's disease as many have delayed onset of puberty. Two of the children in McLain's study who exhibited catch-up growth were aged 17 at the time of surgery. Growth is not the only issue in the developing adolescent who requires a period that is free of disease symptoms to develop normally, interact with peers and perform well at school. Disease refractory to medical therapy can be of two types. The first is that which does not respond to medical therapy at all, and the other is that which does but only with unacceptable side effects such as growth failure as a consequence of active disease and steroid therapy. Relapse or disease at a new site is common after bowel resection. The best outcome is following limited small bowel or ileo-caecal resection (Right hemicolectomy) (Davies et al 1990).

Scott & Hughes 1994 reported the views of 70 adults who had ileocolonic resections. All felt better after surgery, and 74% thought that in retrospect surgery should have been carried out earlier. Reasons given for earlier surgery included the severity of symptoms pre-operatively, feeling of well being after the resection, the reduced need for drugs and the ability to eat normally. This was an adult study and therefore growth was not an issue.

Discussion

The aim of therapy in Crohn's disease is to induce disease remission thereby controlling disease symptoms and allowing linear and catch-up growth to occur. The options for therapy include corticosteroids, enteral nutrition and surgery. Clearly if a stricture is present then surgery is appropriate. Enteral nutrition is an effective inducer of remission in appropriate cases and avoids the potentially toxic effects of corticosteroids. Which diet should be used is not yet resolved and requires further study. Enteral nutrition has an additional role as maintenance therapy and as an adjunct to other therapies in children with Crohn's disease.

References

Axelsson, C., Jarnum, S. (1977) Assessment of the therapeutic value of an elemental diet in chronic inflammatory bowel disease. *Scand J Gastroenterologyp*, 12, 89–95.

Beattie, R.M., Camacho-Hubner, C., Wacharasindhu, S. et al. (1998) Responsiveness of IGF-1 and IGFBP-3 to therapeutic intervention in children with Crohn's disease. *Clinical Endocrinology*, 49, 483–489.

Beattie, R.M., Schiffrin, E.J., Donnet-Hughes, A., Huggett, A.C., Domizio, P., MacDonald, T.T., Walker-Smith, J.A. (1994) Polymeric nutrition as primary therapy in children with small bowel Crohn's disease. *Aliment Pharmacol Ther*, 8, 609–615.

Beattie, R.M., Walker-Smith, J.A. (1994) Treatment of active Crohn's disease by exclusion diet-selected summary. *J Paed Gastr Nutr*, 19(4), 235–236.

Beattie, R.M., Walker-Smith, J.A., Murch, S.H. (1995) Indications for investigation of chronic gastrointestinal symptoms. *Arch Dis Child*, 73, 354–355.

Beattie, R.M. (2000) Therapy of Crohn's disease in Childhood. *Paediatric Drugs*, 2(3), 193–203.

Belli, D.C., Seidman, E., Bouthillier, L., Weber, A.M., Roy, C.C., Plentincx W., Beaulieu, M., Morin, C.L. (1988) Chronic intermittent elemental diet improves growth failure in children with Crohn's disease. *Gastroenterol*, 94, 603–610.

Brain, C.E., Savage, M.O. (1994) Growth and puberty in chronic inflammatory bowel disease. *Baillière's Clin Gastroenterol*, 8, 83–100.

Chong, S.K.F., Bartram, C., Campbell, C.A., Williams, C.B., Blackshaw, A.J., Walker-Smith, J.A. (1982) Chronic Inflammatory bowel disease in childhood. *BMJ*, 284, 101–104.

Chong, S.K., Blackshaw, A.J., Boyle, S., Williams, C.B., Walker-Smith, J.A. (1985) Histological diagnosis of inflammatory bowel disease in childhood. *Gut*, 26, 55–59.

Cosgrove, M., Jenkins, H. (1997) Experience of percutaneous endoscopic gastrostomy in children with Crohn's disease. *Arch Dis Child*, 76, 141–143.

Davies, G., Evans, C.M., Shand, W.S., Walker-Smith, J.A. (1990) Surgery for Crohn's disease: Influence of site of disease and operative procedure on outcome. *Br J Surg*, 77, 81–94.

Fernandez-Banares, F., Cabre, E., Gonzalez-Huix, F., Gassull, M.A. (1994) Enteral Nutrition as primary therapy in Crohn's disease. *Gut*, 1, S55–S59.

Fernandez-Banares, F., Esteve-Copmas, M., Gassul, M.A. (1995) How effective is enteral nutrition in inducing remission in active Crohn's disease: A metanalysis of the randomised clinical trials. *JPEN*, 19, 356–364.

Friedmann, M., Strang, L.B. (1966) Effect of long term corticosteroids and corticotrophin on the growth of children. *Lancet*, ii, 568–572.

Giaffer, M.H., North, G., Holdsworth, C.D. (1990) Controlled trial of polymeric versus elemental diet in treatment of active Crohn's disease. *Lancet*, 335, 816–819.

Gorard, D.A., Hunt, J.B., Payne-James, J.J. et al. (1993) Initial response and subsequent course of Crohn's disease treated with elemental diet or prednisolone. *Gut*, 34, 1198–1202.

Griffiths, A.M., Ohlsson, A., Sherman, P.M. et al. (1995) Meta-analysis of enteral nutrition as a primary treatment of active Crohn's disease. *Gastroenterol*, 108, 1056–1067.

Imes, S., Pinchbeck, B., Thomson, A.B. (1988) Diet counselling improves the clinical course of patients with Crohn's disease. *Digestion*, 39, 7–19.

Kirschener, B.S., Klich, J.R., Kalman, S.S., deFavaro, M.V., Rosenberg, I.H. (1981) Reversal of growth retardation in Crohn's disease with therapy emphasising oral nutritional restitution. *Gastroenterol*, 80, 10–15.

McLain, B.I., Davidson, P.M., Stokes, K.B., Beasley, S.W. (1990) Growth after gut resection for Crohn's disease. *Arch Dis Child*, 65, 760–762.

Mansfield, J.C., Giaffer, M.H., Holdsworth, C.D. (1995) Controlled trial of oligopeptide versus amino acid diet in treatment of active Crohn's disease. *Gut*, 36, 60–65.

Markowitz, J., Grancher, K., Rosa, E. et al. (1993) Growth failure in paediatric inflammatory bowel disease. *J Paed Gastro Nutr*, 16, 373–380.

Modigliani, R., Mary, J., Simon, J. et al. (1991) Clinical, biological and endoscopic picture of attacks of Crohn's disease. *Gastroenterol*, 98, 811–818.

Murch, S.H., Lamkin, V.A., Savage, M.O. et al. (1991) Serum concentrations of tumour necrosis factor alpha in childhood chronic inflammatory bowel disease. *Gut*, 32, 913–917.

Murch, S.H., Walker-Smith, J.A. (1994) Medical management of chronic inflammatory bowel disease. *Baillière's Clin Gastroenterol*, 8, 133–148.

O'Morain, C., Segal, A.W., Levi, A.J. (1980) Elemental diets in the treatment of acute Crohn's disease. *BMJ*, 281, 1173–1175.

O'Morain, C., Segal, A.M., Levi, A.J., Valmann, H.B. (1983) Elemental diet in acute Crohn's disease. *Arch Dis Child*, 53, 44–47.

Papadopoulou, A., Rawashdeh, M.O., Brown, G.A. et al. (1995) Remission following an elemental diet or prednisolone in Crohn's disease. *Acta Paediatr*, 84, 79–83.

Pearson, M., Teahon, K., Levi, A.J. et al. (1993) Food intolerance and Crohn's disease. *Gut*, 34, 783–787.

Polk, D.B., Hattner, J.A.T., Kerner, J.A. (1992) Improved growth and disease activity after intermitttent administration of a defined formula diet in children with Crohn's disease. *JPEN*, 16, 499–504.

Raouf, A.H., Hildrey, V., Daniel, J. et al. (1991) Enteral feeding as sole treatment for Crohn's disease: Controlled trial of whole protein v amino acid based feed and a case study of dietary challenge. *Gut*, 32, 702–707.

Riordan, A.M., Hunter, J.O., Dickinson, R.J. et al. (1993) Treatment of active Crohn's disease by exclusion diet: East Anglian Multicentre controlled trial. *Lancet*, 342, 1131–1134.

Rigaud, D., Cones, J., Le Quintrec, Y. et al. (1991) Controlled trial comparing two types of enteral nutrition in treatment of active Crohn's disease: Elemental v polymeric diet. *Gut*, 32, 1492–1497.

Ruuska, T., Savilahti, E., Maki, S. et al. (1994) Exclusive whole protein enteral diet versus prednisolone in the treatment of acute Crohn's disease in children. *J Paed Gastr Nutr*, 19, 175–180.

Sanderson, I.R., Udeen, S., Davies, P.S.W., Savage, M.O., Walker-Smith, J.A. (1987) Remission induced by elemental diet in small bowel Crohn's disease. *Arch Dis Child*, 61, 123–127.

Scott, N.A., Hughes, L.E. (1994) Timing of ileocolonic resection for symptomatic Crohn's disease — the patients view. *Gut*, 35, 656–657.

Sedgewick, D.M., Barton, J.R., Hamer-Hodges, D.W. et al. (1991) Population based study of surgery in juvenile onset Crohn's disease. *Brit J Surg*, 78, 171–175.

Seidman, E., Griffiths, A.M., Jones, A., Issenman, R. (1993) The Canadian paediatric Crohn's disease study group: Semi-elemental diet versus prednisolone in the treatment of active Crohn's disease. *Gastroenterol*, 104, A778.

Siedmann, E. (1997) Nutritional therapy for Crohn's disease: Lessons from the Ste.-Justine Hospital experience. *Inflammatory Bowel Diseases*, 3, 49–53.

Siedmann, E., Jones, A., Issenman, R. et al. (1993) Relapse prevention/growth enhancement in paediatric Crohn's disease: Multicentre randomised controlled trial of intermittent enteral nutrition versus alternate day prednisolone. *J Paed Gastro Nutr*, 23, 344.

Thomas, A.G., Taylor, F., Miller, V. (1993a) Dietary intake and nutritional treatment in Crohn's disease. *J Paed Gastro Nutr*, 17, 75–81.

Thomas, A.G. et al. (1993b) Insulin-like growth factor-1, insulin-like growth factor binding protein-1, and insulin in childhood Crohn's disease. *Gut*, 34, 944–947.

Van der Hulst, R.J.W., Van Kreel, B.K., Von Meyenfeldt, M.F. et al. (1993) Glutamine and the preservation of gut integrity. *Lancet*, 341, 1363–1365.

Wilschanski, M., Sherman, P., Pencharz, P. et al. (1996) Supplementary enteral nutrition maintains remission in paediatric Crohn's disease. *Gut*, 38, 543–548.

33

Nutritional support in cystic fibrosis

Michael R. Green

Introduction

Cystic fibrosis (CF) is a single gene disorder inherited in autosomal recessive fashion with an incidence of approximately 1:2000 in Western Europe. The commonest CF gene mutation (ΔF 508) results in the loss of a phenylalanine residue in the first nucleotide binding fold of the gene product, the cystic fibrosis transmembrane conductance regulator (CFTR). Defective chloride transport across epithelial cell membranes results in clinical problems in the chest, with the production of tenacious sputum, leading to recurrent infection. In the pancreas, failure of bicarbonate and water secretion, and ultimately of enzyme synthesis, results in malabsorption leading to malnutrition. The pathophysiology of malnutrition in CF is outlined in Table 33.1.

Historical background

Pancreas

The exocrine pancreatic ductules are impermeable to chloride (Quinton 1983). Inspissated acinar secretions cause ductular dilatation with subsequent formation of periductular fibrous tissue (Imrie et al 1979, Sturgess 1984). Destruction of acinar tissue itself also begins before birth, and is documented by a serial decline

Table 33.1 — Pathophysiology of malnutrition in CF

Reduced appetite due to chest disease
Malabsorption
    Exocrine pancreas
        Failure of bicarbonate and water secretion
        Failure of enzyme synthesis
    Biliary tree
        Intraluminal sequestration of bile acids
        with depletion of bile acid pool
        Stool losses leading to abnormal
        glycine:taurine ratio
    Bowel
        Small bowel enteropathy
        Other specific disease entities, e.g., coeliac
        disease, cow's-milk protein intolerance,
        gastro-oesophageal reflux, Crohn's disease
Increased energy requirements
    Related to degree of respiratory insufficiency
    Energy losses in stool and sputum

in blood immunoreactive trypsin levels (Heeley & Bangert 1992). These processes lead to deficiencies of bicarbonate and pancreatic lipases, which contribute to fat malabsorption leaving the infant to rely on the activity of breast milk and lingual lipases (which represent up to 90% of the total lipolytic activity in the acidic duodenal environment) (Dutta et al 1982).

The bile acid pool is depleted following adsorption to dietary residues (Leroy et al 1986). Both glycine and taurine are lost in the stool, but only glycine can be endogenously synthesized and micellar solubilization of fat is further impaired.

Small bowel

Deficiencies of phospholipid and essential fatty acids that are essential for cell membrane integrity may impair the absorptive phase of fat digestion (Innis 1992). Mucous glycoprotein structure is abnormal, and mucosal hydrolase and transport systems may be altered, affecting the absorption of carbohydrate and amino acids. Decreased lactase activity (Morin et al 1976) and abnormal passive permeability have been demonstrated (Leclercq-Fourcart et al 1987, Murphy et al 1989).

Energy requirements

Children with CF have increased energy expenditure (Shepherd et al 1988, Giradet et al 1994). It is unclear whether there is an intrinsic defect in energy metabolism at molecular level (O'Rawe et al 1990, Fried et al 1991), but there is no doubt that the child with overt respiratory symptoms employs additional energy in combating high microbial loads, mounting inflammatory responses and replacing protein and energy lost in sputum and faeces. These are quite apart from the adverse effect of the associated decline in appetite.

Practice and procedures

Nutritional assessment

Adequate nutritional status cannot be achieved nor maintained without regular assessment by a paediatric dietitian with specific experience in CF (Table 33.2). In order to consolidate this advice, a clinical nurse specialist can also provide invaluable support and advice to the family (Nicholson 1992).

Table 33.2 — Nutritional assessment

Anthropometry
Weight
Length/Height
Head circumference
Mid-upper-arm circumference
Skin-fold thicknesses

Laboratory
Full blood count
Biochemistry with serum protein
3–5 day quantitative fat balance study
Serum fat-soluble vitamin levels
Ferritin
Consider trace elements

A careful assessment of nutritional status is essential at the time of diagnosis and at least yearly intervals thereafter. During infancy, growth parameters should be assessed at each monthly clinic visit and this followed by specific dietary advice. Clinical evaluation includes measurement of body weight, length, and head circumference during infancy together with measurements of mid-upper-arm circumference and skin-fold thicknesses, all of which should be plotted on appropriate centile charts. The annual review blood tests include full blood count and film together with liver function tests and serum proteins. More specific laboratory nutritional assessment includes quantitative fat balance studies (i.e., a 3-day faecal fat collection for estimation of fat content in association with a 5-day dietary record of intake). Fat excretion is normally < 5% of dietary intake, but in children with CF one is aiming to achieve at least 85% fat absorption in order to ensure normal growth. In units where quantitative estimation of faecal fat is not possible, the semi-quantitative method of fat microscopy on spot stool specimens may be used (Walters 1990). Serum levels of the fat-soluble vitamins A, D and E require measuring annually. Trace elements such as zinc and selenium are not measured routinely, but may be indicated in the child who is found to be severely malnourished.

The infant

Human milk

As in healthy infants, breastfeeding is recommended for the baby with CF who is clinically well. The advantages of human milk are discussed later, but there are however one or two theoretical problems with breastfeeding. Human milk has a lower protein content than that of infant formulae and may therefore not fully meet the needs of the infant with CF who has increased losses in the stool and possibly sputum together with increased demands for growth. There have been a few reports of hypoproteinaemia and electrolyte depletion associated with exclusive breast-feeding (Laughlin et al 1981). It is important, therefore, in the infant who is breastfed but who is not gaining weight appropriately to monitor protein levels and also sodium balance. If urinary sodium output is very low in spite of normal serum levels, then the weight may respond to sodium supplementation.

Infant formulae

Infants with CF who are not breastfed can thrive perfectly satisfactorily on standard modified cow's-milk formulae in volumes of up to 200 mL/kg/day (Holliday et al 1991). There seems to be no real indication for the use of semi-elemental feeds in infants without more specific gastrointestinal problems.

Weaning

Depending on the individual growth pattern, the introduction of solid food should be considered at 3 months. Weaning should follow an entirely normal pattern, but the parents should be encouraged to give a normal-to-high fat intake in order to ensure adequate growth.

Pancreatic enzyme supplementation

Pancreatic enzymes as enteric-coated microsphere preparations are required from the time of diagnosis in all but those few children who have no objective evidence of fat malabsorption. The starting dose is empirically determined, using between one-third and one-half of the contents of a capsule with each milk feed. This provides about 1500–2500 units of lipase for Pancrease (Cilag) and 2700–4000 units for Creon (Solvay). The microspheres can be mixed with either a little water, milk or fruit puree and given from a spoon. Once weaning has occurred, the microspheres can be mixed with some semi-solid food taken from a spoon. It is reasonable to divide the dose between the beginning and mid-point of the meal, and in infancy this prevents unnecessary administration if the child subsequently refuses to eat most of what is offered to him. Over 4 years, the suggested starting dose is 1–2 capsules per meal.

Following the recognition of the association between colonic strictures and the use of high-strength pancreatic enzymes, the US Food and Drug Administration Authority (March 1995) recommends that infants receive between 2000–4000 units of lipase/120 mL of formula or with each breast feed (or 450–900 units lipase/g fat). Weaned infants and children under 4 years of age should receive approximately 1000 units/kg/meal. The suggested starting dose in children over 4 years of age when fat intake declines naturally is 500 units/kg/meal. The requirements of children already established on therapy should be reviewed at this age. The maximum recommended is 2500 units lipase/kg/meal, with half of this dose for snacks. The UK Committee on Safety of Medicines (May 1995) recommends a maximum lipase intake of 10,000 IU/kg/day.

Special circumstances

Energy supplementation is necessary where there is inadequate weight gain despite adequate control of fat malabsorption and normal sodium balance. Glucose polymers such as Maxijul (Scientific Hospital Supplies), Polycal (Nutricia Clinical) or Caloreen (Clintec), together with a 50% fat emulsion for example Calogen (SHS), are used. The addition of energy supplements requires careful monitoring by the paediatric dietitian. The addition of 5 g glucose polymer and 3 mL of a 50% fat emulsion/100 mL of normal infant formula provides approximately 100 kcal/100 mL. There is also a combined carbo-hydrate and fat supplement, Duocal (SHS). Duocal should be added in 1 g increments/100 mL of feed, and 7 g/100 mL provides 100 kcal/100 mL. Pancreatic enzyme doses may need to be reviewed with the addition of extra fat into the feed.

Infants who present with meconium ileus and require surgery may post-operatively develop a temporary disaccharide intolerance. The stools should be tested for reducing substances and if positive then protein hydrolysate milks such as Pregestimil (Bristol-Myers), Nutramigen (Bristol-Myers), Pepti-Junior (Cow & Gate) or Prejomin (Milupa) are indicated (Farrell et al 1987). These milks contain a higher proportion of fat as medium-chain triglycerides, but pancreatic enzyme supplementation is still required. If there has been major intestinal resection, a modular feed using comminuted chicken meat (Cow & Gate) as the protein source with additional carbohydrate, fat, vitamins and minerals may be required if hydrolysed protein formulae are not tolerated. Very occasionally, children may require total parenteral nutrition in the early post-operative period.

Gastro-oesophageal reflux is more prevalent in CF (Scott et al 1985), and treatment follows the standard regimen. Infants who have persistent diarrhoea or fail to gain weight despite seemingly-adequate diet and pancreatic enzyme supplementation with normal metabolic status should undergo jejunal biopsy to exclude coeliac disease.

The older child

Beyond infancy, a normal feeding pattern with normal-to-high fat and protein intake should be encouraged. The diet should include full-cream milk, butter, full-fat cheese, meat and eggs, together with liberal snack foods. It is unusual for the infant with CF to require nasogastric feeding, but even so there is a great emphasis on weight gain. As they grow, many children develop feeding problems and enter the cycle of food refusal. It is important to try and resolve these difficulties, and the involvement of a trained clinical psychologist should be considered at a very early stage.

Where manipulation of the diet is failing to maintain adequate nutritional status, as judged by the objective parameters already discussed, then supplementary sources of energy should be considered. Before embarking on this road, it is essential to ensure that fat absorption has been optimized. If significant mal-absorption is demonstrated, then a higher dose of pancreatic enzyme supplementation may be required. If the doses are on the high side already, then the addition of an acid suppression agent such as an H_2 antagonist or a proton-pump inhibitor may improve the absorption of fat. On occasion, it is worth simply changing the enzyme preparation on purely empirical grounds.

High-energy liquid supplements such as Scandishake (SHS), Fresubin (Fresenius) or Provide (Fresenius) are useful. These preparations are available in many different flavours, and it is important to ensure variety in order to maintain adherence to the advised regimen. During periods of energy supplementation in this manner, the child should continue to see the dietitian at frequent intervals in order to reinforce the advice for a diet containing high-energy foods. If these measures fail to produce an adequate growth pattern or nutritional status, then enteral feeding should be considered. The available routes are nasogastric tube feeding and surgically- or endoscopically-placed gastrostomy. There seems to be no difference in fat absorption between enterally-administered elemental or whole protein feeds, and most centres choose a polymeric feed such as Nutrison Paediatric (Nutricia Clinical) or Paediasure (Abbott) in children under 6 years and Nutrison Standard (Nutricia Clinical) for those over 6 years. The enteral feed is given as an overnight infusion of roughly 50% of total energy requirements, leaving the child free during the day time. Pancreatic enzymes are required with these feeds. Half of the total requirement should be given at the beginning and, if feasible, the other half should be given as the child is going to sleep. If it cannot be given at night, it should be given in the morning. Most children with CF who actually require enteral feeding are approaching their teens and adherence is improved by offering at least 1 night a week off the feed. Whatever feeding regimen is employed it should be continued for prolonged periods in order to maintain improvement in nutritional status (Dalzell et al 1992).

Vitamin supplementation

Depletion of the fat-soluble vitamins A, D and E has been detected from within a few months of birth (Sokol et al 1989), and these should therefore be given routinely from the time of diagnosis (Table 33.3). Vitamin A deficiency is associated with failure to thrive, anaemia, blindness and hyperkeratosis. Although bone demineralization can occur in children with CF, rickets is rarely seen probably because dermal synthesis accounts for more than 80% of normal vitamin D requirements (Hahn et al 1979). Vitamin E is a powerful antioxidant, and haemolytic anaemia has been reported in a few newly-diagnosed infants (Farrell et al 1977). Prolonged deficiency is associated with a peripheral neuropathy, but in CF this rarely occurs without advanced liver disease. Clinically-obvious vitamin K deficiency presenting with early haemorrhage is very unusual in infants with CF, and supplementation is not routinely recommended unless there is evidence of liver disease (Scott-Jupp et al 1991).

Table 33.3 — Standard vitamin supplementation

Fat-soluble vitamins	
A	4000–8000 IU/day
D	400–800 IU/day
E	50–200 mg/day
K	Not given routinely

Water-soluble vitamins

B group and C not malabsorbed but given as part of daily multivitamin supplement

Subject to annual monitoring of vitamin levels.

The doses of fat-soluble vitamins should be at least twice the estimated average requirement (EAR). Vitamin A is usually given in a dose of between 4000–8000 IU. Between 400–800 IU of vitamin D are required. Vitamin E requirements increase with age, starting with 50 mg daily during infancy and rising to 200 mg daily by the teenage years. Because there is no single vitamin preparation to provide all three vitamins in satisfactory quantities, a multivitamin preparation such as Abidec (Warner-Lambert) is used together with additional vitamin E. It is essential to monitor serum levels of all three vitamins on at least an annual basis and to alter the doses accordingly. Those infants and young children with poorly-controlled malabsorption, poor dietary adherence or liver disease and those who have had bowel resection are most at risk from vitamin deficiency. The water-soluble vitamins (B group and C) are not usually deficient, but are given as part of the multivitamin supplement.

Minerals and trace elements

Sodium supplementation in doses of 1–2 mmol/kg/day in infancy and up to 40 mmol/day in older children are required in hot weather. Iron absorption is usually normal in infancy, but ferritin levels should be monitored as part of the annual review. Zinc and selenium levels may be monitored, but supplementation is rarely required. Essential fatty acids are required for neuro-development and cell membrane integrity and may be malabsorbed in the presence of steatorrhoea. However, signs of essential fatty acid deficiency such as desquamation, poor wound healing and thrombocytopenia are rarely seen in CF, and supplementation beyond that recommended for inclusion in modern standard formulae milks is unnecessary (Aggett et al 1991).

Discussion

Enough is now known about the ontogeny of the pancreatic defect and of other factors contributing to enhanced nutritional requirements in CF to enable us to recognize and treat early infancy as a critical period. Significant intestinal malabsorption is seen in the majority of infants within a few months of birth, and ultimately in 95% of children with CF. It is accepted that the earlier CF is detected the better the ultimate outcome (Dankert-Roelse et al 1989, Wilcken & Chalmers 1985). Many infants are already malnourished by the time of diagnosis, but if neonatal screening programmes identify disease at an early

Table 33.4 — Proposed stepwise approach to nutritional supplementation

1. 'Normal' CF diet — high fat and protein
2. Energy supplementation if growth inadequate in spite of optimal fat absorption and metabolic status:
   a. Glucose polymers and fat emulsion,
   b. High-energy liquid supplements,
   c. Enteral feeds.

stage, many can achieve normal weight-for-age by 12 months (Weaver et al 1994). Specific improvements in nutritional status have been demonstrated (Greer et al 1991) as well as decreased morbidity with the use of prophylactic Flucloxacillin from the time of diagnosis (Weaver et al 1994). Despite careful management, faecal energy losses can be as high as 10% of energy intake (Murphy et al 1991), and it is suggested that children with CF require 20–50% more energy than the estimated actual requirement for age. The major objectives of treatment, following early diagnosis, therefore are the prevention of pulmonary infection and to ensure optimal growth and nutrition.

Very close monitoring of anthropometric measurements, fat malabsorption and biochemical status is essential whichever milk is chosen early in life. The theoretical advantages of using human milk include an optimal essential amino acid and fatty acid content. The presence of taurine is particularly important because of its role in bile acid conjugation (Roy et al 1977). Human milk also contains a wide range of protective and trophic factors. In addition, it contains amylase (Lindberg & Skeud 1982) and lipase, which at least partly compensates for diminished pancreatic secretion (Jensen et al 1982). It has been demonstrated in normal infants that both fat and carbohydrate absorption are more efficient from human milk than from artificial formulae (Alemi et al 1981). Perhaps as important as any of these objective benefits is the psychological bond created between the breastfeeding mother and infant.

Similar principles apply beyond infancy, and these objective parameters should be used proactively to encourage adequate nutritional intake. First, a high-fat and protein diet should be taken moving on to high-energy supplementation or enteral feeding when growth is seen to be failing (Table 33.4). Energy supplementation is not without problems. The appetite for a normal diet is reduced, and with continuous feeding there is a risk of hyperglycaemia, which necessitates close blood glucose monitoring.

The advent of neonatal screening methods with serum immunoreactive trypsin and genotyping on dried-blood spots has given us the opportunity to identify children with CF very early in life and thus to be able to intervene with physiotherapy, prophylactic antibiotics and most importantly careful nutritional management (Green & Weaver 1994). Optimizing nutritional status and anticipating nutritional needs in childhood is known to improve outcome. With the input of an experienced paediatric dietitian this is now an achievable goal in this chronic disease.

Acknowledgements

My grateful thanks to Linda Wilson for her helpful comments and to Sally Collins for her patience in the preparation of the manuscript.

References

Aggett, P.J., Haschke, F., Heine, W. et al. (1991) ESPGAN Committee on Nutrition. Committee Report. Comment on the content and composition of lipids in infant formulas. *Acta Paediatr Scand*, 80, 887–896.

Alemi, B., Hamosh, M., Scanlon, J.W., Salzman-Mann, C., Hamosh, P. (1981) Fat digestion in very low-birth-weight infants: effect of addition of human milk to low-birth-weight formula. *Pediatrics*, 68, 484–489.

Dalzell, A.M., Shepherd, R.W., Dean, B., Cleghorn, G.J., Holt, T.L., Francis, P.J. (1992) Nutritional rehabilitation in cystic fibrosis: A 5 year follow-up study. *J Pediatr Gastroenterol Nutr*, 15, 141–145.

Dankert-Roelse, J.E., te Meerman, G.J., Martijn, A., ten Kate, L.P., Knol, K. (1989) Survival and clinical outcome in patients with cystic fibrosis, with or without neonatal screening. *J Pediatr*, 114, 362–367.

Dutta, S.K., Hamosh, M., Abrams, C.K., Hamosh, P., Hubbard, V.S. (1982) Quantitative estimation of lingual lipase activity in the upper small intestine in adult patients with pancreatic insufficiency. *Gastroenterol*, 82, 1047.

Farrell, P.M., Bieri, J.G., Fratantoni, J.F., Wood, R.E., di Sant'Agnese, P.A. (1977) The occurrence and effects of human vitamin E deficiency. A study in patients with cystic fibrosis. *J Clin Invest*, 60, 233–241.

Farrell, P.M., Mischler, E.H., Sondel, S.A., Palta, M. (1987) Predigested formula for infants with cystic fibrosis. *J Am Diet Assoc*, 87, 1353–1356.

Fried, M.D., Durie, P.R., Tsui, L-C., Corey, M., Levison, H., Pencharz, P.B. (1991) The cystic fibrosis gene and resting energy expenditure. *J Pediatr*, 119, 913–916.

Girardet, J.P., Tounian, P., Sardet, A. et al. (1994) Resting energy expenditure in infants with cystic fibrosis. *J Pediatr Gastroenterol Nutr*, 18, 214–219.

Green, M.R., Weaver, L.T. (1994) Early and late outcome of CF screening. *J Roy Soc Med*, 87(suppl 21), 5–10.

Greer, R., Shepherd, R., Cleghorn, G., Bowling, F.G., Holt, T. (1991) Evaluation of growth and changes in body composition following neonatal diagnosis of cystic fibrosis. *J Pediatr Gastroenterol Nutr*, 13, 52–58.

Hahn, T.J., Squires, A.E., Halstead, L.R., Strominger, D.B. (1979) Reduced serum 25-hydroxy vitamin D concentration and disordered mineral metabolism in patients with cystic fibrosis. *J Paediatr*, 94, 38–42.

Heeley, A.F., Bangert, S.K. (1992) The neonatal detection of cystic fibrosis by measurement of immunoreactive trypsin in blood. *Ann Clin Biochem*, 29, 361–376.

Holliday, K.E., Allen, J.R., Waters, D.L., Gruca, M.A., Thompson, S.M., Gaskin, K.J. (1991) Growth of human milk-fed and formula-fed infants with cystic fibrosis. *J Pediatr*, 118, 77–79.

Imrie, J.R., Fagan, D.G., Sturgess, J.M. (1979) Quantitative evaluation of the development of the exocrine pancreas in cystic fibrosis and control infants. *Am J Pathol*, 95, 697–708.

Innis, S.M. (1992) Plasma and red blood cell fatty acid values as indexes of essential fatty acids in the developing organs of infants fed with milk or formulas. *J Pediatr*, 120(suppl), S78–S86.

Jensen, R.G., Clark, R.M., de Jong, F.A., Hamosh, M., Liao, T.H., Mehta, N.R. (1982) The lipolytic triad: Human lingual, breast milk, and pancreatic lipases: Physiological implications of their characteristics in digestion of dietary fats. *J Pediatr Gastroenterol Nutr*, 1, 243–255.

Laughlin, J.J., Brady, M.S., Eigen, H. (1981) Changing feeding trends as a cause of electrolyte depletion in infants with cystic fibrosis. *Pediatrics*, 68, 203–207.

Leclercq-Foucart, J., Forget, P.P., Van Cutsem, J.L. (1987) Lactulose-rhamnose intestinal permeability in children with cystic fibrosis. *J Pediatr Gastroenterol Nutr*, 6, 66–70.

Leroy, C., Lepage, G., Morin, C.L., Bertrand, J.M., Dufour-Larue, O., Roy, C.C. (1986) Effect of dietary fat and residues on fecal loss of sterols and on their microbial degradation in cystic fibrosis. *Dig Dis Sci*, 31, 911–918.

Lindberg, T., Skude, G. (1982) Amylase in human milk. *Pediatrics*, 70, 235–238.

Morin, C.L., Roy, C.C., Lasalle, R., Bonin, A. (1976) Small bowel mucosal dysfunction in patients with cystic fibrosis. *J Pediatr*, 88, 213–216.

Murphy, J.L., Wootton, S.A., Bond, S.A., Jackson, A.A. (1991) Energy content of stools in normal healthy controls and patients with cystic fibrosis. *Arch Dis Child*, 66, 495–500.

Murphy, M.S., Sheldon, W., Brunetto, A. et al. (1989) Active and passive sugar absorption in pancreatic insufficiency. *J Pediatr Gastroenterol Nutr*, 8, 189–194.

Nicholson, K. (1992) The CF Nurse Specialist and Neonatal Screening: Child Care And Research in East Anglia. In: Davis, T.J. (ed.) *Role of the Cystic Fibrosis Nurse Specialist*, pp. 32–38. Abingdon: Medicine Group.

O'Rawe, A., Dodge, J.A., Redmond, A.O.B., McIntosh, I., Brock, D.J.H. (1990) Gene/energy interaction in cystic fibrosis. *Lancet*, 335, 552–553.

Quinton, P.M. (1983) Chloride impermeability in cystic fibrosis. *Nature*, 301, 421–422.

Report of the Pancreatic Enzyme working party. Committee a Safety of Medicines May (1995). London England.

Roy, C.C., Weber, A.M., Morin, C.L. et al. (1977) Abnormal biliary lipid composition in cystic fibrosis. Effect of pancreatic enzymes. *N Engl J Med*, 297, 1301–1305.

Scott-Jupp, R., Lama, M., Tanner, M.S. (1991) Prevalence of liver disease in cystic fibrosis. *Arch Dis Child*, 66, 698–701.

Scott, R.B., O'Loughlin, E.V., Gall, D.G. (1985) Gastrooesophageal reflux in patients with cystic fibrosis. *J Pediatr*, 106, 223–227.

Shepherd, R.W., Vasques-Velasquez, L., Prentice, A., Holt, T.L., Coward, W.A., Lucas, A. (1988) Increased energy expenditure in young children with cystic fibrosis. *Lancet*, i, 1300–1303.

Sokol, R.J., Reardon, M.C., Accurso, F.J. et al. (1989) Fat soluble vitamin status during the first year of life in infants with cystic fibrosis identified by screening of newborns. *Am J Clin Nutr*, 50, 1064–1071.

Sturgess, J.M. (1984) Structural and developmental abnormalities of the exocrine pancreas in cystic fibrosis. *J Pediatr Gastroenterol Nutr*, 3(suppl 1), S55–S66.

US Cystic Fibrosis Foundation/Food and Drug Administration Conference. March (1995).

Walters, M.P., Kelleher, J., Gilbert, J., Littlewood, J.M. (1990) Clinical monitoring of steatorrhoea in cystic fibrosis. *Arch Dis Child*, 65, 99–102.

Weaver, L.T., Green, M.R., Nicholson, K. et al. (1994) Prognosis in cystic fibrosis treated with continuous flucloxacillin from the neonatal period. *Arch Dis Child*, 70, 84–89.

Wilcken, B., Chalmers, G. (1985) Reduced morbidity in patients with cystic fibrosis detected by neonatal screening. *Lancet*, ii, 1319–1321.

34

Nutritional support in inborn errors of metabolism

Marilyn Bernard, Lauren Furuta and Clifford Lo

Introduction

Inborn errors of metabolism are disorders caused by genetic defects that produce an interference in the normal flow of metabolic processes. They result from variations in the structure and function of enzymes or other proteins. The aim of treatment is to correct the biochemical abnormality and may include the following:

1. Restriction of the accumulated substrate;

2. Enhancement of mutant enzyme by supplying larger doses of co-enzyme;

3. Provision of alternate pathways for the accumulated substrate.

Historical background

The first inborn error of metabolism to be successfully managed nutritionally was phenylketonuria (PKU). In 1953, Bickel et al documented that restriction of phenylalanine lowered blood concentrations of phenylalanine and prevented the severe manifestations associated with untreated PKU. Since then, the development of diet therapies for other inborn errors has occurred relatively swiftly (Table 34.1).

Nutritional evaluation involves assessment of growth, nutrient intake and biochemical parameters. Treatment of most metabolic disorders requires the restriction of at least one nutrient or dietary component. However, adequate energy intake is essential for both normal growth and the prevention of unnecessary catabolism. Most disorders require the use of a specialized semi-synthetic formula (or medical food) to meet the nutritional requirements. For disorders of protein metabolism, specialized nitrogen-free foods (pastas, breads, baked products) are typically needed to provide adequate calories.

Practice and procedures

Disorders of amino acid metabolism

Hyperphenylalaninaemias

Phenylketonuria (PKU) is caused by a defect in the enzyme phenylalanine hydroxylase, which causes the inability to convert the amino acid phenylalanine to tyrosine (Fig. 34.1). Phenylalanine and its metabolites accumulate in the blood and other body tissues.

Untreated, PKU eventually progresses to damage to the brain and central nervous system, most likely due to competition between elevated phenylalanine and other amino acids for transport into the brain, hypomyelination and impaired development of central nervous system white matter (Hackney 1968).

In *classical PKU*, very little or no phenylalanine hydroxylase is present. Blood phenylalanine levels are > 20 mg/dl. Phenylalanine and its metabolites, phenylpyruvic acid and phenylacetic acid, are excreted in the urine. The blood tyrosine level may be normal or low. Dietary treatment is essential to prevent mental retardation and other features of untreated PKU, which include pale complexion from decreased melanin production, eczema and a musty odour of urine and skin.

Atypical PKU is caused by a diminished quantity of phenylalanine hydroxylase. The untreated blood level of phenylalanine is between 10–20 mg/dl. Phenylalanine metabolites may not be present in the urine. Tyrosine levels are normal. Dietary treatment is needed but may not be as restrictive as the classical PKU diet.

Benign hyperphenylalaninaemia is characterized by mildly-elevated phenylalanine levels. The optimal phenylalanine level is < 6 mg/dl while consuming a normal diet. It is not necessary to treat this disorder. Phenylalanine levels may be a concern for women as they reach their child-bearing years.

Rare defects in tetrahydrobiopterin (BH4), the co-factor for phenylalanine hydroxylase, can also cause elevated phenylalanine levels. Metabolism of tyrosine and tryptophan are dependent on this co-factor, so a defect in BH4 also leads to neurological problems from neurotransmitter deficiencies. Treatment involves early diagnosis by urine studies, supplementation with a combination of neurotransmitter precursors, BH4 and folinic acid (Kaufman 1986), and in some cases a reduced phenylalanine diet.

Dietary management of hyperphenylalaninaemias
Restriction of phenylalanine beginning in infancy results in the lowering of phenylalanine levels and the prevention of mental retardation. The dietary treatment allows for a prescribed amount of phenylalanine, which is an essential amino acid, to allow appropriate growth and development while maintaining phenylalanine levels at 2–6 mg/dl (Cockburn et al 1993). Tolerance for dietary phenylalanine varies with the severity of the enzyme defect (Table 34.2). Special medical formulas

Table 34.1 — Dietary treatment of metabolic disorders

Disorder	Enzyme Deficiency	Biochemical Features	Nutritional Therapy/Adjunct Treatment
Amino Acid Disorders			
Hyperphenylalaninaemias			
'Classic' PKU	Phenylalanine Hydroxylase	Blood phe > 20 mg/dl Inc phenylketones in urine Mental retardation if untreated	Restrict Phe Increase Tyr
'Atypical' PKU	Phenylalanine Hydroxylase	Blood phe 10–20 mg/dl Mental retardation if untreated; less severe than in classical	Restrict Phe +/– Increase Tyr
Mild Hyperphenylalaninaemia	Phenylalanine Hydroxylase	Blood phe < 10 mg/dl	Not necessary
Tyrosinaemias			
Tyrosinaemia type 1 (Hereditary)	Fumarylacetoacetic Acid Hydroxylase Maleylacetoacetic Acid Isomerase (in some cases)	Inc blood/urine Tyrosine and +/– Methionine	Restrict Phe and Tyr +/– Restrict Met Liver transplant NTBC
Tyrosinaemia type II	Tyrosine Aminotransferase	Inc blood/urine/CSF Tyr Inc urine phenolic acids	Restrict Phe and Tyr
Other amino acid disorders			
Homocystinuria	Cystathionine-β-Synthase	Inc blood/urine Hcy Inc blood Met Dec blood cystine and cystathionine	+/– Pyridoxine (Vit. B6) supplement (if responsive) Restrict protein, Met Supplemental L-cystine
Maple syrup urine disease	Branched Chain Ketoacid Dehydrogenase Complex	Inc blood Leu, Ile, Val	Restrict Leu, Ile, Val +/– Thiamin (if responsive)
Isovaleric acidaemia	Isovaleryl-CoA Dehydrogenase	Inc blood/urine isovaleric acid Inc urine N-isovaleryl glycine and 3-hydroxy-isovaleric acid	Restrict Ile or protein +/– Carnitine supplement Glycine supplement
Propionic acidaemia	Propionyl-CoA Carboxylase	Inc blood ammonia Inc blood propionic acid	Restrict Met, Val, Ile, Leu Restrict odd-chain fatty acids +/– L-amino acid supplements Carnitine +/– Biotin supplement (if responsive)
Methylmalonic acidaemia	Methylmalonyl-CoA Mutase or Cobalamin Reductase	Inc blood/urine methylmalonic acid	Restrict Met, Val, Ile, Leu +/– Cobalamin supplement (if responsive) +/– Carnitine

PKU – phenylketonuria, Phe – phenylalanine, Tyr – tyrosine, Met – methionine, CSF – cerebral spinal fluid, NTBC – 2- (2-nitro-4-trifluoromethyl benzoyl)-1,3-cyclohexanedione, Hcy – homocysteine, Leu – leucine, Ile – isoleucine, Val – valine.

Table 34.1 — (cont'd)

Disorder	Enzyme Deficiency	Biochemical Features	Nutritional Therapy/Adjunct Treatment
Glutaric acidaemia type I	Glutaryl-CoA Dehydrogenase	Inc urine dicarboxylic acids, glutaric acid, glutarylcarnitine Metabolic acidosis +/– Dec carnitine	Carnitine and riboflavin supplements Low-protein diet (Res Lys and Try)
Glutaric acidaemia type II	Multiple Acyl-CoA Dehydrogenase	Hypoglycaemia (non-ketotic) Metabolic acidosis Abnormal urine organic acids	Low-protein and fat diet +/– riboflavin and carnitine (Treatment often unsuccessful)
Urea cycle defects Carbamyl phosphate synthetase deficiency	Carbamyl Phosphate Synthetase	Inc blood ammonia and glutamine	Low-protein diet Sodium benzoate Sodium phenylacetate +/– citrulline Liver transplant
Ornithine transcarbamylase deficiency	Ornithine Transcarbamylase	Inc blood ammonia, glutamine, glutamic acid, alanine	Low-protein diet Sodium benzoate Sodium phenylacetate +/– citrulline Liver transplant
Citrullinaemia	Argininosuccinate Synthetase	Inc blood citrulline, ammonia, alanine	Low-protein diet Arginine supplement Sodium benzoate Liver transplant
Argininosuccinic (AS) aciduria	Argininosuccinate Lyase	Inc blood AS, citrulline, ammonia	Low-protein diet Arginine supplement Sodium benzoate Liver transplant
Argininaemia	Arginase	Inc blood arginine +/– inc ammonia	Low-protein diet Liver transplant
Carbohydrate Disorders Galactosaemia	Galactokinase or GAL-1-Phosphate Uridyltransferase (GALT)★ or Uridine Diphosphate (UDP)-GAL-4-Epimerase	Inc blood/urine galactose	Galactose-restricted diet
Hereditary fructose	Fructose-1-Phosphate Aldolase	Inc blood/urine fructose	Fructose, sucrose, and sorbitol-free diet
Pyruvate dehydrogenase complex deficiency	Pyruvate Dehydrogenase Complex	Normal or low lactate: pyruvate ratio Increased alanine (following carbohydrate intake)	Ketogenic Diet (+/– long-term success) +/– DCA (dichloral-acetate)

Lys – lysine, GAL – galactose, GALT – galactose-l-phosphate uridyl transferase, MCT – medium chain triglycoride.

Table 34.1 — (cont'd)

Disorder	Enzyme Deficiency	Biochemical Features	Nutritional Therapy/Adjunct Treatment
Fatty Acid Oxidation Disorders			
LCAD deficiency VLCAD deficiency	Long-Chain Acyl-CoA-Dehydrogenase Very Long-Chain Acyl-CoA-Dehydrogenase	Features common to fatty acid oxidation disorders: 1. Metabolic decompensation associated with fasting	Low-fat diet (15% energy) Res long-chain fatty acids Avoid fasting +/− MCT oil supplement Carnitine supplement +/− Essential fatty acids
MCAD deficiency	Medium-Chain Acyo-CoA-Dehydrogenase	2. Chronic involvement of fatty-acid-dependent tissues (cardiac, skeletal) 3. Episodes of hypoketotic hypoglycaemia 4. Alterations in plasma or tissue concentrations of carnitine.★★	Low-fat diet (20–25% energy) Res medium-chain fatty acids Avoid fasting Carnitine supplement
SCAD SCHAD	Short-Chain Acyl-CoA-Dehydrogenase Short-chain Hydroxyacyl-CoA Dehydrogenase		Low-fat diet (20–25% energy) Res medium-chain fatty acids Avoid fasting Carnitine supplement
HMG-CoA lyase deficiency	3-Hydroxy-3-Methylglutaryl Lyase	Abnl urine organic acids (3-hydroxy-3-methylglutaric acid) Abnl methylglutaryl acid	Low fat (~25% energy) Mild protein restriction (~75–100% minimum requirements) Avoid fasting +/− Carnitine supplement

★most common.
★★Hale et al (1992).

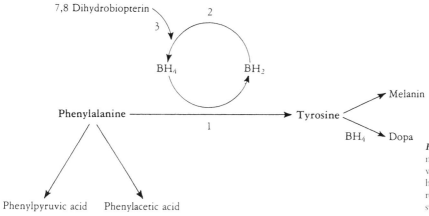

Figure 34.1 — Phenylalanine metabolism. From Rohr et al (1985), with permission (1) phenylalanine hydroxylase (2) dihydropteridine reductase (3) tetrahydropteridine synthetase.

Table 34.2 —Values for determining initial phenylalanine prescription

Plasma phenylalanine (Umol/L)	(mg/dl)	Dietary phenylalanine (mg/kg)
≤ 605	≤ 10	70
605–1211	11–20	55
1212–1816	21–30	45
1817–2421	31–40	35
> 2421	> 40	25

From Acosta & Yanicelli (1997), with permission.

that contain all the amino acids except phenylalanine are required for assuring an adequate protein intake. The medical formulas are supplemented with vitamins and minerals.

The diet of an infant with PKU consists of a prescribed amount of regular formula or breastmilk combined with a PKU formula (Table 34.3). The appropriate phenylalanine requirement is determined by the initial phenylalanine level and subsequent levels once diet is initiated. Breastfeeding is encouraged, but must be managed closely to avoid excess phenylalanine

Table 34.3 — Formulas available* for the treatment of amino acid disroders

PKU
XP Analog, XP Maxamaid, XP Maxamum, Periflex (SHS)
Lofenalac, Phenylfree, PKU 1, PKU 2, PKU 3 (Mead Johnson Nutritional)
Phenex-1, Phenex-2 (Ross Laboratories)
Phenylade (Foodtec Manufacturing Inc.)

Tyrosinaemia Type I
XPHEN, TYR, MET Analog (SHS)
Tyromex-1 (Ross Laboratories)

Tyrosinaemia Type II
Low Phe/Tyr Diet Powder, TYR 1, TYR 2 (Mead Johnson Nutritionals)
Tyrex-2 (Ross Laboratories)
XPHEN, TYR Maxamaid (SHS)

Homocystinuria (Vitamin B6 non-responsive)
XMET Analog, XMET Maxamaid, XMET Maxamum (SHS)
Ketonex-1, Ketonex-2 (Ross Laboratories)
MSUD Diet Powder, MSUD 1, MSUD 2 (Mead Johnson Nutritionals)

Maple Syrup Urine Disease
MSUD Analog, MSUD Maxamaid, MSUD Maxamum (SHS)
Ketonex-1, Ketonex-2 (Ross Laboratories)
MSUD Diet Powder, MSUD 1, MSUD 2 (Mead Johnson Nutritionals)

Propionic Acidaemia, Methylmalonic Acidaemia
XMET, THRE, VAL, ISOLEU Analog; XMET, THRE, VAL, ISOLEU Maxamaid; XMET, THRE, VAL, ISOLEU Maxamum (SHS)
Propimex-1, Propimex-2 (Ross Laboratories)
OS 1, OS 2 (Mead Johnson Nutritionals)

Glutaric Acidaemia Type 1
XLYS, TRY Analog; XLYS, TRY Maxamaid; XLYS, TRY Maxamum (SHS)
Glutarex-1, Glutarex-2 (Ross Laboratories)

Disorders of Leucine Metabolism
XLEU Analog, XLEU Maxamaid (SHS)
I-Valex-1, I-Valex-2 (Ross Laboratories)

Urea Cycle Disorders
Cyclinex-1, Cyclinex-2 (Ross Laboratories)
UCD 1, UCD 2 (Mead Johnson Nutritionals)

*Available in the United States. SHS – Scientific Hospital Supply, Phen – phenylalanine, Tyr – tyrosine, met – methionine, msud – maple syrup urine disease, Thre – threonine, Val – valine, Isoleu – isoleucine, Lys – lysine, Try – tryptophan, Leu – leucine, UCD – urea cycle defect.

Table 34.4 — Nutrient requirements of infants and children with PKU

Age	Phenylalanine	Tyrosine	Protein	Calories
0 to < 3 months	25–70 mg/kg	300–350 mg/kg	3.5–3 g/kg	120 kcals/kg
3 to < 6 months	20–45 mg/kg	300–350 mg/kg	3.5–3 g/kg	120 kcals/kg
6 to < 9 months	15–35 mg/kg	250–300 mg/kg	3–2.5 g/kg	110 kcals/kg
9 to < 12 months	10–35 mg/kg	250–300 mg/kg	3–2.5 g/kg	105 kcals/kg
1 to < 4 years	200–400 mg/day	1700–3000 mg/day	30 g/day	900–1800/day

From Acosta & Yanicelli (1997), with permission.

ingestion. The practical method of management consists of alternating between breastfeedings and special formula feedings. Phenylalanine levels are measured once per week, and the diet is adjusted accordingly to keep blood levels in the appropriate range.

As the child ages, solid foods are introduced. The allowed foods include only those that are naturally low in protein such as vegetables, fruits and some grain products. Special food products that have been modified to be low in protein are an important source of calories, bulk and variety. Resources are available to help estimate the phenylalanine content of foods (Evans 1994, Schuett 1995). Guidelines for phenylalanine and other nutrient requirements are described in Table 34.4.

The diet for PKU was originally discontinued during early childhood around age 5 years. It has now been determined that this practice was detrimental to some children's development. The current recommendation is to continue phenylalanine restriction throughout life (Koch et al 1987, Potocnik & Widhalm 1994).

Tyrosinaemia type 1

Tyrosinaemia type 1, also known as hereditary tyrosinaemia, is a defect of tyrosine metabolism and is detected by elevated tyrosine levels in plasma and urine and by an increase in urinary phenolic acids. The affected enzyme, fumarylacetoacetate hydrolyase (FAH), is at the terminal end of the tyrosine metabolism pathway and is responsible for converting fumaryl-acetoacetic acid to fumaric acid and acetoacetic acid. The block leads to an accumulation of succinylacetone in the blood and urine (Fig. 34.2).

Clinical symptoms in the early stages of the disease include vomiting, diarrhoea, failure to thrive and abdominal distension. Complications that may develop

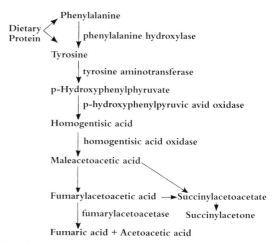

Figure 34.2 — Tryosine metabolism. From Rohr et al (1985), with permission.

include hepatomegaly, splenomegaly, ascites, oedema and haemorrhagic tendencies.

The pathogenesis of tyrosinaemia type I is complex and involves the following: depletion of glutathione, accumulation of succinylacetone, inhibition of certain enzymes (including one in the porphyrin pathway), eventual hepato-cellular degeneration, nodular cirrhosis or hepatoma. Elevated serum alpha–fetoprotein is a marker of the hepatic complications. Renal complications include tubular reabsorption impairment and Fanconi's syndrome (Kvittingen 1986).

The use of the drug NTBC (2-(2-nitro-4-trifluoromethylbenzoyl)-1,3-cyclohexanedione) inhibits the enzyme pHPPD (hydroxyphenylpyruvic acid dioxygenase), which is an hepatic enzyme associated with the presence of succinylacetone. Clinically, NTBC has been shown to prevent acute porphyric episodes and decrease the rate of progression of liver cirrhosis and Fanconi's syndrome (Lindstedt et al 1992).

Liver transplantation has successfully improved the outcome for persons with tyrosinaemia type I. Although long-term data on patients with liver transplants is not yet available, transplants seem to cure liver manifestations and prevent the development of hepatomas and further neurological crises.

Dietary management of tyrosinaemia type I

The goal of dietary management is to provide a diet restricted in both phenylalanine and tyrosine. Adequate protein is provided through special formulas (medical foods) that do not contain phenylalanine, tyrosine or methionine (see Table 34.3). Total phenylalanine and tyrosine should be restricted adequately so that blood tyrosine levels are between 30–100 µmol/L. For patients on NTBC therapy, serum tyrosine are often markedly elevated; an acceptable level is approximately < 500 µmol/L (Linsdedt et al 1992).

When the diagnosis is made, all tyrosine and phenylalanine should be eliminated from the diet for 24–48 hours. Specialized amino acid formulas are used to provide tyrosine and phenylalanine-free protein, calories, vitamins and minerals. Tyrosine and phenylalanine, from either breastmilk or regular infant formula, are gradually introduced. The phenylalanine and tyrosine combined in infants' diets are usually restricted to approximately 65–155 mg/kg. Clinical improvement and short-term outlook for patients with tyrosinaemia type I has improved since NTBC therapy has been available.

Tyrosinaemia type II

Tyrosinaemia type II (also known as oculocutaneous tyrosinaemia, tyrosine amino transferase deficiency, and Richner-Hanhart syndrome (Mitchell 1995)) is an autosomal recessive inherited disorder caused by a deficiency in tyrosine aminotransferase (TAT). It is characterized by greatly-elevated concentrations of blood and urine tyrosine and by increases in urinary phenolic acids, N-acetyltyrosine and tyramine. Features of disease include eye, skin, and neurological signs.

Eye features include hyperlacrimation, photophobia, redness and pain. Painful hyperkeratotic plaques occur on the soles of the feet and palms of the hands. Neurological abnormalities include mental retardation and, rarely, seizures. Dietary control may help improve the skin and eye lesions.

Dietary management of tyrosinaemia type II

The goals of dietary management are similar to type I tyrosinaemia. Methionine restriction is not necessary.

Special medical foods are available to provide adequate protein, vitamins and minerals (see Table 34.3). Phenylalanine and tyrosine are restricted so that tyrosine levels are maintained at approximately ≤ 20 mg/dl (Ney et al 1983). Because this diagnosis is usually made later in life, instituting the diet may be difficult in a person who already has defined food likes and dislikes.

Homocystinuria

Elevated homocysteine may be caused by several different defects involving methionine metabolism. The classic form of homocysteinaemia is caused by impairment of the enzyme cystathionine synthase, a vitamin B6-dependent enzyme in the methionine-to-cysteine pathway, which converts homocysteine to cystathionine (Fig. 34.3). Both homocysteine and methionine are elevated. Homocysteine may also be re-methylated back to methionine. The primary mode of re-methylation occurs through the transfer of a methyl group from N5-methyltetrahydrofolate (THF) to homocysteine. Co-factors for this reaction are B12 and folate dependent; abnormalities in the co-factors result in elevated homocysteine with normal methionine levels. Another re-methylation pathway uses betaine, which is derived from choline, as the methyl donor.

Patients with the classic form of homocystinuria who are untreated or poorly controlled develop clinical manifestations over time. These include dislocation of the ocular lens (ectopia lentis), skeletal malformations with Marfanoid features, mental retardation and vascular complications involving atherosclerosis with a predisposition to thromboembolic events.

Dietary management of homocystinuria

Dietary methionine should be restricted to levels that maintain adequate growth. Restriction may be achieved by either limiting methionine or limiting protein and supplementing with a methionine-free metabolic formula (see Table 34.3). Cystine becomes a conditionally-essential nutrient because its synthesis is impaired. The cystine requirement in infants starts at approximately 300 mg/kg and is adjusted based on serum levels. Methionine intake in infants is started at 15–30 mg/kg. Blood levels initially should be monitored frequently to determine the adequacy of the nutritional regimen.

Treatment that is started during infancy usually prevents the development of mental retardation and skeletal abnormalities. However, dislocation of the ocular lens is usually detected regardless of treatment, occurring

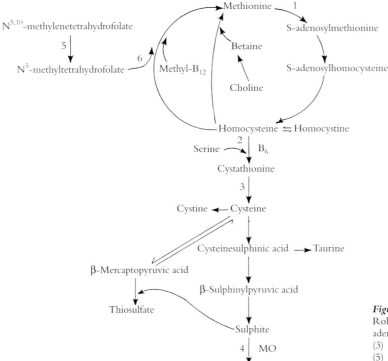

Figure 34.3 — Methionine metabolism. From Rohr et al (1985), with permission. (1) methionine adenosyltransferase (2) cycstathionine β-synthase (3) cystathionase (4) sulphite oxidase (5) $N^{5,10}$-methyltetrahydrofolate-homocysteine methyltransferase.

by the fourth decade in nearly all treated patients (Andria & Sebastio 1996). Approximately 50% of patients with homocystinuria respond to large doses (50–1000 mg) of pyridoxine hydrochloride, which is a co-factor for cystathionine B-synthase. Improvement is usually noted after approximately 10 days of therapy (Seashore et al 1972). If responsive, individuals may be treated with B6 supplementation and little or no dietary methionine restriction. Lifelong treatment is recommended to minimize the development of vascular complications.

Maple syrup urine disease

Maple syrup urine disease (MSUD; Branched-chain Ketoaciduria) is caused by a deficiency of the enzyme complex branched chain alpha-ketoacid dehydrogenase. The enzyme is common to the degradative pathways of the branched-chain amino acids—leucine, valine and isoleucine. Thiamine is the co-enzyme. The block results in increased levels of the amino acids and their keto-derivatives in blood, urine and cerebral spinal fluid. The accumulation and presence of alloisoleucine, the stereoisomer of isoleucine, is diagnostic of MSUD (Fig. 34.4).

MSUD patients can be divided into five types based

on their presentation and their response to thiamine. The five phenotypes are classic, intermediate, intermittent, thiamine-responsive, and dihydrolipoyl dehydrogenase (E3) deficient (Chuang & Shih 1995).

Classic MSUD presents in the first week of life with symptoms including feeding difficulties, lethargy, metabolic acidosis and the distinctive maple-syrup odour in the urine, sweat, and earwax. Neurological impairment may progress to seizures, apnoea and death within 10 days of life.

The intermediate and intermittent forms have an increased amount of functional enzyme. Patients with intermediate MSUD may have failure to thrive and developmental delay. Alloisoleucine, branched-chain amino acids (BCAA) and branched-chain keto acids (BCKA) are persistently elevated, but acidosis is uncommon. Patients with intermittent MSUD have normal BCAAs but become susceptible to elevated levels during periods of illness or stress. The features of thiamine-responsive MSUD are similar to the intermediate form. Pharmacological doses of thiamine (100–150 mg/day) along with a protein-restricted diet result in lowered amounts of BCAA and BCKA (Duran & Wadman 1985).

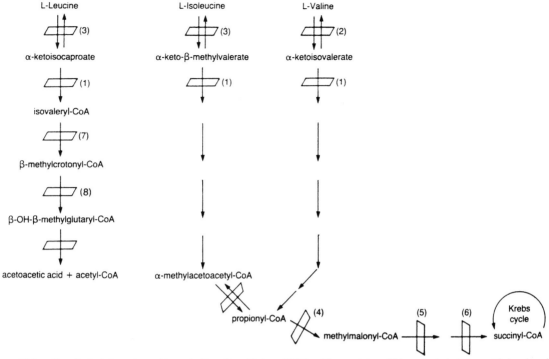

Figure 34.4 — Branched-chain amino acid metabolism. From Trahms (1992), with permission. (1) branched-chain ketoacid decarboxylase (2) valine aminotransferase (3) leucine – isoleucine aminotransferase (4) propionyl CoA reductase (5) methylmalonyl CoA racemase (6) methylmalonyl CoA mutase (7) isoraleryl CoA dehydrogenase (8) beta-methylcroteryl CoA carboxylase.

Dihydrolipoyl dehydrogenase (E3) deficiency is extremely rare and mimics the clinical phenotype of intermittent MSUD with the additional feature of severe lactic acidosis. Attempts at treatment with protein restriction and vitamins (thiamine, biotin and lipoic acid) have not yet been successful (Chuang & Shih 1995).

High levels of leucine and its ketoacid, alpha-ketoisocaproic acid, appear to be the neurotoxic agents in the disorder (Chuang & Shih 1995). Leucine levels tend to be more greatly elevated than the others and respond to dietary restriction more slowly because leucine is the predominant BCAA in most animal and plant proteins (Berry et al 1991).

Dietary management of maple syrup urine disease

Treatment involves both long-term dietary management and aggressive therapy during acute metabolic decompensation. Early diagnosis and initiation of a BCAA-free diet before the age of 10–14 days is essential to reduce the risk of permanent neurological damage or death.

The goal of acute therapy is to correct the acidosis and normalize the amino acid concentrations. Initial

measures may include peritoneal dialysis, renal dialysis or parenteral nutrition (Berry et al 1991). When the clinical status has stabilized, oral feedings using special formulas without BCAA are given.

Long-term dietary therapy requires the restriction of leucine, isoleucine and valine so that only the amount necessary for normal growth and development are provided. Blood levels of amino acids (especially leucine) must be monitored. Because the leucine concentration of natural protein is greater than isoleucine or valine concentrations, supplements of these two amino acids may be needed to maintain normal serum levels. Special BCAA-free formulas are required to fulfil the total protein requirements (see Table 34.3).

Organic acidaemias: Propionic acidaemia and methylmalonic acidaemia

Propionic acidaemia (PPA) and methylmalonic acidaemia (MMA) share similar metabolic pathways, clinical features and treatment. Both disorders are due to defects in methionine, threonine, valine, isoleucine, odd-chain fatty acid and eventually propionate metabolism (Fig. 34.5). The metabolic defect occurs

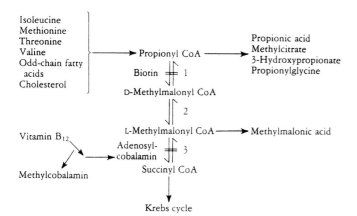

Figure 34.5 — Propionate and methylmalonate metabolism. From Rohr et al (1985), with permission. (1) propionyl CoA carboxylase (2) methylmalonyl CoA racemase (3) nethylmalonyl CoA mutase.

in the enzyme propionyl-CoA carboxylase or methyl-malonyl-CoA mutase. Methylmalonyl-CoA mutase is vitamin B12 dependent, therefore poor activity may also be caused by defects in formation of the B12 co-factor. Metabolic acidosis with hyperammonaemia and ketonuria are features of episodic decompensation, usually precipitated by excessive protein intake, constipation or infection.

Hyperammonaemia is a result of the abnormal organic acid, propionate (propionyl-CoA) or methylmalonate (methylmalonyl-CoA), which interfere with the urea cycle by inhibiting formation of N-acetylglutamate, the co-factor for carbamoyl phosphate synthetase, early in the urea cycle (Petrowski et al 1987). Hyper-glycinaemia is common and may be due to prolonged intake of excess protein or inhibited glycine cleavage due to isoleucine metabolites (Hillman et al 1973). The exact mechanism of increased glycine is unknown. The organic acids identified in the urine include methylcitrate and 3-hydroxypropionate for PPA and methylmalonic acid for MMA.

Dietary Management of PPA and MMA

The goals of dietary therapy can be divided into acute episode management and long-term management. During the acute phase, the goals are to maintain biochemical balance by aggressively treating the ketoacidosis. Large amounts of fluid and protein-free calories (up to 50% above normal intake) are given either enterally if tolerated or intravenously. Sodium bicarbonate may also be required to treat the acidosis.

Long-term management aims to prevent ketoacidosis and reduce accumulation of the metabolites. Protein intake from natural sources should be restricted to approximately 50% of the recommended amount for age. However, natural protein tolerance is highly individual and requires frequent monitoring of urine

organic acids and ketones, as well as of blood amino acids and ammonia. Amino acid supplementation, in the form of both a metabolic formula and individual amino acids, is usually required (see Table 34.3). Nutritional management may be complicated by food refusal, apparent lack of appetite and frequent vomiting. Aggressive nutrition support (i.e., feeding tube) should be considered if an adequate nutrient intake cannot be achieved with oral feedings.

Some cases of MMA respond to therapeutic doses of Vitamin B12, which is a component of a co-enzyme required for the conversion of methylmalonyl-CoA to succinyl-CoA.

Urea cycle defects

Each of the six enzymes in the urea cycle has a known defect (Table 34.5). The urea cycle, which occurs in the liver, is responsible for converting ammonia to urea (Fig. 34.6). If a deficiency occurs in any one of the enzymes, ammonia accumulates in the blood and all the cells of the body.

The clinical signs include poor feeding, vomiting, lethargy, hypotonia, stupor and bleeding diatheses, convulsions, coma, shock and death. Infection or increased protein intake often precede development of clinical features. Infants who survive the adverse effects of elevated ammonia are often mentally retarded. However, successful control of the metabolic crisis and prevention of the prolonged hyperammonaemia may prevent the adverse outcome during the neonatal period (Maestri et al 1991). Besides the neonatal period, there are other ages when symptoms are likely to occur. These include later in infancy when high-protein formula or milk is introduced, during infection and during puberty (possibly caused by lowered compliance to diet or medication) (Treem 1994).

Table 34.5 — Urea cycle disorders

Disorder	Defective enzyme	Biochemical findings	Location: mitochondria/ cytoplasm
NAGS deficiency	N-acetyglutamate synthase (NAGS)	dec citrulline	Mitochondria
CPS deficiency	Carbamylphosphate synthetase (CPS)	dec citrulline, dec arginine	Mitochondria
OTC deficiency	Orntihine transcarbamylase (OTC)	dec citrulline, inc orotic acid, dec arginine	Mitochondria
Citrullinaemia	Argininosuccinate synthetase	inc, inc citrulline, inc orotic acid, dec arginine	Cytoplasm
Argininosuccinic aciduria	Argininosuccinate lyase	citrulline, inc orotic acid, dec arginine, inc argininosuccinic acid	Cytoplasm
Arginase deficiency	Arginase	Normal citrulline, inc orotic acid inc arginine	Cytoplasm

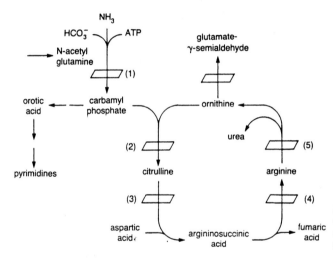

Figure 34.6 — Urea cycle, nitrogen metabolism. From Trahms (1992), with permission. (1) carbamyl phosphate synthetase (2) ornithine carbamyl transferase (3) argininosuccinic acid synthetase (4) argininosuccinic aid lyase (5) arginase.

Dietary management of urea cycle disorders

The goal of dietary management is control of blood ammonia levels with a maintenance of adequate plasma concentrations of amino acids. This is accomplished with a combination of protein restriction, supplementation with individual amino acids and use of medication (sodium phenylacetate or sodium phenylbutyrate) to help decrease accumulated nitrogenous metabolites by providing alternate pathways for nitrogen excretion. The use of an essential amino acid formula may be beneficial for maintaining adequate plasma amino acid levels while on a protein-restricted diet.

Typical diets will consist of 1–1.5 g protein/kg/day during the first few years of life. L-arginine (Brusilow et al 1979), L-citrulline, sodium phenylacetate and/or sodium phenylbutyrate may be prescribed to help increase nitrogen excretion (Batshaw 1994). Ideally, the diet should be provided as small frequent meals with the protein evenly divided throughout the day to help avoid large post-prandial protein loads. Many children with urea cycle disorders are finicky eaters with poor appetites. Attention must be given not only to adequate protein intake but also to adequate calorie intake to prevent catabolism. During illness, higher-calorie low-protein foods (e.g., popsicles, juice, soda, Koolaid) should be encouraged. If the patient is unable to consume any calories, hospitalization to provide calories intravenously may be necessary. Plasma amino acids and blood ammonia should be monitored. Initially, levels are checked once or twice per week until plasma concentrations stabilize. Once the patient is stable, levels may be checked every 2–3 months.

Fatty acid oxidation defects

Fatty acid oxidation defects are inborn errors of fat metabolism. There are currently at least 13 known defects (Tyni et al 1995, Roe & Coates 1995). Common features include acute metabolic decompensation associated with fasting, hypoketotic hypoglycaemia, involvement of cardiac or skeletal muscle and alterations of plasma or tissue carnitine. The disorders may be divided into categories of transport defects and disorders of the beta-oxidation pathway.

Transport defects include carnitine uptake deficiency (CUD), carnitine palmitoyl transferase deficiency (CPT I), CPT II, and translocase deficiency (Trans). These enzymes are involved with transporting fatty acids from the cytoplasm into the mitochondria.

Disorders of beta-oxidation include long-chain acyl-CoA dehydrogenase (LCAD), medium-chain acyl-CoA dehydrogenase (MCAD), short-chain acyl-CoA dehydrogenase (SCAD), long-chain 3-hydroxyacyl-CoA dehydrogenase (LCHAD), and short-chain 3-hydroxyacyl-CoA dehydrogenase (SCHAD). MCAD deficiency is the most common disorder of fatty acid oxidation and has been associated with sudden infant death syndrome (Brackett et al 1994).

The primary treatment for all the disorders is to avoid prolonged fasting. Infants < 1 year should not fast longer than 6 hours; children between the ages of 1 and 4 years may fast for up to 12 hours (Hale et al 1992). Uncooked cornstarch has been used to help delay the onset of fasting. The prescribed dose (usually 1.5–2 gm/kg body weight) may be added to formula at night (Dionsi Vici et al 1991).

Because fatty acids become available when fat stores are mobilized or when dietary fat is consumed, dietary fat restriction may be beneficial. Long-chain fats are often limited to 10–20% of total calories. Linoleic and linolenc acid should provide 3% and 0.5% respectively of total daily calories (Acosta & Yanicelli 1997).

Medium-chain triglycerides oil may be a useful adjunct calorie source in defects involving long-chain fatty acids. Care should be taken to avoid excess calorie intake, which would lead to storage as long-chain fats in the adipose tissue.

Disorders of carbohydrate metabolism

Galactosaemia

Galactosaemia may be caused by a defect in one of

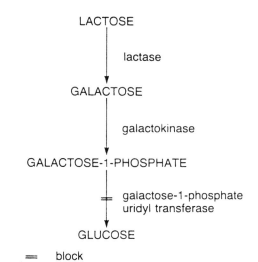

= block

Figure 34.7 — Galactose metabolism. From Trahms (1992), with permission.

three different enzymes necessary for galactose metabolism (Fig. 34.7). A deficiency of galactose-1-phosphate uridyl transferase (GALT) activity results in the most common form of galactosaemia. Galactose, galactitol, and galactose-1-phosphate accumulate in blood and tissues. Early features of untreated galactosaemia appear in infancy and include hypoglycaemia, jaundice, failure to thrive, vomiting and E coli sepsis. The symptoms appear after an infant has begun consuming milk sugar from formula or breast milk. Without treatment, death from E coli sepsis of meningitis occurs within the first 1–2 weeks of life (Elsas et al 1993). If the infant survives, long-term features of the disease include mental retardation, liver cirrhosis and cataracts.

Early detection and elimination of galactose from the diet can prevent death and reduce the risk of cataracts. Many states include galactosaemia in their newborn screening programmes. However, dietary treatment does not seem to guarantee a normal clinical outcome. Neurological impairment and sub-optimal intellectual development has been reported (Fishler et al 1972, Komrower 1982). Most females have ovarian failure (Kaufman et al 1981). The reason for these poor outcomes has not been definitively determined. Theories include foetal damage *in utero* or before intervention, endogeneous production of galactose (Berry et al 1995), or inadequate or excess galactose intake.

Dietary management of galactosaemia

A galactose-restricted diet should begin as soon as the

infant is diagnosed. Soy formula should replace cow's-milk based formulas or human milk. It should be noted that starch components of soy in soy formula naturally contain some galactose. However, the enzyme α-galactosidase, required to release the galactose from the soy, is not found in humans. Generally, milk-free foods form the base of the diet. Hidden sources of lactose must also be avoided. This is accomplished by reading labels and avoiding ingredients such as whey, casein, non-fat dry milk, milk solids, lactose, hydrolysed protein, lactoglobulin, lactalbumin, caseinate and soy flour. Organ meats must be avoided because they are a storage site for galactose.

Given the poor outcome even amongst those patients that are compliant with the traditional diet, it has been suggested that additional sources of galactose, more-recently discovered, may be resulting in a chronic galactose intake. These foods include several fruits, vegetables, legumes, nuts and cereals (Acosta & Gross 1995).

The effect of dietary restriction can be monitored by measuring the post-prandial erythrocyte GAL-1-P concentration or filter paper whole blood samples. A well-treated patient should maintain levels < 3.0 mg/dl (Wenz 1993).

Glycogen storage disease

At least 12 different types of glycogen storage diseases (GSD) have been identified. Abnormalities of the biochemical pathways involved in glycogenolysis and glycogen synthesis result in deposition of excess glycogen, abnormal structure of the compound, or both. The liver and muscle are the major sites of glycogen deposition. Common signs and symptoms include hypoglycaemia, hepatomegaly, muscle weakness and cramping and fatigue. This section focuses on the type of GSD that respond to nutritional therapy.

GSD Ia (von Gierke's disease)

GSD Ia results from a deficiency of glucose-6-phosphatase, the last enzyme in the pathways involved in the production of glucose from either gluconeogenesis or glycogenolysis. GSD Ib, a clinical variant of Ia, results from a defect in the glucose-6-phosphate transport protein and responds to the same nutritional intervention as does Ia. Biochemical abnormalities seen in GSD I include lactic acidaemia, hypoglycaemia, hyperlipidaemia and hyperuricaemia.

DIETARY MANAGEMENT FOR GSD I. Because endogenous glucose production is limited, a constant source of exogenous glucose is necessary to maintain a normal plasma glucose concentration and prevent hypoglycaemia. Historically, treatment for hypoglycaemia included portacaval shunts and total parenteral nutrition (Folkman et al 1972) or continuous enteral tube feedings (Burr et al 1974, Greene et al 1980). More recently, uncooked cornstarch (UCS) (Chen et al 1984, Chen et al 1993) has been widely used to provide a source of continuous glucose. UCS is effective in maintaining normoglycaemia and improving metabolic abnormalities (Wolfsdorf et al 1990b) and growth retardation (Wolfsdorf et al 1990c). Side effects may include diarrhoea and flatulence until acclimated to the cornstarch and excessive weight gain (Chen et al 1993). Continuous nocturnal tube feedings of glucose and intermittent doses of UCS are the two dietary manipulations most commonly used to manage GSD I.

The UCS doses are calculated using 1.75–2.5 g/kg body weight per dose (Chen et al 1984) or by calculating estimated glucose production rate using the following equation (Wolfsdorf & Crigler 1994): $y = 0.0014(x^3) - 0.214(x^2) + 10.411(x) 9.084$ where y = mg glucose/minute and x = body weight in kg.

UCS is mixed in cool water or other sugar-free flavoured fluid for oral consumption (Chen et al 1984). Doses are given at 3–5 h intervals during the day and 4–5 h intervals at night (Wolfsdorf & Crigler 1994); after puberty, large doses at bedtime, designed to prevent hypoglycaemia for at least 7 h may be attempted. The dose and schedule may be adjusted according to blood glucose monitoring results (Wolfsdorf & Crigler 1997).

Infants should be fed every 2–4 h with a glucose-containing formula. Tube feedings of the same formula are often necessary, later in infancy, to ensure normoglycaemia, particularly at night (Fernandes et al 1988, Wolfsdorf et al 1990a). Introduction to UCS may be attempted at approximately 8 months of age. Gradual introduction to UCS is recommended to induce enzyme activity (for example 1 teaspoon per feeding), because pancreatic amylase activity may be insufficient to digest necessary cornstarch dosages (Wolfsdorf et al 1990a).

Alternatively, nocturnal nasogastric or gastrostomy feedings may be used to provide adequate glucose during an overnight fast combined with frequent daytime oral feedings (Greene et al 1976, Greene et al 1980). The formula should contain the minimun dose of glucose necessary to maintain blood glucose levels

Table 34.6 — Dietary therapies for other types of glycogen storage diseases

Type[a]	Affected enzyme	Dietary therapy	Reference
IV	Brancher enzyme	Frequent meals, UCS or tube feedings[b]	Greene et al 1988
VI	Liver phosphorylase	High carbohydrate, frequent feedings[c]	Scriver et al 1995
IX	Phosphorylase kinase	Night-time snack[d]	Wolfsdorf

[a]No nutritional therapies are either known or indicated for glycogen storage disease types II, V, VII or X.
[b]Liver transplant is the only present effective treatment. Dietary therapy is indicated to prevent hypoglycaemia and to improve growth and muscle strength prior to transplant.
[c]Treatment is indicated only if symptomatic with hypoglycaemia.
[d]In rare cases of hypoglycaemia, a night-time snack is indicated to prevent hypoglycaemia.

$\geq$ 70 mg/dl. Although proven effective, tube feedings also pose significant risk of hypoglycaemia in the case of pump malfunction or other case of interrupted feeding (Leonard & Dunger 1978). Patients should eat immediately after the overnight feeding has been discontinued.

The diet usually contains 60–70% of calories as carbohydrate (the majority of which is complex), 20% as fat, and the remainder as protein. Because patients are unable to metabolize either galactose or fructose the diet should be limited in dairy products, fruits and simple carbohydrates. However universal agreement on the degree of limitation has not been reached (Goldberg & Slonim 1993). Dietary restrictions are likely to necessitate the use of multivitamins and calcium supplements.

GSD III (Debrancher deficiency; Limit dextrinosis; Cori or Forbes disease)

Patients with *GSD III* are able to degrade glycogen only partially due to a deficiency of amylo-1, 6-glucosidase enzyme activity. This enzymatic deficiency results in the accumulation of abnormal glycogen in the liver. Unlike GSD I, these patients are able to synthesize glucose via gluconeogenesis. The clinical characteristics are similar to GSD I with distinguishing features including fasting ketosis, less significant hypoglycaemia and hyperlipidaemia and absence of lactic acidaemia and hyperuricaemia.

DIETARY MANAGEMENT FOR GSD III. Frequent daytime meals and snacks are recommended to maintain normoglycaemia. As in GSD I, either UCS (Gremse et al 1990) or nocturnal tube feedings (Borowitz & Greene 1987) is recommended to prevent hypoglycaemia during the night.

A high-protein diet to provide increased substrate for gluconeogenesis has been advocated to help reverse myopathy and prevent growth retardation. A diet consisting of 20–25% protein with approximately one-quarter to one-third given as a high-protein nocturnal tube feeding reversed myopathy in GSD III patients with severe muscle wasting disease (Slonim et al 1984). Dietary therapies for other types of glycogen storage diseases are outlined in Table 34.6.

Discussion

The treatment of many inborn errors of metabolism is often nutritional, involving alterations in protein, carbohydrate, fat or energy intake. Dietary manipulations should be undertaken with a physician who is familiar with the disorders and an experienced dietician. The goal should be not only to prevent adverse outcomes but also to assist families and patients to incorporate their special diets into a lifestyle that is as normal and as healthy as possible.

References

Acosta, P.B., Gross, K.C. (1995) Hidden sources of galactose in the environment. *Eur J Pediatr*, 154(suppl 2), S87–S92.

Acosta, P.B., Yanicelli, S. (1997) *The Toss Metabolic Formula System Nutrition Support Protocols*, 3rd edn. Columbus: Toss Products Division/Abbott Laboratories.

Andria, G., Sebastio, G. (1996) *Inborn Metabolic Diseases — Diagnosis And Treatment*. Berlin: Springer.

Batshaw, M.L. (1994) Inborn errors of urea synthesis. *Annals of Neurol*, 35, 133–141.

Berry, G.T. et al. (1991) Branched-chain amino acid-free parenteral nutrition in the treatment of acute metabolic decompensation in patients with maple syrup urine disease. *NEJM*, 324, 175–179.

Berry, G.T. et al. (1995) Endogenous synthesis of galactose in normal men and patients with hereditary galactosaemia. *Lancet*, 346, 1073–1074.

Bickel, H. et al. (1953) The influence of phenylalanine intake on the chemistry and behavior of a phenylketonuric child. *Lancet*, 2, 812–813.

Borowitz, S.M., Greene, H.L. (1987) Cornstarch therapy in a patient with type III glycogen storage disease. *J Pediatr Gastroenterol Nutr*, 6, 631–634.

Brackett, J.C. et al. (1994) A novel mutation in medium chain acyl-CoA dehydrogenase causes sudden neonatal death. *J Clin Invest*, 94, 1477–1483.

Brusilow, S.W. et al. (1979) New pathways of nitrogen excretion in inborn errors of urea synthesis. *Lancet*, 2, 452–454.

Brusilow, S.W., Maestri, N.E. (1996) Urea cycle disorders: diagnosis, pathophysiology, and therapy. *Adv Ped*, 43, 127–170.

Burr, I.M., O'Neill, J.A., Karzon, D.T., Howard, L.J., Greene, H.L. (1974) Comparison of the effects of total parenteral nutrition, continuous intragastric feeding, and portacaval shunt on a patient with type I glycogen storage disease. *J Pediatr*, 85, 792–795.

Chen, Y.T., Bazzarre, C.H., Lee, M.M., Sidbury, J.B., Coleman, R.A. (1993) Type I glycogen storage disease: Nine years of management with cornstarch. *Eur J Pediatr*, 152(suppl 1), S56–S59.

Chen, Y.T., Cornblath, M., Sidbury, J.B. (1984) Cornstarch therapy in type I glycogen-storage disease. *N Engl J Med*, 310, 171–175.

Chuang, D.T., Shih, V.E. (1995) Disorders of Branchid Chain in Amino Acid and Keto Acid Metabolism. In: Scriver, C.R., Beaudet, A.L., Slyws Valle, D. (eds) The metabolic and Molecular Bases of Inherited Disease, 7th edn. New York: McGraw-Hill. Ch 34, 1239–1278.

Cockburn, F. et al. (1993) Recommendation on the dietary management of phenylketonuria—Report of Medical Research Council Working Party on Phenylketonuria. *Arch Dis Child*, 68, 426–427.

Dionisi Vici, C. et al. (1991) Progressive neuropathy and recurrent myoglobinuria in a child with a long-chain 3-hydroxyacyl-coenzyme A dehydrogenase deficiency. *J Ped*, 118, 744–746.

Duran, M., Wadman, S.K. (1985) Thiamine-responsive inborn errors of metabolism. *J Inher Metab Dis*, 8(suppl 1), 70–75.

Elsas, L.J. et al. (1993) Galactosemia—A molecular approach to the enigma. *Inter Ped*, 8, 101–109.

Evans, J.M. et al. (1994) *PHE for Three*, 2nd edn. Portland: Oregon Health Sciences University.

Fernandes, J., Leonard, J.V., Moses, S.W., Odievre, M., di Rocco, M., Schaub, J., Smit, G.P.A., Ullrich, K.,

Durand, P. (1988) Glycogen storage disease: Recommendations for treatment. *Eur J Pediatr*, 147, 226–228.

Fishler, K. et al. (1972) Intellectual and personality development in children with galactosemia. *Pediatrics*, 50, 412–419.

Folkman, J., Philippart, A., Tze, W.J., Crigler, J. (1972) Portacaval shunt for glycogen storage disease: Value of prolonged intravenous hyperalimentation before surgery. *Surgery*, 72, 306–314.

Goldberg, T., Slonim, A.E. (1993) Nutrition therapy for hepatic glycogen storage diseases. *J Am Diet Assoc*, 93, 1423–1430.

Gremse, D.A., Bucuralas, J.C., Batistreri, W.F. (1990) Efficacy of cornstarch therapy in type III glyeogen storage disease. *Am J Clin Nutr*, 52, 671–674.

Greene, H.L., Ghishan, F.K., Brown, B., McClenathan, D.T., Freese, D. (1988) Hypoglycemia in type IV glycogenosis: Hepatic improvement in two patients with nutritional management. *J Pediatr*, 112, 55–58.

Greene, H.L., Slonim, A.E., Burr, I.M., Moran, J.R. (1980) Type I glycogen storage disease: Five years of management with nocturnal intragastric feeding. *J Pediatr*, 96, 590–595.

Greene, H.L., Slonim, A.E., O'Neill, J.A., Burr, I.M. (1976) Continuous nocturnal intragastric feeding for management of type I glycogen-storage disease. *N Engl J Med*, 294, 423–425.

Hackney, I.M. et al. (1968) Phenylketonuria: Mental development, behavior, and termination of low phenylalanine diet. *Pediatrics*, 72, 646–655.

Hale, D.E. et al. (1992) Fatty acid oxidation disorders: a new class of metabolic diseases. *J Ped*, 121, 1–11.

Hillman, R.E. et al. (1973) Inhibition of glycine oxidation in cultured fibroblasts by isoleucine. *Pediat Res*, 7, 945–947.

Kaufman, F.R. et al. (1981) Hypergonadotropic hypogonadism in female patients with galactosemia. *NEJM*, 304, 994–998.

Kaufman, S. (1986) Unsolved problems in diagnosis and therapy of hyperphenylalaninemia caused by defects in tetrahydrobiopterin metabolism. *J Pediatr*, 109, 572–578.

Koch, R. et al. (1987) The effect of diet discontinuation in children with phenylketonuria. *Eur J Pediatr*, 146(suppl 1), A12–A16.

Komrower, G.M. (1982) Galactosaemia—thirty years on the experience of a generation. *J Inher Metab Dis*, 5(suppl 2), 96–104.

Kvittingen, E.A. (1986) Hereditary tyrosinemia type I: An overview. *Scand J Clin Lab Invest*, 46(suppl 184), 27–34.

Leonard, J.V., Dunger, D.B. (1978) Hypoglycaemia complicating feeding regimens for glycogen-storage disease. *Lancet*, 2, 1203–1204.

Linstedt, S. et al. (1992) Treatment of hereditary tyrosinaemia type 1 by inhibition of 4-hydroxyphenylpyruvate dioxygenase. *Lancet*, 340, 813–817.

Maestri, N.E. et al. (1991) Prospective treatment of urea cycle disorders. *J Pediatr*, 119, 923–928.

Mitchell, G.A., Lambert, M., Tanguay, R.M. (1995) Hypertyrosinemia. In: Scriver, C.R., Beaudet, A.L., Sly, W.S., Valle, D. (eds) The metabolic and molecular Bases of Inherited Disease, 7th ed. New York: McGraw-Hill, 28, 1077–1106.

Ney, D. et al. (1983) Dietary management of oculocutaneous tyrosinemia in an 11-year-old child. *Amer J Dis Child*, 137, 995–1000.

Petrowski, S. et al. (1987) Pharmacologic amino acid acylation in the acute hyperammonemia of propionic acidemia. *J Neurogen*, 4, 87–96.

Potocnik, U., Widhalm, K. (1994) Long-term follow-up of children with classical phenylketonuria after diet discontinuation: A review. *J Amer Col Nutr*, 13, 232–236.

Roe, C.R., Coates, P.M. (1995) Mitoihandrial Fatty Acid Oxidation Disorders. In: Scriver, C.R., Beaudet, A.L., Slyws Valle, D. (eds) The Metabolic and Molecular Bases of Inherited Disease, 7th ed. New York: McGraw-Hill. Ch 45, 1501–1534.

Rohr, F. et al. (1985) Inborn Errors of Metabolism. In: Walker, W.A., Watkins, J.B. (eds.) *Nutrition in Pediatrics*. Boston: Little, Brown and Company.

Schuett, V.E. (1995) *Low Protein Food List for PKU*. Burnaby: Hemlock Printers Ltd.

Seashore, M.R. et al. (1972) Studies of the mechanism of pyridoxine-responsive homocystinuria. *Pediat Res*, 6, 187–196.

Slonim, A.E., Coleman, R.A., Moses, W.S. (1984) Myopathy and growth failure in debrancher enzyme deficiency: Improvement with high-protein nocturnal enteral therapy. *J Pediatr*, 105, 906–911.

Trahms, C.M. (1992) Nutritional Care And Metabolic Disorders. In: Mahan, L.K., Arlin, M. (eds.) *Krause's Food, Nutrition and Diet Therapy*, 8th edn. Philadelphia: WB Saunders Ch 41, 699–716.

Treem, W.R. (1994) Inherited and acquired syndromes of hyperammonemia and encephalopathy in children. *Sem Liv Dis*, 14, 236–257.

Tyni, T. et al. (1995) Long-chain 3-hydroxyacyl-coenzyme A dehydrogenase deficiency with the G1528C mutation—Clinical presentation of thirteen patients. *J Pediatr*, 130, 67–76.

Wenz, E. (1993) *Pediatric Nutrition in Chronic Diseases and Developmental Disorders*. New York: Oxford University Press.

Wolfsdorf, J.I., Crigler, J.F. (1994) Glycogen Storage Diseases. In: Lavin, N. (ed.) *Manual of Endocrinology And Metabolism* 37, pp. 505–516, 2nd edn. Boston: Little, Brown and Company.

Wolfsdorf, J.I., Crigler, J.F. (1997) Cornstarch regimens for nocturnal treatment of young adults with type I glycogen storage disease. *Am J Clin Nutr*, 65, 1507–1511.

Wolfsdorf, J.I., Keller, R.J., Landy, H., Crigler, J.F. (1990) Glucose therapy for glycogenosis type I infants: Comparison of intermittent uncooked cornstarch and continuous overnight glucose feedings. *J Pediatr*, 117, 384–391.

Wolfsdorf, J.I., Plotkin, R.A., Laffel, L.M.B., Crigler, J.F. (1990a) Continuous glucose for treatment of patients with type I glycogen-storage disease: Comparison of the effects of dextrose and uncooked cornstarch on biochemical variables. *Am J Clin Nutr*, 52, 1943–1950.

Wolfsdorf, J.I., Rudlin, C.R., Crigler, J.F. (1990b) Physical growth and development of children with type I glycogen-storage disease: Comparison of the effects of long-term use of dextrose and uncooked cornstarch. *Am J Clin Nutr*, 52, 1051–1057.

35

Childhood obesity: Diagnosis, incidence and strategy for change

Ruth M. Ayling

Introduction

Energy stored within the body is the difference between energy intake and energy expended. *Obesity* is the metabolic abnormality that results when excess energy has been accumulated as fat. It is one of the most prevalent diseases in Western society.

Historical background

Definition

Clinically, the diagnosis of obesity is usually made by observation, but there are, as yet, no firmly-established criteria for the definition of obesity in childhood. In adults the most commonly-used measurement is the *Body Mass Index* (BMI), originally used by Quetelet (1835). This is obtained by dividing the weight (kg) by the square of the height (m^2). Using this index, a normal weight-for-height in adults has been proposed as a BMI of 20–24.9, grade 1 obesity as 25–29.9, grade 2 as 30–40 and grade 3 as > 40 (Garrow 1981). In children, BMI is defined as greater than the eighty-fifth centile of age and corresponds to 120% of ideal body weight, equivalent to a BMI of 30 in adults. BMI is more difficult to use in children as the norms change with age and gender. For example the eighty-fifth centile for boys is > 23 at age 12–14 years and > 24.3 at age 15–17 years. For girls, the corresponding figures are 23.4 and 24.8 (Harlan 1993). Populations with different adult heights do tend to have similar BMI by early adulthood (Rolland-Cachera 1993). However, BMI does not measure fatness directly and makes no allowances for variation in framesize—it cannot distinguish the 'overweight' from the 'overfat'. Skin-fold measurements using special callipers have been used to assess obesity in children, having good correlation with estimation of body fat from accurate techniques such as underwater weighing (Harsha et al 1978). Four sites can be used—triceps, subscapular, biceps and suprascapular skin folds (Durnin & Wormersley 1974). The triceps skin fold is measured at a point that is equidistant from the tip of the acromion and the olecranon and that correlates best with *percentage* body fat. The subscapular skin fold, measured just below the tip of the inferior angle of the scapular, correlates best with total body fat.

Measurements of body-fat distribution in adults have shown a correlation between the abdominal distribution of adipose tissue and risk for type 2 diabetes mellitus and for cardiovascular disease. However, the female-type gluteofemoral-fat distribution is less closely associated (Bjorntorp 1992, Van der Kooy & Siedell 1993). The waist:hip ratio (WHR) is a useful measurement for obtaining information on body-fat distribution in adults, but until sexual maturity gluteofemoral-fat distribution is not fully developed, especially in females. Hence, use of WHR has not been shown to be strongly associated with other measures and outcomes of obesity in children. A large number of techniques exist for assessing body composition, for example isotope dilution, electrical impedance and total body electrical conductivity. These may prove increasingly useful for clinical use as well as for research purposes.

Incidence

With no absolute diagnostic criteria it is hard to estimate the prevalence of obesity. In addition, many of those affected do not see obesity as a medical problem and therefore do not present to seek help. Current UK data is hard to obtain. The US National Health and Nutrition Examination Survey (NHANES III 1990) reported that 34% of the US adult population, 65–75 million people, were obese. This was an increase from 25% during the previous 10 years. In children, 22% of the paediatric population aged 6–19 years were found to have a BMI > the eighty-fifth centile, an increase from 15% 10 years before. The prevalence of 'super-obesity' (i.e., those above the ninety-fifth centile) had increased even more rapidly. Such detailed UK data is hard to find. A prevalence rate for obesity of 1.5 (USA versus UK) has been found in adults (Van Itallie 1996), suggesting the problem may be of a smaller magnitude in the United Kingdom at the present time.

A major concern is that obese children will become obese adults. Childhood obesity results in almost one-third of adult obesity, and adults who were obese as children are more likely to have severe obesity (Dietz 1994). A 22-year review found that 26–41% of obese pre-school children became obese adults, and 42–62% of obese school-age children became obese adults (Serdula et al 1993). Therefore in many cases, obesity is a chronic disease.

Family and social variables are important in the aetiology of obesity, for example larger families tend to have a lower prevalence of obesity and older parents tend to have fatter children (Dietz 1993). Parental neglect has been shown to predict a risk of obesity in young adulthood, independent of the child's age, BMI in childhood, gender and social background (Hellmich 1992). Socio-economic class has a relation to obesity whilst race is a complicated variable due to overlap with socio-economic group. Dietary and lifestyle patterns are initiated in childhood, and dietary-fat intake and a sedentary lifestyle are correlated with increased cholesterol, obesity and hypertension in children (Cunnane 1993). The composition of the diet itself may be a factor in obesity. The fat intake may be linked to obesity even when total energy intake is not increased (Gutin & Manos 1993). Children who consume diets higher in total saturated and monounsaturated fats have been shown to have greater body fatness (Gazzaniga & Burns 1993). Other lifestyle factors include the amount and type of exercise taken. Obesity in childhood is directly related to the hours of television watched per day (Dietz & Gortmaker 1985). This is not only due to the decreased time spent engaged in physical activity whilst watching but also due to the increased opportunity for snacking. As well, television commercials prompt consumption of foods with high-calorie content (Dietz 1991).

Studies of families show that if both parents are obese more than two-thirds of their children will be obese; if only one parent is obese the risk of obesity in their children is about one-third; if neither parent is obese the risk is about 10%. Twin studies have shown a greater discordance in the weight of non-twin sibling pairs and fraternal twins than identical twins, even when raised in different households (Borjeson 1976, Stunkard et al 1986). These studies suggest that both genetic and environmental factors may be involved in the aetiology of obesity.

The *ob* gene was the first rodent gene for obesity to be discovered (Zhang et al 1994), its product being named leptin from the Greek word for thin. Leptin is a hormone produced in adipocytes. It is thought to act via receptors in the hypothalamus, to inhibit food intake and to increase energy expenditure. In strains of *ob/ob* obese mice, there are mutations in the *ob* gene that abolish leptin synthesis. Administration of leptin to these mice led to weight loss (Weigle et al 1995). Leptin was also able to cause weight loss in lean and over-fed normal mice (Campfield et al 1995). Leptin deficiency has now been described, most recently in children due to mutation in the *ob* gene (Montague

et al 1997). Obesity genes may have offered a survival advantage in the past, for example in times of famine, but now that food sources are abundant their expression results in obesity.

It has been suggested that there are certain critical periods in childhood during which the development of obesity is associated with an increased risk of persistent obesity and its complications. These have been identified as gestation and early infancy, around the age of 5–7 years and during adolescence. Studies of 19-year-old men who had been exposed to famine in the third trimester *in utero* showed the prevalence of obesity was lower than in those exposed in the first two trimesters (Ravelli et al 1976). Studies of infants of diabetic mothers also suggest that the third trimester may be a critical period for the development of obesity (Pettit et al 1983). Long-term follow-up studies have now shown associations between low birth weight and increased risk of hypertension, impaired glucose tolerance, diabetes mellitus and cardiovascular disease in adulthood (Barker et al 1989, Barker et al 1990, Hales et al 1991). Thus, the morbidity usually associated with obesity may be dissociated from the effects of pre-natal nutritional over-exposure.

BMI increases in the first year of life, decreases and then increases at about 5 years of age. This is known as 'the period of adiposity rebound'. Children whose adiposity rebound began early were found to have greater BMI and skin-fold thickness in adolescence and adult life than those in whom it was average or late (Rolland-Cachera et al 1984, Rolland-Cachera 1987). The third critical period is adolescence, the effect at this time being greater in females (Dietz 1994).

The majority of children with simple obesity have associated tall stature, advanced bone age and may have early onset of puberty. Children who have an underlying endocrine cause for their obesity tend to have short stature accompanied by delay in bone age and puberty. Endocrine disorders may result in obesity. In growth hormone deficiency and Cushing's syndrome, obesity tends to be of a centripetal distribution. The polycystic ovary syndrome manifests in the post-pubertal period and is associated with obesity, mild androgen excess, increased ratio of leutinizing:follicle stimulating hormone, and hyper-insulinism. Obesity can also be associated with abnormalities of the hypothalamic region, often secondary to hyperphagia and with a number of rare syndromes. Disorders rarely found to be the cause of obesity are shown in Table 35.1, they account for < 1% of clinical cases in children.

Table 35.1 — Rare associations of obesity in childhood

Endocrine
- Hypothyroidism
- Cushing's Syndrome
- Growth hormone deficiency
- Hypopituitarism
- Hypothalamic dysfunction

Dysmorphic syndromes
- Prader-Willi
- Laurence-Moon-Biedl
- Pseudohypoparathyroidism
- Carpenter's

Table 35.2 — Complications of obesity in childhood

Psychological
- Loss of self-esteem
- Depression

Cardiovascular
- Hypertension
- Hyperlipidaemia

Neurological
- Pseudotumour cerebri

Gastrointestinal
- Cholelithiasis
- Hepatic steatosis

Endocrine
- Early puberty
- Hyperinsulinism and insulin resistance

Musculoskeletal
- Slipped capital femoral epiphysis
- Valgus deformities

Dermatological
- Acanthosis nigricans

Practice and procedures

Complications

Psychological disturbances are a common complication of obesity, and it has been estimated that up to 10% of obese children may become clinically depressed (Klish 1998). Other complications in children can involve the cardiovascular, gastrointestinal, musculoskeletal, respiratory, endocrine and nervous systems. Complications of obesity are shown in Table 35.2.

The complications of childhood obesity extend into adult life. A 7-year follow-up of adolescents with a BMI > ninety-fifth centile showed that overweight girls had completed fewer years of school, were less likely to be married and had lower household incomes, after correction for baseline aptitude scores and socio-economic status (Gortmaker et al 1993). There are some long-term follow-up studies of cohorts of obese children. In a 40-year follow-up of obese Swedish children, overall mortality, cardiovascular disease and digestive disease occurred earlier than in a non-obese reference population (Dietz & Robinson 1993). A 55-year follow-up (The Third Harvard Growth Study) showed mortality to be higher in men who were overweight in adolescence compared with lean controls. Morbidity from chronic illness was also increased in those who were obese adolescents (Must et al 1992).

Treatment

The epidemiology of childhood obesity may help to identify a proportion of those at risk of becoming obese. For those at risk, close attention to the rate of weight gain in early life may allow intervention.

Once it has become established, obesity requires treatment, and the goals of this treatment are the achievement and maintenance of weight loss without detrimental effects to health or growth. Before commencing a treatment programme, a child should undergo a medical examination so that rare causes of obesity are not overlooked. The presence of complications should also be sought.

Education is essential for the success of any weight reducing programme and should be provided for the whole family. The education may need to include aspects of parental food preparation strategies and parental obesity (Epstein et al 1994). It should also include a simple explanation of the pathophysiology of obesity and an outline of the objectives of the treatment proposals suggested.

Treatment options for obesity include caloric restriction, exercise, behaviour modification, drug therapy and surgery (Table 35.3), although the last two are not favoured in children. A team approach involving medical, psychology and dietetic staff is useful, and the most successful programmes are those that incorporate diet, exercise and behavioural modification (Keller & Stevens 1996).

Caloric restriction

Only a small daily caloric excess can lead to obesity.

Table 35.3 — Treatment of obesity in childhood

Education
Caloric restriction
    Moderate reduction
    Very restrictive

Exercise
    To increase activity as part of lifestyle change

Behavioural modification
    Self monitoring
    Contingency training
    Positive reinforcement
    Cognitive restructuring

Drug treatment
    Not recommended

Surgery
    Not recommended

For example as little as 40 kcal/day can result in a gain of over 2 kg over one year. It has long been suggested from energy balance studies that obese children do not appear to have a greater caloric intake than lean children (Johnson et al 1956, Hampton et al 1967). However, this work assessed energy intake using weighed records, which are known to be subject to inaccuracies. Indirect calorimetry and studies of energy expenditure were then performed with conflicting results (Griffiths et al 1990, Fontvieille 1992), so there are as yet no convincing data to suggest that low energy expenditure is a major cause of obesity. The majority of obese children therefore require a diet, or 'eating plan', that is deficient in only a moderate amount of energy. This can then be used as the foundation upon which new eating patterns are laid. Very restrictive diets should be used for the treatment of extremely-obese adolescents or for children or adolescents with serious complications of obesity such as pseudotumour cerebri or sleep apnoea. A virtually carbohydrate free, very-high protein (~2 g/kg/day ideal body weight) diet can be used. Vegetables should be freely available and multivitamins and mineral supplements are required. Potassium supplements may need to be given. Diets of this type should be very carefully monitored as serious side effects include cardiac arrythmias, orthostatic hypotension, protracted nitrogen loss, impaired growth and gallstones (Dietz & Schoeller 1982).

Exercise

The effect of exercise on weight reducing programmes has been known for a long time (Christakis et al 1966,

Seltzer & Mayer 1970). Ideally, to maximize weight loss, the exercise should be aerobic and of moderate intensity, but the incorporation of lesser degrees of exercise as part of a lifestyle change may be a more important benefit by helping to maintain any weight loss achieved. Exercise also tends to have a beneficial effect on unfavourable lipoproteins in obese children. In 10 obese adolescents after an exercise programme, triceps skin folds decreased by 25% and total cholesterol, low-density lipoproteins and triglycerides decreased by 14%, 13% and 33% respectively (Jacogson 1993).

Behavioural modification

This can be a useful component of a weight loss programme. Effective techniques include self-monitoring, contingency training, positive reinforcement and cognitive re-structuring. It is known that obese and non-obese children tend to underestimate caloric intake (Bandini et al 1990), but the degree of under-reporting is greater in obese children. Self-monitoring is best achieved by the use of a food diary, recording not only what was eaten but also the circumstances in which it was consumed. Contingency training then helps the family to identify 'danger times' and to plan strategies to try to avoid food intake. Positive reinforcement should be frequent throughout the programme, and cognitive re-structuring aims to change negative attitudes to positive ones and build self-esteem. Some children may benefit from participating in a support group. Commercial programmes used by adults are generally not aimed at children and they lack a behavioural component. School-based programmes have been used successfully in some areas (Resnicow 1993).

Drug treatment

The use of drugs in the treatment of obesity is not generally recommended, particularly in children. Experience with the available agents has been acquired principally in adults. Amphetamine-based drugs are rarely prescribed, and dexfenfluramine hydrochloride (Adifax) and fenfluramine hydrochloride (Ponderax), which are serotonin-based anorexiants, have now been withdrawn due to an association with cardiac valvulopathy (Bowen et al 1997). Sibutramine hydrochloride (a serotonin and norepinephrine re-uptake inhibitor) and Orlistat (a gastrointestinal lipase inhibitor) have recently become available, although neither is advised in children. An injected leptin preparation has been reported to have some effect on lowering body weight in obese volunteers (Amgen Press Release 1997), but the use of leptin in children at present is not an option except in those very few patients with disorders of leptin physiology. There are no studies evaluating the use of drugs without a weight-reducing diet, and on those occasions when pharmacotherapy is considered, it should always be within the framework of lifestyle intervention.

Surgery

Surgical treatments for obesity include jaw-wiring, liposuction, jejuno-ileostomy gastroplasty, and gastric bypass. However, surgery is not recommended in children unless obesity is associated with major complications. Jejuno-ileostomy bypasses part of the small intestine, leading to a degree of malabsorption so that food intake must be curtailed for symptomatic relief. Complications of malabsorption may be severe and the procedure is now virtually obsolete.

In a series of nine children treated with gastric bypass surgery, three with Prader-Willi syndrome and three others regained weight and three maintained near ideal body weight (Deitz 1993). Gastric banding, which can be performed via a laparoscopic technique, has been carried out successfully in children (O'Brien et al 1999). Stereotactic surgery for obesity has been attempted in a very limited capacity (Quaade 1974), but as the necessary skills develop perhaps it could be applied as a treatment for obesity to areas of the brain known to cause aphagia.

Discussion

Obesity should be thought of as a chronic disease. It is an important public health problem with far-reaching adverse effects and its prevalence is increasing. Whilst in a small number of cases there are genetic and metabolic factors pre-disposing to obesity, effort should be focused on fostering a healthy lifestyle from early childhood with due regard to both the quality and quantity of food consumed and the amount of activity undertaken.

References

Amgen press release, Amgen Inc., thousand oaks, CA, USA.

Bandini, L.G., Schoeller, D.A., Cyr, H.N., Dietz, W.H. (1990) Validity of reported energy intake in obese and non-obese adolescents. *Am J Clin Nut*, 52, 421–425.

Barker, D.J.P, Bull, A.R., Osmond, C., Simmonds, S.J. (1990) Fetal and placental size and risk of hypertension in adult life. *Br Med J*, 301, 259–262.

Barker, D.J., Winter, P.D., Osmond, C., Margetts, B.,

Simmonds, S.J. (1989) Weight in infancy and death from ischaemic heart disease. *Lancet*, 2, 577–580.

Bjorntorp, P. (1992) Regional Obesity. In: Bjorntorp, P., Brodoff, B.N. (eds.) *Obesity*. Philadelphia: Lippincott.

Borjeson, M. (1976) The aetiology of obesity in children. A study of 101 twin pairs. *Acta Paediatr Scand*, 65, 279–287.

Bowen, R., Glicklich, A., Khan, M. et al. (1997) Cardiac valvulopathy associated with exposure to fenfluramine or dexfenfluramine: US Department of Health and Human Services Interim Public Health Recommendations. *MMWR Morb Mortal Wkly Rep*, 46, 1061–1066.

Campfield, L.A., Smith, F.J., Guisez, Y., Devos, R., Burn, P. (1995) Recombinant mouse OB protein: Evidence for a peripheral signal linking adiposity and central neural networks. *Science*, 269, 546–549.

Christakis, G., Sajecki, S., Hillman, R.W., Miller, E., Blumenthal, S., Archer, M. (1966) Effect of a combined nutrition education and physical fitness program on the weight of obese high school boys. *Fed Proc*, 25, 15–19.

Cunnane, S.C. (1993) Childhood origins of lifestyles-related risk factors for coronary heart in adulthood. *Nutr Hlth*, 9, 107–115.

Dietz, W. (1991) Factors associated with childhood obesity. *Nutrition*, 7, 290–291.

Dietz, W.H. (1993) Therapeutic stragies in childhood obesity. *Horm Res*, 39(suppl 3), 86–90.

Dietz, W.H. (1994) Critical periods in childhood for the development of obesity. *Am J Clin Nut*, 59, 955–959.

Dietz, W.H., Gortmaker, S.L. (1985) Do we fatten our children at the television set? Obesity and television viewing in children and adolescents. *Pediatrics*, 75, 807–812.

Dietz, W.H., Robinson, T.N. (1993) Assessment and treatment of childhood obesity. *Pediatr Rev*, 14, 337–343.

Dietz, W.H., Schoeller, D.A. (1982) Optimal dietary therapy for obese adolescents: Comparison of protein plus glucose and protein plus fat. *J Pediatr*, 100, 638–644.

Durnin, J.V., Womersley, J. (1974) Body fat assessed from total body density and its estimation from skinfold thickness. *Br J Nutr*, 32, 77–97.

Epstein, L.H., Mckenkie, S.J., Valoski, A., Klein, K.R., Wing, R.R. (1994) Effects of mastery criteria and contingent reinforcement for family-based child weight control. *Addic Behav*, 19, 315.

Fontvieille, A.M., Dwyer, J., Ravussin, E. (1992) Resting metabolic rate and body composition of Pima Indian and Caucasian children. *Int J Obesity Relat Metab Disord*, 16, 535–542.

Garrow, J.S. (1981) Indices of adiposity. *Nutr Abst Rev*, 53, 697–708.

Gazzaniga, J.M., Burns, T.L. (1993) Relationship between diet composition and body fatness with adjustment for resting energy expenditure and physical activity in preadolescent children. *Am J Clin Nutr*, 8, 21–28.

Gortmaker, S.L., Must, A., Perrin, J.M., Sobol, A.M., Dietz, W.H. (1993) Social and economic consequences of overweight in adolescence and young adulthood. *N Eng J Med*, 329, 1008–1012.

Griffiths, M., Payne, P.R., Stunkard, A.J., Rivers, J.P., Cox, M. (1990) Metabolic rate and physical development in children at risk of obesity. *Lancet*, 336, 76–78.

Gutin, B., Manos, T.M. (1993) Physical activity in the prevention of childhood obesity. *Ann Y Acad Sci*, 699, 115–126.

Hales, C.N., Barker, D.J., Clark, P.M., Cox, L.J., Fall, C., Osmond, C., Winter, P.D. (1991) Fetal and infant growth and impaired glucose tolerance at age 64. *Br Med J*, 303, 1019–1022.

Hampton, M.C., Hueneman, R.L., Shapiro, L.R. et al. (1967) Caloric and nutritional intake of teenagers. *J Am Diet Assoc*, 50, 385–396.

Harlan, W.R. (1993) Epidemiology of childhood obesity. A national perspective. *Ann NY Acad Sci*, 699, 1–5.

Harsha, D.W., Frerichs, R.R., Berensen, G.S. (1978) Densitometry and anthropometry of black and white children. *Hum Biol*, 50, 261–280.

Hellmich, N. (1992) Today's kids weigh in heavier. *USA Today*, 25, IL.

Jacobson, M.S., Copperman, N., Haas, T., Shenker, I.R. (1993) Adolescent obesity and cardiovascular risk: A rational approach to management. *Ann NY Acad Sci*, 699, 220–229.

Johnson, M.L., Burke, B.S., Mayer, J. (1956) Relative importance of inactivity and overeating in the energy balance of obese high school girls. *Am J Clin Nutr*, 4, 37–44.

Keller, C., Stevens, K.R. (1996) Assessment, etiology and intervention in obesity in children. *Nurse Practioner*, 21, 31–42.

Klisch, W.J. (1998) Childhood obesity. *Pediatr Rev*, 9, 312–315.

Montague, C.T., Farooqi, I.S., Whitehead, J.P., Soos, M.A., Rau, H., Wareham, N.J., Seweter, C.P., Digby, J.E., Mohammed, S.N., Hurst, J.A., Cheetham, C.H., Earley, A.R., Barnett, A.H., Prins, J.B., O'Rahilly, S. (1997) Congenital leptin deficiency is associated with severe early onset obesity in humans. *Nature*, 387, 903–908.

Must, A., Jacques, P.F., Dallal, G.E., Bajema, C.J., Dietz, W.H. (1992) Long-term morbidity and mortality of overweight adolescents: A follow-up of the Harvard Growth Study of 1922–1935. *N Eng J Med*, 327, 1350–1355.

NHANES 111 National health and nutrition examination survey (1988–1994). Department of health and human services, national centre for health statistics. National Technical Information Service. Springfield VA. USA.

O'Brien, P.E., Brown, W.A., Smith, A., McMurrick, P.J., Stephens, M. (1999) Prospective study of a laparoscopically placed adjustable gastric band in the treatment of morbid obesity. *Br J Surg*, 86, 113–118.

Pettitt, D.J., Baird, H.R., Aleck, K.A., Bennett, P.A., Knowler, W.C. (1983) Excessive obesity in offspring of Pima Indian women with diabetes during pregnancy. *N Eng J Med*, 308, 242–245.

Quaade, F. (1974) Stereotaxy for obesity. *Lancet*, 1, 267.

Quetelet, A. (1835) *Sur l'homme et Le Development de Ses Facultes, Ou Essai de Physique Sociale*. Paris: Bachelier.

Resnicow, K. (1993) School-based obesity prevention: Population versus high risk interventions. *Ann NY Acad Sci*, 699, 154–166.

Rolland-Cachera, M.F. (1993) Body composition during adolescence: Methods, limitations and determinants. *Horm Res*, 39(suppl), 25–40.

Rolland-Cachera, M.F., Deheeger, M., Bellisle, F., Sempe, M., Guilloud-Bataille, M., Patoise, E. (1984) Adiposity rebound in children: A simple indicator for predictor of obesity. *Am J Clin Nut*, 39, 129–135.

Rolland-Cachera, M.F., Deheeger, M., Guilloud-Bataille, M., Avois, P., Patois, E., Sempe, M. (1987) Tracking the development of adiposity from one month of age to adulthood. *Ann Hum Biol*, 14, 219–229.

Seltzer, C.C., Mayer, J. (1970) An effective weight control programme in a public school. *Am J Public Health*, 60, 679–689.

Serdula, M.K., Ivery, D., Coates, R.L., Freedman, D.S., Williamson, D.F., Byers, T. et al. (1993) Do obese children become obese adults? A review of the literature. *Prev Med*, 22, 167–177.

Stunkard, A.J., Sorensen, T.I., Hanis, C., Teasdale, T.W., Chakraborty, R., Schull, W.J., Schulsinger, F. (1986) An adoption study of human obesity. *N Eng J Med*, 314, 193–198.

Van der Kooy, K., Seidell, J.C. (1993) Techniques for the measurement of visceral fat: A practical guide. *Int J Obes Relat Metab Disord*, 17, 187–196.

Van Itallie, T.B. (1996) Prevalence of obesity. *Endocrinol Metab Clin North Am*, 25, 887–905.

Weigle, D.S., Bukowski, T.R., Foster, D.C., Holderman, S., Kramer, J.M., Lasser, G., Lofton-Day, C.E., Prunkard, D.E., Raymond, C., Kuijper, J.L. (1995) Recombinant *ob* protein reduces feeding and body weight in the *ob/ob* mouse. *J Clin Invest*, 96, 2065–2070.

Zhang, Y., Proena, R., Maffei, M., Barone, M., Leopold, L., Freidman, J.M. (1994) Positional cloning of the mouse obese gene and its human homologue. *Nature*, 372, 425–432.

36

Failure to thrive: Home-based interventions

Maura MacPhee

Abbreviations

FTT   Failure to Thrive
NOFTT   Non-organic Failure to Thrive
OFTT   Organic Failure to Thrive

Introduction

Failure to thrive (FTT) typically describes infants and children under the age of 2 years who do not maintain an expected rate of growth over time. In all cases of FTT, there are physiological alterations due to malnutrition or the lack of necessary calories to sustain adequate growth for age and gender (Maggioni & Lifshitz 1995). Specific criteria have evolved to identify infants and children with FTT using standardized growth charts. Accepted criteria, such as weight decreasing by two major growth centiles, emphasize a disproportionate decrease in weight gain compared with height growth. Some infants and children may also manifest decelerated growth for height and head circumference as well as delays in developmental skills (Zenel 1997).

FTT has been categorized as organic, non-organic or mixed aetiology. Fifty percent of all FTT cases are non-organic (NOFTT), 25% are organic (OFTT) and the remaining cases are mixed (Mitchell et al 1980, Homer & Ludwig 1981). Organ-system dysfunction or a major illness are the causes of OFTT. Psychosocial factors such as impaired interactions between the caregiver and child account for NOFTT (Chatoor et al 1984, Lobo et al 1992, MacPhee et al 1994). The aetiology can be ascertained 75% of the time from the history and 25% of the time from the physical examination (Accardo 1982). Laboratory tests rarely contribute to a diagnosis, although they can be helpful when establishing a baseline physiological assessment of the infant's or child's malnourished status (Zenel 1997).

Early identification and intervention are critical for children under the age of 2 years when rapid growth is occurring, particularly maturation of the brain and the central nervous system (Frank & Zeisel 1988). Early malnutrition is related to persistent fine motor and gross motor dysfunctions found in later life (Henry 1992). Studies have also shown that intellectual and emotional problems are common in FTT children (Drotar & Sturm 1988, Drotar & Sturm 1992). There is evidence that early intervention can modify or prevent deleterious outcomes (Hutcheson et al 1997).

The exact prevalence of FTT is not known. In the United States, FTT has accounted for 3–5% of hospital admissions (Berwick 1980), and in outpatient urban and rural settings, FTT has been reported in 10–20% of infants and small children (Mitchell et al 1980, Drotar 1985). In the United Kingdom, one study showed that 5% of children < 5 years of age might have been affected by problems associated with FTT (Hampton 1996).

The focus of this chapter is on assessment techniques for identifying infants and children at risk for FTT and on home-based interventions to manage the most commonly encountered problems associated with FTT. Except in cases where the child is at risk for abuse or where outpatient management has failed, managing these children in the hospital is not efficacious. There are case management guidelines for hospitalized children with FTT (MacPhee & Hoffenberg 1996), but this chapter discusses what can be done in community-based clinics and homes where the environment is more natural to the child and where the caregivers have a greater sense of control (Wright & Talbot 1996).

Although it is important to consider underlying organic problems and to instigate appropriate referrals to paediatric specialists, the majority of FTT cases are primarily due to non-organic reasons such as chaotic home environments, lack of resources, and caregiver and child dynamics that create feeding difficulties. These non-organic issues can be successfully managed in community-based or home-based programmes, and they are best managed via multi-disciplinary team members who can address specific concerns and the needs of the child's family members (Hobbs & Hanks 1996). This chapter, therefore, pertains predominantly to NOFTT management or to mixed aetiology cases where there are non-organic components that can be successfully serviced through a home-based approach.

Historical background on home-based interventions

Research on home-based interventions with FTT children has had mixed outcomes. Haynes et al (1984) devised a 6-month lay home visitor programme for families of FTT children, and compared developmental outcomes over a period of 3 years with outcomes of non-intervention families matched for similar environmental variables. Developmental assessments did not differ between groups. Drotar & Eckerle (1989) found no effects of home visitation between a group of infants with FTT and a control group where the trained home visitors were professionals such as nurses, social workers and psychologists.

Black et al (1995) reported significant, positive cognitive outcomes for infants and toddlers with FTT after an intervention strategy that utilized clinic-based follow-up and a 12-month lay home visitor programme. The researchers also noted wide variability in family characteristics. They postulated that there may be specific risk factors that moderate the effects of home-based interventions.

Some research has shown better intervention results amongst the highest-risk families. For instance, Olds et al (1986) found home-based intervention was only successful amongst first-time mothers who were highest risk (i.e., low income, unmarried, adolescent). Other studies, however, have shown that home-based interventions were more effective amongst families with more resources and for children with less severe symptomatology (Jessop & Stein 1991).

There have been attempts to classify risk factors in order to determine what types of families and children would benefit most from home-based intervention (Sameroff et al 1993). Sameroff et al (1993) developed a cumulative risk score that combines demographic and psychological components. More recently, Hutcheson et al (1997) separated maternal negativity factors (i.e., depression, hostility, anxiety) from demographic risk factors to determine their moderating effects on home-based intervention for FTT children. In their study, all the families attended a multi-disciplinary growth clinic; half the families received 1-h weekly visits from lay home visitors that lasted for a year. The home-based intervention effectively reduced the amount of cognitive decline in children whose mothers had lower levels of depression, anxiety and hostility. The researchers concluded that interventions may be most effective for families 'who are neither desperately chaotic and unable to cope with the challenges of a child with a chronic health problem, nor those who are highly competent and may not need the intervention' (Hutcheson et al 1997, p. 663). The researchers also found 'sleeper effects'. Significant effects occurred 1 year post-intervention. Other research has shown that intervention strategies may not appear until later (Achenbach et al 1993), and predictive factors may shift as children develop and mature. For instance, Drotar & Sturm (1989) found

that infant nutritional status lost its value as a predictor of cognitive outcomes and that family and child variables became more important over time.

In the United Kingdom, The Children's Society has been working with FTT children under 3 years of age. A multi-disciplinary team works with families in their homes to address children's specific feeding difficulties. Interventions are described as 'modifying maternal behaviour and responses during the act of feeding by counselling, modelling, and carefully structured feeding situations' (Hampton 1996, p. 263). Two-thirds of 108 children satisfactorily gained weight, and 93% of the caregiver participants described their relationship with project professionals as good or excellent.

There are many maternal, child and environmental risk factors that can influence the physical, cognitive and emotional outcomes of infants and small children with FTT. Despite the need for more research to determine which risk factors most predict and affect outcomes for children with FTT, experience has shown that certain assessment techniques and interventions are effective in home-based settings. These specific techniques and interventions are addressed in the following section.

Practice and procedures

Assessment

Table 36.1 provides a summary of the key procedures to be included in the assessment of an infant or child with FTT.

Physical examination and growth measurements

Growth measures

Referrals for FTT evaluation are usually based on deficient weight gain or decline. It is critical to use standardized approaches to obtain infants' growth measurements, and to plot these data on standardized growth curves. Schwartz & Abegglen (1996) provide a detailed overview of growth measures. Although FTT can arise in older infants and toddlers, it should be detected as early as possible to prevent developmental problems. Health care providers also have more frequent access to infants during well-baby examinations. For infants, birth weight should be regained by the 2-week visit, and there should be a steady weight gain thereafter of about 30 grams daily. During infancy, failure to gain weight over a 2-month period constitutes FTT (Weston & Berman 1991).

Table 36.1 — Summary of assessments

Physical examination and growth measures

Weight, height, head circumference with well-child examinations—plotted on standardized growth curves with corrections for prematurity. Thorough head-to-toe assessment to detect signs of organic disease, malnutrition, abuse and neglect. Laboratory tests and procedures—minimize.

History taking

'A Typical Day' (See Fig. 36.1).
History of present illness—What the family thinks contributed to the growth failure.
Past medical history—Perinatal and post-natal history from mother's perspective. Obtain history of alcohol, drug, cigarette use after establishing rapport.
Family history—Genogram, and list of family strengths and weaknesses. Social services may be required to address risk factors such as lack of income and transportation.

Nutrition assessment

3-day calorie count—helps determine caregivers' perspective of child's caloric intake.
Feeding assessment—observe caregiver-child feeding dynamics more than once.

Developmental assessment

Screen for motor, cognitive, language, social delays. Refer for any suspicious delays.

A thorough physical examination and history are critical to distinguishing between organic and non-organic FTT. Laboratory tests and procedures may help determine the degree of malnourishment and provide a baseline assessment of the child's physiological status, but expensive laboratory work-ups rarely add to aetiologic determination.

Growth measures need to be corrected for prematurity during the first 2 years of life, and certain growth patterns may be indicative of organic problems, intrauterine growth retardation, familial or genetic inheritance patterns, and changes in growth velocity that are normal—a phenomenon known as 'factitious failure to thrive' (Lifshitz et al 1991). Maggioni & Lifshitz (1995) provide an excellent discussion of growth parameter assessment.

Physical examination

The physical examination should include a thorough head-to-toe assessment. Signs of malnutrition, organic disease or illness, and abuse should be noted. Gahagan & Holmes (1998) provide an examination outline for FTT children, and Zenel (1997) presents an algorithm for detecting underlying organic problems with FTT based primarily on physical assessment and history.

This is also an opportunity to observe the level of activity and the affect of the infant. The caregivers' attentions to the infant provide clues to the quality of caregiver-infant interactions. Schwartz & Abegglen (1996) have constructed a useful table of adaptive and maladaptive infant behaviours for which to watch in FTT situations.

History taking

'A typical day'

It is important to search for physical, psycho-social and environmental risk factors that may distinguish whether the FTT is organic, non-organic or of mixed origin. A thorough history is 'the most important investigative technique in the evaluation' (Gahagan & Holmes 1998, p. 172). An intensive history can be exhaustive and intimidating to caregivers; it is important to establish a rapport with families before focusing on personal issues as well as growth and development issues that may be sensitive topics. Families may get defensive or sense that they have failed as caregivers when their child is not growing. The history-taking process, therefore, has to be broached as a collaborative effort 'to help the child get better'. Figure 36.1 is an example of an 'icebreaker' used by one multi-disciplinary team (The Children's Hospital of Denver). The caregivers are initially asked to fill out a 'typical day' form for the infant or child. This visually displays when the child is sleeping, playing and eating. When parents have a hard time indicating what the child is doing, this also provides information about the potential quality of the relationship. Knowing about the child's typical day from the adults' perspective is valuable information that supports observational data on caregiver-child interactions. This cursory information also helps the health care provider determine how many times the child is fed: this form can initiate a detailed nutritional assessment. What the caregivers choose to share about their infant or child in the centre section of the form is also insightful and can help target a diagnosis. For instance, if the parent is concerned about the infant arching and crying during a feeding, the possibility of an organic component (gastro-oesophageal reflux) needs to be explored.

If there are concerns for the caregivers' literacy level, any questionnaires or informational forms should be done as an interview. It is very important to establish a caring, non-threatening professional-caregiver relationship in order to obtain vital information about

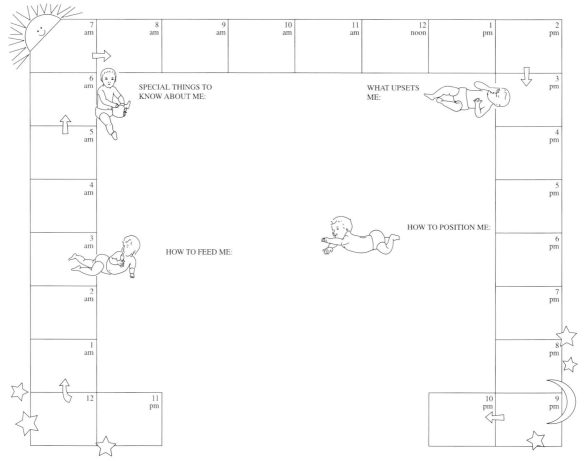

Figure 36.1 — 'Typical day' form. This form should be completed by the primary caregivers of the failure-to-thrive infant or child. It provides an overview to the eating, playing and sleeping behaviours of the child from the caregivers' perspective. It also provides an outline for more focused history taking. Families feel included in the search for 'why the child is not growing'. This form can serve as an icebreaker and the initiation of a collaborative relationship between professionals and family members.

the child and family and to ensure compliance with treatment planning and interventions.

History of present illness

The starting point of the formal history taking should be the caregivers' perception of the present illness or what they think is contributing to the child's poor growth. Some families may deny a problem. In such an instance, it is helpful to show the caregivers the child's growth chart and explain the significance of the child's weight decline. Other families have ready-made explanations for the growth problem, such as 'We're all small people'. It is important to show respect for the families' opinions, and to use the growth curves in an illustrative fashion. Gahagan & Holmes (1998) provide

some other, excellent suggestions for how to proceed with a FTT history.

The past medical history

The past medical history should review the perinatal history, and in addition to gleaning information on potential pregnancy complications, the provider should attend to the mother's affect. Post-partum depression may require more intensive professional support. In addition, the mother's perceptions of the pregnancy and her expectations of motherhood may indicate unrealistic hopes or fears that would benefit from professional education and counselling.

A history of alcohol, drugs and cigarette smoking

should be pursued in a sensitive fashion after rapport has been established. Most parents are willing to share this information when they understand why professionals need such information to diagnose and treat their children. Gahagan & Holmes (1998) give other suggestions for addressing potentially sensitive topics during history taking.

A post-natal history should re-address the caregivers' perceptions of why the infant is not growing. Caregiver perceptions of growth failure should be re-visited throughout the history and examination to detect shifts in stories that may divulge more aetiologic cues. Parents of OFTT children can usually provide detailed accounts of concerning behaviours or signs in their infants. Parents of NOFTT infants tend to provide more diffuse, ambiguous accounts of their infants' behaviour (MacPhee & Hoffenberg 1996).

Family history

Some providers choose to use genograms to map out a family history with notable medical and surgical problems (Gahagan & Holmes 1998). If possible, it is helpful to review the growth curves and development patterns for siblings.

Once a rapport has been established with the caregiver(s), the strengths and weaknesses of the family should be explored. A family-systems approach works best in the presence of multiple risk factors. MacPhee (1995) and Dunst et al (1988) offer concrete examples of how to interview and manage families from a systems perspective.

It is important to note that with NOFTT in particular, dysfunctional and chaotic family environments are often implicated (Hutcheson et al 1997). Some researchers have found high rates of parental patho-psychology with NOFTT children (Duniz et al 1996), and other studies have shown that mothers of NOFTT children often have been abused and have residual emotional and psychological problems (Weston et al 1993). These familial-parental risk factors are some of the most difficult to assess and to manage.

In addition, FTT can occur in any socio-economic setting, but poverty is a significant risk factor for FTT. Depending on the family's circumstances, a social worker can obtain a history of financial status and assist the family with obtaining relevant services. These families may have difficulty problem-solving, but the family should be encouraged to develop their own self-sufficiency skills (Dunst et al 1988).

The nutritional assessment

3-day calorie count

A 3-day diet history can be completed at home by the family, and caloric intake can be calculated by a dietitian. If calorie counts are adequate for growth, an organic aetiology should be investigated more closely. The diary should be closely examined for unusual feeding patterns or 'ideal' feeding patterns (i.e., what the caregiver thinks the provider expects to see) that might indicate NOFTT. Moores (1996) provides a detailed discussion of how this method should be used for home-based interventions.

Feeding assessment

An assessment of the feeding relationship between the child and caregiver(s) provides a mirror to the overall quality of their relationship. Interactional feeding difficulties are common with NOFTT. Arvedson (1997) provides an overview of common FTT feeding disorders, assessment approaches and interventions. From a home-based standpoint, it is important for providers to observe actual feedings in the home under their natural circumstances (i.e., what the child typically eats, where the child typically eats, who typically feeds the child and when feedings typically occur). Feeding observations should be as unobtrusive as possible, and several observations should be completed as part of the FTT evaluation.

Some professionals videotape feedings for later analysis, and to provide feedback to families (Hobbs & Hanks 1996). There are standardized feeding assessment tools (Barnard 1978, Chatoor et al 1989) that require provider training, and there is a standardized screening tool (MacPhee & Schneider 1996) that assists professionals with identifying positive and negative feeding behaviours for infants, toddlers and caregivers. The screening tool is intended to highlight areas to praise and areas to pursue with role modelling, education and other types of support. Because it is fairly concise, it can be completed after an observation, which is less intimidating to the caregivers. If organic problems are suspected, occupational therapists have detailed assessment tools to evaluate oral-motor feeding problems.

Developmental assessment

FTT infants and children are at risk for developmental delays. OFTT children tend to have motor delays, whereas NOFTT children have delays that also encompass cognitive, social and language domains. For home-based and clinic settings, developmental

Table 36.2 — Summary of important home-based interventions

The team approach

Begin with a few, key health care professionals. Add specialists as needed.

Nutritional interventions

Catch-up growth based on a dietitian's individualized dietary plan. Family collaboration is critical to success.

Psycho-social considerations

Support of caregivers—unconditional, positive emotional support is most important. May need assistance with finances, other material resources. Education, coaching, modelling to provide a nurturant environment for child.

Respite care for child when more intensive counselling/therapies are required for caregivers.

A family-systems approach is necessary to guarantee the commitment of the child's primary caregivers. Instrumental support (financial aid, transportation), informational support (education, coaching, modelling), and emotional support are important considerations for families of children with FTT.

---

screening tools such as the Denver II can be used from birth to 6 years of age (Frankenburg 1994). If developmental delays are apparent, children can be referred for more extensive developmental assessment.

Home-based interventions

Table 36.2 includes a summary of home-based interventions that should be considered for infants and children with FTT.

The team approach

Because of the complexity of FTT situations, the multi-disciplinary team approach is recommended (MacPhee et al 1994, Hobbs & Hanks 1996, Wright & Talbot 1996). It is best for a few key team members such as the nurse, the physician, and the dietitian to begin work with the family. Other team members can be utilized as needed. As mentioned by Wright & Talbot (1996), it is important to be the 'least intrusive' as possible, especially when working with families in their own homes.

Nutritional interventions

The dietary plan—'catching up'

The team and family should work together to design a feeding plan that enhances oral intake during the day. The dietitian can create an individualized dietary plan to promote 'catch-up' growth for the FTT child. Pipes & Trahms (1993) provide information on age-specific protein and energy requirements for catch-up growth in FTT infants and children, and Stevenson (1992) gives an excellent review of how to serve and prepare foods for different-aged children who are malnourished. Children with FTT often require supplements of vitamins, iron, and zinc (Frank & Zeisel 1988).

Because the food volume may be overwhelming to a child with FTT, enteral feeding supplements may be necessary. There are many approaches for combining oral and enteral feedings to ensure adequate caloric intake for catch-up growth. One approach for older infants and toddlers is to offer three meals and three snacks throughout the day. If adequate calories are not orally consumed, enteral feedings can be given while the child is sleeping. They should be discontinued within at least 2 hours of the first oral feeding, although more time between enteral-oral feedings is preferred to 'develop an appetite'. When the volume of night-time enteral feedings is too great for the child to manage physiologically, bolus enteral feedings may be done after each oral feeding during the day.

When malnutrition is severe, re-feeding should be slowly advanced. There is always the risk of mal-absorption difficulties with diarrhoea and vomiting. Depending on the severity of the malnutrition and growth declines, several months of accelerated growth may be required before the child re-attains age-appropriate growth parameters, and some chronic FTT children never achieve catch-up growth (Frank & Zeisel 1988).

The mealtime environment

Feeding is a social occasion (Satter 1990), and it is important to socially-model mealtimes. A pleasant, non-distracting environment should be created with other family members eating with the FTT infant or child. Structured meals and snacks are equally important. Some older infants and children are used to 'grazing,' and they eat small quantities of food throughout the day. Insufficient calories are consumed through grazing, and important hunger and satiety cues are depressed by persistent snacking (Satter 1995).

Although the child should not be the focus of a meal (too much attention can be distracting), verbal praise for eating is a strong, positive reinforcement for children. Some parents use reinforcers such as reading books, playing games, or blowing bubbles during meals to encourage their children to take bites of food. Unfortunately, this type of reinforcement actually distracts from the meal and results in less oral intake. The social time with the family and gentle verbal praise should be adequate reinforcers for eating behaviour. In addition, it is important to have structured playtime after meals to help the child clearly distinguish between these two types of social interactions with family members.

Table 36.3 contains a summary of important feeding time 'do's and don'ts'. Satter (1995) describes other developmental considerations for feeding infants and toddlers with FTT. Outpatient regimens that use behavioural approaches are presented by Babbitt et al (1994) and Hampton (1993). Arvedson (1997) summarizes different treatment approaches for FTT feeding disorders.

Psycho-social interventions

There are key caregiver behaviours that promote normal development and normal feeding behaviours in infants and children. These are discussed by Satter (1990) and Greenspan & Lourie (1981). Unfortunately, FTT infants and children often come from dysfunctional family environments where important developmental behaviours are not supported (Hutcheson et al 1997). Drotar (1991) found that these families often have ineffective coping skills. The families' coping strategies must be enhanced, and family

Table 36.3 — Do's and don'ts for meal times

Do's	Don'ts
Feed only at scheduled times. For infants, specify #* ounces of formula every #* hours during the day. For toddlers, provide 3 meals and 2–3 snacks during the day.	Graze or snack. Fill up on water or juices.
Feed at consistent times, same place. Children need consistency and structure to meals. Distractions should be minimized.	Play games, tell stories, sing songs or use toys during meals. Do not leave on the television.
Make meals and snacks a social time, an enjoyable time.	Stare at the child or threaten the child with punishment for not eating. Avoid anxiety.
Encourage normal development. When it is time, older infants and toddler need to learn how to feed themselves. They will make messes—Be prepared!	Let child throw food. When children get tired of eating, they may throw their food. When they indicate the meal is done, say, 'We are done eating.' Let them help with the clean up. Toddlers like to help.
Give the right amount of food and the right kinds of food. For older infants and toddlers, offer solids first and then liquids. *Solids*: Offer 1 Tablespoon of solid food for every year of age. Offer 3 types of solid foods at one time. Use finger foods, and offer favourite, nutritious foods. *Liquids*: Your toddler needs # ounces of milk or high-calorie drinks through the day.	Substitute water or juice for milk. The phyician may allow so many ounces of water or juice per day, and this should be concretely specified in the meal plan.
Allow enough time to eat and enough time to digest food between meals. Allow 30 minutes for meals and 15 minutes for snacks. Some children are slow eaters: allow them a little more time. Permit 2 h between meals/snacks.	Make your child sit at the table until the food is gone. Feeding times should not drag on—this is punishment. Do not give in to them if they come back in 30 minutes and demand food. Let them know that a meal is over. They will have to wait until the next meal/snack for another chance to eat and drink. Be firm but kind about meal rules!

These guidelines will help the infant or child learn how to follow their body's natural hunger and fullness cues in a supportive, social environment. These rules will also help children learn how to eat right and to eat well for the rest of their lives.
* = number of.

problems and concerns must be addressed before FTT situations can be resolved. Needy caregivers therefore often require more care than their infants and children (Patterson & Geber 1991). Health care providers must be prepared to provide material support (i.e., concrete resources, such as financial aid and transportation), informational support (i.e., how to parent effectively), and most importantly, unconditional emotional support (MacPhee et al 1994).

There will be family situations where the caregivers need considerable therapy to function adaptively with their children (Duniz et al 1996). In such situations, nursery care or day care outside the home can provide appropriate developmental stimulation and structured, social feeding times for the children. Hampton (1996) stated, 'Highly-stimulating nursery type provision was helpful in assisting children to achieve some catch-up growth in their developmental milestones' (p. 261).

Discussion

Basic interventions such as teaching basic nurturant techniques, coaching and role modelling (Sullivan 1991) may be sufficient to aid many families with infants and children with FTT. There are however, many more families who will require intensive professional support and community resources. Success or failure often depends on the adequacy of supportive services in the community.

Prevention of FTT is ideal, but because of the multi-factorial nature of FTT, it is hard to know which risk factors most demand early intervention. As stated by Schwartz & Abegglen (1996), 'Anything that facilitates the mother-infant relationship during pregnancy, delivery, and the first few months of infancy may decrease the risk of NOFTT' (p. 32).

Although FTT practitioners often focus on the caregiver-child interactional process (MacPhee et al 1994) or the family system (MacPhee 1995), other models include a broader perspective of other environmental and societal influences that affect children's growth outcomes (Reifsnider 1995). Reducing the numbers of children with growth retardation and other negative sequelae is a key health status objective for the Surgeon General of the United States. This requires policy at national levels. As stated by Kleinman (1991), 'Improving the way we treat children is a first step toward a more just society' (p. 1992).

To ensure healthy outcomes for our children, careful screening and assessment are essential. In the case of FTT, we can effectively screen for growth parameter changes by closely monitoring weight, height and head circumference during the critical first 2 years of life. To screen for interactional difficulties, we can observe the dynamics between caregivers and their children. We know the warning flags of neglect and abuse.

We also know that families and children do better in their own environments. Our attentions, therefore, should be turned to interventions that support families and children in their homes so that they can manage their lives more effectively. Ultimately, the paybacks to society are worth the cost and the effort.

References

Accardo, P. (1982) *Failure to Thrive in Infancy And Early Childhood: A Multi-Disciplinary Team Approach*. Baltimore: University Park Press.

Achenbach, T., Howell, C., Aoki, M., Rauh, V. (1993) Nine-year outcome of the Vermont intervention program for low birthweight infants. *Pediatrics*, 91, 45–55.

Arvedson, J. (1997) Behavioral issues and implications with pediatric feeding disorders. *Sem Speech Lang*, 18, 51–69.

Babbitt, R., Hoch, T., Coe, D., Cataldo, M., Kelly, K., Stackhouse, C., Perman, J. (1994) Behavioral assessment and treatment of pediatric feeding disorders. *J Dev Behav Pediatr*, 15, 278–291.

Barnard, K. (1978) *Nursing Child Assessment Feeding Scales*. Seattle, WA: University of Washington.

Berwick, D. (1980) Nonorganic failure-to-thrive. *Pediatr Review*, 1, 265–270.

Black, M., Dubowitz, H., Hutcheson, J., Berenson-Howard, J., Starr, R. (1995) A randomized clinical trial of home intervention for children with failure to thrive. *Pediatrics*, 95, 807–814.

Chatoor, I., Menvielle, E., Getson, P., O'Donnell, R. (1989) *Observational Scale for Mother-Infant Interaction During Feeding*. Washington, DC: Children's Medical Center.

Chatoor, I., Schaeffer, S., Dickson, L., Egan, J., Conners, K., Leong, N. (1984) Pediatric assessment of nonorganic failure to thrive. *Pediatr Ann*, 13, 844–850.

Drotar, D. (1985) Research and practice in failure to thrive: The state of the art. Zero to Three. *Bull Nat Cent Clin Infant Prog*, 5, 1–4.

Drotar, D. (1991) The family context of nonorganic failure to thrive. *Amer J Orthopsych*, 61, 23–33.

Drotar, D., Eckerle, D. (1989) The family environment in nonorganic failure to thrive: A controlled study. *J Pediatr Psychol*, 14, 245–257.

Drotar, D., Sturm, L. (1988) Prediction of intellectual development in young children with early histories of nonorganic failure to thrive. *J Ped Psychiatr*, 13, 281–296.

Drotar, D., Sturm, L. (1989) Influences of the home environment of preschool children with early histories of nonorganic failure to thrive. *J Dev Behav Pediatr*, 10, 229–235.

Drotar, D., Sturm, L. (1992) Personality development, problem-solving, and behavior problems among preschool children with early histories of nonorganic failure to thrive: A controlled study. *Dev Behav Pediatr*, 13, 266–273.

Duniz, M., Scheer, P., Trojovsky, A., Kaschnitz, W., Kvas, E., Macari, S. (1996) Changes in psychopathology of parents of NOFT infants during treatment. *Eur Child Adoles Psych*, 5, 93–100.

Dunst, C., Trivette, C., Deal, A. (1988) *Enabling And Empowering Families*. Cambridge: Brookline Books.

Frank, D., Zeisel, S. (1988) Failure to thrive. *Pediatr Clin North Am*, 35, 1187–1205.

Frankenburg, W. (1994) Preventing developmental delays: Is developmental screening sufficient? Developmental screening and the Denver II. *Pediatrics*, 93, 586–589.

Gahagan, S., Holmes, R. (1998) A stepwise approach to evaluation of undernutrition and failure to thrive. *Pediatr Clin North Am*, 45, 169–187.

Greenspan, S., Lourie, R. (1981) Developmental structuralist approach to classification of adaptive and pathologic personality organizations: Infancy and early childhood. *Am J Psychiatry*, 138, 725–735.

Hampton, D. (1993) Failure to thrive—tackling feeding problems: A community-based approach. *Health Visitor*, 66, 407–408.

Hampton, D. (1996) Resolving the feeding difficulties associated with nonorganic failure to thrive. *Child: Care, Health and Development*, 22, 261–271.

Haynes, C., Cutler, C., Gray, J., Kempe, R. (1984) Hospitalized cases of failure to thrive: The scope of the problem and short-term lay visitor home intervention. *Child Abuse and Neglect*, 8, 229–242.

Henry, J. (1992) Routine growth monitoring and assessment of growth disorders. *J Pediatr Health Care*, 6, 291–301.

Hobbs, C., Hanks, H. (1996) A multidisciplinary approach for the treatment of children with failure to thrive. *Child: Care, Health and Development*, 22, 273–284.

Homer, C., Ludwig, S. (1981) Categorization of etiology of failure to thrive. *Am J Dis Child*, 135, 848–851.

Hutcheson, J., Black, M., Talley, M., Dubowitz, H.,

Howard, B., Starr, R., Thompson, S. (1997) Risk status and home intervention among children with failure-to-thrive: Follow-up at age 4. *J Pediatr Psychol*, 22, 651–668.

Jessop, D., Stein, R. (1991) Who benefits from a pediatric home care program? *Pediatrics*, 88, 497–505.

Kleinman, L. (1991) Health care in crisis. *J Am Med Assoc*, 265, 1991–1992.

Lifshitz, F., Moses-Finch, N., Ziffer-Lifshitz, J. (1991) *Children's Nutrition*. Boston: Jones & Bartlett.

Lobo, M., Barnard, K., Coombs, J. (1992) Failure to thrive: A parent-infant interaction perspective. *J Pediatr Nurs*, 7, 251–261.

MacPhee, M. (1995) The family systems approach and pediatric nursing care. *Pediatr Nurs*, 21, 417–425.

MacPhee, M., Hoffenberg, E. (1996) Nursing case management for children with failure to thrive. *J Pediatr Health Care*, 10, 63–74.

MacPhee, M., Mori, C., Goldson, E. (1994) Change in the hospital setting: Adopting a team approach for nonorganic failure-to-thrive. *J Pediatr Nurs*, 9, 218–225.

MacPhee, M., Schneider, J. (1996) A clinical tool for nonorganic failure-to-thrive feeding interactions. *J Pediatr Nurs*, 11, 29–39.

Maggioni, A., Lifshitz, F. (1995) Nutritional management of failure to thrive. *Pediatr Clin North Am*, 42, 791–809.

Mitchell, W.G., Gorrell, R.W., Greenberg, R.A. (1980) Failure-to-thrive: A study in a primary care setting. *Pediatrics*, 65, 971–977.

Moores, J. (1996) Non-organic failure to thrive—dietetic practice in a community setting. *Child: Care, Health and Development*, 22, 251–259.

Olds, D., Henderson, C., Chamberlin, R., Tatelbaum, R. (1986) Preventing child abuse and neglect: A randomized trial of nurse intervention. *Pediatrics*, 78, 65–78.

Patterson, J., Geber, G. (1991) Preventing mental health problems in children with chronic illness or disability. *Children's Health Care*, 14, 96–102.

Pipes, P., Trahms, C. (1993) Nutrition: Growth and Development. In: Pipes, P., Trahms, C. (eds.) *Nutrition in Infancy and Childhood*, 1, pp. 1–29, 5th edn. St. Louis: Mosby.

Reifsnider, E. (1995) The use of human ecology and epidemiology in nonorganic failure to thrive. *Pub Health Nurs*, 12, 262–268.

Sameroff, A., Seifer, R., Baldwin, A., Baldwin, C. (1993) Stability of intelligence from preschool to adolescence: The influence of social and family risk factors. *Pediatrics*, 79, 343–350.

Satter, E. (1990) The feeding relationship: Problems and interventions. *J Pediatr*, 117, S181–S189.

Satter, E. (1995) Feeding dynamics: Helping children to eat well. *J Pediatr Health Care*, 9, 178–184.

Schwartz, R., Abegglen, J. (1996) Failure to thrive: An ambulatory approach. *Nurse Practitioner*, 21, 19–35.

Stevenson, M. (1992) Nutritional Care of Slow Growing And Underweight Children. In: Rokusek, C., Heinrichs, E. (eds.) *Nutrition And Feeding for Persons with Special Needs*, 5, pp. 139–152, 2nd edn. Vermillion, SD: University of South Dakota.

Sullivan, B. (1991) Growth-enhancing interventions for nonorganic failure to thrive. *J Pediatr Nurs*, 6, 236–242.

Weston, J., Berman, S. (1991) Failure to Thrive. In: Berman, S.

(eds.) *Pediatric Decision Making*, 14, pp. 396–399, 2nd edn. Philadelphia: Decker.

Weston, J., Colloton, M., Halsey, S., Covington, S., Gilbert, J., Sorrentino-Kelly, L., Renoud, S. (1993) A legacy of violence in nonorganic failure to thrive. *Child Abuse and Neglect*, 17, 709–714.

Wright, C., Talbot, E. (1996) Screening for failure to thrive—what are we looking for? *Child: Care, Health and Development*, 22, 223–234.

Zenel, J.A. (1997) Failure to thrive: A general pediatrician's perspective. *Pediatr Rev*, 18, 371–378.

37

Approaches to breastfeeding: The role of hospitals, professionals and governments in promoting breastfeeding

Cheryl Levitt

Introduction

'Immunization is preventive medicine par excellence. If a new vaccine became available that could prevent a million or more child deaths a year, and that was moreover cheap, safe and administered orally, required no cold chain, it would become an immediate public health imperative. Breastfeeding can do all this and more, but it requires its own 'warm chain' of support—that is, skilled care for mothers to build their confidence and show them what to do, and protection from harmful practices. If this warm chain has been lost from the culture, or is faulty, then it must be made good by health services.' (Editorial 1994)

Breastfeeding is undoubtably the best start for new-born babies and there is abundant evidence for its effectiveness. Unfortunately, many countries in both the developing and developed world have a long way to go to ensure that their babies are breastfed. The World Health Organization (WHO) recommends that all infants should be exclusively breastfed for the first 4–6 months, and weaning should occur in the second year (Innocenti Declaration 1990).

Physicians and other health professionals, their professional organizations, hospitals and governments have an important role to play in protecting, promoting and supporting breastfeeding. This chapter outlines the historical background to breastfeeding deterrents and some advocacy strategies that could be undertaken as a comprehensive public health initiative to improve breastfeeding rates. These approaches are based on international programmes led by the World Health Organization (WHO) and United Nations' Childrens' Fund (UNICEF), evidence found in the medical literature, and experiences reported in the United States and Canada as well as to a lesser extent some other countries.

The advantages of breastfeeding

Human breast milk is the unique and superior form of infant nutrition against which all substitute feeding methods must be measured with regard to growth, health, development and other effects (American Academy of Pediatrics 1997). There is compelling evidence from extensive recent studies that breast-feeding has many advantages and benefits to babies, mothers, families and society. Breastfeeding enhances health; nutrition; immunology; development; psychological, social and economic factors; and the environment.

Epidemiological evidence demonstrates that breast-feeding also decreases the risk of acquiring a number of acute and chronic diseases.

Effect on babies

Breast milk reduces the severity and incidence of otitis media (Kovar et al 1984, Paradise et al 1994), bacteraemia, bacterial meningitis (Takala et al 1989), diarrhoea (Kovar et al 1984, Dewey et al 1995), respiratory infection (Wright et al 1995), botulism (Arnon 1984), urinary tract infection (Piscane et al 1992) and necrotizing enterocolitis (Lucas & Cole 1990).

Human milk may protect against insulin-dependent diabetes mellitus (Gerstein 1994), Crohn's disease, ulcerative colitis (Rigas et al 1993), sudden infant death syndrome (Ford et al 1993), lymphoma (Shu et al 1995), allergies (Saarinen & Kajosaari 1995), and other chronic digestive diseases (Greco et al 1988). Breast milk may enhance childhood cognitive development (Lucas et al 1992).

Effect on mothers

For mothers, breastfeeding promotes uterine involution and reduces post-partum haemorrhaging. It delays menstruation, reduces menstrual blood flow in the first post-partum months (Chua et al 1994) and delays ovulation, thus increasing child spacing (Kennedy & Visness 1992). Recent research demonstrated that lactating women have an earlier return to pre-pregnant weight (Dewey et al 1993), improved bone re-mineralization post-partum (Melton et al 1993), and reduced osteoporotic hip fractures in the post-menopausal period (Cumming & Klineberg 1993). Breastfeeding reduced the risk of ovarian cancer (Rosenblatt & Thomas 1993) and pre-menopausal breast cancer (Newcomb et al 1994).

Effect on society

Society benefits socially and economically from breastfeeding, through improved health outcomes, reduced costs of feeding and reduced employee absenteeism for care attributable to child illness. The 1993 cost of purchasing infant formula for the first year after birth was estimated to be US$855. If maternal caloric intake is taken into account and cost adjustments made, a cost of > US$400 per child can be expected during the first year. (Tuttle & Dewey 1996, American Academy of Pediatrics 1997).

Contraindications of breastfeeding

Although breastfeeding benefits the vast majority of mothers and babies, there are some situations in which it is contraindicated. These include the infant with galactosaemia (Wilson 1990), maternal drug use (American Academy of Pediatrics 1994), and the infant whose mother has untreated active tuberculosis or is infected with the human immunodeficiency virus (HIV) (American Academy of Pediatrics 1995). In 1997, the Joint United Nations (UN) Programme on HIV/AIDS and two of the six co-sponsoring agencies, WHO and UNICEF, issued a joint policy statement on HIV and Infant Feeding (UNAIDS et al 1997) and initiated the development of guidelines. A broad consensus on a public health approach that is based on universally-recognized human rights' standards has been reached. Details of the recent 1999 technical consultation in Geneva can be viewed on the website http://www.unaids.org/highband/document/mother-to-child/index.html.

Historical background

Until the nineteenth century most babies were breast-fed. Health professionals, manufacturers of breast milk substitutes and hospitals have all played a role in influencing breastfeeding practices.

Physicians' role

Physicians began to influence infant feeding practices during the nineteenth and twentieth century in Europe and the United States. Motivated by the desire to help women balance their responsibilities, their influence included separating mothers from their babies at birth, restricting the frequency and duration of breastfeeding, recommending nipple washing, and supplementing artificial feeds before and after breastfeeding. These practices had a deleterious effect on many women's ability to breastfeed. Women turned to artificial alternatives and the commercial baby food industry expanded (Palmer 1993).

The breast-milk substitute industry

The manufacturing of formula has had a major impact on breastfeeding practices. Profit by sales has led these companies to use marketing strategies that target pregnant women and new mothers to influence them to use a breast-milk substitute. Once a substitute has been introduced, breastfeeding ability may be undermined.

The role of hospitals

Hospitals have also played a role in influencing breastfeeding practices. Women initiate breastfeeding immediately after birth and health professionals working in hospitals have a profound influence on their choice of breastfeeding versus supplementation and/or formula feeding. The practices of hospital-based health professionals influence other staff that work in the hospitals and ultimately affect the whole community they serve.

Practice and procedures

Health professionals, hospitals, professional organizations and governments can individually and together alter their practices and procedures to protect, promote and support breastfeeding. Significant advances can occur through initiatives designed to implement the international programmes promoted by WHO and UNICEF. Other initiatives include: 1) improving the knowledge, attitudes and skills of health professionals; 2) undertaking rigorous scientific research to evaluate what aspects of these strategies are most effective; 3) ensuring support from professional organizations; and 4) influencing government to enact protective legislation to support ethical marketing practices and work-place breastfeeding and to provide appropriate resources to ensure the best possible nutritional start for infants.

The International Code

The International Code on Marketing of Breast-Milk Substitutes was devised in 1981 by WHO to protect mothers and health care workers from commercial pressure by manufacturers (World Health Organization 1981) (Table 37.1). It was endorsed by the infant formula manufacturers. It forbids provision of free samples to mothers or health facilities (except for professional research) because of the negative effect that these practices have on breastfeeding (Margen et al 1991). It also forbids inducements to health care workers because recipients are more likely to promote a particular product rather than breastfeeding (Chren & Landefeld 1994).

When the International Code was adopted by the World Health Assembly in 1981 it was recognized that it may require clarification or even revision. Accordingly, resolutions have been adopted every 2 years since 1982. These subsequent resolutions have

Table 37.1 — 10 important provisions of the International Code on Marketing of Breast-Milk Substitutes

1. No advertising of breast-milk substitutes to the public;
2. No free samples of breast-milk substitutes/related products to mothers;
3. No promotion of breast-milk substitutes/related products in health facilities;
4. No company mothercraft nurses to advise mothers;
5. No gifts or personal samples to health care workers;
6. No words or pictures idealizing artificial feeding, including pictures of infants on the labels of the product;
7. Information to health workers must be scientific and factual;
8. All information on artificial feeding, including the labels, should explain the benefits of breastfeeding and the costs and hazards associated with artificial feeding;
9. Unsuitable products, such as sweetened condensed milk, should not be promoted for babies;
10. All breast-milk substitute products should be of a high quality and take into account the climatic and storage conditions of the country where they are used.

Table 37.2 — 10 steps to successful breastfeeding

1. Have a written breastfeeding policy that is routinely communicated to all health care staff;
2. Train all health care staff in skills necessary to implement this policy;
3. Inform all pregnant women about the benefits and management of breastfeeding;
4. Help mothers initiate breastfeeding within half an hour of birth;
5. Show mothers how to breastfeed and how to maintain lactation even if they should be separated from their infants;
6. Give newborn infants no food or drink other than breastmilk, unless medically indicated;
7. Practice rooming-in so that mothers and infants can remain together 24 h a day;
8. Encourage breastfeeding on demand;
9. Give no artificial teats, pacifiers, or soothers to breastfed infants;
10. Foster the establishment of breastfeeding support groups and refer mothers to them on discharge from hospitals or clinics.

From WHO/UNICEF (1989).

equal status to the International Code and close many of the loopholes exploited by the baby-food industry. In 1994, the World Health Assembly passed a resolution that called on member countries to ensure that the practice of distributing free 'gift' samples of formula through physicians' offices and other health care facilities was stopped (World Health Assembly 1994).

The baby-friendly hospital initiative

In 1989, WHO/UNICEF proposed to address the influence of hospitals on breastfeeding practices and issued a joint statement that described ten steps to successful breastfeeding (WHO/UNICEF 1989). These Ten Steps are internationally relevant to developed and developing countries and outline the policies and practices that should be implemented in hospitals in order to protect, promote, and support breastfeeding (Table 37.2).

In 1990, as a follow-up to the joint statement, the Innocenti Declaration was produced and adopted by participants at the WHO/UNICEF policy makers'

meeting in Innocenti, Italy (Innocenti Declaration 1990). It called for all governments to develop national breastfeeding policies and set appropriate targets for the 1990s. The next year, the WHO/UNICEF Baby Friendly Hospital Initiative (BFHI), a global initiative and structured method of promoting, protecting, and supporting breastfeeding, was developed as a strategic programme to combine the essential principles of the International Code, the Ten Steps and the Innocenti Declaration (World Health Organization & United Nations Children's Fund 1991). The BFHI has two objectives, as outlined below by James Grant, the late Executive Director of UNICEF:

To transform maternal and child care practices at the health care facility level by fully implementing the Ten Steps. Hospitals are targeted in this effort as they are the main sources of 'misinformation' and 'mis-leadership' regarding infant and young child feeding and have been instrumental in the trend away from breastfeeding.

To eliminate the most detrimental practice inducing mothers away from breastfeeding: the free or low-cost distribution of infant formula through hospitals and maternity facilities. The availability of these supplies encourages routine bottle feeding and the separation of infants from mothers. As the Ten Steps are fully implemented, the need for breast-milk substitutes at health care facilities will substantially diminish (Grant 1992).

At the time of writing, more than 14,000 hospitals worldwide have been certified as 'Baby-Friendly'. Some countries have enacted legislation. Developing countries such as China and Brazil have extensive implementation of the BFHI. In the Scandinavian countries considerable progress has been made in implementing the BFHI and breastfeeding initiation, as well as continuation rates have increased significantly. In the United States 26 hospitals have BFHI status. In Canada, only 1 hospital has attained BFHI status. In Canada, not a single hospital has yet attained this certification.

Overcoming the barriers to implementing the BFHI

A recent study of 104 (80 respondents) breastfeeding support groups undertaken by the Breastfeeding Committee for Canada and UNICEF (1997) provides some insight into what strategies might help overcome the barriers to the BFHI. Respondents reported problems with professional attitudes, lack of professional skills and knowledge, parents' knowledge and beliefs, lack of hospital resources, institutional policies and practices and the marketing practices of formula companies. Respondents, from their experience, recommended broad strategies to implement the BFHI successfully, including working together, social marketing and community-wide initiatives, professional education, diligence in monitoring and advocacy, and support from professional organizations and provincial and federal governments.

Administrators in hospitals have difficulty addressing the economic costs of introducing the BFHI. Breast-milk substitute manufacturers target hospitals as a prime marketing location to promote their products to new mothers. Many millions of dollars (usually associated with obligations to distribute the formula as gifts) are offered to hospitals as incentives to promote a single product. The money is used to fund research and clinical programmes. In Canada, a study of hospitals providing maternity services demonstrated that almost all (81.9%) had formula contracts (Levitt et al 1995). These days, where health care is subjected to major financial difficulties, hospital administrators find it difficult to find new funds to support breastfeeding.

The WHO in collaboration with Wellstart International

has developed an innovative teaching resource consisting of a collection of eight training modules, complete with slides and handouts, for use in a short course intended to help administrators and policy makers promote breastfeeding in health facilities (WHO & Wellstart International 1996).

Improving the knowledge, attitudes and skills of health professionals

Many primary care physicians believe their training in breastfeeding management has been inadequate, and they lack confidence in their breastfeeding management abilities (Freed et al 1995). In a recent study of paediatricians in the Unites States, breastfeeding exclusively for the first month after birth was recommended by only 65% of respondents. A majority agreed with or had neutral opinions about the statement that breastfeeding and formula feeding are equally acceptable methods for feeding infants. Reasons given for not recommending breastfeeding included medical conditions with known treatments that did not preclude breastfeeding. The majority of paediatricians (72%) were unfamiliar with the contents of the BFHI (Shandler et al 1999).

Professionals who are not well informed provide not only inaccurate but also inconsistent information to women and families, further confusing them when they might already be experiencing some difficulties.

In the United States, new initiatives to address physicians' poor knowledge and skills in managing breastfeeding include the new American Academy of Pediatrics (APP) Policy Statement on Breastfeeding (1997) and the development of a practice parameter on breastfeeding. More physicians' continuing-education programmes are being offered by national and regional organizations. Materials and training courses from agencies such as Wellstart International are available for the education of all health care professionals.

Education should begin at the most formative stage. School curricular, health science education, post-graduate education and continuing-education programmes should ensure that breastfeeding knowledge, attitudes and skills are effectively taught.

Undertaking research to evaluate the impact of the BFHI and other strategies

Since 1992 many studies on the Ten Steps have been

undertaken. An ambitious randomized controlled trial of the BFHI, called the Promotion of Breastfeeding intervention trial (PROBIT) study, is presently being undertaken as a partnership between Canadian researchers, WHO and collaborators in Belarus (Kramer 2000). In 1998, WHO published an analysis on the evidence for the Ten Steps to successful breastfeeding (World Health Organization 1998). The study reported that the evidence for most of the Ten Steps is substantial, even when each step is considered separately, despite the inherent difficulties of randomization.

Steps 1 and 2 on policy and training are necessary requirements for the implementation of the BFHI. Eighteen hours of training seems to be an absolute minimum and longer is necessary for improved skills and attitudinal change. Three steps have very strong evidence. These are: steps 3 (antenatal education), 5 (showing mothers how to breastfeed), and 10 (continuing support after discharge).

There is good evidence for step 4 (early contact), and highly-suggestive evidence for step 7 (rooming-in) and step 8 (demand feeding). Step 6 (the use of supplement feeds) and step 9 (the use of pacifiers) are closely related. Studies on these have demonstrated a strong association between their use and the early cessation of breastfeeding.

Studies on the BFHI programme elements that relate to the International Code (World Health Organization 1981) have shown that the provision of commercial discharge packs adversely effects breastfeeding. In addition, discontinuing the provision of formula in maternity facilities has been shown to be one of the most cost-effective health interventions known (World Health Organization 1998).

Ensuring support from professional organizations

Professional organizations, because of their prestige and expertise, have tremendous influence over society and governments. They can play a role in promoting breastfeeding by ensuring that they speak up in support of breastfeeding, by endorsing the International Code of Marketing of Breast-Milk Substitutes, by facilitating knowledge and skill development of their members through conferences and continuing education events, by publishing articles in their journals and newsletters and by developing innovative programmes.

Two examples of innovative office-based programmes have emerged recently in Canada and the United

Table 37.3 — 10 steps to a baby-friendly office

1. Support, promote, and protect breastfeeding by appropriately informing women about infant feeding;
2. Establish a baby-friendly office policy in collaboration with your colleagues and office staff and inform all new staff of this policy;
3. Eliminate the practice of distributing free formula to women from your office;
4. Ensure that your patient education materials and magazines do not advertise breast-milk substitutes;
5. Display baby-friendly posters to promote breastfeeding;
6. Provide a relatively private area where infants can be breastfed;
7. Do not refer pregnant women to formula-company-run pre-natal or post-natal classes;
8. Eliminate the practice of free breast-milk substitute/related product sample distribution to health professionals and office staff;
9. Advocate to ensure that your hospital is a baby-friendly hospital;
10. Support mothers who need to work outside their home to continue to breastfeed by advocating for baby-friendly workplaces.

States. In Canada, 'Ten Steps to a Baby-Friendly Office' was developed as a tool to promote breastfeeding support by family physicians (Levitt et al 1997) (Table 37.3). In the Unites States, the American Academy of Pediatrics has recently been funded for an innovative educational initiative called 'Breastfeeding Promotion in the Pediatricians' Office'.

Influencing government

Influencing government to enact protective legislation to support ethical marketing practices and breastfeeding in the workplace as well as to provide appropriate resources to ensure the best possible nutritional start for infants is very important. Governments are perceived to have expertise, objectivity and financial resources. In many countries, government fund sectors of the health care system that support health care for the very poor, for maternity services and for infant care.

'Model laws' to assist legislators are available from WHO/UNICEF (Sokol 1997). Supplemental funds to support National Breastfeeding Committees to oversee BFHI implementation, research incentives for breastfeeding, partnerships with professional organizations and Non Governmental Organization (NGOs) and other initiatives are all important strategies that governments can undertake to promote breast-feeding.

In 1969, the International Labour Organization of Geneva advocated lactation breaks at work and suggested provision of suitable facilities in the work-place. Employers were encouraged to allow flexible hours and privacy to nursing mothers. Governments should respect women's rights to breastfeed in the work-place through legislative initiatives designed to protect their rights. Part-time employment (< 35 h/week or a maximum of 7 h/day) is an effective strategy to help mothers combine breastfeeding and employment (Fein & Roe 1998).

Government can also provide resources to assist in promoting, supporting and protecting breastfeeding. This includes: 1) funding a National Breastfeeding Committee to oversee the BFHI and accreditation of hospitals; 2) supporting research in breastfeeding as a priority; 3) funding demonstration projects that demonstrate improvement in breastfeeding in the community; and 4) publicly marketing breastfeeding.

Discussion

Breastfeeding is the single most important, cost-effective, public health initiative that would ensure that infants have the best nutritional beginnings. Unfortunately, many barriers exist in both the developing and developed world to the protection, promotion and support of breastfeeding. Overcoming these barriers is possible. It involves a broad range of approaches, including education of health professionals, research into the most appropriate clinical tools and practices, implementation of the WHO/UNICEF BFHI, professional organization advocacy and support, and governmental legislation and regulation. These together form a 'warm chain' to support breastfeeding.

References

American Academy of Pediatrics, Committee on Drugs. (1994) The transfer of drugs and other chemicals into human milk. *Pediatrics*, 93, 137–150.

American Academy of Pediatrics, Committee on Pediatric Aids. (1995) Human milk, breastfeeding, and transmission of human immunodeficiency virus in the United States. *Pediatrics*, 96, 977–979.

American Academy of Pediatrics. (1997) Breastfeeding and the Use of Human Milk Work Group on Breastfeeding. Policy Statement (RE9729). *Pediatrics*, 100, 1035–1039.

Arnon, S.S. (1984) Breast feeding and toxigenic intestinal infections: Missing links in crib death? *Rev Infect Dis*, 6, S193–S201.

Breastfeeding Committee for Canada, UNICEF. (1997) *Survey To Assess The Current Status of Baby-Friendly Hospital Initiative/Baby-Friendly Initiative (BFHI/BFI) Activities in Canada and To Determine Future Needs*. Available from the Breastfeeding Committee for Canada, PO Box 65114, Toronto, Ontario, Canada. (http://www.geocities.com/HotSprings/Falls/1136/index.html#Baby Friendly Initiative)

Chren, M.M., Landefeld, C.S. (1994) Physicians' behaviour and their interactions with drug companies: A controlled study of physicians who requested additions to a hospital drug formulary. *JAMA*, 271, 684–689.

Chua, S. et al. (1994) Influence of breastfeeding and nipple stimulation on postpartum uterine activity. *Br J Obstet Gynaecol*, 101, 804–805.

Cumming, R.G., Klineberg, R.J. (1993) Breastfeeding and other reproductive factors and the risk of hip fractures in elderly woman. *Int J Epidemiol*, 22, 684–691.

Dewey, K.G. et al. (1993) Maternal weight-loss patterns during prolonged lactation. *Am J Clin Nutr*, 58, 162–166.

Dewey, K.G. et al. (1995) Differences in morbidity between breast-fed and formula-fed infants. *Pediatrics*, 126, 696–702.

Editorial. (1994) A warm chain for breastfeeding. *Lancet*, 344, 1239–1241.

Fein, S.B., Roe, B. (1998) The effect of work status on initiation and duration of breastfeeding. *Amer J Pub Health*, 88, 1042–1046.

Ford, R.P.K. et al. (1993) Breastfeeding and the risk of sudden infant death syndrome. *Int J Epidemiol*, 22, 885–890.

Freed, G.L. et al. (1995) National assessment of physicians' breastfeeding knowledge attitudes, training and experience. *JAMA*, 273, 472–476.

Gerstein, H.C. (1994) Cow's milk exposure and type 1 diabetes mellitus. *Diabetes Care*, 17, 13–19.

Grant, J. (1992) *Parameters for Involvement of The Infant Formula Industry with The Baby Friendly Hospital Initiative*. Letter to WHO/UNICEF Regional Directors, CF/EXD/1992–2018.

Greco, L. et al. (1988) Case control study on nutritional risk factors in celiac disease. *J Pediatr Gastroenterol Nutr*, 7, 395–399.

Innocenti Declaration. (1990) *On the Protection, Promotion And Support of Breast Feeding*. Adopted at the WHO/

UNICEF policy makers' meeting on "Published by Breastfeeding in the 1990s: a global initiative." Held at Spedale degli Innocenti, Italy. Document 10017, New York, UNICEF.

Kennedy, K.I., Visness, C.M. (1992) Contraceptive efficacy of lactational amenorrhoea. *Lancet*, 339, 227–230.

Kovar, M.G. et al. (1984) Review of the epidemiologic evidence for an association between infant feeding and infant health. *Pediatrics*, 74, S615–S638.

Kramer, M.S., Chalmers, B., Hodnett, E.D. et al (2000) Promotion of breastfeeding intervention trial (PROBIT): A cluster-randomized trial in the republic of Belarus. Design, follow-up and data validation. *Adv Exp Med Bio* 478, 327–345.

Levitt, C. et al. (1995) Survey of Routine Maternity Care and Practices in Canadian Hospitals: Ottawa: Health Canada and Canadian Institute of Child Health.

Levitt, C. et al. (1997) Our strength for tomorrow: Valuing our children. Part 2: Unborn and newborn babies. *Can Fam Phys*, 43, 1585–1589.

Lucas, A. Cole, T.J. (1990) Breast milk and neonatal necrotising enterocolitis. *Lancet*, 336, 1519–1523.

Lucas, A. et al. (1992) Breast milk and subsequent intelligence quotient in children born premature. *Lancet*, 339, 261–264.

Margen, S. et al. (1991) *Infant Feeding in Mexico: A Study of Health Facility And Mother's Practices in Three Regions*. Washington: Nestlé Infant Formula Audit Commission.

Melton, L.J. et al. (1993) Influence of breastfeeding and other reproductive factors on bone mass later in life. *Osteoporos Int*, 3, 76–83.

Newcomb, P.A. et al. (1994) Lactation and a reduced risk of premenopausal breast cancer. *N Engl J Med*, 330, 81–87.

Palmer, G. (1993) *Politics of Breastfeeding*. London: Pandora Press.

Paradise, J.L. et al. (1994) Evidence in infants with cleft palate that breast milk protects against otitis media. *Pediatrics*, 94, 853–860.

Pisacane, A. et al. (1992) Breast-feeding and urinary tract infection. *Pediatrics*, 120, 87–89.

Rigas, A. et al. (1993) Breast-feeding and maternal smoking in the etiology of Crohn's disease and ulcerative colitis in childhood. *Ann Epidem*, 3, 387–392.

Rosenblatt, K.A., Thomas, D.B. (1993) WHO Collaborative Study of Neoplasia and Steroid Contraceptives. *Int J Epidemiol*, 22, 192–197.

Saarinen, U.M., Kajosaari, M. (1995) Breastfeeding as prophylaxis against atopic disease: Prospective follow-up study until 17 years old. *Lancet*, 346, 1065–1069.

Schanler, R.J., O'Connor, K.G., Lawrence, R.A. et al (March 1999) Pediatricians' Practices and Attitudes Regarding Breastfeeding Promotion. *Pediatrics*, 103, 3, 35.

Shu, X-O. et al. (1995) Infant breastfeeding and the risk of childhood lymphoma and leukaemia. *Int J Epidemiol*, 24, 27–32.

Sokol, E. (1997) *The Code Handbook. A Guide to Implementing The International Code of Marketing of Breast-milk Substitutes.* Published by IBFAN Sdn Bhd, Malaysia. In Collaboration with Stichting ICDC, International Code Documentation Centre, Netherlands.

Takala, A.K. et al. (1989) Risk factors of invasive *Haemophilus influenzae* type B disease among children in Finland. *Pediatrics*, 115, 694–701.

Tuttle, C.R., Dewey, K.G. (1996) Potential cost savings for Medi-Cal, AFDC, food stamps, and WIC programs associated with increasing breast-feeding among low-income Hmong women in California. *J Am Diet Assoc*, 96, 885–890.

UNAIDS, WHO, UNICEF. (1997) HIV and Infant Feeding: A Policy Statement Developed Collaboratively by UNAIDS, WHO and UNICEF.

Wilson, M.H. (1990) Feeding The Healthy Child. In: Oski, F.A., DeAngelis, C.D., Feigin, R.D. et al. (eds.) *Principles and Practice of Pediatrics*, pp. 533–553. Philadelphia: JB Lippincott.

World Health Assembly. (1994) Forty-Seventh World Health Assembly. WHA 47.5 Agenda item 19.

World Health Organization. (1981) International Code on Marketing of Breast-Milk Substitutes. Document WHA34/1981/REC/1, Annex 3, Geneva.

World Health Organization, Geneva, (1998). Vallenas C and Savage F. Evidence for the ten steps to successful breast-feeding. Child Health and Development, Family and Reproductive Health, Division of Child Health and Development. WHO/CHD/98.9.101.

WHO/UNICEF. (1989) *Protecting, Promoting And Supporting Breastfeeding; The Special Role of Maternity Services.* Geneva: WHO.

World Health Organization, United Nations Children's Fund. (1991) *The Baby-Friendly Hospital Initiative: A Global Effort to Give Babies The Best Possible Start.* Geneva: WHO.

WHO, Wellstart International. (1996) *Short Course for Administrators and Policy Makers.* Geneva: WHO.

Wright, A.L. et al. (1995) Relationship of infant feeding to recurrent wheezing at age 6 years. *Arch Pediatr Adolesc Med*, 149, 758–763.

38

Formula feeds: Attributes and disadvantages

Christine A. Northrop-Clewes

Abbreviations

COMA	Committee on Medical Aspects of Food Policy
DHA	Docosahexanoic acid
DHSS	Department of Health and Social Security
EC	European Commission
EPA	Eicosapentanoic acid
ESPGAN	European Society of Paediatric Gastroenterology and Nutrition
FA	Fatty acid
MAFF	Ministry of Agriculture, Fisheries and Food
ONS	Office for National Statistics
OPCS	Office of Population Censuses and Surveys
PUFA	Polyunsaturated fatty acids
RE	Retinol equivalents
RNI	Relative nutrient intake
SIgA	Secretory Immunoglobulin A
SNF	Solids-not-fat
TBARs	Thiobarbituric acid reactive substances
UNICEF	United Nations Children's Fund
WHO	World Health Organisation

Introduction

Human milk is the preferred way to feed all infants including premature and sick newborns. Breast milk is species-specific, and it is different from all other substitute feeding options. To date, the breastfed infant has been the 'gold standard' against which all alternative feeding methods have been measured with regard to growth, health, development and other long- and short-term benefits (American Academy of Pediatrics 1997). However, breastfeeding may not always be justified. For example when considering vitamin requirements, it has been suggested that greater consideration needs to be given to differences in bioavailability of vitamins in breast milk compared to formula feeds, the influence of season, stage of lactation and stated composition (Powers 1997).

Historical background

The history of infant feeds

At the time of the hunter-gatherer (more than 12,000 years ago) lactational failure would have resulted in 100% infant mortality unless, within the small social group, a wet nurse could have been found or a substitute milk used. However, in the absence of domesticated animals there would have been little possibility of this. When agricultural-based societies developed, about 500–600 generations ago, people began to settle in permanent villages and towns and the likelihood of finding a milk substitute if lactation failed was increased. However, with the development of urbanization, overcrowded and unhygienic conditions quickly followed and this led to high infant mortality (Cuthbertson 1999). Howarth (1905) quotes infant death rates of 70 breastfed and 198 hand-fed infants per 1000 live births in Derby, United Kingdom between the years 1900–1903.

Wet nursing

Wet nurses have served as surrogate mothers since the earliest of times. Plato advocated the rearing of all children in creches by wet nurses and, in fact, the wealthier Greeks and Romans hired slaves to wet-nurse. However, the Roman philosophers were opposed to wet nursing because they recognized the strong attachment between the wet nurse and infant, which was seen as a threat to the natural mother (Baumslag & Michels 1995a).

High illegitimacy rates in Europe during the eleventh and twelfth centuries led to vast foundling hospitals where women nursed their own child plus three or four other infants at a time, but mortality rates were high (56–99%). In eighteenth century England, women in affluent households hired wet nurses, usually women of low social class, which allowed wealthy women to produce a child as often as once a year because the contraceptive effect of breastfeeding was circumvented. Large numbers of children meant that the family could acquire wealth, power and influence by advantageous marriages. However, by 1910 the wet nurse had almost disappeared and artificial feeding became popular as an alternative to breastfeeding (Mettler 1982).

Dry nursing

Until the nineteenth century, artificial feeding was very much a recipe for disaster. Although a wide variety of products and feeding methods were tried, failure was the most frequent outcome (Baumslag & Michels 1995b). In 1880, the general state of public health in the United Kingdom began to improve with the introduction of water chlorination, improved methods of sewage disposal and stricter regulation of dairy herd housing and feeding (Baumslag & Michels

1995b). At this time, artificial feeding (dry nursing) with 'paps,' a mixture of cereals and cows' milk with added water or barley water, became possible, and although inadequate and unhygienic about two-thirds of infants survived.

Development of the first commercial infant formulas

In the mid-nineteenth century, when more detailed analytical information became available, a more scientific approach to infant formulae was adopted (Mettler 1982). Dried full-cream milk powder was first made by Grimwade in 1847 by vacuum concentration of milk at low temperature (71°C), forming a dough-like mass that, when cool, set as a solid and could be ground to a powder (Barber & Page 1982). Although commercially available from the 1860s, milk powder was largely replaced by 'patent' or 'proprietary' infant foods that began to be manufactured around 1860–1870 and were made of dried, cooked and malted cereal to be mixed with milk or water. During the 1870s, 'tinned' sweetened condensed milk made from skim milk, a by-product from butter factories, became easily available to those who could afford it (Cuthbertson 1994). The increase in scurvy, especially in the better-off families, was attributed to the use of such 'proprietary' foods (Barlow 1894). The addition of fresh foods into the diet such as milk and meat juices or even more effective vegetable or fruit juices resolved the scurvy. Poor families continued to use potato in their 'paps' and were not so affected by scurvy.

Development of infant formulas in the twentieth century

In 1902, Just and Hatmaker devised the roller-drying process for cheap and effective production of full-fat dried milk products that became the basis for artificial infant foods for the first seven decades of the twentieth century (Cuthbertson 1994). The first roller-dried infant foods were marginally deficient in ascorbic acid, vitamins A and D and iron. However, supplements of fruit or vegetable juices, cod liver oil and iron were found to eliminate the problems of scurvy, rickets and anaemia. Vitamin D was added into infant foods in the mid-1920s, as soon as odourless preparations became available and tests for vitamin D were developed (Jephcott & Bacharach 1926). In 1931, ferric ammonium citrate was added to milk powders to combat iron-deficiency anaemia (Mackay & Goodfellow 1931). Destabilization of ascorbic acid was caused by roller-drying and the technology to add

crystalline ascorbic acid to the dry infant milk was not developed until the 1960s, but once added the vitamin C was retained without deterioration (Cuthbertson 1994).

Although roller-dried foods had been available since 1904, the commonest infant-feeding regimen up until the Second World War still depended on diluted fresh cows' milk with added sugar. During and after the war, roller-dried full-cream milk formulations were increasingly used so that by the 1960s fresh milk was rarely used (Whitehead & Paul 1987). At this time, many believed that breastfeeding and bottle-feeding were equally as good and that brands of infant food hardly differed from each other except in price and packaging.

Problems of simple roller-dried infant milks

Vitamin D

In 1953, Lightwood and Stapleton reported that even an essential nutrient such as vitamin D could be harmful in excess. At that time, needlessly-high concentrations of vitamin D were added to infant foods and supplements, resulting in the majority of infants receiving 40–100 µg vitamin D/day. A small minority of infants showed evidence of idiopathic hypercalcaemia, a condition which almost completely disappeared after 1957 when the vitamin D content of milk formula was reduced to 1 µg/100 ml and to 15 µg/100 g in cereal weaning foods.

Phosphate/calcium in formulas

Neonatal hypocalcaemia can result in neonatal convulsions, a condition found to be associated with the use of certain milk formulations (Oppe & Redstone 1968). Barltrop & Oppe (1970) showed neonatal hypocalcaemia to be related to the phosphate content of the infant food, which could be controlled either by a decrease in phosphate or an increase in calcium content of the milk formulation.

High-electrolyte formulas

Taitz & Byers (1972) noticed a high incidence of dangerous hypertonic dehydration in babies with gastroenteritis in the United Kingdom. The use of over-concentrated feeds coupled with needlessly-high levels of protein and electrolytes (especially sodium) in the full-cream milk powders was shown to be the cause. Calculation of the effects of food and water intakes and insensible water losses on renal loads clearly indicated a very significant decrease in the risk from dehydration when low-electrolyte formulas were used (Shaw et al 1973). Infant food manufacturers responded rapidly to the need for low-electrolyte infant foods so that by 1974 no high-electrolyte infant formulas were sold, except for the UK government's subsidized National Dried Milk which was withdrawn from the market in 1977.

Low-electrolyte infant formulas

The first of the low-electrolyte formulas were produced by approximately halving the solids-not-fat (SNF) of the dried milk moiety of the food and replacing it with carbohydrate. The reduction in solids of the SNF led to reductions in several other nutrients (e.g., water-soluble vitamins and trace elements). The shortfalls were made up to the levels found in the unmodified milks or to concentrations suggested by various bodies such as Codex Alimentarius Commission (1976), European Society of Paediatric Gastroenterology and Nutrition (ESPGAN) (1977) and the UK Department of Health and Social Security (DHSS) (1980a).

DHSS reports

The problems highlighted above led to the commissioning by the DHSS of a series of reports on topics related to infant nutrition (DHSS 1974, 1977, 1980a, 1980b, 1981). The reports led to the publication of nutritional guidelines for the composition of artificial milks intended for use by the infant (DHSS 1980a). In addition, recommendations were made as to how novel formulations might be tested without unnecessarily inhibiting or delaying the application of new findings for the manufacture of improved products (Cuthbertson 1994).

Practice and procedures

The WHO/UNICEF international code

The minimum international requirement for breast-milk substitutes in all countries

At about the same time as the publication of the UK DHSS nutritional guidelines, the WHO/UNICEF International Code of Marketing of Breast-Milk Substitutes was adopted by a Resolution (WHA 34.22) of the World Health Assembly in 1981. In the code, it states it is the right of every child and pregnant and lactating woman to be adequately nourished as a means of attaining and maintaining health. In addition, it recognizes that the health of infants and young

children cannot be isolated from women's health and nutrition, socio-economic status and role as mothers. The report promulgated the ideas that: 1) breastfeeding is an unequalled way of providing ideal food for the healthy growth and development of infants; 2) it forms a unique biological and emotional basis for the health of both mother and child; 3) the anti-infective properties of breast milk help to protect infants against disease; and 4) there is an important relationship between breastfeeding and child spacing. Breastfeeding is therefore an important aspect of primary health care in all countries and cultures. However, if mothers do not breastfeed, or do so partially, then there is a legitimate market for infant formula and for suitable ingredients from which to prepare it. All these products should be made accessible to those who need them through commercial or non-commercial distribution systems, but they should not be marketed or distributed in ways that may interfere with the protection or promotion of breastfeeding. The code recognizes that inappropriate feeding practices lead to infant malnutrition, morbidity and mortality in all countries and that improper practices in the marketing of breast-milk substitutes and related products can contribute to these major public health problems. The forty-ninth World Health Assembly in 1996 stressed the continued need to implement the above code and all subsequent relevant resolutions of the World Assembly, including the Innocenti Declaration (1990) and the World Declaration and Plan of Action for Nutrition (1992).

European directive

In 1986, the European Commission submitted a specific directive (77/94/EEC) and laid down compositional and labelling requirements for infant formulas and follow-up milks and gave the following definitions:

1. 'Infant formula' shall mean foodstuffs intended for particular nutritional use by infants during the first 4–6 months of life, satisfying by themselves the nutritional requirements of this category of persons.

2. 'Follow-up milks' shall mean foodstuffs intended for particular nutritional use by infants aged > 4 months and constituting the milk element in a progressively diversified diet of this category of persons.

Article 3 of the directive continued by saying that 'infant formula shall be manufactured from food ingredients whose suitability for particular nutritional use by infants from birth has been established by generally accepted scientific data'. A similar statement was made for follow-up milks.

Table 38.1 — Approximate composition of colostrum, mature human milk, cows' milk and a typical modern milk formula

	Colostrum	Human milk	Cows' milk	Modern[1] formula
Energy (kJ/L)	[2]	2856	2730	2800
(kcal/L)	[2]	680	650	670
Protein (g/L)	100	9	31	15
Whey	840	600	200	210
Casein (g/kg TP)[3]	160	300	800	789
Lactose (g/L)	53	70	49	72
Fat (g/L)	32	42	38	36
Poly- & mono-unsaturated FA (g/kg total FA)	590	470	250	498
Sodium (mM)	21	6.5	20	10
Chloride (mM)	17	12	30	15
Calcium (mM)	8	9	30	16.5
Phosphate (mM)	5	5	30	13.5
Iron (µM)	28	12.5	9	12.5
Vitamin A (µg/L)[4]	1260	600	540	600
Vitamin C (mg/L)	70	38	10	80
Vitamin D (µg/L)	18	0.4	0.3	10

[1] Adapted from Poskitt (1994).
[2] Energy content is difficult to determine because much of the protein is not absorbed.
[3] total protein.
[4] 1 µg retinol equals 1 retinol equivalent.
Abbreviations: FA, fatty acid. The concentrations of nutrients in cow and human milk vary enormously so the values are approximations. The formula milk data is from a typical manufacturer's nutrition-information leaflet.

Modern infant formulas

The great majority of modern infant formulas used throughout the world for normal infants are based on protein derived solely from cows' milk. There are two types:

1. *Group 1*: milks with protein supplied solely from cows' milk SNF (i.e., 'casein dominant').

2. *Group 2*: milks with the casein:non-casein protein ratio adjusted with demineralized whey to resemble more closely that in human milk (i.e., 'whey dominant').

A small minority of infants are lactose intolerant and therefore cannot be given cows' milk-protein-based formulas. In these cases, formulas in which processed soya is the protein source are used (see *Protein* below).

The Office of Population Censuses and Surveys (OPCS) (Martin & White 1988) survey (1985) indicated that 82% of bottle-feeding mothers in the United Kingdom gave whey-dominant formula at birth, but only 43% were still using this formulation at 4–6 months. However, there appeared to be no firm evidence upon which to base such a choice as no important differences had been highlighted between the whey and casein-dominant formulas.

Table 38.1 indicates concentrations of the major nutrients in cows', human and a modern infant formula milk. The concentrations of nutrients in cow and human milk vary enormously so the values are approximations; the formula milk data is from a manufacturers nutrition information leaflet.

Composition of human versus cows' milk formula

Protein

Casein is the part of milk that is precipitated at 20°C and that has an acid pH of 4.5. Casein is formed from various compounds bonded together into micellar formation as a 'calcium caseinate complex' with associated phosphate, magnesium and citrate ions. The casein micelles of cows' milk are larger than those of human milk and form large flocculates in the upper bowel when fresh cows' milk is given to young infants (Jelliffe & Jelliffe 1978, Hambraeus 1991). In the past, intestinal obstruction secondary to undigested casein curds obstructing the small intestine (i.e., inspissated curd syndrome) was not uncommon in young infants fed neat cows' milk or unmodified cows' milk formula. Heat treatment in the preparation of casein-predominant formulas affect micellar formation making the curds 'less tough' hence young infants are able to digest the casein of modern formulas readily. However, inspissated curd syndrome is still seen when curd-predominant formulas are given to infants with poor gastrointestinal function, particularly premature infants (Poskitt 1994).

Whey protein is the protein that remains in the supernatant after extraction of casein and makes up about 70% of the protein in human milk (Schanler & Cheng 1991). The amino acid composition of human whey is different to that of cows' milk. Cows' milk-based formulas, in which the total protein and whey content have been modified to be similar to human milk, still have a different overall amino acid composition.

Human milk whey protein is predominantly α-lactoalbumin, lactoferrin (see *iron* below), secretory immunoglobulin (sIgA) and enzymes, especially lysozyme and bile-stimulated lipase. α-lactalbumin binds calcium and may increase its bioavailability (Hambraeus 1991). The immunological functions of breast milk, including the protective roles of sIgA, have been known for some time. Convincing epidemiological data shows that the risk of dying from diarrhoea in developing countries is reduced 14–24 times in breastfed infants (Hanson et al 1993). A protective effect against many infectious diseases is also seen in industrialized countries (Wold & Hanson 1994, Newman 1995). By mechanisms which are still unclear, evidence also suggests that breastfeeding promotes post-natal development of secretory immunity and enhanced secretory as well as systemic immune response to oral and parenteral vaccines (Brandtzaeg 1998). However, several pro-spective studies have reported that an early physiological increase in salivary IgA (and IgM) is more prominent in formula-fed than breastfed infants (Brandtzaeg 1998), although this difference apparently disappears after weaning. Other studies suggest that breastfeeding

for only 3 weeks, in comparison to formula-feeding, reduces salivary IgA antibody levels to cows' milk proteins. Therefore, it seems that although breastfeeding may initially reduce salivary sIgA antibody levels, it boosts them at a later stage of infancy (up to 8 months) (Brandtzaeg 1998).

Cows' milk whey proteins are mainly lactoglobulins. β-lactoglobulin is one of the proteins responsible for cows' milk-protein intolerance. Cows' milk-protein intolerance is now more widely recognized, but whether this is a real increase in prevalence or due to higher concentrations of β-lactoglobulin in modern formula, better diagnosis of the disease or some other factor is not known.

Carbohydrate

Lactose is the predominant carbohydrate in both human and cows' milk. The presence of lactose in milks facilitates calcium and magnesium absorption, however the reason why is not clear. The lactose content of human milk is higher than that of cows' milk, however the lack of facilitated absorption of calcium with cows' milk may be overcome by the overall higher levels of calcium in cows' milk. Other carbohydrates occurring naturally in milks are oligosaccharides, nucleotide sugars (present in high concentrations in breast milk in free and bound forms), and lipid- and protein-bound carbohydrates.

Modern formulas do have added carbohydrate, which may be lactose and/or other carbohydrates, to increase their energy content.

Early studies reported differences in the gut microflora of breastfed and formula-fed infants, that is breastfed infants had microflora dominated by bifidobacteria, which resulted in a lower incidence of infant-related diseases such as enterocolitis (Heavy & Rowland 1999). Free nucleotides were added to formula feeds because it was thought that they would enhance the growth of bifidobacteria. However, in a study by Balmer et al (1994), infants who were fed a whey-based formula supplemented with nucleotide monophosphate salts were found to have *Escherichia coli* as the dominant micro-organism in their faecal flora. More recent studies suggest there is now little difference between the gut microflora of breastfed and formula-fed infants of industrialized countries, although differences are seen between Asian and Western countries perhaps due to ecological variation (Heavy & Rowland 1999).

Preliminary results from *in vitro* studies now indicate nucleotides may play an important role in gut maturation of the foetus, especially proliferation, differentiation and apoptosis of the mucosal epithelium.

The nonimmunological factors of human milk have recently become of interest, including glycoproteins, glycolipids and lactose-derived oligosaccharides. Oligosaccharides are added to adult foods as *prebiotics*, that is non-digestible food ingredients that beneficially affect the host by selectively stimulating the growth and/or activity of one or a limited number of bacteria in the colon and thus improving health (Gibson et al 1995). Human milk contains more than 130 oligosaccharides, which are based on 5 monosaccharide residues including sialic acid, N-acetyl-glucosamine, fucose, glucose and galactose. It is thought that oligosaccharides bind with sugar receptors on epithelial cells and so prevent bacterial adhesion (Heavy & Rowland 1999). Brand Miller et al (1994) noted that the total concentration of oligosaccharides decreased throughout lactation, and the relative concentrations of the individual oligosaccharides varied. They also noticed that milk from two mothers with pre-term infants was twice as high in oligosaccharide components as full-term milk and may therefore be of benefit to the more immature gut of the premature infant.

Probiotics (i.e., live microbial food supplements which are beneficial to health) are also being used to promote infant health. *Lactobacillus GG* given to infants (4–45 months) in the form of fermented milk and freeze-dried reconstituted powders shortened the duration of diarrhoea compared to controls (Isolauri et al 1991). However, when given to premature infants, it failed to show any clinical benefits although it successfully colonized the gut. More research is needed to establish whether pre- and probiotics have a beneficial role in infant health.

Fat

Human milk contains the essential fatty acids, linoleic acid (18:2, n-6) and linolenic acid (18:3 n-3) and the very long-chain polyunsaturated fatty acids (PUFA), arachidonic acid (20:4 n-6), eicosapentanoic acid (EPA) (20:5 n-3) and docosahexanoic acid (DHA) (22:6 n-3). Linoleic and linolenic acids are not inter-convertible and are the parents of the n-3 and n-6 series of fatty acids. They play important roles in providing PUFA, which act as components of cellular membranes and are particularly important in eye and brain development. They are also precursors of other metabolites such as prostacyclins and prostaglandins. Cows' milk contains more saturated fat than human milk, less of the essential fatty acids and no PUFA. In the late 1970s and early 1980s the butterfat of cows' milk formula was partially or completely replaced by vegetable oils in novel infant foods made to meet the recommendations of Codex Alimentarius Commission (1976), DHSS (1980a) and ESPGAN (1977). The new formulations were prepared by manufacturers to meet the levels of linoleic acid required by the advisory bodies. However, the oils had lower relative proportions of linolenic acid than breast milk or even the butterfat of cows' milk. DHA has an important role in normal brain function and in the retinal pigment epithelium in the eye, and depletion of tissue DHA occurs when diets have low levels of n-3 fatty acids and high levels of n-6. That is, the degree of deficiency is mostly determined by the ratio of linoleic:linolenic acid. The linolenic content of vegetable oil is low with linoleic:linolenic ratios varying from 50:1 in corn oil to 150:1 in safflower oil, resulting in the depression of the conversion of linolenic acid to DHA by competitive inhibition of the D-6-desaturase enzyme. The need for linolenic acid was not recognized until the 1990s ESPGAN (1991), thus many formulas used from the mid-1970s until the early 1990s may have provided much less of the n-3 essential fatty acids than would now be advised (Cuthbertson 1999). ESPGAN (1991) now recommend a linoleic:linolenic ratio of between 5:1 and 15:1 and that PUFA are added in amounts typical of human milk levels (i.e., n-6 and n-3 PUFA approximately 1% and 0.5%, respectively).

A study of the fatty acid composition of the brains of sudden-death infants show higher concentrations of DHA in those who received breast milk than those only given formula (Farquharson et al 1992). In addition, Lucas et al (1992) attributed better developmental outcome at 8-years follow-up in premature infants given some breast milk at birth. Three independent studies are now underway to determine the effects of formulas containing arachodonic acid (AA) and DHA in comparison with breast milk on neurological development in term and pre-term infants (Cuthbertson 1999).

Human milk has high levels of cholesterol (100–159 mg/L). It is speculated that giving infants high dietary cholesterol early in life equips them for metabolizing cholesterol efficiently, thus reducing the risks of hypercholesterolaemia and arteriosclerosis in later life (Poskitt 1994).

Carnitine is absent from cows' milk but present in high concentrations in human milk. Newborn infants can synthesize carnitine, but when growth and fat deposition are rapid it is possible that endogenous carnitine synthesis may limit rates of metabolism. Lower levels of plasma carnitine have been found in normal full-term formula-fed infants but no clinical effects have been identified (Hamosh 1991).

PUFAs are major substrates for lipid peroxidation and have been associated with enhanced oxidative injury. In a study by Granot et al (1999) breastfed infants were found to have 2.5-fold higher thiobarbituric acid reactive substances (TBARs) in plasma than formula-fed infants. TBARs are a reflection of the quantity of PUFA in the tissue and plasma lipids, which reflect dietary intake, as well as the levels of antioxidants and oxidative stress. However, breast milk is regarded as optimal infant nutrition, so it is difficult to understand why it would contain potentially harmful factors. One hypothesis may be that oxygen reactive species hold the balance between beneficial and detrimental effects, that is the presence of lipids susceptible to oxidation by scavenging oxygen radicals may provide a substrate for cellular antioxidant protection at the early stages of development when other antioxidant defences may be less effective (Granot et al 1999).

Vitamins

The consensus approach to the estimation of infant vitamin requirements is to calculate approximate intakes in breastfed infants. Breast milk provides an adequate source of vitamins and would therefore seem to be a reasonable method of estimation (Powers 1997). However, differences in the composition of milk from the left or right breast, differences in the fore and hind milks, diurnal and seasonal variation as well as the stage of lactation may all introduce variation into the estimated vitamin concentration (Powers 1997). Other problems include vitamin stability, for example vitamin C and riboflavin (Bates et al 1985, Fritz et al 1987), and method of extraction and detection, for example folate and vitamin A. Of greatest practical importance is the bioavailability of vitamins in breast milk. A major determinant of bioavailability is the efficiency of absorption, which can be affected by factors such as current nutrient status, nutrient digestion and gastrointestinal integrity. There are virtually no comparative studies of the bioavailability of vitamins in formulas and human milk but there are some *in vitro* data that suggest there may be differences for some vitamins (Powers 1997).

Table 38.2 summarizes the range of concentrations of vitamins in formula for term infants (0–6 months) compared to levels in breast milk. Table 38.3 describes the estimated daily vitamin intakes from

formulas compared with the current UK and US recommendations. Potential problems associated with the recommendations are discussed below.

Thiamin

Few data are available on requirements for thiamin in infancy, however thiamin requirements are closely related to energy intake. The relative nutrient intake (RNI) (see Table 38.3) was set by the UK Committee on Medical Aspects of Food Policy (COMA) panel (DHSS 1991) and is based on levels reported in breast milk. Levels in formulas (see Table 38.2) may be in excess of needs but the lack of reported toxic effects and concerns about the shelf life of the product have encouraged the use of the higher levels.

Riboflavin

Levels in formulas for term infants are comparable with breast milk (see Table 38.2). However, there are concerns that there may be transient riboflavin deficiency around the time of weaning, resulting in morphological and kinetic changes in the duodenal epithelium (Powers 1997). Deficiency at a critical time in gastrointestinal development may prevent normal development of the gastrointestinal tract. The possibility of long-term damage justifies further research when considering recommendations for riboflavin levels in formulas (Powers 1997).

B_{12}

The RNI of B_{12} (see Table 38.3) is based on a study showing normalization of abnormal methylmalonate excretion in breastfed infants of vegetarians (Specker et al 1990). B_{12} from formulas (see Table 38.2) is generous compared with breast milk because of the less efficient absorption from formulas; breast milk contains B_{12}-binding proteins which are thought to facilitate absorption (Trugo & Sardinha 1994).

Folate

Most folate is stored late in the third trimester of pregnancy, therefore the pre-term infant may have low folate stores at birth. Increased demands due to the rapid growth of the pre-term infant may lead to folate deficiency, and as many as two-thirds of pre-term infants may develop low serum folate levels between 1–3 months of age. Overall, there is very little margin of safety at the lower recommended concentrations of folate in formulae (see Table 38.2). Factors that may increase the requirement for folate in all infants include haemolytic anaemia, which may occur as a result of inadequate vitamin E intake or when certain drugs are used (e.g., methotrexate or 5-fluoracil). In addition, concurrent illnesses that lead to anorexia,

Table 38.2 — Range of concentrations of vitamins in formula for term infants from birth to 6 months compared to levels in human milk

Vitamin	Formula[1]/L	Human milk[2]/L
Thiamin (mg)	0.39–1	0.14–0.28
Riboflavin (vitamin B_2)(mg)	0.53–1.5	0.4–2.87[3]
Niacin (mg)	3.4–9	1.8–3.9
Pyridoxine (vitamin B_6)(mg)	0.33–0.65	0.23–0.4[4]
Folic acid (µg)	33–110[5]	30–137
Vitamin B_{12} (µg)	0.33–2.2	0.23–1.8
Ascorbic acid (vitamin C) (mg)	66–90	33–110
Pantothenic acid (mg)	2–4	2.6
Biotin (µg)	10–20	5.2
Vitamin A (mg retinol equivalents (RE))	0.6–1[6]	0.49–0.77
Vitamin E (mg α-tocopherol equivalents)	4.6–10	1.1–8
Vitamin D (µg)	10–11	13–17[7]
Vitamin K (µg)	26–100	13–130[8]

[1]Information supplied by the following companies, whose formulas are available in the United Kingdom: Boots, Cow and Gate, Farleys, SMA, Milupa (the energy content of the formulas range from 65–75 kcals/100 mL; the protein content between 1.3–1.6 g/100 mL).
[2]*Lower limit*: the lowest average concentration reported in human milk from apparently healthy women with ideally biochemical or clinical evidence of a healthy baby. Upper limit: the highest concentration in human milk (after supplementation, in the absence of any biochemical evidence of excess in the baby).
[3]Lower limit based on intakes in Gambian infants sufficient to normalize biochemical deficiency.
[4]Lower limit based on average in human breast milk of mothers consuming the reference nutrient intake.
[5]Folate may be less available from formula than human milk. This intake in formula is associated with normal erythrocyte morphology in term infants.
[6]Lower limit based on recommendations by Olson (1987).
[7]Intake sufficient to maintain plasma 25-hydroxyvitamin D_3 above 20 µg/L.
[8]Based on upper level in breast milk in unsupplemented women from industrialized countries.
Adapted from Powers (1997).

Table 38.3 — Estimated daily vitamin intakes from formulas compared with current recommendations.

Vitamin	Intake from formulas	UK RNI	USA RDI
Thiamin (mg)	0.29–0.75	0.2	0.3
Riboflavin (mg)	0.4–1.13	0.4	0.4
Niacin (mg)	2.55–6.75	3	6
Pyridoxine (mg)	0.25–0.49	0.2	0.3
Folic acid (µg)	25–83	50	25
Vitamin B_{12} (µg)	0.98–1.65	0.3	0.3
Ascorbic acid (mg)	50–68	25	30
Pantothenic acid (mg)	1.5–3	1.7[4]	2[4]
Biotin (µg)	7.5–11.3	n/a	10[4]
Vitamin A (µg RE)	450–750	350	375
Vitamin D (µg)	7.5–11	8.5	7.5
Vitamin E (mg)	3.5–7.5	> 2.35[4]	3
Vitamin K (µg)	19.5–75	n/a	5

[1]Estimated from levels in formula (table 2) with a consumption of 750 ml of milk daily.
[2]DHSS (1991)
[3]National Research Council (1989)
[4]Estimated safe and adequate intake (Powers 1997)

such as gastroenteritis, may place the infant in negative folate balance. Folate supplements have proved useful in treating subjects with homocysteinaemia, and if infant screening for this disorder was introduced there would be implications for folate intakes (Powers 1997).

Vitamin C

Concentrations of plasma vitamin C found in some premature infants are high enough to interfere with the antioxidant ferroxidase (Fe 2^+ to Fe 3^+) activity usually exhibited by caeruloplasmin (Powers 1997). Low plasma antioxidant activity has been identified as an important predictor of poor outcome in premature infants, however the relevance to term babies has not been evaluated (Silvers et al 1994). Commercial formulas for term infants contains levels of vitamin C comparable with breast milk, but because of the concerns over the possible effects of high plasma concentrations, it has been suggested that there might be a case for setting safe upper limits of intake during infancy (Powers 1997).

Vitamin A

Infants are born with very low hepatic stores of retinol and are dependent on their diet to build up their stores and to have adequate circulating levels of vitamin A for normal growth and development. The recommendations of the FAO/WHO Expert Group (2001, in press) re-confirmed the recommendations made in 1988 that 0.35 mg retinol equivalents (RE)/day were adequate for the first year of life. Commercial formulas for term infants in the United Kingdom provide 0.6–1 mg/RE/day (see Table 38.2), which is comparable with that provided in the milk of well-nourished but unsupplemented mothers. Excess vitamin A has toxic effects, but safe upper limits for infants are still to be evaluated. β-Carotene is added to some formulas for pre-term infants because it might help to protect against oxidative damage.

Vitamin E

Vitamin E requirement is highly influenced by the PUFA content of the tissues, which in turn is influenced by dietary intake. The DHSS (1991) recommended 0.4 mg tocopherol equivalents/g PUFA for infant milk formulas.

Minerals and trace elements

In the manufacture of demineralized whey, the concentration of the minerals and trace elements are reduced to very low levels and these are subsequently adjusted to levels which are close to human milk. All

Table 38.4 — Example of the mineral and trace element content of casein-based infant formula

Minerals/trace elements	Per 100 ml prepared formula
Sodium (mg)	25
Calcium (mg)	76
Phosphorus (mg)	46
Iron (mg)	0.7
Magnesium (mg)	8
Zinc (mg)	0.5
Iodine (µg)	9.1
Potassium (mg)	97
Chloride (mg)	63
Copper (µg)	30
Manganese (µg)	8

infant formulas have higher levels of iron to compensate for the relatively poor absorption of iron compared to that from human milk (see *iron* below). Not all trace elements reach levels found in human milk (e.g., zinc and selenium), and absorption may also be reduced where they are present in bound forms (DHSS 1988). Table 38.4 gives a summary of typical concentrations of minerals and trace elements found in casein-based formula.

Iron

The appropriate level of iron supplementation of infant formulas is still under discussion (Hernell & Lönnerdal 1996). In Europe, formulas generally contain 7 mg/L (see Table 38.4) (1 mg/100 kcal), but in the United States 12 mg/L (1.8 mg/100 kcal) is used. Both levels are effective in preventing iron deficiency and anaemia during the first 6 months of life. However, studies by Hernell & Lönnerdal (1996) suggest that a whey-predominant milk-based infant formula containing only 2 mg iron/L would result in satisfactory iron status up to 6 months of age, which suggests that the fortification level of such formulas could be reduced.

Iron is usually added as ferrous sulphate and its absorption can be improved by the addition of 100–200 mg/L of vitamin C. The widespread consumption of iron and vitamin C fortified formulas in the United States is regarded as the reason for the dramatic fall in the prevalence of anaemia in the last 30 years (Yip 1994).

Lactoferrin is a major iron-binding protein in human milk and is thought to facilitate iron absorption.

However, Davidsson et al (1994) found, using stable isotopes, that the mean iron absorption in breastfed infants 3–10 months old was 11%, but when the lactoferrin was removed from the breast milk the mean iron absorption increased to 20%. Therefore the authors found no support for an enhancing effect of lactoferrin on iron absorption in this age group. However in one 2-month-old infant, iron absorption was highest from whole breast milk, supporting a hypothesis by Brock (1980) that the biological role of lactoferrin changes from early to late infancy. The method by which iron is taken up and transferred across the mucosal cell is beginning to be understood in adults (Powell et al 1999), but the role of lactoferrin at mucosal level in infants is not yet elucidated. A specific receptor on the brush border membrane of the infant gut may facilitate cellular uptake of lactoferrin and iron, which may in turn regulate iron metabolism, but further studies at the cellular and molecular levels are still needed.

Finally, *in vitro* lactoferrin has been shown to prevent multiplication in the gut of many facultative and obligate anaerobes that are iron-dependent. This has not been confirmed *in vivo* (Roberts et al 1992).

Copper

Pre-term breast milk contains high concentrations of copper (0.8 mg/L), which decreases by 25% in the first 4 weeks post-partum. The recommended daily dose for term infants 0–6 months of age is 0.1–0.6 mg/L.

Soya-based infant formulas

Concern has been expressed that phytoestrogens present in soya-based infant formulas may affect the sexual development and future fertility of infants. However, some babies cannot tolerate formulas based on cows' milk, so if they are not being breastfed they may be fed soya-based infant formulas as an alternative. Other infants are fed soya-based formula for ethical or cultural reasons. About 2% of all babies in the United Kingdom are fed soya-based infant formulas (MAFF 1998). Soya-based formulas have not been reported to cause adverse effects in infants, but in 1996 it was noted that phytoestrogens had been shown to have effects on the menstrual cycle of women on a Western diet. It was recommended that research should be undertaken to determine whether the use of infant formulas carries any risk to the sexual development and future fertility of infants. In 1998, the Committee on Toxicity of Chemicals in Food, Consumer Products and the Environment (COT) (MAFF 1998) were

reassured that the levels of phytoestrogens in soya infant formulas (18–41 mg/L) were similar to data published from other countries. It endorsed advice by the Department of Health that women who have been advised by health professionals to feed soya-based formulas should continue to do so.

Commercial promotion of infant formula

The commercial promotion of processed milks as breast-milk substitutes began as early as the second half of the nineteenth century in Western countries and as early as the 1920s in some developing countries with large expatriate communities, such as Malaysia and the Caribbean. By the 1950s advertisements were increasingly directed at the local population of Malaysia and the Caribbean. In Nigeria, widespread promotion of processed infant foods occurred in the 1960s, and by the 1970s there were over 40 brands of milk and milk-based products and 11 brands of feeding bottle on the market. In 1981, the WHO Code of Marketing of Breast Milk Substitutes was passed (see p 413). By 1988, only a few countries had ratified the code; however, 70 countries, including Malaysia, India and some Caribbean countries, are awaiting legislation or have partly enacted the Code. The result of the enactment of the Code means that the advertising of infant formulas in the mass media and direct contact of company personnel with mothers is prohibited. As a consequence of this, there has been an increase in the advertising of follow-on milks, and hospitals continue to request and accept excessive quantities of formula donated by the companies (King & Ashworth 1994). Subsequent resolutions to the Code (every 2 years since 1982) have tried to close many of the loopholes exploited by the baby-food industry.

Infant mortality

Between 1900 and 1903, Howarth (1905) noted that infant mortality amongst artificially-reared babies was 198 live births/1000 compared to 70/1000 amongst infants who were breastfed. By 1998, infant mortality in the United Kingdom was 5.7/1000 live births (Office for National Statistics 1998) a fall of over 90% in < 100 years. The dramatic reduction in mortality was probably due to major modifications in housing, water supply, sewage disposal, food production and storage together with advances in medicine and education in the United Kingdom, a typical situation in the Western world. In contrast, however, in many developing countries infant mortality is still high (e.g., in Pakistan it is 95/1000 live births), and the question of using artificial milk feeds in such societies has to be considered as a separate issue (UNICEF 1998).

Developing countries

The many advantages of breast milk over other foods for early infant feeding and the hazards of artificial milks and bottle feeding, especially in developing countries, are well established (Jelliffe & Jelliffe 1988). In developing countries beset by poverty and adverse living conditions, breastfeeding is vital for infant health. Because access to modern contraceptive methods may also be limited, breastfeeding plays an important role in child spacing, which benefits both maternal and child health. In addition, the purchase of imported milk products has a negative economic impact at both the household and national level (King & Ashworth 1994).

Despite the many benefits of breastfeeding, a decline in its use has been observed throughout the world. Breastfeeding in developing countries is associated with lower income, lower social class and rural living. The greatest decline in breastfeeding has been amongst the urban elite mothers who have higher levels of education and more likely to be employed in the modern sector. In some societies, feeding infant formula is associated with being modern and progressive, whereas breastfeeding is regarded as 'primitive' and backward (King and Ashworth 1987).

Women's work roles may be incompatible with exclusive breastfeeding, and supplements are often provided at an early age while the mother is working in the fields (Carballo & Pelto 1991). In a review of 16 developing-world studies comparing infant feeding practices amongst working and non-working mothers, eight reported no difference between the two groups, four found reduced breastfeeding in those who were working and four were inconclusive. King & Ashworth (1994) suggest that in some contexts the positive economic effects of maternal employment may offset the negative effect of reduced breastfeeding.

In a number of countries, institution-based measures have implemented supportive practices such as ensuring early and frequent suckling, encouragement and informed advice and avoidance of formula endorsement. An outcome of many programmes is that many infants who would previously have been formula fed are now successfully breastfed.

Table 38.5 — Infant feeding 1980–1995

	England & Wales			
	1980	**1985**	**1990**	**1995**
Prevalence of breastfeeding up to 9 months %[1]				
Birth	67	65	64	68
1 week	58	56	54	58
2 weeks	54	53	51	54
6 weeks	42	40	39	44
4 months	27	26	25	28
6 months	23	21	21	22
9 months	12	11	12	14
Duration of breastfeeding — % those starting initially[2]				
Birth	100	100	100	100
1 week	88	87	85	86
2 weeks	81	81	80	81
6 weeks	63	61	62	65
4 months	40	40	39	42
6 months	34	33	33	32
9 months	18	17	18	21

[1]Prevalence of breastfeeding. The proportion of babies still breastfed at 9 months, even if the babies were also receiving infant formula or solid food.
[2]Duration of breastfeeding. Length of time that mothers who breastfed initially continue to do so even if they were also giving their baby other foods.
From Office for National Statistics (1995).

Infant Feeding Survey (Office for National Statistics 1995)

Many Western mothers could breastfeed their babies but for economic or social reasons choose not to. In 1995 the fifth national survey of infant feeding practices was carried out in the United Kingdom. Thirty-two percent of mothers in England and Wales gave infant formula from birth (Table 38.5). By 4 months, 72% of all mothers were using formula exclusively; of those who initially started breastfeeding, 58% had changed to formula milks (Table 38.5). Almost half (46%) of mothers in Great Britain who were breastfeeding at 6–10 weeks were also giving infant formula. This was significantly higher than 1990 (39%) and 1985 (34%). The most common type of formula used for babies 6–10 weeks was whey-dominant (60%) but by 4 months of age 54% of mothers were giving casein-dominant formulas. The relative importance of whey-dominant formulas in the early weeks has increased in the last decade (ONS 1995).

Discussion

When women decide to feed formula rather than breastfeed, they often see it as a choice between two infant foods. However, breastfeeding is much more than a means of providing calories to a newborn, it is a natural extension to the process of pregnancy and child birth. Breastfed babies are healthier and have lower mortality rates, particularly in developing countries. Evidence also suggests that they have far less chronic illness later in life (Baumslag & Michels 1995c).

It is only in the last century that artificially-fed infants have had a good chance of survival. Before then, poor hygienic practices resulted in high mortality rates. Infant formulas are improving all the time but do still lack many of the factors present in human milk. It is probable that the role of most of these factors is more physiological than nutritional (e.g., carnitine, cholesterol, nucleotides, PUFA, enzymes and non-protein nitrogen), and it is probably desirable that at least some of them be added to formulas, however, it might not be practical.

The composition of formula continues to be modified and adapted but it is unlikely that it will ever reproduce the individuality of a mother's own milk or the changing composition of breast milk, which caters for the changing needs of the growing, maturing infant.

References

American Academy of Pediatrics (1997) Policy statement. Breast feeding and the use of human milk (RE9729). *Pediatrics*, 100, 1035–1039.

Balmer, S.E., Hanvey, L.S., Wharton, B.A. (1994) Diet and faecal flora in the newborn nucleotides. *Arch Dis Childhood*, 70, 137–140.

Barber, H.J., Page, J.E. (1982) Grimwade and The Desiccated Milk Company, pp. 352–353. Chemistry and Industry.

Barlow, T. (1894) Infantile scurvy and its relation to rickets. *Lancet*, ii, 1075–1080.

Barltrop, D., Oppe, T.E. (1970) Dietary factors in neonatal calcium homeostasis. *Lancet*, ii, 1333–1335.

Bates, C.J., Liu, D.S., Fuller, N.J., Lucas, A. (1985) Susceptibility of riboflavin and vitamin A in breast milk to photodegradation and its implications for the use of banked breast milk in infant feeding. *Acta Paediatr Scand*, 74, 40–44.

Baumslag, N., Michels, D.L. (1995a) Wet Nursing, Surrogate Feeding And Healing Qualities of Breast Milk. In: Baumslag, N., Michels, D.L. (eds.) *Milk, Money And Madness:The Culture And Politics of Breastfeeding*, 2, pp. 39–64, 1st edn. Westport, Connecticut: Bergin & Garvey.

Baumslag, N., Michels, D.L. (1995b) Artificial Feeding. In: Baumslag, N., Michels, D.L. (eds.) *Milk Money And Madness: The Culture And Politics of Breastfeeding*, 4, pp. 113–143, 1st edn. Westport, Connecticut: Bergin & Garvey.

Baumslag, N., Michels, D.L. (1995c) Artificial Feeding. In: Baumslag, N., Michels, D.L. (eds.) *Milk Money and Madness*, xxi–xxxi, 1st edn. Westport, CT: Bergin & Garvey.

Brand Miller, J., Bull, S., Miller, J., McVeagh, P. (1994) The oligosaccharide composition of human milk: Temporal and individual variations in monosaccharide components. *J Pediatr Gastroenterol Nutr*, 9, 371–376.

Brandtzaeg, P. (1998) Development and basic mechanisms of human gut immunity. *Nutr Rev*, 56, S5–S18.

Brock, J.H. (1980) Lactoferrin in human milk: Its role in iron absorption and protection against enteric infection in the newborn infant. *Arch Dis Childhood*, 55, 417–421.

Carballo, M., Pelto, G. (1991) Social and Psychological Factors in Breast-Feeding. In: Falkner, F. (ed.) *Infant Feeding and Child Nutrition: Issues and Perspectives*, pp. 177–192. Boca Raton, FL: CRC Press.

Codex Alimentarius Commission (1976) *Recommended International Standards for Foods for Infants and Children*. Rome: WHO/FAO.

Cuthbertson, W.F.J. (1994) Infant Foods from Victorian Times to The Present Day. In: Walker, A.F., Rolls, B.A. (eds.) *Infant Nutrition*, 1, pp. 1–34, 1st edn. London: Chapman & Hall.

Cuthbertson, W.F.J. (1999) Evolution of infant nutrition. *BJN*, 81, 359–371.

Davidsson, L., Kastenmayer, P., Yuen, M., Lonnerdal, BO., Hurrell, R.F. (1994) Influence of lactoferrin on iron absorption from human milk in infants. *Pediatr Res*, 35, 117–124.

Department of Health and Social Security. (1974) *Present Day Practice in Infant Feeding. Reports on Health and Social Subjects No 9*. London: HMSO.

Department of Health and Social Security. (1977) *The Composition of Mature Human Milk. Reports on Health and Social Subjects No 12*. London: HMSO.

Department of Health and Social Security. (1980b) *Present Day Practice for Infant Feeding. Reports on Health and Social Subjects No 20*. London: HMSO.

Department of Health and Social Security. (1980a) *Present*

Day Practice in Infant Feeding. Reports on Health and Social Subjects No 20. London: HMSO.

Department of Health and Social Security. (1981) *The Collection and Storage of Human Milk.* London: HMSO.

Department of Health and Social Security. (1988) *Present Day Practice in Infant Feeding: Reports on Health and Social Subjects No 32.* London: HMSO.

Department of Health and Social Security. (1991) *Dietary Reference Values for Food Energy And Nutrients for the United Kingdom. Report of The Panel on Dietary Reference Values of The Committee on Medical Aspects of Food Policy.* London: HMSO.

European Society of Paediatric Gastroenterology and Nutrition (ESPGAN). (1977) Guidelines on infant nutrition. I. Recommendations for the composition of an adapted formula. *Acta Paediatr Scand,* 262(Suppl),

European Society of Paediatric Gastroentology and Nutrition (ESPGAN) (1991) Committee on Nutriton. Comment on the content and composition of lipid in infant formula. *Acta Paediatrica Scandinavica 80.*

Farquharson, J., Cockburn, F., Patrick, W.A., Jamieson, C.E., Logan, R.W. (1992) Infant cerebral cortex phospholipid fatty-acid composition and diet. *Lancet,* 340, 810–813.

Fritz, I., Said, H., Harris, C., Murrell, J., Greene, H.L. (1987) A new sensitive assay for plasma riboflavin using high performance liquid chromatography. *J Am College Nutr,* 6, 49–449.

Gibson, G.R., Beatty, E.R., Wang, X., Cummings, J.H. (1995) Selective stimulation of Bifidobacteria in the human colon by oligofructose and inulin. *Gastroenterol,* 108, 975–982.

Granot, E., Golan, D., Rivkin, L., Kohen, R. (1999) Oxidative stress in healthy breast fed versus formula fed infants. *Nutr Res,* 9, 869–879.

Hambraeus, L. (1991) Human Milk: Nutritional Aspects. In: Brunser, O. et al. (eds.) *Clinical Nutrition of The Young Child,* pp. 289–301, New York: Raven Press.

Hamosh, M. (1991) Lipid Metabolism. In: Hay, W.W. (ed.) *Neonatal Nutrition And Metabolism,* pp. 122–142. St Louis: Mosby Year Books.

Hanson, L.Å., Ashraf, R., Carlsson, B. et al (1993) *Child Health And the Population Increase.* Göteborg: University of Göteborg and the Nordic School of Public Health.

Heavy, P.M., Rowland, R. (1999) The gut microflora of the developing infant: Microbiology and metabolism. *Microbial Ecol Health Dis,* 11, 75–83.

Hernell, O., Lönnerdal, B. (1996) Iron Requirements and Prevalence of Iron Deficiency in Term Infants during The First 6 Months of Life. In: Hallberg, L., Nils-Georg, A. (eds.) *Iron Nutrition in Health and Disease,* 13, pp. 129–136. London: John Libbey & Company Ltd.

Howarth, W.J. (1905) The influence of feeding on the mortality of infants. *Lancet,* 210–213.

Innocenti Declaration (1990) *WHO/UNICEF Policymakers' Meeting on BreastFeeding in The 1990s: A Global Initiative.* New York: UNICEF.

Isolauri, E., Juntunen, M., Rautanen, T., Sillanaukee, P., Koivula, T. (1991) Lactobacillus strain promotes recovery from acute diarrhea in children. *Pediatr,* 88, 90–97.

Jelliffe, D.B., Jelliffe, E.F.P. (1978) *Human Milk in The Modern World.* Oxford: Oxford University Press.

Jelliffe, D.B., Jelliffe, E.F.P. (1988) *Programmes to Promote Breast-Feeding.* New York: Oxford University Press.

Jephcott, H., Bacharach, A.L. (1926) A rapid and reliable test for vitamin D. *Biochem J,* 20, 1351–1355.

King, J., Ashworth, A. (1994) Patterns and determinants of infant feeding practice world wide. In: Walker, A.F., Rolls, B.A.(eds) *Infant Nutrition,* 3, 61–91.

Lightwood, R., Stapleton, T. (1953) Idiopathic hypercalcaemia. *Lancet,* 255–256.

Lucas, A., Morley, R., Cole, T.J., Lister, G., Leeson-Payne, C. (1992) Breast milk and subsequent intelligence quotient in children born preterm. *Lancet,* 339, 261–264.

Mackay, H.M., Goodfellow, R. (1931) Medical Research Council Special Report Series No 157 London HMSO. London: HMSO.

Martin, J., White, A. (1988) Infant feedings 1985 office of population censuses and surveys. London *HMSO.*

Ministry of Agriculture, Fisheries and Food (1998) Food surveillance: Soy-based Infant formulae. Information Bulletin 102 November.

MAFF. (1998) Food Surveillance: Soya-Based Infant Formulae. http://www.maff.gov.uk/food/bulletin/1998/no102/soya.htm.

Mettler, A.E. (1982) Infant formula. *Acta Paediatr Scand Suppl,* 299, 58–76.

Newman, J. (1995) How breast milk protects newborns. *Scientific American,* 273, 58–61.

Office for National Statistics. (1995) *Infant Feeding 1995.* London: The Stationery Office.

Office for National Statistics (1998) Mortality statistics: Childhood, Infant and Perinatal. Series DH3, No 31, Table 2: UK and Constituent Countries p2. London: The stationery office.

Olson, J.A. (1987) Recommended dietary intakes (RDI) of vitamin A in humans. *AJCN* 45, 704–716.

Oppe, T.E., Redstone, D. (1968) Calcium and phosphorus levels in healthy newborn infants given various types of milk. *Lancet,* 1045–1048.

Poskitt, E.M.E. (1994) Use of Cow's Milk in Infant Feeding. In: Walker, A.F., Rolls, B.A. (eds.) *Infant Nutrition*, 7, pp. 163–185, 1st edn. London: Chapman & Hall.

Powell, J.J., Jugdaohsingh, R., Thompson, R.P.H. (1999) The regulation of mineral absorption in the gastrointestinal tract. *Proc Nutr Soc*, 58, 147–153.

Powers, H.J. (1997) Vitamin requirements for term infants: Considerations for infant formulae. *Nutr Res Rev*, 10, 1–33.

Roberts, A.K., Chierici, R., Sawatzki, G., Hill, M.J., Volpato, S., Vigi, V. (1992) Supplementation of an adapted formula with bovine lactoferrin: 1. Effects on the infant faecal flora. *Acta Paediatr*, 81, 119–124.

Schanler, R.J., Cheng, S.F. (1991) Infant Formulas for Enteral Feeding. In: Hay, W.W. (ed.) *Neonatal Nutrition And Metabolism*, pp. 303–334. St Louis: Mosby Year Books.

Shaw, J.C.L., Jones, A., Gunther, M. (1973) Mineral contents of brands of milk for infant feeding. *BMJ*, 2, 12–15.

Silvers, K.M., Gibson, A.T., Powers, H.J. (1994) High plasma vitamin C concentrations at birth associated with low antioxidant status and poor outcome in premature infants. *Arch Dis Childhood*, 71, F40–F44.

Specker, B.L., Black, A., Allen, L., Morrow, F. (1990) Vitamin B_{12}: Low milk concentrations are related to low serum concentrations in vegetarian women and to methymalonic aciduria in their infants. *AJCN*, 52, 1073–1076.

Taitz, L.S., Byers, H.D. (1972) High calorie osmolar feeding and hypertonic dehydration. *Arch Dis Childhood*, 47, 257–260.

Trugo, N.M.F., Sardinha, F. (1994) Cobalamin and cobalamin-binding capacity in human milk. *Nutr Res*, 14, 23–33.

UNICEF (1998) *State of the World's Children – Child Malnutrition and Women's Rights*, 1, 7–90 Oxford and New York: Oxford University Press for UNICEF.

US National Research Council (1989) Recommended Dietary Allowances, pp 195–205, 10th edition, Washington DC: National Academy Press.

Whitehead, R.G., Paul, A.A. (1987) *Changes in Infant Feeding Practice in Britain During The Last Century*. London: Medical Research Council Environmental Epidemiology Unit Scientific Report: Infant Nutrition and Cardiovascular Disease.

WHO/UNICEF (1981) The WHO/UNICEF International code of marketing Breastmilk substitutes. World Health Assembly Geneva, Switzerland.

World Declaration and Plan of Action for Nutrtion (1992) Medical Research Council Special Report Series no 157, London, HMSO.

World Declaration and Plan of Action for Nutrition (1992) Adopted at International Conference of Nutrition, Rome, Italy.

Wold, A.E., Hanson, L.Å. (1994) Defense factors in human milk. *Curr Opin Gastroenterol*, 10, 652–658.

Yip, R. (1994) Iron deficiency: Contemporary scientific issues and international programmatic approaches. *J Nutr*, 124, 1479S–1490S.

39

The role of colonic fermentation in infants[1]

Carlos H. Lifschitz

[1]This work is a publication of the USDA/ARS Children's Nutrition Research Center, Department of Pediatrics, Baylor College of Medicine, Houston, TX. This project has been funded in part with federal funds from the US Department of Agriculture, Agricultural Research Service, under Co-operative Agreement number 58-6250-1-003. The contents of this publication do not necessarily reflect the views or policies of the US Department of Agriculture, nor does mention of trade names, commercial products, or organizations imply endorsement from the United States.

Introduction

At birth, the colonic function of the human infant is immature. The development of the colonic function (i.e., water absorption and carbohydrate fermentation) is related in part to that of the bacterial flora. Both in infants and adults, a variable proportion of dietary carbohydrate is not absorbed in the small bowel and arrives in the colon where it undergoes bacterial fermentation. The products of this fermentation are short-chain fatty acids (SCFAs), principally acetate, propionate, and butyrate (Cummings & Macfarlane 1997), together with gases such as CO_2, hydrogen (H_2), and methane (CH_4) (Fig. 39.1). A fraction of these products are absorbed through the colonic mucosa into the circulatory system; butyrate is utilized by the epithelial cells of the colon (Roediger 1992); the rest is expelled through the anus as stools or flatus (Levitt & Engel 1975).

Biochemistry of carbohydrate fermentation

The term *short-chain fatty acid* is really a misnomer as these acids, although indeed have a short chain of carbons, are not really fatty but are chemically closer to carbohydrates than to fat (Wrong 1995). The term *volatile fatty acids* is not, however, a better descriptor of its characteristics. The name comes from the fact that originally these acids were measured by steam-distillation following acidification of the intestinal contents and, therefore, were volatile. More modern methods of separation such as gas-liquid chromatography resulted in that name being abandoned. Acetate, propionate and butyrate are moderately-strong acids, with an average pK value of 4.8. In the intestine, they exist as negatively-charged anions and not as free acids. When ionized, SCFAs are not volatile.

When carbohydrate arrives in the colon, fermentation reactions occur. As a result, colonic lumenal pH decreases while the concentrations of ammonia, short- and long-chain fatty acids, and bile acids increase. The bacteria capable of fermenting carbohydrate are mainly anaerobes or facultative aerobes (Mcfarlane & Gibson 1995). The process of carbohydrate fermentation requires for the colonic bacterial flora to be present in a high enough concentration and that the lumenal pH be in accordance to the bacterial pK (6 or greater). Therefore, it is obvious that newborns are incapable of carbohydrate fermentation to the level achieved by older infants and adults. Another situation in which carbohydrate fermentation is decreased or even

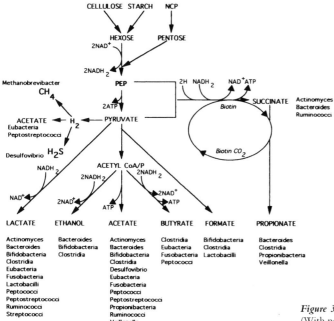

Figure 39.1 Colonic carbohydrate metabolism by the fecal flora. (With permission from MacFarlane, 1995).

abolished is during treatment with broad-spectrum antibiotics (Gilat et al 1978) or when large amounts of carbohydrate are malabsorbed daily because the lumenal pH fails below the bacterial pK (Perman 1981). The not uncommon finding of reducing substances in the stools of infants during the first few days of life due to the presence of intact carbohydrate can be explained by the fact that a fraction of the dietary carbohydrate that is malabsorbed by the small bowel cannot be fully fermented and transformed into SCFAs. This is also reflected by the low breath H_2 levels (Stevenson 1982). Similarly, despite the fact that the infants are malabsorbing carbohydrate, the faecal pH may be 6 or higher. Special types of bacteria are necessary to produce propionate, H_2 and CH_4, and to the extent that they are needed, not every individual is capable of producing them (see Fig. 39.1) (Strocchi 1982). For example, CH_4 is generally not produced in the first years of life. Rutili et al (1996) studied faecal samples from children between 3 months and 5 years for the presence of methanogenic bacteria. Methanobacteria were not detected in faecal samples obtained from children under 27 months, of age. At 27 months, only one subject harboured methanobacteria; the number of methanobacteria hosts subsequently increased with age, with an incidence of 40% at 3 years and 60% at 5 years. The appearance of methanobacteria was not directly related to the introduction of particular foods in the child's diet. These dietary changes could give rise to some physical-chemical modifications of the enteric lumen, thus causing the conversion of the intestinal flora to an adult pattern and, in most subjects, the development of methanobacteria.

SCFAs are known to enhance intestinal growth and function in animal models of resection (Tappenden 1997) and in humans with ulcerative colitis (Breuer et al 1997). As well, they may play an important role in the intestine after surgery (Tappenden 1997). Of the products of fermentation of carbohydrate, butyrate contributes to the energy needs of the colonic epithelial cell (Roediger 1992). The process of carbohydrate fermentation and absorption of its products is known as 'colonic scavenging'. Acetate and to a lesser extent propionate are absorbed into the system and, at least in ruminants, contribute a significant amount to the energy needs of the host (Martin 1994). SCFAs and butyrate in particular have effects on epithelial cells. Butyrate inhibits proliferation and promotes differentiation of several colonic epithelial cell lines (Basson et al 1996), alters cell morphology (Scheppach 1997) and even influences synthesis and secretion of

several proteins (Frankel et al 1994). SCFAs promote cell migration (Wilson 1997). The preferential substrate for the *colonocyte*, the cell that constitutes the mucosal lining of the colon, is butyrate.

Fitch & Fleming (1999) determined the influence of substrate concentration and substrate interactions on SCFA metabolism in an animal model. When the luminal concentrations of butyrate were increased 20-fold, linear increases in total C resulted, but CO_2 production from butyrate increased as a function of concentration only up to a certain point and was stable at higher butyrate concentrations, indicating a saturation process in the capacity of the colon to further utilize butyrate. The presence of a mixture of alternative substrates in the lumen had no influence on the metabolism of butyrate to CO_2, but significantly reduced the metabolism of acetate to CO_2. When compared with young (4-month-old) animals, transport of butyrate was significantly lower for aged (48-month-old) animals. These results show that important aspects of SCFA transport and metabolism are not predicted from data using isolated colonocytes but require study using an *in vivo* model.

Because it was not known whether colonocytes in the newborn can metabolize butyrate, this was examined in the newborn and infant rat colon (Krishnan & Ramakrishna 1998). Isolated colonocytes from rats of different perinatal ages were incubated with ^{14}C-labelled butyrate or glucose *in vitro*. Complete oxidation was estimated by the production of ^{14}C-labelled CO_2, whereas intermediate metabolites were measured enzymatically. Oxidation of butyrate was highest in newborns, declining at day 10 and even further in adult rats. Glucose oxidation was also highest at birth, with a minor increase at approximately day 20 (weaning period) before decreasing to adult levels. Butyrate oxidation was substantially higher than was glucose oxidation in all age groups. The authors concluded that neonatal rat colon epithelial cells resemble adult colonocytes in their preference for butyrate as a metabolic substrate, indicating a constitutive expression of this property.

Of interest is the fact that the normal microflora of the large intestine synthesizes biotin and that the colon is capable of absorbing intraluminally introduced free biotin. To understand the mechanism of biotin absorption in the large intestine and its regulation, Said et al (1998) used a human-derived, non-transformed, colonic-epithelial cell line. The initial rate of biotin uptake was found to be temperature and energy dependent, Na^+ dependent saturable as a function of concentration, and competitively inhibited by the vitamin pantothenic acid. These results point to the functional existence of a Na^+-dependent, specialized, carrier-mediated system for biotin uptake in colonic-epithelial cells. This system is shared with pantothenic acid.

Role of the colonic flora

The fate of dietary carbohydrate in the infant and the adult is that, even under physiological conditions, a certain proportion of the ingested carbohydrate, particularly complex ones such as starches, escape complete digestion by pancreatic and mucosal enzymes and thus absorption by the small bowel, therefore arriving in the large bowel. In the case of most infants, until cereals are introduced into the diet, the carbohydrate incompletely absorbed is lactose. Recent studies indicate that the fraction of carbohydrate malabsorbed by breastfed infants could be the oligosaccharides present in breast milk (Brand-Miller et al 1998). In the presence of a functioning colonic flora, the unabsorbed carbohydrate is fermented according to a series of well-defined reactions that depend on the type of bacteria present (see Fig. 39.1). The composition of the colonic flora depends on such things as the way the infant was delivered (Long & Swenson 1977, Groniund et al 1999), whether they were term or pre-term (Long 1977, Sakata 1985), the diet (Langhendries et al 1985, Lundequist et al 1985, Balmer et al 1989, Kleessen et al 1995) and ill-defined influences. The introduction of additional food items results in changes in the bacterial enzyme activity (Mykkanen et al 1997). By the eighth post-natal day, Bacteroides fragilis can be isolated from the stool of more than 50% of formula-fed, term infants delivered vaginally (Wilson 1997). Possibly because of contamination that occurs during passage through the birth canal, infants delivered vaginally have significantly higher faecal isolates of anaerobic bacteria and Bacteroides fragilis in particular than those delivered by cesarean section (Fig. 39.2). Moreover, in the study by Long & Swenson (1977), it was demonstrated that gestational age also affects colonization of the bowel, so that by 7 days of age, pre-term infants have significantly less anaerobic bacteria isolated from stools than those born full term. This finding could be related to the fact that term infants are larger and spend a longer time in contact with maternal fluids in the birth canal. The type of feeding also played a role in determining the establishment of the faecal flora, an effect that becomes apparent by the

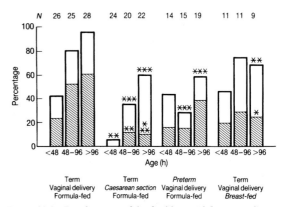

Figure 39.2 Development of the fecal bacterial flora according to the time of birth and type of delivery. Anaerobic bacteria, white bars, *Bacteroides Fragilis*, Hatched bars. (With permission from Lifschitz, 1995).

seventh day of life. By the third day of life both breast-fed and formula-fed infants have similar bacterial counts of *Bacteroides fragilis*, other anaerobic bacteria, aerobic gram-negative bacilli and streptococci. By the end of the first week, however, only 22% of breastfed infants have *Bacteroides fragilis* isolated from the stools compared to 61% of the formula-fed counterparts.

The faecal flora is also affected by iron supplementation (Balmer & Wharton 1991). In a study that compared the prevailing bacteria in the faecal flora of infants, it was seen that in contrast to breastfed infants in whom bifidobacteria predominated and in whom counts of *E. coli* were low and other bacteria were rarely present, infants who were fed an Fe-fortified cow-milk formula had high counts of *E. coli* and low counts and isolation frequency of bifidobacteria. In addition, many other kinds of bacteria were frequently isolated in the Fe-supplemented, formula-fed infants. Other studies have demonstrated that stools of breastfed infants who have also received formula or cow milk acquire certain characteristics not observed in samples from exclusively breastfed infants (Balmer, 1989, 1991). Such differences include higher faecal pH and production of propionate, a SCFA which is virtually absent in faeces of exclusively breastfed infants (Lifschitz 1990).

The role of the colon on carbohydrate scavenging in the newborn has been the attention of several studies. In one of them, sequential studies of breath H_2 excretion in response to lactose feeding were carried out in 22 premature infants during the first 7 weeks of life (MacLean & Fink 1980). Seventy-five percent of infants excreted H_2 in breath during the first 2 weeks; 100% did so by the end of the third week. The peak

H_2 concentration and the 5-hour mean breath H_2 excretions were significantly related to lactose intake per day. Calculations using the 5-hour mean H_2 excretion allowed the authors to estimate that 66% or more of ingested lactose entered the colon and was fermented. Throughout the studies, stool patterns and rates of weight gain of the infants were normal. In another study, Kien et al (1987) measured carbohydrate energy absorption and breath H_2 concentration in 12 premature infants at 28–32 weeks gestational age and 2–4 weeks post-natal age. Infants received one of two formulas that differed only in carbohydrate source: one contained 100% lactose (LAC) and the other 50% lactose:50% glucose polymers (LAC + GP). In 11 of the 12 infants studied, there was evidence of extensive colonic fermentation as suggested by the breath H_2 levels. An approximate 100% increase in lactose intake in the LAC group was associated with a similar increase in breath H_2 concentration. None of the infants exhibited diarrhoea or vomiting or developed delayed gastric emptying. The mean ± standard deviation calculated carbohydrate energy absorption was, respectively, 86 ± 5% and 91 ± 3% in the LAC and the LAC + GP groups. The authors concluded that colonic bacterial fermentation may be critical to energy balance and to the prevention of osmotic diarrhoea in premature infants fed lactose. From these and other studies it can be concluded that premature infants normally malabsorb substantial amounts of lactose. The elevation of breath H_2 observed in these infants, however, apparently represents a successful adaptation of the colonic microflora to this physiological malabsorption and should not be cause to modify the diet of an infant who is clinically well.

With the purpose of identifying aspects of the process of carbohydrate fermentation that could differ between breastfed and formula-fed infants, the authors performed an *in vitro* study of carbohydrate fermentation by the faecal flora of both of the above groups of infants (Lifschitz et al 1990). The authors incubated faecal samples from breastfed and formula-fed infants under different conditions: pH 6.8 and 5.5, with and without the addition of lactose, to simulate the faecal pH observed in cases of complete carbohydrate absorption in the small bowel in the former and that of malabsorption in the latter. The effect of acid pH on bacterial fermentation and changes in carbohydrate fermentation in relation to the age of the infant were also studied. At pH 6.8, which is within the normal range, addition of lactose resulted in a significant increase in the production of SCFAs and larger amounts of lactose, glucose and galactose compared

with what was found in incubates to which no lactose was added. Irrespective of the diet, when stools were incubated at pH 5.5, which is the pH found in stools of infants with carbohydrate malabsorption, SCFA production was significantly lower compared to what occurred at pH 6.8. At the acid pH, accumulation of glucose and galactose in the incubate of faeces of formula-fed infants increased significantly compared to what occurred at the alkaline pH. In contrast, incubates at pH 5.5 of stools from breastfed infants resulted in a greater proportion of lactose as a result of a decrease in the amount of lactose hydrolysed. The decrease in lactose hydrolysis in breastfed infants resulted in a lower osmolality of the incubate which, if it also were to occur *in vivo*, could provide a partial explanation for the fact that stool output in cases of carbohydrate malabsorption such as in acute gastro-enteritis is milder in this population. This is an example of how diet may affect the way that malabsorbed carbohydrate is handled by the colon.

Edwards et al (1994) measured the concentration of faecal SCFA in babies fed breast milk or infant formula from birth. Their study corroborated the knowledge that breastfed infants have significantly lower faecal pH values at week 2 and 4 than formula-fed infants. These authors found no difference, however, in the amount of faecal water between the two dietary groups. As opposed to Lifschitz et al (1990), Edwards et al found that the concentration of SCFA was not different between the two groups. However, in agreement with Lifschitz et al they demonstrated higher faecal concentration of propionic, as well as N-butyric and isovaleric acids, and also confirmed the predominance of lactic and acetic acid in the faeces of breastfed infants. Of interest is the fact that breastfed infants produce very little N-butyrate, a SCFA that is known to be the preferential nutrient of the mature colonocyte.

As the infant matures and the faecal flora develops, new metabolic products appear in faeces. Norin et al (1985) used the concept of microflora-associated characteristics (MAC), which they defined as the identification of an anatomical structure or biochemical or physiological function in the host that is influenced by the microflora. Several of these MACs were identified. Only in the second year of life could intestinal bacteria convert bilirubin to urobilin, degrade mucin and convert cholesterol. Tryptic activity was not demonstrated in meconium, was present in faeces from all children studied up to 21 months of age and, for reasons that are not apparent, absent in 6 out of 15 children in the age group of 46–61 months. The relevance of this study is that it demonstrated that the establishment of the full metabolic capacity of the bacterial flora is a considerably extended process. Another indicator of maturation of the faecal flora can be exemplified by the fact that most infants and young children cannot produce CH_4, as stated before (Rutili et al 1996).

It is known that SCFA play a role in water homeostasis in the colon. However, because of the inaccessibility of this organ, precise data in humans is difficult to obtain. The transport of sodium has been studied in the infant colon (Jenkins et al 1993). Absorption of SCFA and its effects on water and sodium conservation by the colon were studied in pigs and shown to be age-dependant (Murray et al 1989). Maximal absorption of SCFA was seen at birth, followed by a rapid decline over 72 h to a lower and relatively stable level. Water and sodium absorption increased with age and the addition of SCFA to the experimental perfusion solution resulted in further enhancement in the first 2 weeks of life. After the fourteenth day of life, sodium absorption continued to be enhanced by addition of SCFA, but water absorption remained unchanged from control levels, suggesting that although lumenal SCFA levels may be limited early in life, their presence has stimulatory effects on the absorption of sodium and water in the colon of newborns. The development of the faecal flora has very important practical implications such as regulation of water absorption in the colon. The capacity of the colon to compensate for the excessive arrival of fluid as it occurs in gastroenteritis was studied by Argenzio et al (1984). In this study, maximal water absorption capacity was compared between 3-day-old and 3-week-old pigs infected with transmissible gastroenteritis virus. The older animals exhibited a compensatory response to the excess water inflow to the colon and were able to increase up to six-times the capacity to absorb fluids compared to the younger animals to the point that diarrhoea was completely prevented. Moreover, the 3-week-old pigs were able to ferment to SCFA all carbohydrate that arrived in the colon completely, whereas in the younger pigs carbohydrate passed through the colon unchanged and appeared in faeces. This study demonstrated that development of microbial digestion together with rapid SCFA absorption is a primary feature responsible for the colonic compensation observed as a factor of age.

As stated before, broad-spectrum antibiotic treatment results in a considerable decrease of the colonic bacterial flora and consequently the capacity to ferment dietary carbohydrate that arrives in the colon and may explain the diarrhoea that frequently occurs in infants treated with such drugs (Bhatia et al 1986). Whenever the amount of carbohydrate arriving in the colon is relatively large, colonic fermentation (which can be monitored by the production of H_2) and SCFA become clinically relevant. This can be the case with gastroenteritis or a large amount of carbohydrate and/or carbohydrates that cannot be completely digested such as when a relatively large amount of certain fruit juices or beverages containing a high concentration of carbohydrate are administered (Smith 1995). Although much has been said about fruit juice and carbohydrate malabsorption, the authors have demonstrated that at lower, reasonable volumes of juice intake, carbohydrate absorption is not a problem (Lifschitz 1999).

Excessive colonic fermentation as a consequence of carbohydrate malabsorption or by a characteristic of the faecal flora has been considered to be one of the causes of infantile colic. Moore et al (1988) performed breath H_2 tests following a lactose challenge in infants with colic. They concluded that amongst the infants that they studied, colicky infants produced more H_2 in both the fasted state and after the ingestion of formula. The authors considered that lactose malabsorption, differences in colonic bacterial fermentation conditions, or a difference in the way that the H_2 produced was handled (i.e., absorbed vs. excreted by flatus) could explain the differences observed between colicky and non-colicky infants. Another study, however, failed to demonstrate a significant difference in the amount of H_2 produced by colicky and non-colicky babies (Hyams et al 1989).

Over the years, multiple studies have addressed the potential positive effects of colonization with *Lactobacillus* species (e.g., *GG*). *Lactobacillus* is considered to be a pro-biotic, that is a living organism capable of exerting health benefits beyond inherent basic nutrition. An interesting example is the effect of *Lactobacillus GG* on shortening the duration of acute diarrhoea in children (Isolauri et al 1991).

As an interesting concept in the process of development of the colon, it is known that the faeces of 40–70% of newborn infants harbor *Clostridium difficile* and toxin B (Cooperstock et al 1983) in concentrations similar to those found in adults with pseudomembranous colitis. However, most newborn infants experience no symptoms. Possible explanations for this state of asymptomatic carrier in infants include: 1) absence of enterotoxin A, the toxin responsible for pathogenesis; 2) absence of colonic receptors; and 3) diminished inflammatory response. Again, differences were found based on the type of nutrition: infants fed formula were nearly four times more likely to carry *Clostridium difficile* than were those exclusively breastfed (62% versus 16%). Breastfed infants who were also receiving formula or solids had an intermediate rate of colonization (35%) (Cooperstock et al 1983).

Discussion

Fermentation of carbohydrate in the large bowel results in the production of acids and gas. It may also result in increased water in the lumen of the bowel. The products of carbohydrate fermentation play an important role in assuring the welfare of the colonocytes. SCFAs are known to enhance intestinal growth and function in animal models of resection and in humans with inflammatory bowel disease. As well, they may play an important role in the intestine after surgery. Butyrate, one of the SCFAs produced during the fermentation of dietary fibre, is a potent inducer of differentiation of tumour cells, and it has been speculated that it may account for the protective effects of certain types of fibre for colonic tumourigenesis. In the infant under physiological conditions, particularly if breastfed, a moderate amount of carbohydrate arrives in the colon and is fermented by the bacterial flora. The fact that fermentation of carbohydrate takes place and is almost complete is evidenced by the finding of H_2 breath, the lack of reducing substances in stools and an increased amount of SCFAs although faecal pH remains above 5.5. Whenever the amount of carbohydrate arriving in the colon exceeds the capacity of the bacterial flora to ferment it, carbohydrate appears in the stool. Another possibility is that when the amount of SCFA produced is greater than that which can be absorbed by the colon, faecal pH falls. This is particularly true for lactic acid, which diffuses through the colonic mucosa less well than the other acids. Infants with an incompletely developed colonic flora or those receiving antibiotics, which destroy the flora, may not be able to handle excessive amounts of non-absorbed dietary carbohydrate and develop diarrhoea. Older infants produce gas in the colon when fermentation of carbohydrate takes place, which leads to discomfort, irritability or even crying spells. However, a certain amount of SCFA may be necessary for the welfare and regulation of cell proliferation of the colonocytes. It is therefore important to determine the right amount, if any, of non-absorbable carbohydrate that infants may ingest without developing symptoms.

References

Argenzio, R.A., Moon, H.W., Kemeny, L.J., Whipp, S.C. (1984) Colonic compensation of transmissible gastro-enteritis in swine. *Gastroenterology*, 86, 1501–1506.

Balmer, S.E., Scott, P.H., Wharton, B.A. (1989) Diet and faecal flora in the newborn: Casein and whey proteins. *Arch Dis Child*, 64, 1678–1684.

Balmer, S.E., Wharton, B.A. (1991) Diet and faecal flora in the newborn: Iron. *Arch Dis Child*, 66, 1390–1394.

Basson, M.D., Turowski, G.A., Rashid, Z., Hong, F., Madri, J.A. (1996) Regulation of human colonic cell line proliferation and phenotype by sodium butyrate. *Dig Dis Sci*, 41, 1989–1993.

Bhatia, J., Prihoda, A.R., Richardson, C.J. (1986) Parenteral antibiotics and carbohydrate intolerance in term neonates. *Am J Dis Child*, 144, 111–113.

Brand-Miller, J.C., McVeagh, P., McNeil, Y., Messer, M. (1998) Digestion of human milk oligosaccharides by healthy infants evaluated by the lactulose hydrogen breath test. *J Pediatr*, 133, 95–98.

Breuer, R.I., Soergel, K.H., Lashner, B.A., Christ, M.L., Hanauer, S.B., Vanagunas, A., Harig, J.M., Keshavarzian, A., Robinson, M., Sellin, J.H., Weinberg, D., Vidican, D.E., Flemal, K.L., Rademaker, A.W. (1997) Short chain fatty acid rectal irrigation for left-sided ulcerative colitis. A randomised, placebo controlled trial. *Gut*, 40, 485–491.

Cooperstock, M., Riegie, L., Woodruff, C.W., Onderdonk, A. (1983) Influence of age, sex, and diet on asymptomatic colonization of infants with *Clostridium difficile*. *J Clin Microbiol*, 17, 830–833.

Cummings, J.H., Macfarlane, G.T. (1997) Role of intestinal bacteria in nutrient metabolism. *J Parenter Enteral Nutr*, 21, 357–365.

Edwards, C.A., Parrett, A.M., Balmer, S.E., Wharton, B.A. (1994) Faecal short chain fatty acids in breast-fed and formula-fed babies. *Acta Paed*, 83, 459–462.

Fitch, M.D., Fleming, S.E. (1999) Metabolism of short-chain fatty acids by rat colonic mucosa in vivo. *Physiol*, 277, G31–G40.

Frankel, W., Lew, J., Su, B., Bain, A., Kiurfeld, D., Einhorn, E., MacDermott, R.P., Rombeau, J. (1994) Butyrate increases colonocyte protein synthesis in ulcerative colitis. *J Surg Res*, 57, 210–214.

Gilat, T., Ben Hur, H., Geiman-Malachi, E., Terdiman, R., Peled, Y. (1978) Alterations of the colonic flora and their effect on the hydrogen breath test. *Gut*, 19, 602–605.

Groniund, M.M., Lehtonen, O.P., Eerola, E., Kero, P. (1999) Fecal microflora in healthy infants born by different methods of delivery. Permanent changes in intestinal flora after cesarean delivery. *J Pediatr Gastroenterol Nutr*, 28, 19–25.

Hyams, J.S., Geertsma, M.A., Etienne, N.L., Treem, W.R. (1989) Colonic hydrogen production in infants with colic. *J Pediatr*, 115, 592–594.

Isolauri, E., Juntunen, M., Rautanen, T., Sillanaukee, P., Koivula, T. (1991) A human *Lactobacillus* strain (*Lactobacillus* casei sp strain GG) promotes recovery from acute diarrhea in children. *Pediatrics*, 88, 90–97.

Jenkins, H.R., Schnackenberg, U., Milia, P.J. (1993) *In vitro* studies of sodium transport in human infant colon: The influence of acetate. *Pediatr Res*, 34, 666–669.

Kien, C.L., Liechty, E.A., Myerberg, D.Z., Mullett, M.D. (1987) Dietary carbohydrate assimilation in the premature infant: Evidence for a nutritionally significant bacterial ecosystem in the colon. *Am J Clin Nutr*, 46, 456–460.

Kleessen, B., Bunke, H., Tovar, K., Noack, J., Sawatzki, G. (1995) Influence of two infant formulas and human milk on the development of the faecal flora in newborn infants. *J Acta Paediatr*, 84, 1347–1356.

Krishnan, S., Ramakrishna, B.S. (1998) Butyrate and glucose metabolism in isolated colonocytes in the developing rat colon. *J Pediatr Gastroenterol Nutr*, 26, 432–436.

Langhendries, J.P., Detry, J., Van Hees, J., Lamboray, J.M., Darimont, J., Mozin, M.J., Secretin, M.C., Senterre, J. (1985) Effect of a fermented infant formula containing viable bifidobacteria on the fecal flora composition and pH of healthy full-term infants. *Acta Paediatr Scand*, 74, 45–51.

Levitt, M.D., Engel, R.R. (1975) Intestinal gas. *Adv Intern Med*, 20, 151–165.

Lifschitz, C.H. (1995) Colonic short-chain fatty acids in infants and children. In: Cummings, J.H., Rombeau, J.L., Sakata, T. (eds). Physiological and clinical aspects of short-chain fatty acids. 525–535. Cambridge University Press.

Lifschitz, C.H. (1999) Carbohydrate absorption from fruit juices in infants. *Pediatrics*.

Lifschitz, C.H., Wolin, M.J., Reeds, P.J. (1990) Characterization of carbohydrate fermentation in feces of formula-fed and breast fed infants. *Pediatr Res*, 27, 165–169.

Lifschitz, C.H. (2000) Carbohydrate absorption from fruit juices in infants.

Long, S.S., Swenson, R.M. (1977) Development of anaerobic fecal flora in healthy newborn infants. *J Pediatr*, 91, 298–301.

Lundequist, B., Nord, C.E., Winberg, J. (1985) The composition of the faecal microflora in breastfed and bottle fed infants from birth to eight weeks. *Eur J Pediatr*, 144, 186–190.

Macfarlane, G.T., Gibson, G.R. (1995) Microbiological Aspects of The Production of Short-Chain Fatty Acids in The Large Bowel. In: Cummings, J.H., Rombeau, J.L., Sakata, T. (eds.) *Physiological and Clinical Aspects of Short-Chain Fatty Acids*, 401–425. Cambridge University Press.

MacLean, Jr., W.C., Fink, B.B. (1980) Lactose malabsorption by premature infants: Magnitude and clinical significance. *J Pediatr*, 97, 383–388.

Martin, S.A. (1994) Nutrient transport by ruminal bacteria: A review. *J Anim Sci*, 72, 3019–3031.

Moore, D.J., Robb, T.A., Davidson, G.P. (1988) Breath hydrogen response to milk containing lactose in colicky and noncolicky infants. *J Pediatr*, 113, 979–984.

Murray, R.D., McCiung, H.J., Li, B.U.K., Ailabouni, A. (1989) Stimulatory effects of short-chain fatty acids on colonic absorption in newborn piglets *in vivo*. *J Pediatr Gastroenterol Nutr*, 8, 95–101.

Mykkanen, H., Tikka, J., Pitkanen, T., Hanninen, O. (1997) Fecal bacterial enzyme activities in infants increase with age and adoption of adult-type diet. *J Pediatr Gastroenterol Nutr*, 25(3), 312–316.

Norin, K.E., Gustafsson, B.E., Lindblad, B.S., Midtvedt, T. (1985). The establishment of some microflora associated biochemical characteristics in feces from children during the first years of life. *Acta Paediatr Scand*; 74(2), 207–212.

Perman, J.A., Modler, S., Olson, A.C. (1981). Role of pH in production of hydrogen from carbohydrates by colonic bacterial flora. Studies in vivo and in vitro. *J Clin Invest*; 67, 643–650.

Sakata, H., Yoshioka, H., Fujita, K. (1985) Development of the intestinal flora in very low birth weight infants compared to normal full-term newborns. *Eur J Pediatr*. 144(2), 186–190.

Stevenson, D.K. (1989) Breath hydrogen in preterm infants. *Am J Dis Child*; 143(11), 1262–1263.

Rutili, A., Canzi, E., Brusa, T., Ferrari, A. (1996) Intestinal methanogenic bacteria in children of different ages. *New Microbiol*; 19(3), 227–243.

Said, H.M., Ortiz, A., McCloud, E., Dyer, D., Moyer, M.P., Rubin, S. (1998) Biotin uptake by human colonic epithelial NCM460 cells: a carrier-mediated process shared with pantothenic acid. *Am J Physiol*; 275-(5 pt 1), C1365–1371.

Scheppach, W., Muller, J.G., Boxberger, F., Dusel, G., Richter et al (1997) Histological changes in the colonic mucosa following irrigation with short-chain fatty acids. *Eur J Gastroenterol Hepatol*; 9(2), 163–168.

Smith, M.M., Davis, M., Chasalow, F.L., Lifschitz, F. (1995) Carbohydrate absorption from fruit juice in young children. *Pediatrics*; 95(3), 340–344.

Strocchi, A., Levitt, M.D. (1992) Factors affecting hydrogen production and consumption by human fecal flora. The critical roles of hydrogen tension and methanogenesis. *J Clin Invest*; 89(4), 1304–1311.

Tappenden, K.A., Thomson, A.B., Wild, G.E., McBurney, M.I. (1997) Short-chain fatty acid-supplemented total parenteral nutrition enhances functional adaptation to intestinal resection in rats. *Gastroenterology* 112(3), 792–802.

Wilson, A.J., Gibson, P.R. Short-chain fatty acids promote the migration of colonic epithelial cells in vitro (1997) *Gastroenterology*; 113(2), 487–496.

Index